D1707978

STROKE

A Practical Approach

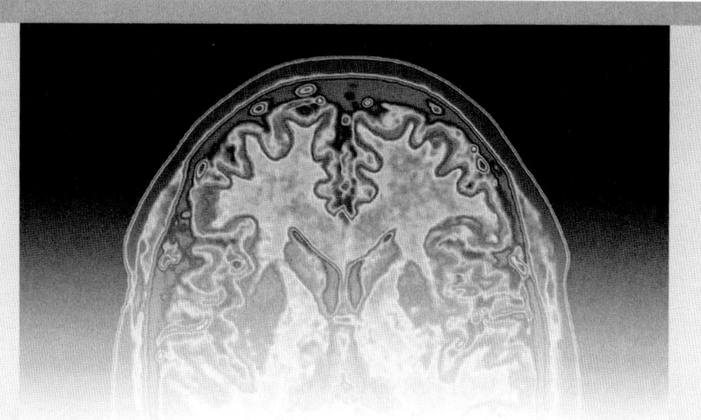

STROKE

A Practical Approach

James D. Geyer, MD, FAASM

Clinical Associate Professor
Neurology and Sleep Medicine
College of Community Health Sciences
University of Alabama
Medical Director
Clinical Neurophysiology Laboratories and Sleep Center
Alabama Neurology and Sleep Medicine
Tuscaloosa, Alabama

Camilo R. Gomez, MD

Division of Critical Care Neurology
Alabama Neurological Institute
Birmingham, Alabama

Wolters Kluwer | Lippincott Williams & Wilkins
Health

Philadelphia • Baltimore • New York • London
Buenos Aires • Hong Kong • Sydney • Tokyo

Acquisitions Editor: Frances DeStefano
Managing Editor: Leanne McMillan
Project Manager: Alicia Jackson
Senior Manufacturing Manager: Benjamin Rivera
Marketing Manager: Brian Freiland
Designer: Stephen Druding
Cover Designer: Stephen Druding
Production Service: Spearhead Global, Inc.

530 Walnut Street
Philadelphia, PA 19106 USA
LWW.com

Printed in the USA

Library of Congress Cataloging-in-Publication Data
Stroke : a practical approach / [edited by] James D. Geyer, Camilo R. Gomez.
p. ; cm.
Includes bibliographical references.
ISBN 978-0-7817-6614-2
1. Cerebrovascular disease—Handbooks, manuals, etc. I. Geyer, James D. II. Gomez, Camilo R.
[DNLM: 1. Stroke. WL 355 S9207 2009]
RC388.5.S846 2009
616.8'1—dc22 2008024285

10 9 8 7 6 5 4 3 2 1

To my wife Stephenie and my daughters Sydney and Emery.
Thank you for your help and understanding.

—JG

It is not the critic who counts, not the man who points out how the strong man stumbled, or where the doer of deeds could have done better. The credit belongs to the man who is actually in the arena; whose face is marred by the dust and sweat and blood; who strives valiantly; who errs and comes short again and again; who knows the great enthusiasms, the great devotions and spends himself in a worthy course; who at best, knows in the end the triumph of high achievement, and who, at worst, if he fails, at least fails while daring greatly; so that his place shall never be with those cold and timid souls who know neither victory or defeat.

—Theodore Roosevelt

CONTRIBUTORS

Nadeem Akhtar, MD
Internal Medicine
University of Alabama at Birmingham Health System
Birmingham, Alabama

Nader Antonios, MD
Assistant Professor
Department of Neurology
University of Florida College of Medicine
Vascular Neurologist
Department of Neurology
Shands Hospital
Jacksonville, Florida

José Biller, MD, FACP, FAHA, FAAN
Professor of Neurology and Neurological Surgery
Chairman
Department of Neurology
Loyola University Chicago
Stritch School of Medicine
Maywood, Illinois

Lorenzo Blas, MD
Stroke Fellow
Department of Neurology
Mount Sinai School of Medicine
Mount Sinai Hospital
New York, New York

Alan Blum, MD
Professor
Family Medicine
Director
The Center for the Study of Tobacco and Society
University of Alabama School of Medicine
Tuscaloosa, Alabama

Murray E. Brandstater, MD, PhD
Professor and Chairman
Physical Medicine and Rehabilitation
Loma Linda University
Chief, Physical Medicine and Rehabilitation Service
Loma Linda Medical Center
Loma Linda, California

Rebecca Brashler, LCSW
Assistant Professor
Physical Medicine and Rehabilitation and Medical Humanities and Bioethics
Feinberg School of Medicine
Northwestern University
Director of Inpatient Care Management
Rehabilitation Institute of Chicago
Chicago, Illinois

Paul R. Carney, MD
Professor
Departments of Pediatrics and Neurology
University of Florida
Chief, Departments of Pediatrics and Neurology
Shands Hospital
Gainesville, Florida

R. Webster Crowley, MD
Resident
Department of Neurological Surgery
University of Virginia School of Medicine
Charlottesville, Virginia

Rima M. Dafer, MD
Associate Professor
Department of Neurology
Loyola University Chicago
Stritch School of Medicine
Departments of Neurology and Neurological Surgery
Loyola University Health System
Maywood, Illinois

Stephenie C. Dillard, MD
Neurology and Sleep Medicine
College of Community Health Sciences
University of Alabama
Tuscaloosa, Alabama

Joseph Drabick MD, FACP
Professor of Medicine
Department of Medicine-Hematology/Oncology
Pennsylvania State University
Milton S. Hershey Medical Center
Hershey, Pennsylvania

Aaron S. Dumont, MD
Assistant Professor
Departments of Neurological Surgery and Radiology
University of Virginia School of Medicine
Co-Director Cerebrovascular and Skull Base Surgery
Comprehensive Stroke Center
Department of Neurological Surgery
University of Virginia Health System
Charlottesville, Virginia

Azadeh Farin, MD
Resident Physician
Department of Neurosurgery
University of Southern California
Los Angeles, California

John M. Field, MD
Professor of Medicine and Surgery
Heart and Vascular Institute
College of Medicine
Pennsylvania State University
Hershey, Pennsylvania

Michael J. Fogli, MD
Consulting Cardiologist
Cardiovascular MRI Department
Oklahoma Heart Institute
Tulsa, Oklahoma

Jennifer A. Frontera, MD
Assistant Professor
Departments of Neurosurgery and Neurology
Mount Sinai School of Medicine
Co-Director, Neuro-intensive Care Unit
Departments of Neurosurgery and Neurology
Mount Sinai Hospital, New York, New York

James D. Geyer, MD, FAASM
Clinical Associate Professor
Neurology and Sleep Medicine
College of Community Health Sciences
University of Alabama
Medical Director
Clinical Neurophysiology Laboratories and Sleep Center
Alabama Neurology and Sleep Medicine
Tuscaloosa, Alabama

Steven L. Giannotta MD, FACS
Professor and Chairman
Department of Neurosurgery
Keck School of Medicine
University of Southern California
Los Angeles, California

Camilo R. Gomez, MD
Division of Critical Care Neurology
Alabama Neurological Institute
Birmingham, Alabama

Sameer Gupta, MD
Resident
Department of Internal Medicine
Pennsylvania State College of Medicine
Milton S. Hershey Medical Center
Hershey, Pennsylvania

Maxim D. Hammer, MD
Assistant Professor of Neurology
Department of Neurology
University of Pittsburgh Medical Center
Attending Physician
The Stroke Institute
University of Pittsburgh Medical Center
Pittsburgh, Pennsylvania

Jason Heil, MD
Clinical Instructor
Department of Neurology
University of Cincinnati; Resident
Department of Neurology
University Hospital
Cincinnati, Ohio

Monica M. Henderson, RN, RPSGT
Sleep Health Coordinator
Alabama Neurology and Sleep Medicine
Tuscaloosa, Alabama

Dara G. Jamieson, MD
Associate Professor
Department of Neurology
Weill Cornell Medical College
Associate Neurologist
Department of Neurology
New York-Presbyterian Hospital
New York, New York

Tudor G. Jovin, MD
Assistant Professor of Neurology
Department of Neurology
University of Pittsburgh Medical Center
Attending Physician
The Stroke Institute
University of Pittsburgh Medical Center
Pittsburgh, Pennsylvania

Neal F. Kassell, MD
Department of Neurological Surgery
University of Virginia School of Medicine
Charlottesville, Virginia

Brett Kissela, MD
Associate Professor
Vice Chair of Graduate Medical Education and Hospital Services
Department of Neurology
University of Cincinnati
Cincinnati, Ohio

Giuseppe Lanzino, MD
Associate Professor
Departments of Neurosurgery and Radiology
Chief
Cerebrovascular Section
University of Illinois College of Medicine at Peoria
Peoria, Illinois

Kenneth Lichstein, PhD
Professor and Chair
Psychology Department
University of Alabama
Tuscaloosa, Alabama

Geoffrey S.F. Ling, MD, PhD
Director
Critical Care Division
Department of Anesthesiology and Critical Care Medicine
Uniformed Services University of the Health Sciences
Bethesda, Maryland

Irene Malaty, MD
Clinical Lecturer
Neurology Department
University of Florida and Physician
Shands Hospital
Gainesville, Florida

Marc Malkoff, MD
Director
Neurovascular and Neurocritical Care Programs
Division of Neurology
Barrow Neurological Institute
Phoenix, Arizona

Edward T. Martin, MD, FACC, FAHA, FACP
Professor
Department of Medicine
University of Oklahoma
Director
Cardiovascular MRI Department
Oklahoma Heart Institute
Tulsa, Oklahoma

Stephan A. Mayer, MD
Associate Professor
Department of Neurology
Columbia University
Director
Neuro ICU
Department of Neurology
New York-Presbyterian Hospital
New York, New York

W. Alvin McElveen, MD, FAAN
Chairman
Neurosciences Committee
Blake Medical Center
Bradenton, Florida

Chad M. Miller, MD
Assistant Professor
Department of Neurosurgery
UCLA Medical Center
Los Angeles, California

Babak B. Navi, MD
Chief Resident
Neurology Department
New York-Presbyterian Hospital
New York, New York

Daniel C. Potts, MD
Alabama Neurology and Sleep Medicine
Tuscaloosa, Alabama

Stylianos Rammos, MD
Resident
Neurological Surgery Department
University of Illinois College of Medicine at Peoria
St. Francis Hospital
Peoria, Illinois

Kerri S. Remmel, MD, PhD
Associate Professor
Chief
Vascular Neurology
Department of Neurology
University of Louisville School of Medicine
Louisville, Kentucky

Ronald G. Riechers II, MD
Assistant Professor
Department of Neurology
Uniformed Services University of Health Sciences
Bethesda, Maryland
Staff Neurologist
Department of Neurology
Walter Reed Army Medical Center
Washington, D.C.

Fred Rincon, MD
Clinical Fellow
Neurological Intensive Care and Stroke Department
Neurological Institute
Columbia University
Clinical Assistant
Department of Neurology
New York-Presbyterian Hospital
New York, New York

Matthew A. Saxonhouse, MD
Assistant Professor
Department of Pediatrics
University of Florida
Assistant Medical Director
Neonatal Intensive Care Unit
Shands Children's Hospital
Gainesville, Florida

Alan Z. Segal, MD
Associate Professor of Clinical Neurology
Department of Neurology
Weill Cornell Medical College
Associate Attending Neurologist
Department of Neurology
New York-Presbyterian Hospital
New York, New York

A. Robert Sheppard, MD
Associate Professor
Department of Internal Medicine
University of Alabama School of Medicine
Director of Hospital Services
DCH Regional Medical Center
Tuscaloosa, Alabama

Scott Silliman, MD
Associate Professor
Department of Neurology
University of Florida College of Medicine
Director
Comprehensive Stroke Program
Shands Hospital
Jacksonville, Florida

Shanthi Sivendran, MD
Resident
Department of Medicine
Pennsylvania State University
Milton S. Hershey Medical Center
Hershey, Pennsylvania

Michael A. Sloan, MD, MS, FAAN, FACP
Professor
Departments of Neurology and Neurosurgery
University of South Florida
Director
Stroke Program
Department of Medicine
Tampa General Hospital
Tampa, Florida

Gene Sung, MD, MPH
Director
Neurocritical Care and Stroke Division
Department of Neurology
University of Southern California
Los Angeles, California

David J. Teeple, MD
Division of Neurology
Barrow Neurological Institute
St. Joseph's Hospital and Medical Center
Phoenix, Arizona

Julie C. Tsikhlakis, RN
Sleep Health Coordinator
Alabama Neurology and Sleep Medicine
Tuscaloosa, Alabama

Anna Wanahita, MD
Co-Medical Director
St. John Stroke Center
Director
St. John Stroke Service
St. John Medical Center
Tulsa, Oklahoma

Heather P. Whitley, PharmD, BCPS, CDE
Clinical Assistant Professor
Departments of Pharmacy Practice and Community Practice and Rural Medicine
Harrison School of Pharmacy
Auburn University;
University of Alabama School of Medicine
Tuscaloosa, Alabama
Clinical Pharmacy Specialist
Moundville Medical Clinic
Moundville, Alabama

PREFACE

When we first considered the idea of publishing a book on stroke, we immediately asked ourselves "Why should we do this, if there already are several publications on the subject?" There could only be one answer, "Let's do a different type of book!" So we embarked in a journey that required us to examine the existing publications and discern what, if anything, they were lacking that could constitute our contribution to the subject. It became readily apparent (at least to us) that all the available books on stroke had been written following the mainstream flow of thoughts that one could easily find simply by reviewing the literature. Thus, we decided to approach the subject from a more personal point of view. Together, we have well over forty years of combined clinical practice in neurology, and we viewed our contribution to the field of vascular neurology as a compilation of practical ideas that could be applied at the bedside, for the benefit of stroke patients. *Stroke: A Practical Approach* takes the position that it is not sufficient to quote papers and studies. They must be placed in perspective with a critical look at the limitations and incongruence that often go unrecognized in published results of clinical research.

We live in a time when the medical community has misguidedly oversimplified evidence-based medicine (EBM) into a "randomized clinical trial or bust" philosophy. As a consequence, the pendulum of medical education has swung almost to the extreme of a recipe-driven, nonthinking, logic-defying, guideline-following decision-making practice. In this context, we thought it would be better to present our message from the vantage point of the second component of EBM: clinical expertise! Thus, we hope that the reader will find in these pages some practical opinions that, although certainly developed in the framework of all of the existing evidence, are tempered by our experience in dealing with the day-to-day practice of our specialty. *Stroke: A Practical Approach* is not all-inclusive, and the reader may find some passages to be controversial, even unorthodox, but it is an honest and practical approach to stroke and its management in the field. And so . . .

. . . enjoy the reading and Godspeed!

James D. Geyer
Camilo R. Gomez

ACKNOWLEDGMENTS

he editors would like to recognize the work of the clinicians managing stroke and its aftermath. We hope this book helps with this daunting task.

The editors would also like to thank Leanne McMillan and Fran DeStefano at Lippincott Williams & Wilkins for their support and assistance with the text.

CONTENTS

SECTION I

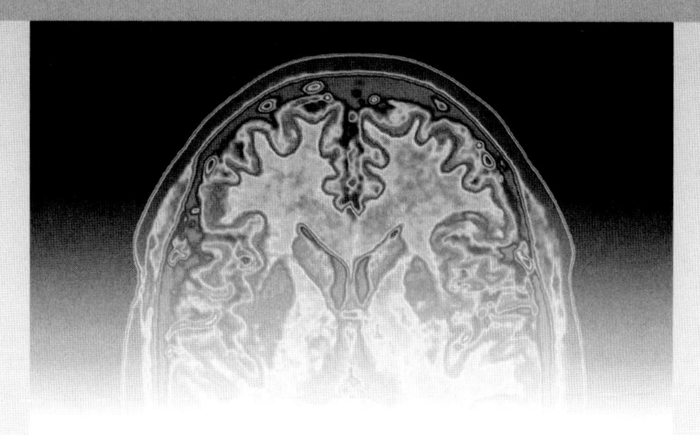

Introduction to Stroke

Stroke Mythology

JAMES D. GEYER AND CAMILO R. GOMEZ

The recent recognition of vascular neurology as a subspecialty of neurology, creating a structure similar to that which relates cardiology to internal medicine, underscores the complexity of our medical field. Still, despite such an evolution, the value of a vascular neurologist is yet to be realized by the medical community. In fact, in a large proportion of community hospitals, neurology is not even considered its own specialty but rather a branch of internal medicine, and the existence of vascular neurology is not a matter of priority. The problem is compounded by the wide acceptance of concepts that, although hardly reasonable or true, are repeated in a somewhat dogmatic way and embraced as if they represented gospel-generated knowledge on the subject of stroke. These concepts, which we view as *stroke myths*, require reflection and critical analysis so that stroke patients are not subjected to inexorable outcomes resulting from the erroneous understanding of their condition. This chapter describes the most important of these stroke myths, followed by an alternative view of their true meaning and an admonishment of their potential deleterious impact on patient care.

GENERAL MYTHS

Physician + Magnetic Resonance Imaging = Neurologist

There is no doubt that the introduction of magnetic resonance imaging (MRI) represents a major advance in our ability to identify and catalog different forms of stroke, and more recently, to noninvasively assess the status of the cerebral vasculature. The technology even allows us to select patients for certain specific therapeutic strategies. There is, however, the perception that MRI provides any physician with all the answers necessary to care for stroke patients. Therefore, although no one would dream of caring for patients with myocardial infarction without the involvement of a cardiologist, most strokes are handled regardless of the availability of a vascular neurologist (or even a neurologist for that matter). This leads to a double standard that shortchanges the stroke patient and his or her access to expert care. Paradoxically, despite the medical community's obsession with evidence-based medicine (see section on Evidence-Based Medicine = Randomized Clinical Trials) the behavior centered on this myth occurs despite extensive evidence of the extent to which stroke patient outcomes are improved by direct neurological care. In our view, the unspoken notion that anyone who can order an MRI is capable of managing stroke patients is an extension of the traditional view of neurology as an eminently diagnostic, rather than therapeutic, specialty. Furthermore, although MRI results are important, when they are taken out of the context of the entire patient microenvironment, they lead at best to therapeutic confusion and, at worst, to erroneous decisions. Another interesting dimension of the use of sophisticated brain imaging, especially MRI, is its incorporation into the decision tree of stroke care. For years we have championed the concept of MRI effectively representing bedside neuropathology, and we argue that the most qualified individual to properly understand the transcendence of the imaging findings is one with extensive knowledge of neuropathology (such as that acquired through systematic sessions of brain cutting), neurophysiology (such as that acquired as part of the study of normal and abnormal behavior of the cerebral circulation and their clinical manifestations), and the natural history of various types of stroke (such as that acquired from the irreplaceable experience of being directly in charge of the care of thousands of these patients). In today's health care environment, it is no longer possible to use the lack of availability of neurologists as an excuse to circumvent expert care. Indeed, telemedicine and all the advances made around it have resulted in a paradigm that allows any stroke patient to have access to neurological care, regardless of location.

Mini Strokes, Cerebrovascular Accidents, and Chaotic Communication

We live in a society in which anyone with access to the Internet thinks they have as much knowledge as any physician regarding the diagnosis and treatment of clinical disorders, including stroke. Such accessibility by patients and families to uncritical and nonauthoritative information, in our experience, leads to more confusion and conflict than is necessary or desirable. The existence of a large segment of our population with partial information, and without the educational framework to assess the relevance or importance of the information itself, forces health care professionals to be extra careful in what they say and how it is said. Invariably, patients and families with clearly erroneous (or sometimes just inaccurate) information have significant difficulties listening to corrective statements because their tendency is to try to fit any new information in the context of what they already think to be true. From this perspective, health care professionals must strive to communicate as clearly and accurately as possible, thereby not compounding the existing problem. In vascular neurology, this represents a major challenge, since one of the inadequacies of our specialty is that of using inappropriate (or out-of-date) nomenclature. For example, it is not unusual for patients and families to relate how they have been told that the patients have had a *mini stroke*—a term that lacks specificity and accuracy. As such, it is impossible to be sure whether *mini* refers to the small size, brief duration, light deficit, or nondisabling long-term impact of an event. These characteristics of stroke are not interchangeable, as anyone who has cared for a patient with a pontine perforator infarction knows: a small infarct, with pronounced motor deficit, and significant chances of disability.

Finally, in our view the preciseness with which we communicate reflects the clarity of our thoughts and the depth of our knowledge. As such, communication between the health care professional and the patient also leaves a lot to be desired, as evidenced by the continued and pervasive use of the term *cerebrovascular accident* (CVA). For more than 20 years we have pointed out why this term is inappropriate (i.e., stroke does not occur by accident, but it occurs in stroke-prone individuals) and inaccurate (i.e., the term does not specify the type of stroke), yet it remains anchored in the mainstream of everyday clinical communication. With this in mind, we take the position that the most important step health care professionals can take toward improving stroke management is to optimize their communication skills, striving toward more precise, concise, and focused discussions with peers as well as patients.

DIAGNOSTIC MYTHS

The "Self-Evident" Cause of Ischemic Stroke

Despite all the educational campaigns, conferences, symposia, and discussions, not a day goes by without a patient presenting to an emergency department with symptoms of ischemic stroke and an electrocardiogram (ECG) showing de novo atrial fibrillation, which is immediately blamed for the event. Largely, such a scenario obviates any critical analysis of concurrent risk factors or a thorough evaluation of the patient. The fallacy of this approach is easy to identify: Having any one risk factor for stroke does not exclude the presence of concurrent ones. The dire consequence is that patients are undiagnosed and only partially treated. How many times have patients been sent home from emergency rooms after having had a normal carotid ultrasound, only to come back a week later with an acute basilar occlusion due to an intracranial stenosis that was never identified because of inadequate testing? An old saying goes, "We find what we look for . . . and we recognize what we know!" In our view, every stroke patient represents a diagnostic mystery that must be investigated in its entirety, allowing for the possibility of concurrent and coexistent risk factors, which we have come to call *double jeopardy*. Both philosophically and practically we view stroke risk factors as functions of one of three categoric dimensions: vascular, cardiac, and hematologic. From this point of view, every stroke patient deserves a critical evaluation, including stratification of the type and number of risk factors present, to be the subject of an all-inclusive secondary prevention strategy that ensures optimal reduction of subsequent stroke risk. Otherwise, any focused preventive strategy is unlikely to sufficiently protect the patient.

Lacunes, Lacunar Infarcts, and Small Vessel Disease

Lacunes, lacunar infarcts, and small vessel disease are among the most misunderstood subjects in vascular neurology, which leads to significant miscommunication. The premise for this myth is the oversimplified belief that every small subcortical infarction should be labeled as *lacunar*, manifesting itself as a *lacunar syndrome*, and is the direct result of *small vessel disease*. In our view, such train of thought demonstrates a lack of understanding of the differences between phenomenology, pathophysiology, and pathology of such conditions. We must state our view on this subject by transporting the reader back to the 19th century, when Durand-Fardel used the term *lacune* for the first time in the medical literature. It is unclear whether the author differentiated these pathological findings as the result of infarction or simply as perivascular dilatations (considering that he also introduced the term *etat criblé* in the same manuscript). Then, 20 years later, Proust published a thesis in which he addressed the subject, for the first time pointing out that three different processes can result in the postmortem finding of lacunes: infarction, hemorrhage, or perivascular disorganization. The years that followed brought with them a series of reports largely emphasizing the clinicopathologic correlation between lacunes and certain specific lacunar syndromes, culminating with a 1965 paper in which Fisher equated lacunes to small deep infarctions. Interestingly, this manuscript concluded by drawing a direct association between hypertension and these deep infarcts.

Each of these communications, with immense historical value, must be placed in the context of the primitive status of the imaging techniques of that era. Inferences were being made by drawing conclusions from the autopsy table and depending on preexisting clinical observations that were often poorly recorded. Nevertheless, reviewing these papers in toto should quickly uncover what has come to be proved by modern, imaging-based studies: (a) not every lacune represents an underlying infarction, (b) lacunar infarction does not have to course with a classic lacunar syndrome, and (c) deep small infarctions have more than one potential pathogenesis. Along these lines, it is our view that the term *lacune* should be reserved for more generic references relative to small brain cavities that can be caused by several processes, only one of which is ischemia due to perforating arterial occlusion. The literature cited earlier also notes that many of the patients who display these lesions at autopsy have not had any previous history of stroke symptoms. Furthermore, the literature on lacunar syndromes shows over and over again the lack of localizing value of such a presentation, as each of these syndromes has been associated with a multitude of lesion locations.

Finally, the most uncritical aspect of this subject is the de facto association of lacunar infarction with small vessel disease. The truth is that such a disease does not exist! In other words, anyone who uses the term should be challenged to describe the etiology, pathogenesis, treatment, and prognosis of that illness. Any answer to such a challenge is bound to represent an inaccurate or incomplete description of another entity the precise name of which has been ignored. Our view is that the term *lacunar infarction* should be reserved for those small deep infarcts secondary to direct occlusion of penetrating small arterioles chronically affected by lipohyalinosis and fibrinoid necrosis (i.e., hypertensive arteriolopathy), satisfying the direct association between the two conditions emphasized by Fisher and others. In turn, we recommend that the term *small vessel disease* should not be used as such, since it carries an inherent lack of specificity. After all, there are many conditions that primarily affect the so-called small vessels, including meningovascular syphilis, granulomatous vasculitis, and lupus. Finally, we recommend that *lacunar infarction* not be used to describe small deep infarcts when the pathogenic mechanism is known to be other than hypertensive arteriolopathy. This is important because the existing literature clearly supports the notion that small deep infarcts are caused by embolism and by hemodynamic compromise.

Cryptogenic Stroke and Relative Ignorance

No term in the stroke nomenclature seems to have gained more popularity in the last decade than *cryptogenic stroke*. It has been the source of reports, publications, discussions, seminars, and clinical trials, and has attracted the attention of other specialists (namely cardiologists through their interest in percutaneously closing patent foramina ovale). This term was introduced in the literature to imply the presence of a stroke without evident cause, or stroke of unknown cause. However, this is probably a misnomer. The term *cryptogenic* can be broken down into two components: *crypto-* from the Latin *crypta* and the Greek term *kruptos* (κρυπτοσ), meaning hidden, and *-genic* from the Latin term *genea*, meaning origin. This term has been applied to conditions of unknown or obscure cause. However, we must point out that these are not equivalent and that an ischemic stroke caused, for example, by excessive factor VIII activity certainly has a cause that is obscure cause but known.

However, it is imperative to consider that the so-called cryptogenicity of any stroke is relative and that it directly results from the extent to which the evaluation for its cause has been carried out. As such, there are those who still think that performing a carotid ultrasound in the emergency room to exclude carotid stenotic pathology is a sufficient evaluation of the patients. Our view is consistent with the experience over the last 30 to 40 years. If one were to review the reports from studies carried out in the 1970s or 1980s, the rate of stroke of unknown etiology was as high as 50% in some series. The reason is simple—diagnostic technology had not come of age. The introduction of computed tomography (CT), MRI, and transesophageal echocardiography (TEE), however, changed all of that, demonstrating a series of causes of stroke that had previously been overlooked. Thus, inadequate evaluation of stroke patients is likely to yield a high number of cryptogenic strokes but this will not be the case when the patients are well evaluated. From this point of view, we also take the position that every patient in the emergency room has a cryptogenic stroke, since no steps for etiologic evaluation have yet been carried out. The level of cryptogenicity decreases concurrently as new answers are found through diagnostic testing.

Patent Foramen Ovale and Cardiogenic Stroke

One the most heated sources of argument at the present time is the best method for managing patients with ischemic stroke and a patent foramen ovale (PFO). The issue of whether to use warfarin, antiplatelet therapy, or percutaneous closure of the PFO is the subject of intense debate. Along these lines, because most PFOs are diagnosed via TEE, many include the PFO as a cardiogenic source of embolism. But is this reasonable?

Our view is that, in most cases, the PFO is a conduit (not the source) for embolism and that the latter originates somewhere in the venous side of the circulation. Therefore, we and others have shown that a stroke patient who is found to have a PFO must have an evaluation of the venous channels, not only of the lower limbs but also of the pelvis. From this perspective, ultrasound of the legs is incomplete and inadequate, and the preferred diagnostic tool is indisputably magnetic resonance venography (MRV). Thus, it seems erroneous to stop at the finding of the PFO, without entertaining a search for a venous source of embolism. The alternative is to have the patient suffer a fatal pulmonary embolism from an overlooked source after being treated without adequate anticoagulation coverage.

THERAPEUTIC MYTHS

Evidence-Based Medicine = Randomized Clinical Trials

The term *evidence-based medicine* (EBM) was coined in the early 1990s by a group of researchers at McMaster University to emphasize the critical need to gauge the existing evidence that supported one or another diagnostic or therapeutic strategy. The realizations that led to the introduction of EBM included the daily need for valid information about diagnosis, therapy, and prevention; the inadequacy of traditional sources of information; the disparity between skills/judgment and up-to-date knowledge/performance; and the shortage of time devoted to finding and assimilating information. However, in their design of this system, Guyat, Sackett, and their collaborators underestimated the prevalence of intellectual laziness and the overwhelming necessity of physicians to oversimplify concepts to apply them to their daily work.

And so comments that rightfully pointed out the superiority of randomized clinical trials (RCTs) as an investigative tool have been changed to the widespread accepted notion that without a clinical trial, it is impossible to correctly apply certain treatments to the patients. One predictable consequence of the fascination with RCTs is the obsession to conduct them regardless of how faulty the design is, irrespective of whether they are the most suitable option to attempt to answer a relevant question, and even if they lead to predictably absurd outcomes. Indeed, many academic careers hinge around conducting RCTs, and young investigators quickly fall prey to this style of thinking, to the point that many abandon independent or imaginative yet logical assessment of the clinical problems at hand. The latter behavior is aggravated by the secondary notion that the results of RCTs under any circumstance will trump the clinical judgment of the expert.

Our view on this subject adheres to the original concepts championed by the fathers of EBM. As such, EBM was always meant to be the integration of the following three components, each of which is equally necessary:

1. Best Research Evidence. This was never meant to imply only RCTs but rather to weigh the strength of the evidence so that it could be better placed in perspective with the other two components. Also, the realization that in certain circumstances it is simply impossible to resort to RCTs and that alternative means of finding answers are acceptable (as long as they are the best possible). Along these lines, there are those who often state that "the plural of anecdote is not data," implying that personal, remembered, and other unpublished accounts are useless. We agree that anecdotes are also forms of information; forms of evidence that should be given their own weight. Furthermore, data alone proves nothing, and the most important scientific theories must be proved through disproving null hypotheses (almost equivalent to *reductio ad absurdum* in mathematics). From this point of view, we answer, "The plural of datum is not proof!"
2. Clinical Expertise. The evidence, including RCTs, is of no use if the professionals who are to use it in patient care do not have the expertise to discern when and where any evidence is applicable. For example, it is only the expert specialist who will be able to look at a particular clinical scenario and take into consideration that the patient in question is sufficiently different from those included in the RCTs as to render the results either partially or completely inapplicable.
3. Patient Values. Finally, no evidence or expertise is sufficient unless the patient (the recipient of the treatment) is taken into consideration. This is of particular importance in an era during which there are powerful forces with a tendency

to dehumanize medicine. As such, the evidence may be strong and the expert may think it is applicable, but the patient's personal circumstances place an additional dimension in the algebraic summation of the clinical encounter.

Finally, we must emphasize another more dangerous consequence of misunderstanding EBM: its impact on education. The widespread acceptance of the notion of RCTs as the ne plus ultra for medical knowledge has resulted in a shift in medical education from systematic discernment and analysis of the clinical problems to memorization of relevant papers reporting pivotal RCTs, without which we do not seem to be able to practice. The problem is aggravated by the proliferation of guidelines, which promote a cookbook approach to management of patients and the spread of intellectual laziness.

Systematic Escalation of Antithrombotic Therapy

Another interesting yet illogical approach to stroke treatment is the following notion: A patient who has a stroke while on aspirin needs clopidogrel, and, if the same patient has another stroke on clopidogrel, warfarin must be prescribed. This practice, which is incredibly common, has absolutely no sound reasoning behind it. To begin with, let us point out that there is no infallible strategy for stroke prevention: Each one has a failure rate. Such a failure rate does not imply that another strategy, perceived to be stronger, is necessarily better. Having said this, the parallel argument includes the common practice of having antithrombotic medications approved by the U.S. Food and Drug Administration (FDA) for use in patients who have "failed" with another. It then becomes a self-fulfilling prophecy, because one could argue that perhaps the best drug should have been used in the first place. Our view is that if stroke patients undergo thorough risk stratification, it is likely that the best preventive strategy will become evident. This should be the one applied, always considering that there is no such thing as an infallible approach. Then, if confronted with patients who on the surface seem to have failed the therapy prescribed, rather than automatically escalating to the next stronger antithrombotic agent (or combination), we must systematically review the existing diagnostic data: Have we covered all possible diagnostic angles? Have we overlooked something? Is there room to reexamine other aspects of the patient? Has there been compliance with the treatment? Only by reviewing the previous steps is it possible to reach sound conclusions about the next. Conversely, simply escalating antithrombotic agents is illogical, unreasonable, and counterproductive.

Brain Hemorrhage Demands Neurosurgical Consultation

There is no more frequent clinical reflex than that of the emergency physician paging neurosurgery upon review of the urgent CT of a patient with a brain hemorrhage. This widely popular practice is paradoxically without foundation in the medical literature, with a few exceptions. In general, the existing evidence (interestingly being ignored) is that craniotomies to evacuate intracerebral hemorrhages are not only unhelpful but also often counterproductive. Yet the neurosurgeons are invariably summoned to care for patients they largely have no interest in. Our view is that most patients with hemorrhagic stroke need a neurologist with expertise in critical/intensive care. In fact, even subarachnoid hemorrhages, once primarily treated by surgical clipping of the aneurysm, are more commonly treated with endovascular therapy by interventional neurologists. In all fairness, there are two exceptional scenarios. The first is the patient with cerebellar hemorrhage for whom a suboccipital craniotomy may be lifesaving. The other is the patient with intraventricular hemorrhage who may require a ventriculostomy. However, in both cases, a neurointensivist is likely to optimally orchestrate the care of the patient.

CONCLUSION

We live in a very difficult health care environment, plagued with miscommunication, misconceptions, misperceptions, and mishaps. Add to this the overregulation and incomprehensible reprioritization of our clinical mission, with the consequent belief by many that patient satisfaction is more important than high-quality outcomes and promoting quality of life. We cannot afford to compound the problems by being uncritical about the information necessary to properly care for patients. We must question concepts that are obsolete, antiquated, inapplicable, suspect, bureaucratic, or simply wrong. Courage and determination at the bedside are likely to benefit patients and to improve the quality of the outcomes. Our views may not be popular, but they are the product of more than 30 years of combined clinical practice.

SELECTED REFERENCES

Ay H, Oliveira-Filho J, Buonanno FS, et al. Diffusion-weighted imaging identifies a subset of lacunar infarction associated with embolic source. *Stroke* 1999; 30(12):2644–2650.

Durand-Fardel M. *Traite du Ramollissement du Cerveau.* Paris: Bailliere; 1843.

Fisher C. Lacunes: Small, deep cerebral infarcts. *Neurology* 1965; 15:774–784.

Furlan AJ. CVA: reducing the risk of a confused vascular analysis. The Feinberg lecture. *Stroke* 2000; 31(6):1451–1456.

Gerraty RP, Parsons MW, Barber PA, et al. Examining the lacunar hypothesis with diffusion and perfusion magnetic resonance imaging. *Stroke* 2002; 33(8):2019–2024.

Jung DK, Devuyst G, Maeder P, et al. Atrial fibrillation with small subcortical infarcts. *J Neurol Neurosurg Psychiatry* 2001; 70(3): 344–349.

Mohr JP. Cryptogenic stroke. *N Engl J Med* 1988; 318(18):1197–1198.

Morgenstern LB, Frankowski RF, Shedden P, et al. Surgical treatment for intracerebral hemorrhage (STICH): A single-center, randomized clinical trial. *Neurology* 1998; 51(5):1359–1363.

Proust A. *Des Differentes Formes de Ramollissement du Cerveau.* Paris: 1866.

Sackett D, Straus S, Richardson WS, et al. *Evidence-Based Medicine: How to Practice and Teach EBM.* New York: Churchill Livingstone; 2000.

Saver JL. Cryptogenic stroke in patients with patent foramen ovale. *Curr Atheroscler Rep* 2007; 9(4):319–325.

Tejada J, Diez-Tejedor E, Hernandez-Echebarria L, et al. Does a relationship exist between carotid stenosis and lacunar infarction? *Stroke* 2003; 34(6):1404–1409.

CHAPTER 2

Stroke Localization

MURRAY E. BRANDSTATER, JAMES D. GEYER, AND CAMILO R. GOMEZ

The pathology of a lesion can be surmised from an analysis of the temporal profile of the clinical presentation, which includes the history and the progression and pattern of recovery of the lesion. Anatomic localization of a lesion can usually be established with reasonable accuracy based on a careful delineation of the neurological deficits. A complete picture of the neurological deficits may not be initially possible if the patient is confused and unable to cooperate fully with the examination. Therefore, repeat examinations of the patient in the early recovery phase help to further define the combination of deficits and assist in establishing the precise localization of the lesion. The following discussion describes in some detail the typical features observed in patients with commonly encountered focal stroke syndromes.

INTERNAL CAROTID ARTERY SYNDROME

The most minor clinical deficits associated with internal carotid artery ischemia are transient ischemic attacks (TIAs) caused by microembolic platelet aggregates carried peripherally from atherosclerotic plaques in the internal carotid or other large arteries. Transient occlusion of the retinal branches of an ophthalmic artery produces sudden, transient loss of vision in one eye—the amaurosis fugax syndrome. Cerebral TIAs take the form of brief motor, sensory, or language deficits.

The clinical consequences of complete occlusion of an internal carotid artery vary from no observable clinical deficit, if there is good collateral circulation, to massive cerebral infarction in the distribution of the anterior and middle cerebral arteries with rapid severe obtundation. The latter presents with head and eyes turned toward the side of the lesion and dense contralateral motor and sensory deficits. Often there is cerebral edema with transtentorial herniation and death. Less extensive infarctions result in partial or total lesions in the distribution of the middle cerebral artery. The anterior cerebral circulation may be preserved through flow from the opposite side via the anterior communicating artery. The first branch of the internal carotid artery is the ophthalmic, and if there is inadequate collateral flow through the orbit from the external carotid artery, there may be ipsilateral blindness from retinal ischemia on the side of the lesion associated with contralateral hemiplegia.

Middle Cerebral Artery Syndromes

The internal carotid artery divides into the middle and anterior cerebral arteries. The middle cerebral artery supplies the lateral aspect of the frontal, parietal, and temporal lobes and the underlying corona radiata, extending as deep as the putamen and the posterior limb of the internal capsule. As the main stem of the middle cerebral artery passes out through the Sylvian fissure, it gives rise to a series of small branches called lenticulostriate arteries, which penetrate deeply into the subcortical portion of the brain and perfuse the basal ganglia and internal capsule. At the lateral surface of the hemisphere, the middle cerebral artery divides into upper and lower divisions, which perfuse the lateral surface of the hemisphere. When the middle cerebral artery is occluded at its origin, a large cerebral infarction develops involving all the structures mentioned earlier. Because of the cerebral edema that usually accompanies such a large lesion with brain displacement, the patient initially shows depressed consciousness, with head and eyes deviated to the side of the lesion, as well as contralateral hemiplegia, decreased sensation, and homonymous hemianopia (see Table 2.1). If the dominant hemisphere is involved, a global aphasia is usually present. As the patient's mental status improves, other features become evident, such as dysphagia, contralateral hemianopia, and in patients with nondominant hemisphere lesions, perceptual deficits and neglect. Patients who survive the acute lesion regain control of head and eye movements, and their normal level of consciousness is restored. However, severe deficits involving motor, visuospatial, and language function usually persist with only limited recovery.

Occlusion of the branches of the middle cerebral artery, except for the lenticulostriate, is almost always embolic in origin, and the associated infarctions are correspondingly smaller and more peripherally located. The superior division of the middle cerebral artery supplies the Rolandic and pre-Rolandic areas, and an infarction in this territory will result in a dense sensorimotor deficit on the contralateral face, arm, and leg, with less involvement of the leg. As recovery occurs, the patient is usually able to walk with a spastic, hemiparetic gait. Little recovery occurs in motor function of the arm. If the left hemisphere is involved, there is usually severe aphasia initially, with eventual improvement in comprehension, although an expressive aphasia is likely to persist. Small focal infarctions from occlusions of branches of the superior division will produce more limited deficits such as pure motor weakness of the contralateral arm and face, apraxia, or expressive aphasia.

TABLE 2.1 Middle Cerebral Artery Syndrome

Contralateral hemiparesis and sensory loss (greater in the upper extremity and face)
Homonymous hemianopia
Aphasia/aprosody
Gaze abnormalities
Extinction
Astereognosis
Apraxia

The inferior division of the middle cerebral artery supplies the parietal and temporal lobes, and lesions on the left side result in severe inhibition of language comprehension. The optic radiation is usually involved, resulting in partial or complete homonymous hemianopia on the contralateral side. Lesions affecting the right hemisphere often result in neglect of the left side of the body. Initially, the patient may completely ignore the affected side and even assert that the arm on his left side belongs not to him but to somebody else. Such severe neglect seen initially often gradually improves but may be followed by a variety of persisting impairments, such as constructional apraxia, dressing apraxia, and perceptual deficits.

The lenticulostriate arteries are branches arising from the main stem of the middle cerebral artery that penetrate into the subcortical region and perfuse the basal ganglia and posterior internal capsule. Several characteristic and rather common isolated syndromes have been described when discrete focal lesions occur. These are frequently referred to as *lacunar strokes*. The most common is a lesion in the internal capsule causing a pure motor hemiplegia. An anterior lesion in the internal capsule may cause dysarthria with hand clumsiness, and a lesion of the thalamus or adjacent internal capsule causes a contralateral sensory loss with or without weakness. The neurological deficits in these lesions often show early and progressive recovery with good ultimate outcome.

Patients with hypertension and diabetes are at risk for recurrent lacunar strokes. Pseudobulbar palsy is a syndrome that develops when multiple small lesions affect the anterior limb of both internal capsules, including the corticobulbar pathways. This syndrome consists of excessive emotional lability and spastic bulbar (pseudobulbar) paralysis, which is characterized by dysarthria, dysphonia, dysphagia, and facial weakness (see Table 2.2). There are often sudden outbursts of inappropriate and uncontrolled crying and laughter, at times blending into each other, without corresponding emotional stimulus. Drooling is often prominent. The term *pseudobulbar* is applied to this syndrome to distinguish it as an upper motor neuron lesion in contrast to a lower motor neuron lesion in the medulla. More widespread and posterior subcortical lacunar infarctions will often produce a dementia, often called multi-infarct dementia.

Anterior Cerebral Artery Syndromes

Branches of the anterior cerebral arteries supply the median and paramedian regions of the frontal cortex and the strip of the lateral surface of the hemisphere along its upper border. There are deep penetrating branches that supply the head of the caudate nucleus and the anterior limb of the internal capsule. Occlusions of the anterior cerebral artery are not common, but when they occur, there is contralateral hemiparesis with relative sparing of the hand and face and greater weakness of the leg. There is associated sensory loss of the leg and foot. Lesions affecting the left side may produce a transcortical motor aphasia characterized by diminution of spontaneous speech but preserved ability to repeat words. A grasp reflex is often present along with a sucking reflex and paratonic rigidity (*gegenhalten*). Urinary incontinence is common. Large lesions of the frontal cortex often produce behavioral changes, such as lack of spontaneity, distractibility, and tendency to perseverate. Patients may have diminished reasoning ability (see Table 2.3).

TABLE 2.2 Bulbar versus Pseudobulbar Signs

	Bulbar	Pseudobulbar
Tongue		
Size	Atrophy	Normal
Movement	Decreased	Decreased
Fasciculation	Present	Absent
Speech	Flaccid	Spastic
Face	Weak	Weak
Emotional lability	Absent	Present
Jaw jerk	Absent	Present
Gag	Absent	Hyperactive
Extraocular movements	Decreased	Decreased

TABLE 2.3 Anterior Cerebral Artery Syndrome

Contralateral hemiparesis and sensory loss (greater in the legs and feet)
Disconnection syndromes
Behavior disturbances (abulia, akinetic mutism)

VERTEBROBASILAR SYNDROMES

The two vertebral arteries join at the junction of the medulla and pons to form the basilar artery. Together, the vertebral and basilar arteries supply the brainstem through the paramedian and short circumferential branches and supply the cerebellum by long circumferential branches. The basilar artery terminates by bifurcating at the upper midbrain level to form the two posterior cerebral arteries. The posterior communicating arteries connect the middle to the posterior cerebral arteries, completing the circle of Willis.

Some general clinical features of lesions in the vertebrobasilar system should be noted. In contrast to lesions in the hemispheres, which are unilateral, lesions involving the pons and medulla often cross the midline and cause bilateral features. When motor impairments are present, they are often bilateral, with asymmetric corticospinal signs, and they are frequently accompanied by cerebellar signs. Cranial nerve lesions are very frequent and occur ipsilateral to the main lesion, producing contralateral corticospinal signs. There may be dissociated sensory loss (involvement of the spinothalamic pathway with preservation of the dorsal column pathway or vice versa), dysarthria, dysphagia, disequilibrium and vertigo, and Horner syndrome. Of particular note is the absence of cortical deficits, such as aphasia and cognitive impairments. Visual field loss and visuospatial deficits may occur if the posterior cerebral artery is involved, but not with brainstem lesions. Identification of a specific cranial nerve lesion allows precise anatomic localization of the lesion.

Lacunar infarcts are common in the vertebrobasilar distribution, arising from occlusion of small penetrating branches of the basilar artery or posterior cerebral artery. In contrast to cerebral lacunes, most brainstem lacunes produce clinical features. There are a variety of characteristic brainstem syndromes associated with lesions at various levels in the brainstem. These brainstem syndromes are not infrequently encountered in patients referred for rehabilitation. The reader is referred to neurological texts for a comprehensive discussion of these lesions.

The lateral medullary syndrome (Wallenberg syndrome) is produced by an infarction in the lateral wedge of the medulla. It may occur as an occlusion of the vertebral artery or the posterior inferior cerebellar artery. The clinical features of this syndrome, along with the corresponding anatomic structures involved, are impairment of contralateral pain and temperature control (spinothalamic tract); ipsilateral Horner syndrome consisting of miosis, ptosis, and decreased facial sweating (descending sympathetic tract); dysphagia, dysarthria, and dysphonia (ipsilateral paralysis of the palate and vocal cords); nystagmus, vertigo, nausea, and vomiting (vestibular nucleus); ipsilateral limb ataxia (spinocerebellar fibers); and ipsilateral impaired sensation of the face (sensory nucleus of the fifth nerve). Patients with this syndrome are frequently disabled initially because of vertigo, disequilibrium, and ataxia, but they often make a good functional recovery.

Occlusion of the basilar artery may result in severe deficits with complete motor and sensory loss and cranial nerve signs from which patients do not recover. Patients are often comatose. Less extensive lesions, however, are compatible with life, and a characteristic syndrome observed occasionally is the locked-in syndrome. The infarction in such cases affects the upper ventral pons, involving the bilateral corticospinal and corticobulbar pathways but sparing the reticular activating system and ascending sensory pathways. Patients have normal sensation and can see and hear but are unable to move or speak. Blinking and upward gaze are preserved, which provides a very limited but usable means for communication. The patient is alert and fully oriented. Some patients do not survive, and those who do are severely disabled and dependent. Some slow progressive improvement and partial recovery may occur in this group of patients, justifying appropriate levels of rehabilitation intervention.

Focal infarctions may occur in the midbrain and affect the descending corticospinal pathway, sometimes also involving the third cranial nerve nucleus (Weber's syndrome), resulting in ipsilateral third nerve palsy and paralysis of the contralateral arm and leg (see Table 2.4).

The posterior cerebral artery perfuses the thalamus through perforating arteries, as well as the temporal and occipital lobes with their subcortical structures, including the optic radiation. An occipital lobe infarction will cause a partial or complete contralateral hemianopia, and when these visual deficits involve the dominant hemisphere, there may be associated difficulty in reading or in naming objects. When the thalamus is involved, there is contralateral

TABLE 2.4 Lacunar Syndromes

1. Pure sensory
   a. Location: Ventral posterior thalamus
   b. Contralateral sensory loss
2. Pure motor
   a. Location: Posterior limb internal capsule, cerebral peduncle, pons, or hemispheric white matter
   b. Contralateral weakness
3. Ataxic hemiparesis
   a. Location: Basis pontis but localizes poorly
   b. Contralateral weakness and ataxia
4. Dysarthria clumsy hand syndrome
   a. Location: Genu of the internal capsule
   b. Contralateral clumsy hand and dysarthria
5. Thalamic dementia
   a. Location: Thalamus
   b. Subcortical dementia
6. Sensorimotor
   a. Location: Thalamus and internal capsule
   b. Contralateral sensory loss and weakness
7. Hemiballismus
   a. Location: Subthalamic nucleus
   b. Contralateral hemiballismus
8. Status lacunaris
   a. Location: multiple widespread lacunes
   b. Parkinsonism, dementia
9. Claude syndrome
   a. Location: midbrain tegmentum, red nucleus, CN III
   b. Ipsilateral CN III palsy
   c. Contralateral ataxia, tremor
10. Benedikt's syndrome
    a. Location: Midbrain tegmentum, red nucleus, CN III, cerebral peduncle
    b. Ipsilateral CN III palsy
    c. Contralateral ataxia, tremor, and weakness
11. Weber's syndrome
    a. Location: ventral midbrain, CN III, cerebral peduncle
    b. Ipsilateral CN III palsy
    c. Contralateral weakness
12. Parinaud's syndrome
    a. Location: Dorsorostral midbrain and posterior commisure
    b. Paralysis of upgaze, convergence-retraction nystagmus, lid retraction, and light near dissociation
13. Nothnagel's syndrome
    a. Location: dorsal midbrain, brachium conjunctivum, CN III, MLF
    b. Ipsilateral ataxia, CN III palsy, and vertical gaze palsy
14. Raymond-Cestan syndrome
    a. Location: mid pons, middle cerebellar peduncle, corticospinal tract
    b. Ipsilateral ataxia
    c. Contralateral weakness
15. One-and-a-half syndrome
    a. Location: PPRF or CN VI and MLF
    b. Ipsilateral horizontal gaze palsy
    c. Contralateral INO
16. Foville's syndrome
    a. Location: PPRF, CN VI, CN VII, corticospinal tract
    b. Ipsilateral horizontal gaze palsy, CN VII palsy
    c. Contralateral weakness, sensory loss, INO
17. Millard-Gubler syndrome
    a. Location: ventral pons, CN VI and VII fascicles corticospinal tracts
    b. Ipsilateral CN VI and CN VII palsy
    c. Contralateral weakness
18. Raymond syndrome
    a. Location: ventral pons, CN VI fascicles, and corticospinal tract
    b. Ipsilateral CN VI palsy
    c. Contralateral weakness

(Continued on following page)

TABLE 2.4 Lacunar Syndromes (continued)

19. Babinski-Nageotte syndrome
    a. Location: dorsolateral pontomedullary junction
    b. Ipsilateral ataxia, facial sensory loss, Horner syndrome
    c. Contralateral weakness, sensory loss in the body vertigo, vomiting, and nystagmus
20. Wallenberg syndrome
    a. Location: dorsolateral medulla, restiform body, CN V, IX, and X
    b. Ipsilateral ataxia, Horner's syndrome, facial sensory loss
    c. Contralateral loss of pain and temperature
21. Cestan-Chenais syndrome
    a. Location: lateral medulla
    b. Ipsilateral ataxia, Horner's syndrome, facial sensory loss
    c. Contralateral hemibody sensory loss and weakness
22. Avellis' syndrome
    a. Location: lateral medulla, CN IX, CN X, lateral spinothalamic tracts
    b. Ipsilateral paralysis soft palate, vocal cords, posterior pharynx
    c. Contralateral hemiparesis and sensory loss
23. Vernet's syndrome
    a. Location: lateral medulla, CN IX, X, and XI
    b. Ipsilateral paralysis palate, sternocleidomastoid (SCM), decreased taste posterior tongue
    c. Contralateral hemiparesis
24. Jackson's syndrome
    a. Location: lateral medulla, CN IX, X, XI, and XII
    b. Ipsilateral paralysis palate, vocal cords, SCM, tongue
    c. Contralateral weakness and sensory loss
25. Preolivary
    a. Location: anterior medulla, CN XII, pyramid
    b. Ipsilateral tongue weakness
    c. Contralateral hemiparesis

CN, cranial nerve; MLF, medial longitudinal fasciculus; PPRF, paramedian pontine reticular formation; INO, intranuclear ophthalmoplegia.

TABLE 2.5 Arterial Vascular and Venous Sinus Distributions

Arterial Vascular Distributions

A. Posterior cerebral artery
   1. Mesencephalic perforating artery
      a. Tectum
      b. Cerebral peduncles
   2. Posterior thalamoperforating artery
      a. Hypothalamus
      b. Subthalamus
      c. Midline and medial thalamic nuclei
   3. Posterior medial choroidal artery
      a. Quadrigeminal plate
      b. Pineal gland
      c. Choroid plexus
      d. Medial dorsal nucleus of the thalamus
   4. Posterior lateral choroidal artery
      a. Choroid plexus
      b. Fornix
      c. Medial dorsal nucleus of the thalamus
      d. Pulvinar
      e. Part of the lateral geniculate body
B. Anterior choroidal artery
   1. Proximal
      a. Optic tract
      b. Genu of the internal capsule
      c. Medial globus pallidus
   2. Lateral
      a. Piriform cortex
      b. Uncus
      c. Hippocampus
      d. Dentate
      e. Tail of the caudate nucleus

Venous Sinus Distributions

A. Superior longitudinal (sagittal) sinus
   1. Location: attached along the falx
   2. Receives flow from superior superficial veins
   3. Empties into the transverse sinus
B. Inferior longitudinal (sagittal) sinus
   1. Location: free margin of the falx
   2. Receives flow from superior superficial veins
   3. Empties into the straight sinus
C. Straight sinus
   1. Location: junction of the falx and tentorium
   2. Receives flow from inferior sagittal sinus and vein of Galen
   3. Empties into the transverse sinus
D. Sigmoid sinus
   1. Location: between transverse sinus and jugular vein
   2. Receives flow from transverse sinus and inferior petrosal sinus
   3. Empties into the sigmoid sinus
E. Cavernous sinus
   1. Location: parasellar area
   2. Receives flow from ophthalmic vein and sphenoparietal sinus
   3. Empties into the superior and inferior petrosal sinuses, among others
F. Superior petrosal sinus
   1. Location: margin of the tentorium along petrous ridge
   2. Receives flow from cavernous sinus, superficial middle cerebral vein and superior cerebellar veins
   3. Empties into the transverse sinus

(Continued)

TABLE 2.5 Arterial Vascular and Venous Sinus Distributions (continued)

Arterial Vascular Distributions	Venous Sinus Distributions
3. Medial a. Cerebral peduncle b. Substantia nigra c. VA nucleus of the thalamus d. VL nucleus of the thalamus e. Red nucleus 4. Distal a. Lateral geniculate body b. Posterior limb of the internal capsule c. Origin of the optic radiations C. Anterior cerebral artery 1. Recurrent artery of Heubner a. Head of the caudate nucleus b. Putamen c. Anterior limb of the internal capsule D. Middle cerebral artery 1. Medial lenticulostriate arteries a. Lateral segment of the globus pallidus 2. Lateral lenticulostriate arteries a. Putamen b. Superior internal capsule c. Caudate d. Corona radiate	G. Inferior petrosal sinus 1. Location: attached along the petrous-occipital suture 2. Receives flow from inferior cerebellar veins, medulla, pons, empties into the jugular bulb

VA; ventral anterior; VL, ventral lateral.

hemisensory loss. A lesion involving the thalamus may cause a syndrome characterized by contralateral hemianesthesia and central pain, although only about 25% of cases of central pain in stroke are caused by lesions of the thalamus. Other lesion sites reported to be associated with central pain are the brainstem and parietal lobe projections from the thalamus. In the thalamic syndrome, patients report unremitting, unpleasant, burning pain affecting the opposite side of the body. The pain usually begins a few weeks after onset of stroke and becomes intractable to conventional medication, including narcotics. It may be partly relieved with tricyclic antidepressants. Examination of the patient reveals contralateral impairment of all sensory modalities, often with dysesthesia. There may be involvement of adjacent structures, such as the internal capsule (hemiparesis, ataxia) or basal ganglia (choreoathetosis) (see Table 2.5)

SELECTED REFERENCES

Geyer JD, Keating JM, Potts DC, et al. *Neurology for the Boards.* 3rd ed. Philadelphia: Lippincott Williams & Wilkins; 2006.

Scott WA. *Magnetic Resonance Imaging of the Brain and Spine.* Philadelphia: Lippincott Williams & Wilkins; 2001.

SECTION II

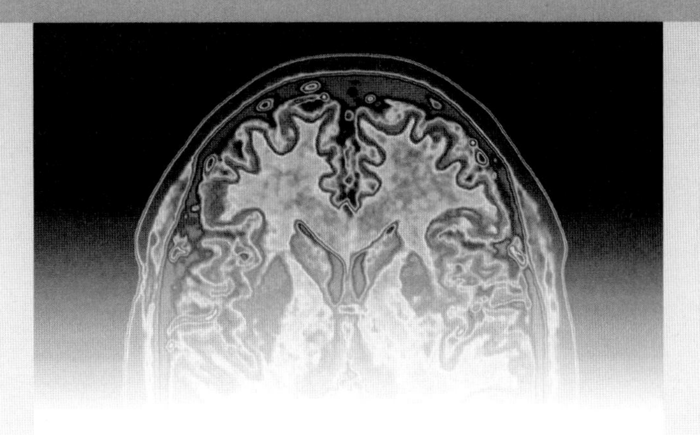

Prevention

CHAPTER 3

Modifiable Risk Factors Associated with Stroke

JAMES D. GEYER, CAMILO R. GOMEZ, A. ROBERT SHEPPARD,
NADEEM AKHTAR, AND MURRAY E. BRANDSTATER

OBJECTIVES

- What are the modifiable factors related to stroke?
- What are the clinical profiles of stroke?

A stroke is a clinical syndrome characterized by the sudden development of a persistent focal neurological deficit secondary to a vascular event. Stroke is a useful clinical term, its sudden onset implying its vascular pathogenesis. The differential diagnosis for a stroke is quite broad but includes seizure, postictal Todd's phenomenon, brain tumor, encephalitis, abscess, trauma, or syncope. For each patient, a pathological diagnosis should be made, such as cerebral infarction or cerebral hemorrhage. The focal brain injuries found in stroke patients will result in a wide range of neurological deficits, such as hemiplegia, hemisensory loss, aphasia, hemianopia, and ataxia. The clinical manifestations should suggest the anatomic localization of the stroke.

EPIDEMIOLOGY

Stroke is the most common serious neurological disorder in the United States, comprising half of all neurological admissions. It is the third leading cause of death after heart disease and cancer. The incidence of stroke in the 1960s was reported to be at around 200 per 100,000 population and still remains high. At present approximately 750,000 new incidents of stroke occur per year in the United States. The incidence of stroke is age related; relatively uncommon before the age of 50 but doubling each decade after the age of 55. After the age of 80, the incidence of stroke may be as high as 2,500 per 100,000. Stroke is more common in men than in women. The incidence of certain stroke subtypes varies among different ethnic groups. While of significant interest for research purposes, these issues do not have as much effect on the evaluation and management of a given stroke patient as do the modifiable risk factors.

Most acute stroke fatalities occur in the first 30 days after onset, with the overall 30-day survival following a new stroke reported to be 70% to 85%. Survival is largely dependent on the type of stroke. The 30-day survival of patients with intracerebral hemorrhage is between 20% and 50%, while it is approximately 85% in patients with cerebral infarction. Death during the first few days following onset is usually attributed to cerebral causes, especially cerebral herniation, but myocardial infarction and arrhythmias are also relatively common. Other complications such as pneumonia and pulmonary embolism also contribute to the 30-day mortality. After the initial 30 days, the death rate declines. The overall mortality from stroke has been declining, reflecting better medical management of patients during the acute phase. It should be noted that long-term survival post stroke is improving; thus, despite reduced incidence, the prevalence of stroke in the population has stayed the same or has increased.

RISK FACTORS AND PREVENTION

There is only limited potential for successful medical treatment to reverse the neurological sequelae of a completed stroke; therefore, interventions aimed at stroke prevention are extremely important. The following sections summarize the risk factors for stroke and describe opportunities for stroke prevention. Age, race, sex, and family history are all important biological indicators of enhanced stroke susceptibility, but these are inherent characteristics and cannot be altered.

Modifiable Risk Factors

Hypertension

Of the modifiable risk factors are listed in Table 3.1, hypertension is the most important for stroke (see Chapter 4). The degree of risk increases with higher levels of blood pressure and becomes particularly strong with levels higher than 160/95 mm Hg. Systolic hypertension and high mean arterial pressure represent parallel risks. In the Framingham Heart Study, a sevenfold increased risk of cerebral infarction was observed in patients who were hypertensive. Hypertension increases the risk of several stroke types including thrombotic, lacunar, hemorrhagic stroke, and subarachnoid hemorrhage. Successful long-term treatment of hypertension results in substantial risk reduction. Early diagnosis and effective management of hypertension limits the secondary changes of hypertensive vascular disease. Treatment of hypertension after a patient has had a stroke is much less effective in reducing the risk of future vascular events.

Heart Disease

Heart disease is an important risk factor for stroke. This in part reflects the common underlying precursors of stroke and heart

TABLE 3.1 Modifiable Risk Factors for Stroke
Hypertension
Heart disease
Ischemic/hypertensive
Valvular arrhythmias
Smoking
Diabetes mellitus
Elevated fibrinogen level
Erythrocytosis
Hyper lipidemia
Obstructive sleep apnea

disease: hypertension and atherosclerosis. The risk of stroke is doubled in individuals who have coronary artery disease, and coronary artery disease accounts for the majority of subsequent deaths among stroke survivors (see Chapter 23).

Atrial Fibrillation

Atrial fibrillation and valvular heart disease increase the risk of cerebral infarction secondary to cerebral emboli (see Chapter 9). Chronic, stable atrial fibrillation increases the risk of stroke by a factor of five. When atrial fibrillation is a manifestation of rheumatic heart disease, the risk of embolic stroke is increased 17-fold. Prevention of embolic stroke in these patients is best achieved by long-term anticoagulation with warfarin. Treatment carries the danger of intracranial hemorrhage, especially in elderly individuals and in those with impaired balance and who are likely to fall. When the risk of hemorrhage appears to be high, aspirin may be used as an alternative to warfarin in patients with nonvalvular atrial fibrillation, although aspirin is much less effective than warfarin in preventing embolism.

Diabetes

Diabetes, as an independent risk factor, doubles the risk of stroke. Unfortunately, good blood sugar control alone does not seem to significantly slow the progression of cerebrovascular disease (see Chapter 5).

Tobacco

Smoking increases the risk of stroke approximately 1.5 times (1.9 times for cerebral infarction). There is clear evidence that smoking cessation reduces the risk of cerebral infarction in addition to reducing the risk of myocardial infarction and sudden death (see Chapter 6).

Lipids

Hyperlipidemia produces a small additional risk for stroke, mainly for individuals younger than 55 (see Chapter 7). Elevated low-density lipoprotein (LDL) cholesterol level is an important risk factor for ischemic heart disease. It is therefore recommended that all patients with cerebrovascular disease and elevated LDL cholesterol level should be treated to reduce serum LDL levels.

Hematological Factors

Elevated fibrinogen levels correlate with a higher risk of stroke (see Chapter 14). Patients who smoke or have hyperlipidemia also have higher fibrinogen levels. Increased hematocrit increases the risk of stroke, most likely secondary to increased blood viscosity. Elevated serum levels of homocystine are associated with premature atherosclerosis and stroke earlier in life. Homocysteinemia can be treated with daily high-dose vitamin therapy, including vitamin B_6 (pyridoxine) and folic acid.

Obstructive Sleep Apnea

Sleep-related breathing disorders are associated with increased vascular risk (see Chapters 13 and 38). The relative risk for stroke is dramatically increased in patients with obstructive sleep apnea. There is significant improvement in the vascular risk when the sleep apnea is effectively treated.

Risk Factors for Recurrent Stroke

The probability of stroke recurrence is highest in the postacute period. For survivors of an initial stroke, the annual risk of a second stroke is approximately 5%, with a 5-year cumulative risk of recurrence of around 25%, although it may be as high as 42%. Risk factors for initial stroke also increase the risk of recurrence, especially hypertension, heart disease, diabetes mellitus, and obstructive sleep apnea. Alcohol abuse is also a risk factor for recurrent stroke.

A number of studies have reported a high mortality for stroke survivors. The reported 5-year cumulative mortality rates depend on the presence of risk factors. Patients with stroke who have hypertension and cardiac symptoms have only a 25% chance of surviving 5 years. Patients with one of these risk factors have a 50% chance of surviving 5 years, and those without heart disease and without hypertension have a 75% chance of surviving 5 years. Leonberg and Elliott were able to achieve 16% reduction in stroke recurrence rate by an energetic and sustained program of control of multiple risk factors. A broad-ranging aggressive risk factor management system is of vital importance to limit morbidity and mortality for the patient and to limit the economic drain related to this condition, especially as the population ages.

CLINICAL PROFILES

Cerebral Thrombosis

Thrombosis of the large extracranial and intracranial vessels usually occurs secondary to atherosclerotic cerebrovascular disease, accounting for approximately 30% of all cases of stroke (see Table 3.2). Atherosclerotic plaques are particularly prominent in the large vessels of the neck and at the base of the brain. In the absence of good collateral flow, occlusion of one of these vessels typically results in a large cerebral infarction. A number of the previously described modifiable risk factors, including hypertension, diabetes, hyperlipidemia, and obstructive sleep apnea can contribute to the development of atherosclerosis. A large vessel such as the internal carotid artery may slowly become stenotic and finally occlude without causing clinical signs or infarction if the slowly progressive stenosis had stimulated the development of sufficient collateral circulation before its occlusion. Conversely, rapid occlusion usually results in a large, devastating infarction (Table 3.2).

A thrombotic occlusion occurs most commonly at night during sleep or during periods of inactivity. Often patients become aware that they have weakness or other impairment only when they attempt to get out of bed. This nocturnal onset is suggestive of an effect of obstructive sleep apnea. The extent of the clinical deficit usually worsens over some hours or several days and then

TABLE 3.2 Causes of Stroke

Cause	%
Large vessel occlusion	32
Cerebral embolism	32
Small vessel occlusion, lacunar	18
Intracerebral hemorrhage	11
Subarachnoid hemorrhage	7

stabilizes, with clinical improvement generally beginning several days after onset.

Cerebral Embolism

Embolism is responsible for about 30% of all cases of stroke. Emboli may arise from thrombi in the heart, or on heart valves or the large extracranial arteries (see Table 3.3). These thrombi develop in the heart at different sites, such as the region of a recent myocardial infarction, an area of myocardial hypokinesis, or the atrium associated with fibrillation. Valvular disease also predisposes to embolic events. The distribution of emboli is not random and is much more common in the middle cerebral artery territory. The embolus is friable and may fragment with a multifocal appearance to the stroke on imaging studies (Table 3.3).

Lacunar Stroke

Lacunar lesions constitute approximately 20% of all strokes. They are small, circumscribed lesions, at most 1.5 cm in diameter but often much smaller. They represent occlusions in the deep penetrating branches of the large vessels that perfuse the subcortical structures such as the internal capsule, basal ganglia, thalamus, and brainstem. However, small, lacunar infarctions may produce severe neurological deficits since the fiber tracts are often densely packed in these areas. It is, however, possible for a lacunar infarction to occur with no overt symptomatology.

Cerebral Hemorrhage

Intracerebral hemorrhages are responsible for 11% of all cases of stroke. Spontaneous intracerebral hemorrhage most commonly occurs at the site of the same small, deep, penetrating arteries, typically associated with lacunar infarctions. These hemorrhages are most likely caused by the rupture of microaneurysms (Charcot-Bouchard aneurysms). Hypertension is the primary modifiable risk factor associated with these events. Most lesions occur in the putamen or thalamus, and in about 10% of patients, the spontaneous hemorrhage occurs in the cerebellum (see Table 3.4).

TABLE 3.3 Sources of Cerebral Embolism

Cardiac
Atrial fibrillation, other arrhythmias
Mural thrombus–recent MI, hypokinesis, cardiomyopathy
Bacterial endocarditis
Prosthetic valve
Nonbacterial valve vegetations/rheumatic heart disease
Atrial myxoma
Large Artery
Atherosclerosis of aorta and carotid arteries
Aneurysm
Paradoxical
Peripheral venous embolism with right-to-left cardiac shunt

TABLE 3.4 Causes of Intracranial Hemorrhage

Primary intracerebral hemorrhage
Ruptured saccular aneurysm
Ruptured arteriovenous malformation
Trauma
Cerebral infarction
Brain tumor
Amyloid angiopathy
Hemorrhagic disorders
Leukemia
Thrombocytopenia
Anticoagulant therapy

Subarachnoid Hemorrhage

Subarachnoid hemorrhage accounts for approximately 7% of all strokes. Subarachnoid hemorrhage of an arterial aneurysm at the base of the brain is associated with bleeding into the subarachnoid space. Aneurysms develop from small defects in the wall of the arteries and slowly increase in size, with eventual hemorrhage. Rebleeding is unfortunately very common, especially in the first several weeks following the initial episode. Within 6 months, 50% of surviving patients will rebleed. The rate of rebleeding in late survivors is 3% per year. Subarachnoid hemorrhage may also result from bleeding from an arteriovenous malformation (AVM).

There are a wide array of modifiable and nomodifiable risk factors for stroke. Comprehensive stroke management requires aggressive management of all potentially modifiable risk factors from smoking to obstructive sleep apnea to hyperlipidemia.

SELECTED REFERENCES

Barnett HJM, Haines SJ. Carotid endarterectomy for asymptomatic carotid stenosis. *N Engl J Med* 1993;328:276–279.

Bonita R. Epidemiology of stroke. *Lancet* 1992;339:342–344.

Booth FW. Effect of limb immobilization on skeletal muscle. *J Appl Physiol* 1982;52:1113.

Diener HC, Cunha L, Forbes C, et al. European stroke prevention study. 2. Dipyridamole and acetylsalicylic acid in the secondary prevention of stroke. *J Neurol Sci* 1996;143:1–13.

Dobkin BH. *Neurologic Rehabilitation*. Philadelphia, PA: FA Davis; 1966.

Dyken ML, Conneally M, Haener AF, et al. Cooperative study of the hospital frequency and character of transient ischemic attacks. 1. Background, organization and clinical survey. *JAMA* 1997;237:882–886.

Feinberg WM, Albers GW, Barnett HJM, et al. Guidelines for the management of transient ischemic attacks. *Stroke* 1994;25:1320–1335.

Foulkes MA, Wolf PA, Price TR, et al. The stroke data bank: design, methods and baseline characteristics. *Stroke* 1988;19:547–554.

Gresham GE, Duncan PW, Stason WB, et al. Post-stroke rehabilitation. Clinical Practice Guideline No 16. Rockville, MD: U.S. Department of Health and Human Services, Public Health Service, Agency for Health Care Policy and Research. AHCPR Publication No. 95–0662, May 1995.

Horner J, Massey EW, Riski JE, et al. Aspiration following stroke: clinical correlates and outcomes. *Neurology* 1988;38:1359–1362.

Kannel WB, Dawber TR, Sorlie P, et al. Components of blood pressure and risk of atherothrombotic brain infarction: the Framingham study. *Stroke* 1976;7:327–331.

Leonberg SC, Elliott FA. Prevention of recurrent stroke. *Stroke* 1981;12:731–735.

Mohr JP, Caplan LR, Melski JW, et al. The Harvard cooperative stroke registry: a prospective study. *Neurology* 1978;28:754–762.

North American Symptomatic Carotid Endarterectomy Trial Collaborators. Beneficial effect of carotid endarterectomy in symptomatic patients with high-grade carotid stenosis. *N Engl J Med* 1991;325: 445–453.

Roth EJ. Medical complications encountered in stroke rehabilitation. *Phys Med Rehabil Clin N Am* 1991;2(3):563–578.

Sacco RL. Risk factors and outcomes for ischemic stroke. *Neurology* 1995;45(Suppl 1):S10–S14.

Sheets RM, Ashwal S, Szer IS. Neurologic manifestations of rheumatic disorders of childhood. In: Swaiman KF, Ashwal S, eds. *Pediatric Neurology: Principles and Practice.* 3rd ed. St Louis, MO: CV Mosby; 1999.

Shinton R, Beevers G. Meta-analysis of relation between cigarette smoking and stroke. *BMJ* 1989;298:789–794.

Stein DG, Brailowsky S, Will B. *Brain Repair* New York: Oxford University Press; 1995.

Steinberg GK, Fabrikant JI, Marks MP, et al. Stereotactic heavy-charged-particle Bragg-Peak radiation for intracranial arteriovenous malformations. *N Engl J Med* 1990;323:96–101.

Stroke Unit Trialists' Collaboration. Collaboration SUT: collaborative systematic review of the randomised trials of organized inpatient (stroke unit) care after stroke. *BMJ* 1997;314:1151–1159.

The National Institute of Neurological Disorders and Stroke rt-PA Stroke Study Group. Tissue plasminogen activator for acute ischemic stroke. *N Engl J Med*1995;333:1581–1587.

Viitanen M, Eriksson S, Asplund K. Risk of recurrent stroke, myocardial infarction and epilepsy. *Eur Neurol* 1988;28:227–231.

Wolf PA, Dawber TR, Thomas HE, Jr, et al. Epidemiologic assessment of chronic atrial fibrillation and risk of stroke: the Framingham study. *Neurology* 1978;23:973–977.

Wolf PA, Kannel WB, Venter J. Current status of risk factors for stroke. *Neurol Clin* 1983;1:317–343.

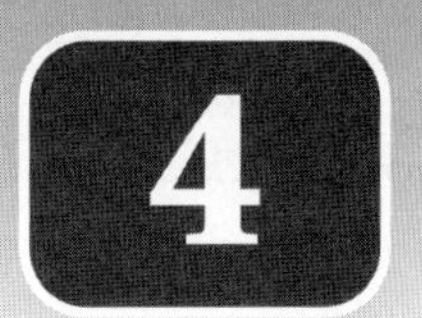

Chronic Hypertension

SAMEER GUPTA AND JOHN M. FIELD

OBJECTIVES

- What are the background and classification of hypertension?
- What is the relationship between blood pressure and the risk of stroke?
- What are the diagnostic criteria for hypertension and for the evaluation of a hypertensive patient?
- What lifestyle modifications and pharmacologic therapy are needed for the treatment of hypertension?
- What is the importance of hypertension treatment in stroke prevention?
- Blood pressure and secondary prevention of stroke

The International Society of Hypertension labels hypertension as the most important modifiable risk factor for stroke. The Seventh Report of the Joint National Commission (JNC 7) defines hypertension as a systolic blood pressure (SBP) >140 mm Hg and a diastolic BP (DBP) >90 mm Hg.

- In the National Ambulatory Medical Care Survey, hypertension has consistently been a leading primary diagnosis in patients presenting in an outpatient setting.
- In 2000, one in four people worldwide were diagnosed with hypertension, with this fraction projected to increase with time.
- The incidence of hypertension in the 18- to 39-year age group is 7%, with prevalence increasing to 64% in patients 60 years and older.
- In the United States, essential hypertension and hypertensive renal disease accounted for nearly 23,000 deaths in 2004. This was a significant increase from 19,000 in 1999.

In the United States alone, in 2001, a total of $55 billion was spent on treating hypertension.

The Framingham risk profile listed increased SBP and hypertension as independent risk factors for stroke. Hypertension is consistently associated with both ischemic and hemorrhagic stroke and also with dementia. This association is stronger for hemorrhagic stroke as compared to ischemic stroke and rises with an increase in BP. With adequate treatment of hypertension this risk decreases. Many patients on active drug therapy for hypertension continue to have poorly controlled BP and may continue to be at an increased risk for stroke (see Fig. 4.1).

CLASSIFICATION OF HYPERTENSION BASED ON ETIOPATHOGENESIS

Hypertension can be classified as either primary or secondary, based on the etiology.

Primary, idiopathic, or essential hypertension is diagnosed when no underlying etiology for increased BP can be identified. Although the exact cause is indeterminate, multiple factors may interplay in the pathogenesis. These include increased sympathetic tone, inability of the kidney to excrete sodium at normal BP, a low renin state, increased peripheral arteriolar resistance, endocrine factors, and genetic predisposition.

Another factor that should be considered in patients with primary hypertension is their ethnic background. It has been observed that certain ethnic and racial groups are at an increased risk for hypertension. Non-Hispanic blacks have a higher prevalence of hypertension as compared to non-Hispanic whites and Mexican Americans. This differentiation may be secondary to multiple factors, including low socioeconomic status, ingestion of a high-sodium and low-potassium diet, and darker skin color. Dyslipidemia, obesity, increased salt intake, and personality traits are also factors that increase the risk for hypertension. Although hypertension is known to run in families, no single gene has been identified as the cause of essential hypertension.

Secondary hypertension is due to an identifiable cause and treatment of the comorbidity will resolve the hypertension. Investigations in search of a probable secondary cause are indicated if an abnormal sign is found on physical examination (e.g., abdominal bruit), or in cases of resistant/refractory hypertension, onset of hypertension in a nonobese patient 30 to 55 years of age with no family history of high BP, or accelerated hypertension (i.e., previously stable and now difficult to control). A list of common causes and screening diagnostic tests is given in Table 4.1.

BLOOD PRESSURE AND STROKE

Earlier classifications of BP used an SBP range from 120 to 129/80 to 84 mm Hg as normal, and a range from 130 to 139/85 to 89 mm Hg as borderline. Patients with borderline hypertension were typically not treated with medication. However, data from multiple

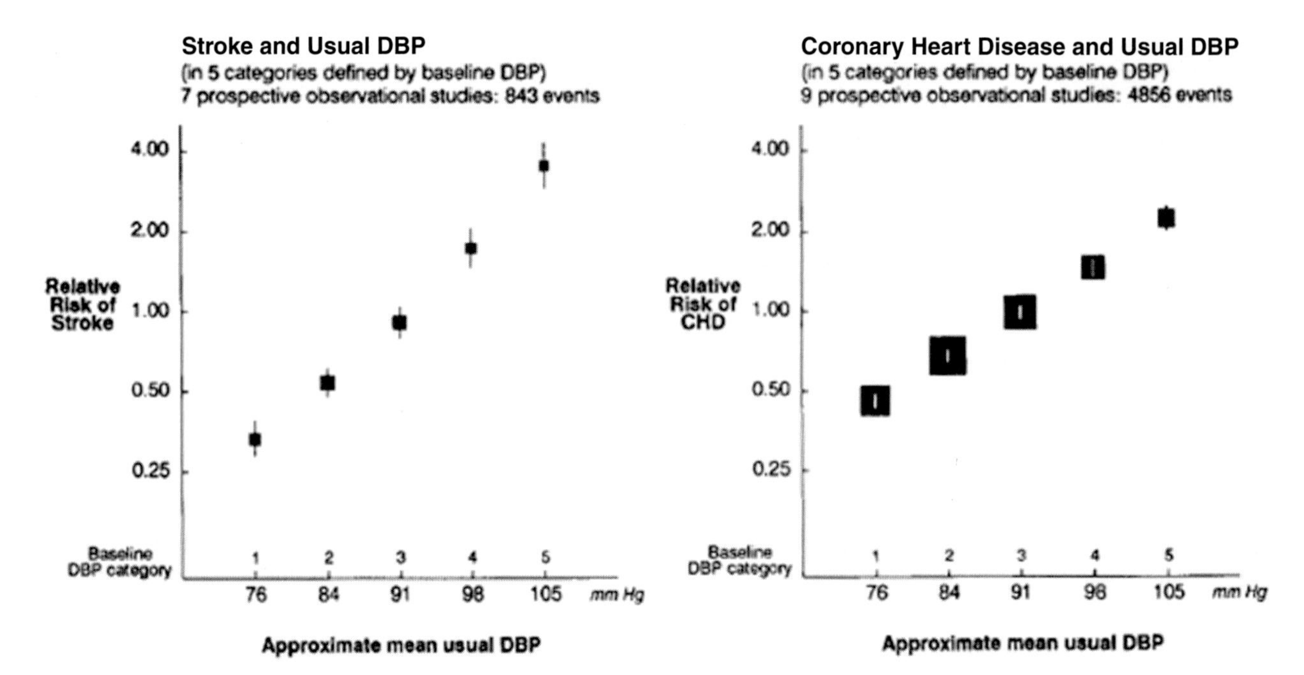

FIGURE 4.1. Relative risks of stroke and of coronary heart disease, estimated from combined results.Estimates of the usual diastolic blood pressure (DBP) in each baseline DBP category are taken from mean DBP values 4 years post baseline in the Framingham Heart study. Solid squares represent disease risks in each category relative to the risk in the whole study population, sizes of squares are proportional to number of events in each DBP category, and 95% confidence intervals for estimates of relative risk are denoted by vertical lines. (Adapted from MacMahon S, Peto R, Cutler J, et al. Blood pressure, stroke, and coronary heart disease. Part 1. Prolonged differences in blood pressure: Prospective observational studies corrected for the regression dilution bias. *Lancet* 1990;335(8692):765–774 with permission.)

observational studies, including the Framingham Heart Study, showed double the risk of cerebrovascular disease (CVD) for BP of 130 to 139/85 to 89 mm Hg when compared to 120/80 mm Hg.

A direct relationship was found to exist between increasing BP and the incidence of stroke. It was noted that 95% of the strokes were in patients who were earlier considered to have normal BP or borderline hypertension (i.e., BP 120 to 139/80 to 89 mm Hg). Also in the Framingham Heart Study, Vasan et al. concluded that patients who are considered normotensive (per previous JNC classification) have a 90% lifetime risk of developing hypertension.

TABLE 4.1 Screening Tests for Identifiable Hypertension

Diagnosis	Diagnostic Tests
Chronic kidney disease	Estimated GFR
Coarctation of the aorta	CT angiography
Cushing's syndrome and other glucocorticoid-excess states including chronic steroid therapy	History, dexamethasone suppression tests
Drug-induced	History, drug screening
Pheochromocytoma	24-hr urinary metanephrine and normetanephrine
Primary aldosteronism and other mineralocorticoid-excess states	24-hr urinary aldosterone level or specific measurements of other mineralocorticoids
Renovascular hypertension	Doppler flow study, magnetic resonance angiography
Sleep apnea	Sleep study with O_2 saturation
Thyroid/parathyroid disease	TSH, serum PTH

GFR, glomerular filtration rate; CT, computed tomography; TSH, thyroid stimulating hormone; PTH, parathyroid hormone.

Adapted from Chobanian AV, Bakris GL, Black HR, et al. The Seventh Report of the Joint National Committee on Prevention, Detection, Evaluation, and Treatment of High Blood Pressure: the JNC 7 report. *JAMA* 2003;289(19):2560–2572, with permission.

TABLE 4.2 Classification of Blood Pressure

Blood Pressure Classification	Systolic Blood Pressure	Diastolic Blood Pressure
Normal	<120	<80
Prehypertension	120–139	80–89
Stage1 hypertension	140–159	or 90–99
Stage 2 hypertension	≥160	or ≥100

As a result, the classification of hypertension was revised in 2003. Patients with BP averaging 120 to 139/80 to 89 mm Hg are considered to be prehypertensive and not normal or borderline. These patients are NOT considered candidates for drug therapy but did warrant the following:

- Lifestyle modification including healthy diet
- Regular exercise and weight reduction strategies
- Low sodium diet

Exceptions include patients with diabetes or kidney disease (e.g., chronic renal failure). In these groups drug therapy can be started if nonpharmacologic measures fail to achieve a BP of <130/80 mm Hg (JNC 7). It is also recommended to recheck BP in 2 years for normotension, 1 year for prehypertension, 2 months for stage 1 hypertension, and earlier for stage 2 hypertension (see. Table 4.2).

DIAGNOSING HYPERTENSION

The rule of halves states that of all the patients with hypertension, only half are aware of their condition. Of the half who are aware, only half are on treatment, and of those in treatment, only half have their BP in control. Although the awareness of BP in the United States has increased from 51% in 1980 to 70% in 2000, only 59% of patients are on treatment and 34% have their BP under control.

Hypertension is diagnosed when the patient's BP is >140/90 mm Hg on two or more visits. Technical aspects are important when measuring the BP. BP is measured with the patient seated quietly for at least 5 minutes, with feet on the floor and arms supported at heart level. Any stimulant, such as caffeine, cigarettes, or exercise, should be avoided at least half an hour before taking the measurement because they may falsely elevate the BP. The patient should be encouraged to measure his or her BP at home to rule out any false elevation (so-called white coat hypertension) that may occur during the outpatient visit.

BP is typically lower in the morning and increases as the day progresses. During sleep BP tends to drop 10% to 20%. Failure of BP to decrease at night is an independent predictor for worse cardiovascular outcomes. Obstructive sleep apnea can increase the nocturnal BP, eliminate the normal nocturnal BP dipping, and eventually lead to daytime hypertension as well.

Ambulatory BP (ABP) monitoring is indicated when the physician suspects episodic hypertension, white coat hypertension, and autonomic dysfunction. It is also indicated if hypotension is suspected in patients taking antihypertensive medications. Cardiovascular risk is related both directly and independently to observed ABP. In this technique a cuff is placed around the arm. The cuff inflates periodically and measures the BP. This is then computed for a 24-hour period and the mean BP, which is a better measure of BP and indicator of hypertension, is calculated. This method, although accurate in cardiovascular risk stratification, is not always used in practice for insurance reasons.

Initial Evaluation

Patients with hypertension need to be evaluated with the following objectives in mind:

- Assessment of lifestyle and other comorbid conditions that may be important in making treatment decisions and prognosis
- Identification of any secondary or correctable cause(s) of hypertension
- Identification of any end-organ damage

The physical examination should include BP measurement in both arms, calculation of body mass index [body weight in kg/(body height in meters)^2], funduscopy (to evaluate for evidence of retinopathy), palpation of the thyroid gland (to rule out any enlargement), auscultation of heart sounds (murmurs, abnormal rhythm or splitting, gallops) and of carotids, abdominal bruit/abnormal pulsations, and palpation for lower-extremity edema.

Laboratory testing before starting therapy should include an electrocardiogram; urinalysis; blood glucose level and hematocrit; serum potassium, creatinine, calcium level, and lipid profile including low-density lipoprotein, high-density lipoprotein, and triglycerides. It is also reasonable to obtain a urine albumin:creatinine ratio. However, extensive testing for source of secondary hypertension is not warranted until BP is difficult to control. IMPORTANT: **DO NOT start aspirin therapy with uncontrolled BP because this could increase the risk of hemorrhagic stroke.**

TREATMENT

To decrease the risk of stroke and cardiovascular mortality with optimal BP control, drug therapy should be started in patients who do not achieve a BP of <140/80 mm Hg with lifestyle modifications.

However, the *big* question is at what point is the BP considered adequately controlled?

There has been considerable debate regarding the goal systolic pressure, diastolic pressure, or pulse pressure. DBP increases up to 50 years of age, plateaus for about a decade, and then decreases. On the other hand, SBP continues to increase with age without a plateau period. Furthermore, there are studies that indicate decreased mortality and stroke in elderly patients treated for isolated systolic hypertension.

These considerations, as well as new data, are reflected in the JNC 7 guidelines. Now, patients with a BP of >140/90 mm Hg are considered hypertensive. The higher pressure category determines the goal, that is, systolic or diastolic. Increased SBP is an important risk factor and requires treatment, especially in the elderly. In patients older than 50 years, SBP is a more accurate marker of BP control than DBP. *When treating isolated systolic hypertension in older patients (>65 years), increased risk of stroke was noted at DBP <65 mm Hg. BP should be treated cautiously in these patients.* If the person has other comorbidities, including diabetes or renal disease, the goal BP is even lower, at <130/80 mm Hg.

Most patients require two or more drugs to achieve adequate BP control. Drug therapy should be combined with lifestyle modification, which is the first-line treatment in all patients.

Lifestyle Modifications

JNC 7 recommends lifestyle modifications as an integral part of treatment of hypertension. Although highly underestimated, this has proven benefits and is the first-line treatment in patients who are pre-hypertensive and those who have first-line hypertension. The American Heart Association (AHA) has stated the following: "in non hypertensive individuals, including those with pre hypertension, dietary changes that lower BP have the potential to prevent hypertension and more broadly to reduce BP and thereby lower risk of BP related clinical complications." The AHA recommends starting lifestyle modifications as an essential part of treatment in all patients with hypertension.

The Dietary Approaches to Stop Hypertension (DASH) diet, which is rich in fruits, vegetables, and low-fat dairy products, has shown to decrease BP in patients with hypertension. These changes are evident as quickly as 2 weeks after starting the diet plan. The PREMIER trial compared the effects of DASH diet and lifestyle changes (weight loss, low sodium diet, increased physical activity, and moderate alcohol consumption) with DASH diet alone. It found following the DASH diet plus lifestyle changes can decrease the prevalence of BP by more than 20%. Some lifestyle modifications and their effects are mentioned in Table 4.3.

Pharmacotherapy

Once a patient is diagnosed as having hypertension, lifestyle modifications are started prior to drug therapy. When lifestyle modifications fail, drug therapy is considered. The 1967 Veterans Affairs (VA) cooperative study was a landmark study that showed the benefits of lowering BP with medications. The group that received active intervention showed a decrease in mortality and complications of hypertension. This was the start of a new era and the beginning of BP screening.

Significant advances have been made in available drugs and treatment strategies. Once initiated, two thirds of the patients will require two or more drugs for optimal control of BP. Data suggests that for every 20/10 mm Hg increase after 115/75 mm Hg, the risk of CVD doubles. If SBP is >20 mm Hg or DBP is >10 mm Hg of goal, therapy is initiated with two drugs, one being a diuretic.

There are various classes of medications for treatment of hypertension. The clinician must be familiar with the various drug options available and have the ability to tailor treatment to specific patients. The list that follows enumerates these drug categories along with some examples of the drugs in each category:

- Diuretics: thiazides (e.g., chlorothiazide), loop diuretics (e.g., furosemide) potassium-sparing diuretics (e.g., amiloride, triamterene)
- β-blockers: atenolol, metoprolol, propranolol
- β-blockers with intrinsic sympathomimetic activity: acebutolol, pindolol
- Angiotensin-converting enzyme inhibitors (ACEI): lisinopril, ramipril, captopril, enalapril
- Aldosterone receptor antagonists: spironolactone
- Angiotensin II receptor blockers (ARB): candesartan, eprosartan, losartan, valsartan
- Calcium channel blockers (CCB)
  - Nondihydropyridines: diltiazem, verapamil
  - Dihydropyridines: amlodipine, nifedipine
- α1-blockers: doxazosin, prazosin
- Centrally α2-agonists and other centrally acting drugs: clonidine, methyl dopa, reserpine
- Direct vasodilators: hydralazine, minoxidil

Therapy for treatment of hypertension has changed significantly over the last few decades. Multiple options are now available that decrease complications and mortality to a varying extent. But which drug therapy should be the first? Some recommendations are given in Table 4.4.

Since the publication of the 1967 VA study, the recommended first-line therapy for treatment of hypertension in patients still remains thiazide diuretics. Multiple trials have consistently shown beneficial effects of treatment with thiazides as compared with any

TABLE 4.3 Lifestyle Modifications to Treat Hypertension

Modification	Recommendation	Approximate SBP Reduction (range)
Weight reduction	Maintain normal body weight (body mass index 18.5–24.9 kg/m^2)	5–20 mm Hg/10 kg
Adopt DASH eating plan	Diet rich in fruits, vegetables, and low-fat dairy products with a reduced content of saturated and total fat	2–8 mm Hg
Dietary sodium reduction	Reduce dietary sodium intake to no more than 100 mmol/d (2.4 g sodium or 6 g sodium chloride)	4–9 mm Hg
Physical activity	Engage in regular aerobic physical activity such as brisk walking (at least 30 min/d, most days of the week)	4–9 mm Hg
Moderate alcohol consumption	Limit consumption to no more than two drinks (e.g., 24 oz beer, 10 oz wine, or 3 oz 80-proof whiskey) per day in most men, and to no more than one drink per day in women and lighter weight persons	2–4 mm Hg

SBP, systolic blood pressure; DASH, Dietary Approach to Stop Hypertension.

Adapted from Chobanian AV, Bakris GL, Black HR, et al., *The Seventh Report of the Joint National Committee on Prevention, Detection, Evaluation, and Treatment of High Blood Pressure: the JNC 7 report. JAMA* 2003; 289(19):2560-72 with permission.

TABLE 4.4 Treatment Protocol of Treatment of Hypertension

BP Classification	Systolic BP (mm Hg)	Diastolic BP (mm Hg)	Lifestyle Modification	Without Compelling Indication	With Compelling Indication
Normal	<120	And <80	Encourage	–	–
Prehypertension	120–139	Or 80–89	Yes	No antihypertensive drug therapy	Drug therapy for compelling indications
Stage 1 hypertension	140–159	Or ≥ 90–99	Yes	Thiazide-type diuretics for most; may consider ACEI, ARB, β-blocker, CCB, or combination	Drugs for compelling indications Other antihypertensive drugs (diuretics, ACEI, ARB, β-blockers, CCB) as needed
Stage 2 hypertension	≥160	Or ≥100	Yes	Two-drug combination for most (usually thiazide-type diuretic and ACEI or ARB or β-blocker or CCB)	Drug(s) for compelling indications Other antihypertensive drugs (diuretics, ACEI, ARB, β-blockers, CCB) as needed

BP, blood pressure; ACEI, angiotensin-converting enzyme inhibitor; ARB, angiotensin II receptor blocker; CCB, calcium channel blocker.
From Chobanian AV, Bakris GL, Black HR, et al. The Seventh Report of the Joint National Committee on Prevention, Detection, Evaluation, and Treatment of High Blood Pressure: The JNC 7 report. *JAMA* 2003;289(19):2560–2572 with permission.

other agent. The Antihypertensive and Lipid-Lowering Treatment to Prevent Heart Attack Trial (ALLHAT) and the Controlled Onset Verapamil Investigation of Cardiovascular Endpoints (CONVINCE) trial showed no further benefit of treatment with an ACEI, CCB, or β-blocker when compared with a diuretic. A meta-analysis of 42 trials showed diuretics to be most effective when compared with other antihypertensive medications. This view was also shared by the AHA and the American Stroke Association (ASA) in their primary prevention guidelines in 2006.

Treatment with a thiazide diuretic is typically started at low doses and titrated upward until the goal BP is reached. Potassium level should be monitored and kept >3.5 mmol per L for optimum benefit. Uric acid level increases with thiazides, but gout is uncommon at therapeutic doses.

ACEIs are widely used to treat hypertension. They not only lower BP, but are also beneficial in heart failure and renal failure, in which they slow the rate of progression. They are also used post myocardial infarction, where they improve survival. A repeat creatinine concentration should be obtained 1 week after starting therapy to rule out decreasing renal perfusion. ACEIs also cause chronic cough in up to 20% of the patients, which may be troublesome and a reason to discontinue treatment. This symptom may begin as early as a few hours to a few days after starting therapy and usually resolves within 3 to 4 weeks of stopping treatment. Other potential side effects are angioneurotic edema, acute renal failure, and hyperkalemia. When side effects warrant discontinuing ACEI, therapy can be started with an ARB.

Beta blockers are also commonly prescribed drugs for treatment of hypertension. The benefits of these drugs also extend beyond BP control and are used in post–myocardial infarction patients, in heart failure, in atrial fibrillation, and in the treatment of thyroid storm. They should not be used in patients with asthma and caution should be used in patients with chronic obstructive lung disease.

If the goal BP is not reached with diuretic alone, a second agent is added on the basis of the presence of comorbid conditions and individual patient consideration (e.g., β-blockers in case of ischemic heart disease and ACEI in case of diabetes). The effects of ACEIs are decreased in African Americans as compared with other ethnic groups and should not be used as monotherapy. The JNC 7 guidelines suggest starting with two agents if the SBP is 20 mm Hg or DBP is 10 mm Hg above goal. Following the American Diabetes Association (ADA) recommendations, ACEI therapy should be initiated for patients with diabetes mellitus who are older than 55 years and at high risk for CVD and β-blockers for those with coronary artery disease.

The Losartan Intervention for Endpoint Reduction in Hypertension (LIFE) study compared losartan (an aldosterone receptor blocker) with a β-blocker and showed decreased risk of stroke and cardiovascular complications in the group treated with an aldosterone receptor blocker. However, the AHA guidelines on primary prevention of stroke published in 2006 do not recommend a specific antihypertensive agent for BP control in primary prevention of stroke. Absolute reduction of BP is more important as compared to specific medication. When treating hypertension, drug therapy is influenced by the other comorbid conditions that are present. For example, in patients with asthma, β-blockers should not be used and other antihypertensives should be tried. A list of some comorbid conditions and the medications of choice is given in Table 4.5. ACEIs, however, are used as antihypertensive drugs of choice in patients with diabetes but are not well established to be beneficial in the prevention of stroke.

TABLE 4.5 Specific Indication for Individual Drug Class

Compelling Indication	Recommended Drug
Heart failure	Diuretic, β-blocker, ACEI, aldosterone antagonist
Post myocardial infarction	β-Blocker, ACEI
High coronary disease risk	Diuretic, β-blocker, ACEI, CCB
Diabetes	Diuretic, β-blocker, ACE I, ARB, CCB
Chronic kidney disease	ACEI, ARB
Recurrent stroke prevention	Diuretic, ACEI

ACEI, angiotensin-converting enzyme inhibitor; CCB, calcium channel blocker; ARB, angiotensin II receptor blocker.
(From Chobanian AV, Bakris GL, Black HR, et al. The Seventh Report of the Joint National Committee on Prevention, Detection, Evaluation, and Treatment of High Blood Pressure: The JNC 7 report. *JAMA* 2003;289(19):2560–2572 with permission.)

SECONDARY PREVENTION

Treating Hypertension after Stroke

Although hypertension is a common finding in acute stroke patients, BP falls spontaneously in a few days following a stroke. These patients may require treatment for their hypertension. The recently updated guidelines for management of patients with acute ischemic stroke discussed broad recommendations for treatment of patients who are candidates for fibrinolytic therapy as well as for acute management of hypertension in other patients with stroke. These are reviewed in Chapters 25 and 36.

The AHA and ASA recommend antihypertensives in all patients who have had a stroke or transient ischemic attack (TIA). A metaregression of trials by Rashid et al., evaluating antihypertensives in secondary prevention of stroke, concluded that the risk of recurrent stroke and TIA is directly related to BP control.

The Perindopril Protection against Recurrent Stroke Study (PROGRESS) trial addressed the issue of whether BP lowering really decreases the risk of recurrent stroke. Patients with a history of TIA or stroke were randomized for treatment with perindopril versus placebo. Indapamide was added as required for optimum BP control. Studies showed a decreased rate of recurrent stroke in patients receiving antihypertensives. This was more in the group receiving both perindopril and indapamide than in the group receiving one medication only. This group had a more significant lowering of BP (12/5 mm Hg vs. 5/3 mm Hg) as compared to the group on perindopril alone.

The Morbidity and Mortality after Stroke, Eprosartan Compared with Nitrendipine for Secondary Prevention (MOSES) trial comparing eprosartan and nitrendipine in secondary prevention of stroke showed a lower rate of recurrent stroke in patients treated with eprosartan for similar lowering in BP.

AHA/ASA recommend starting antihypertensive treatment in *all* patients after a stroke or TIA. Antihypertensives are beneficial for secondary prevention even in patients without hypertension. It is reasonable to start therapy with an ACEI and a diuretic. There is no goal BP, but, as per JNC 7, <120/80 mm Hg is normotensive.

Special consideration must be given to the patient with significant cerebral atherosclerosis. Overly tight BP control can, in some cases with severe stenosis, lead to hypoperfusion and ischemia. The degree and location of stenoses should be considered when prescribing and managing hypertension in the post-stroke patient.

PRACTICAL RECOMMENDATIONS

- Treatment of hypertension in prevention of morbidity, mortality from all causes, and stroke (both primary and secondary) cannot be overemphasized.
- A single reading of high BP does not label a person as hypertensive. Because BP is affected by multiple factors, the patient should be encouraged to check BP at home. Only if multiple readings are high (≥140/90 mm Hg), is the patient diagnosed with hypertension.
- A thorough physical examination as screening for secondary hypertension is invaluable. If any sign for secondary cause of hypertension is found, aggressive testing for the same is warranted.
- Lifestyle modifications, although undervalued, are beneficial in lowering BP and may delay progression to hypertension in previously normotensive individuals.
- If a patient has diabetes or chronic kidney disease, the goal BP should be 130/80 mm Hg.
- Most individuals will require two or more medications for optimum BP control. When treating isolated systolic hypertension in the elderly, caution is advised for DBP <65 mm Hg because of risk of an increased incidence of stroke. Further attempts at lowering SBP maybe stopped for risking further decrease in DBP.
- Drug therapy should always begin with a diuretic. CCB, β-blockers, or ACEIs should be added on an individual patient basis. If the goal BP is >20/10 mm Hg above the goal, treatment is begun with two medications, one being a diuretic. Patients should be warned about signs and symptoms of orthostatic hypotension. No medicine is better than another for primary prevention of hypertension.
- All patients with a history of TIA and stroke should be begun on antihypertensives, even in previously normotensive patients. An ACEI plus a diuretic has been shown to be beneficial in this population.

SELECTED REFERENCES

Appel LJ, Brands MW, Daniels SR, et al. Dietary approaches to prevent and treat hypertension: a scientific statement from the American Heart Association. *Hypertension* 2006;47(2):296–308.

Appel LJ, Champagne CM, Harsha DW, et al. Effects of comprehensive lifestyle modification on blood pressure control: Main results of the PREMIER clinical trial. *JAMA* 2003;289(16):2083–2093.

Balu S, Thomas J III. Incremental expenditure of treating hypertension in the United States. *Am J Hypertens* 2006;19(8):810–816

Black HR, Elliott WJ, Grandits G, et al. Principal results of the Controlled Onset Verapamil Investigation of Cardiovascular End Points (CONVINCE) trial. *JAMA* 2003;289(16):2073–2082.

Burt VL, Whelton P, Roccella EJ, et al. Prevalence of hypertension in the US adult population. Results from the Third National Health and Nutrition Examination Survey, 1988–1991. *Hypertension* 1995;25(3):305–313.

Chalmers J, Todd A, Chapman N, et al. International Society of Hypertension (ISH): Statement on blood pressure lowering and stroke prevention. *J Hypertens* 2003;21(4):651–663.

Chobanian AV, Bakris GL, Black HR, et al. The Seventh Report of the Joint National Committee on Prevention, Detection, Evaluation, and Treatment of High Blood Pressure: The JNC 7 report. *JAMA* 2003; 289(19):2560–2572.

Dicpinigaitis PV. Angiotensin-converting enzyme inhibitor-induced cough: ACCP evidence-based clinical practice guidelines. *Chest* 2006;129(1) (suppl):169S–173S.

Goldstein LB, Adams R, Alberts MJ, et al. Primary prevention of ischemic stroke: A guideline from the American Heart Association/American Stroke Association Stroke Council. Cosponsored by the Atherosclerotic Peripheral Vascular Disease Interdisciplinary Working Group; Cardiovascular Nursing Council; Clinical Cardiology Council; Nutrition, Physical Activity, and Metabolism Council; and the Quality of Care and Outcomes Research Interdisciplinary Working Group. *Circulation* 2006;113(24):e873–e923.

Hajjar I, Kotchen TA. Trends in prevalence, awareness, treatment, and control of hypertension in the United States, 1988-2000. *JAMA* 2003;290(2): 199–206.

Israili ZH, Hall WD. Cough and angioneurotic edema associated with angiotensin-converting enzyme inhibitor therapy. A review of the literature and pathophysiology. *Ann Intern Med* 1992l;117(3):234–242.

Kearney PM, Whelton M, Reynolds K, et al. Global burden of hypertension: analysis of worldwide data. *Lancet* 2005;365(9455):217–223.

Klag MJ, Whelton PK, Coresh J, Grim CE, Kuller LH. The association of skin color with blood pressure in US blacks with low socioeconomic status. *JAMA* 1991;265(5):599–602.

Lewington S, Clarke R, Qizilbash N, et al. Age-specific relevance of usual blood pressure to vascular mortality: a meta-analysis of individual data for one million adults in 61 prospective studies. *Lancet* 2002;360(9349): 1903–1913.

MacMahon S, Peto R, Cutler J, et al. Blood pressure, stroke, and coronary heart disease. Part 1. Prolonged differences in blood pressure: Prospective observational studies corrected for the regression dilution bias. *Lancet* 1990;335(8692):765–774.

ALLHAT Officers and Coordinators for the ALLHAT Collaborative Research Group. Major outcomes in high-risk hypertensive patients randomized to angiotensin-converting enzyme inhibitor or calcium channel blocker vs diuretic: The Antihypertensive and Lipid-Lowering Treatment to Prevent Heart Attack Trial (ALLHAT). *JAMA* 2002;288(23): 2981–2997.

Minino AM, Heron MP, Smith BL. Deaths: Preliminary data for 2004. *Natl Vital Stat Rep* 2006;54(19):1–49.

Nayak B, Burman K. Thyrotoxicosis and thyroid storm. *Endocrinol Metab Clin North Am* 2006;35(4):663–686.

Ong KL, Cheung BM, Man YB, Lau CP, Lam KS. Prevalence, awareness, treatment, and control of hypertension among United States adults 1999-2004. *Hypertension* 2007;49(1):69–75.

PROGRESS Collaborative Group. Randomised trial of a perindopril-based blood-pressure-lowering regimen among 6,105 individuals with previous stroke or transient ischaemic attack. *Lancet* 2001;358(9287): 1033–1041.

Rashid P, Leonardi-Bee J., Bath P. Blood pressure reduction and secondary prevention of stroke and other vascular events: a systematic review. *Stroke* 2003;34(11):2741–2748.

Sacco RL, Adams R, Albers G, et al. Guidelines for prevention of stroke in patients with ischemic stroke or transient ischemic attack: a statement for healthcare professionals from the American Heart Association/ American Stroke Association Council on Stroke. Co-sponsored by the Council on Cardiovascular Radiology and Intervention: the American Academy of Neurology affirms the value of this guideline. *Stroke* 2006;37(2):577–617.

Schrader J, Lüders S, Kulschewski A, et al. Morbidity and mortality after stroke, eprosartan compared with nitrendipine for secondary prevention: principal results of a prospective randomized controlled study (MOSES). *Stroke* 2005;36(6):1218–1226.

SHEP Cooperative Research Group. Prevention of stroke by antihypertensive drug treatment in older persons with isolated systolic hypertension. Final results of the Systolic Hypertension in the Elderly Program (SHEP). *JAMA* 1991;265(24):3255–3264.

Somes GW, Pahor M, Shorr RI, Cushman WC, Applegate WB. The role of diastolic blood pressure when treating isolated systolic hypertension. *Arch Intern Med* 1999;159(17):2004–2009.

Staessen JA, Gasowski J, Wang JG, et al. Risks of untreated and treated isolated systolic hypertension in the elderly: meta-analysis of outcome trials. *Lancet* 2000;355(9207):865–872.

The DASH diet. Dietary approaches to stop hypertension. *Lippincott's Prim Care Pract* 1998;2(5):536–538.

Vasan RS, Larson MG, Leip EP, et al. Impact of high-normal blood pressure on the risk of cardiovascular disease. *N Engl J Med* 2001;345(18): 1291–1297.

Vasan RS, Beiser A, Seshadri S, et al. Residual lifetime risk for developing hypertension in middle-aged women and men: The Framingham heart study. *JAMA* 2002;287(8):1003–1010.

Verdecchia P. Prognostic value of ambulatory blood pressure: Current evidence and clinical implications. *Hypertension.* 2000;35(3): 844–851.

Voko Z, Bots ML, Hofman A, et al. J-shaped relation between blood pressure and stroke in treated hypertensives. *Hypertension* 1999;34(6):1181–1185.

CRITICAL PATHWAY
Treatment of Chronic Hypertension Algorithm

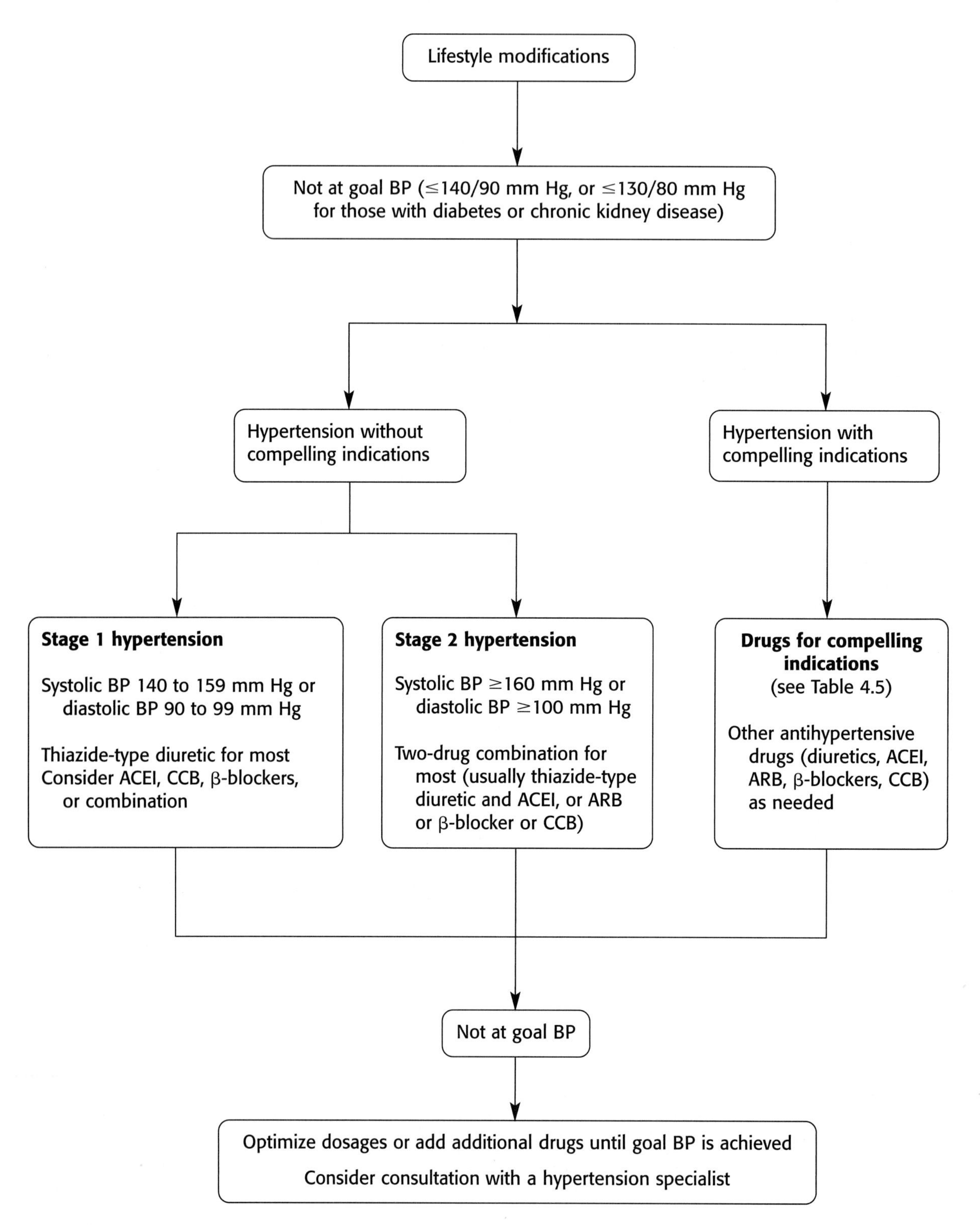

BP, blood pressure; ACEI, angiotensin-converting enzyme inhibitor; CCB, calcium channel blocker; ARB, angiotensin II receptor blockers. (Adapted from Chobanian AV, Bakris GL, Black HR, et al. The Seventh Report of the Joint National Committee on Prevention, Detection, Evaluation, and Treatment of High Blood Pressure: The JNC 7 report. *JAMA* 2003;289 (19):2560–2572.)

CHAPTER

5 Stroke, Diabetes, and the Metabolic Syndrome

JASON HEIL, BRETT KISSELA, JAMES D. GEYER, AND STEPHENIE C. DILLARD

OBJECTIVES

- How does preexisting diabetes affect stroke?
- How should diabetes be treated?
- How does hyperglycemia at stroke presentation affect stroke?
- How should acute hyperglycemia be treated?

The detrimental impact of stroke and diabetes on the health of Americans cannot be overstated. They are, respectively, the third and fifth leading causes of death in the United States, and together they are leading causes of adult disability. Although hypertension is the single most important risk factor for stroke, diabetes is emerging as a major risk factor that contributes significantly to the incidence of stroke. In addition, patients with diabetes who develop heart disease or stroke usually fare worse than their nondiabetic counterparts. This chapter discusses the impact that diabetes and "prediabetes," or insulin resistance, have on ischemic stroke and presents treatment paradigms for the management of diabetic patients to reduce the risk of stroke and for treatment of diabetes during the acute phase of stroke.

As of 2002, the prevalence of diabetes in the United States was 6.7% and that of prediabetes (defined as a fasting blood glucose of 100 to 126 mg per dL) was 2.8%. In the same year, 1.3 million incident cases of type 2 diabetes were diagnosed in patients younger than 20 years and 73,249 deaths were attributed to the disease. The prevalence of diabetes in the United States has been rapidly increasing, paralleling a rise in the rate of obesity. Diabetes is also observed in a disproportionately high prevalence in minority groups, especially African Americans and Mexican Americans. If the current trends continue, it has been predicted that the total number of patients with diabetes will increase from 171 million in 2000 to 366 million in 2030.

Diabetes, both type 1 and type 2, arises when the body can no longer produce adequate insulin levels to maintain glucose homeostasis. Type 1 diabetes results from an autoimmune assault on insulin-producing pancreatic β-cells, causing markedly decreased levels of endogenous insulin. In type 2 diabetes, insulin resistance results when the target cells become less responsive to insulin signaling, forcing the body to produce increased levels of insulin to compensate. It is generally believed that insulin resistance and hyperinsulinemia represent a prediabetic state. Although frank diabetes is not yet present, these patients may demonstrate impaired glucose tolerance characterized by a delay in the restoration of normoglycemia following a glucose challenge. Overt disease occurs when the pancreatic β-cells are no longer able to produce adequate amounts of insulin to meet the rising demand.

No discussion of diabetes would be complete without mention of metabolic syndrome X. The term was first used in the 1950s and the entity began to gain widespread acceptance in the late 1980s. There is some controversy about the diagnostic criteria that define the syndrome, and the standards recommended by the World Health Organization (WHO), the European Group for the Study of Insulin Resistance, and the National Cholesterol Education Program Adult Treatment Panel III are given in Table 5.1. Although there is some disagreement about the specifics, the three groups are in agreement that the syndrome includes insulin resistance and/or elevated fasting glucose levels, central obesity, dyslipidemia, and hypertension. Patients with metabolic syndrome X are at increased risk of developing type 2 diabetes and atherosclerotic vascular disease including heart disease and stroke. Interestingly, some reports have associated metabolic syndrome X with a propensity for hypercoagulability. Many of the studies discussed in the following sections examined the relative risk of stroke in diabetic patients before the widespread acceptance of the concept of a distinct metabolic abnormality linking insulin resistance, hyperlipidemia, and obesity. The potential statistical flaws created by the attempt to determine the relative risk of each of the components of the syndrome are discussed in the next section.

There is also an ill-defined relationship between sleep apnea, type 2 diabetes, and obesity. Obstructive sleep apnea has been shown to produce glucose intolerance, with the severity of the apnea correlating with the degree of insulin resistance. Obstructive sleep apnea is associated with higher blood glucose levels, insulin levels, and glycosylated hemoglobin levels. Unfortunately, treatment of obstructive sleep apnea with continuous positive airway pressure (CPAP) has not resulted in consistent improvement of glucose tolerance. In addition, leptin, a hormone produced by fat cells, is seen in increased levels in obese patients. Males with obstructive sleep apnea have relatively higher levels of leptin than

TABLE 5.1 Recommended Criteria for Diagnosis of Metabolic Syndrome X

World Health Organization (1999)
Requires the presence of diabetes mellitus, impaired glucose tolerance, elevated fasting glucose level, OR insulin resistance AND two of the following:
Blood pressure ≥140/90 mm Hg
Dyslipidemia with triglyceride level ≥150 mg/dL and/or HDL-C level ≤35 mg/dL in men and 40 mg/dL in women
Central obesity with a waist-to-hip ratio >0.90 in men and >0.85 in women, and/or a body mass index >30 kg/m^2
Microalbuminuria with urinary albumin excretion ratio ≥20 mg/min or albumin:creatinine ratio ≥30 mg/g
European Group for the Study of Insulin Resistance (1999)
Requires insulin resistance defined as the top 25% of fasting insulin values among nondiabetic individuals AND two of the following:
Fasting plasma glucose level ≥110 mg/dL
Blood pressure ≥140/90 mm Hg
Dyslipidemia with triglyceride level >180 mg/dL and or HDL-C level <40 mg/dL
Central obesity with a waist circumference ≥94 cm in men and ≥80 cm in women
The National Cholesterol Education Program Adult Treatment Panel III (2001)
Requires three of the following:
Fasting plasma glucose level ≥110 mg/dL
Blood pressure ≥130/85 mm Hg
Dyslipidemia with triglyceride level ≥150 mg/dL or HDL-C level <40 mg/dL in men and <50 mg/dL in women
Central obesity with a waist circumference ≥102 cm in men and ≥88 cm in women

HDL-C, high-density lipoprotein cholesterol.

do males without obstructive sleep apnea. Leptin may increase the production of platelet aggregates, and as a result, may serve as an independent marker for the risk of vascular disease. Studies have shown that leptin levels fall following treatment with CPAP, and therapy for obstructive sleep apnea may not only improve the patient's difficulty with weight gain but also decrease the risk of myocardial infarction and stroke by decreasing the tendency of platelet aggregation.

CLINICAL APPLICATIONS AND METHODOLOGY

It has been estimated that approximately 20% of all strokes in the United States occur in diabetic patients. It should be noted that there does not appear to be a link between insulin resistance/diabetes and hemorrhagic stroke, but insulin resistance has been identified as an independent risk factor for ischemic stroke in multiple studies. The risk is not just limited to patients with frank diabetes. Nondiabetic patients with insulin resistance appear to have an adjusted relative risk for stroke between 1.5 and 2.1. In addition, diabetes is one of the factors most commonly associated with post-stroke mortality, with some studies showing higher mortality in the weeks following the incident stroke and others indicating that mortality is not significantly increased until 1 year or more after stroke.

Epidemiological studies, including both case–control studies and prospective observational cohort studies, have consistently demonstrated a link between insulin resistance and increased stroke risk. The seminal case–control study was done by Gertler et al. in 1975. Mean insulin levels determined by oral glucose tolerance testing in 61 ischemic stroke patients exceeded the levels in 61 healthy age-matched control subjects at all intervals during the oral glucose tolerance test, reaching statistical significance at fasting, 2 hours, and 3 hours.

Pyrola et al. followed up a cohort of 970 Helsinki policemen aged 34 to 64 years who, at the time of baseline testing, were free of diabetes, cerebrovascular disease, and cardiovascular disease. All subjects underwent an oral glucose tolerance test, with plasma insulin and glucose levels measured at 0, 1, and 2 hours. After 22 years, 70 men had suffered a stroke. Hyperinsulinemia at baseline was associated with an increased risk of stroke, but the association was not independent of other risk factors, most notably upper body obesity. The risk factors that independently predicted the increased risk of stroke were upper body obesity, blood pressure, and smoking. When factor analysis was applied to identify whether clustering of risk factors could predict coronary heart disease or stroke risk, three clusters were identified: insulin resistance factor (consisting of body mass index, subscapular skinfold, glucose and insulin levels at baseline, maximal O_2 uptake, mean blood pressure, and triglycerides), lipid factor (cholesterol and triglycerides), and lifestyle factor (physical activity and smoking). Although all three clusters were associated with coronary artery disease, only insulin resistance factor was associated with an increased risk of stroke. Of all variables in the adjusted model, only obesity had a substantial effect on the association between hyperinsulinemia and stroke risk. This underscores the statistical difficulty of accurately assessing the influence of multiple factors when the factors are interrelated, such as in metabolic syndrome X. Researchers may be misled into concluding that stroke risk is associated with obesity, ignoring the role of insulin resistance.

While diabetes is a well-known risk factor for stroke, the magnitude of risk varies widely between studies. In prospective cohorts, the odds ratios for stroke range from 1.41 to 4.89. The Atherosclerosis Risk in Communities (ARIC) study examined fasting plasma insulin levels among 12,728 nondiabetic adults aged 45 to 64 years with no cardiovascular disease at baseline. At the start of the study, waist and hip circumferences were measured and fasting glucose and insulin levels were obtained. The patients were followed up for 6 to 8 years, during which time 191 incidences of strokes occurred. When factors such as age, gender, race, smoking, and education levels were adjusted, the relative risk of ischemic stroke was 3.70 in patients with diabetes, 1.74 in patients with abdominal obesity, and 1.19 for nondiabetic subjects with elevated fasting insulin levels. With adjustment for other stroke risk factors, the relative risks for diabetes, waist-to-hip ratio, and elevated fasting insulin levels were calculated as 2.22, 1.08, and 1.14, respectively.

In 1997, a population-based, case–control study performed in the affluent, mostly white population of Rochester, Minnesota, calculated a population attributable risk of only 5% for diabetes for all ischemic strokes (i.e., diabetes independently accounts for only 5% of all ischemic strokes in this population), an attributable risk less than those of hypertension, ischemic heart disease, and current cigarette smoking. As a result of this and similar studies, diabetes was for many years considered a relatively minor risk factor for stroke. In 2001, the Northern Manhattan Stroke Study (NOMASS) analyzed a population-based, incident case–control study set that included whites, Hispanics, and African-Americans, primarily of Caribbean descent. The goal of this study was to examine the role that race played in the relative risk of stroke. Sacco et al. found that while diabetes did not appear to carry a substantial risk in the white population studied, it accounted for 10% to 14% of strokes among Hispanic and African-American patients.

The Greater Cincinnati/Northern Kentucky Stroke Study (GCNKSS) was a population-based epidemiological study of stroke incidence and mortality that included the residents of the five-county area that comprises the Cincinnati metropolitan area. The population in the region is primarily biracial consisting of approximately 15% African-Americans and the remainder whites, with few other ethnic groups represented. The findings indicated that stroke patients with diabetes were more likely to be younger, African-American, and have a diagnosis of hypertension, myocardial infarction, and/or hypercholesterolemia when compared with nondiabetic controls. Diabetes was shown to carry an increased risk of stroke at all ages, but the risk was more prominent in African-Americans younger than 55 years and in whites younger than 65 years. Although some studies indicate that diabetic patients have a higher mortality in the weeks following a stroke, the GCNKSS found no appreciable difference in survival rate between diabetic and nondiabetic patients with stroke in the first 12 months of follow-up. Given the increased frequency of stroke in the diabetic population, this observation suggests that there are proportionately more patients with diabetes surviving with disability after stroke compared with nondiabetic patients. The GCNKSS recruited a 2,000-person cohort demographically similar to the 2,719 patients with ischemic stroke. The control group was selected by a random digit dialing telephone survey, and the respondents were asked whether they had been diagnosed with conditions known to be risk factors for stroke such as hypertension or diabetes. Population-attributable risks and odds ratios were calculated for each of the risk factors, both alone and in combination. Interestingly, diabetes alone had a higher odds ratio than hypertension alone, but due to the prevalence of hypertension in the population, the population-attributable risk for hypertension was greater than that of diabetes. The odds ratio for stroke in patients with a history of both hypertension and diabetes was substantially greater than that for either condition alone. Diabetes and hypertension, either alone or in combination, accounted for 37% to 42% of the population-attributable risk in both white and African-American subsets of patients (i.e., statistically accounted independently for 37% to 42% of ischemic strokes in this patient population).

Patients with diabetes are at increased risk of morbidity from microvascular complications such as retinopathy, nephropathy, and neuropathy; however, macrovascular complications pose the greatest health risk with 66% to 75% of patients with diabetes ultimately dying from heart disease or stroke. Although diabetic patients are aware of the importance of regular ophthalmologic examinations and scrupulous foot care, surprisingly few are aware of their risk of heart disease and stroke. In a recent survey commissioned by the American Diabetes Association and the American College of Cardiology, >60% of diabetic patients were aware of potential complications such as nephropathy, neuropathy, and retinopathy, but less than one third associated diabetes with an increased risk of heart disease. Results of a telephone survey conducted by random digit dialing in the greater Cincinnati area in 1995 showed that only 57% of the general population could correctly identify one of five established symptoms of stroke (i.e., sudden weakness or numbness, sudden dimness or loss of vision, sudden difficulty speaking or understanding speech, sudden severe headache with no known cause, and unexplained dizziness, unsteadiness, or sudden falls). When asked about their knowledge of stroke risk factors, 57% of patients with hypertension identified hypertension as a risk factor, 35% of current smokers identified smoking as a risk factor, and only 13% of diabetic patients identified diabetes as a risk factor for stroke. The level of awareness of stroke symptoms and risk factors was lowest among older respondents—the population at greatest risk.

Diabetes is emerging as a potent risk factor for stroke, especially in patients younger than 65 years and in some ethnic groups such as African-Americans and Hispanics. Physicians need to be aware of the risk and consciously educate their at-risk patient populations about the signs and symptoms of stroke and the importance of early intervention in acute stroke.

PRACTICAL RECOMMENDATIONS

Management for Stroke Prevention

Recurrent stroke has been shown to occur at a higher frequency in diabetic patients. Since each subsequent stroke is associated with higher mortality and greater residual disability, prevention of future strokes is highly desirable. The U.K. Prospective Diabetes Study (UKPDS) was a large clinical trial that sought to find clinical practices that prevented the macrovascular complications of diabetes such as stroke and heart disease. Surprisingly, while intensive blood glucose control effectively delayed the onset and slowed the progression of diabetic retinopathy, nephropathy, and neuropathy, no significant reduction in the rate of macrovascular complications was detected. In a follow-up study, hypertensive patients were randomized to a group with rigidly controlled blood pressure (<150/<85 mm Hg) or to a group that was allowed to maintain a slightly higher pressure (<180/<105 mm Hg). The patients with the lower blood pressure had a significant reduction in diabetes-related complications, both micro- and macrovascular, which included a 44% reduction in the risk of stroke. The seventh Joint National Committee report (JNC-7) recommends a goal blood pressure for patients with diabetes maintained at <130/80 mm Hg.

For hypertensive patients, the choice of antihypertensive medication may have an impact that extends beyond the effects of maintaining normotensive blood pressures. The Heart Outcomes Prevention Evaluation (HOPE) study examined a subgroup of patients dubbed the MICRO-HOPE substudy group (**MI**croalbuminiuria, **C**ardivovascular and **R**enal **O**utcomes) and sought to evaluate the effectiveness of the angiotensin-converting enzyme (ACE) inhibitor ramipril and vitamin E for the prevention of diabetic nephropathy and cardiovascular disease in patients with diabetes. The study recruited 3,577 diabetic patients who were randomly assigned to receive ramipril or placebo and vitamin E or placebo. Although vitamin E showed no clinical efficacy, the results of ramipril treatment were so striking that the study was terminated 6 months early for safety reasons. Ramipril reduced the risk of myocardial infarction by 22%, stroke by 33%, cardiovascular death by 37%, and total mortality by 24%. The cardiovascular effects persisted even after statistical adjustment for the effects of the decrease in blood pressure.

The "statin" class of lipid-lowering medication has also proved beneficial in the prevention and treatment of vascular complications. The Heart Protection Study looked at the benefits of a 40-mg-per-day dose of simvastatin in 20,536 men and women at high risk of vascular disease. Eligible patients included those with coronary artery disease, other occlusive arterial diseases, and/or diabetes. Roughly 30% of the study participants had diabetes. Patients were randomly assigned to receive simvastatin or placebo. During the 5-year follow-up, patients taking the statin showed a statistically significant reduction in overall morbidity and mortality from coronary disease. There were highly significant reductions in first event rate for myocardial infarction, stroke, and coronary or noncoronary (i.e., carotid artery) revascularization procedures. The rate of reduction was similar for all subtypes of patients including those without coronary disease who had cerebrovascular disease, peripheral artery disease, or diabetes. It was estimated that the addition of simvastatin appeared to reduce the risk of stroke and myocardial infarction and revascularization procedures including bypass and angioplasty of coronary and/or carotid vasculature by 25%, although the calculated benefit was estimated to be closer to one third when noncompliance was taken into account. One of the most notable findings of the study was the lack of evidence for a threshold low-density lipoprotein (LDL) level where the benefits of treatment could first be seen. The trial demonstrated that the benefits of medication were equivalent in patients with nominally elevated LDL and in patients with much greater degrees of hypercholesterolemia. The reduced risk of vascular disease was seen not only in patients with markedly elevated LDL levels but also in patients with baseline LDL cholesterol levels below 116 mg per dL, which decreased to below 77 mg per dL with treatment. Meta-analysis has shown that the benefits reported for simvastatin are similar to those seen with other statin drugs, and the benefits in reducing the rate of stroke and cardiovascular events were independent of measured cholesterol levels.

The Steno-2 study was an open, parallel trial that sought to examine the effects of simultaneously addressing the multiple risk factors for metabolic syndrome X. A total of 160 patients with type 2 diabetes and microalbuminuria were enrolled and followed up for an average of 7.8 years. Eighty were randomized into an intensive, targeted treatment regime that included behavior modification such as smoking cessation, dietary intervention, and pharmacologic therapy targeting hyperglycemia, hypertension, hyperlipidemia, and microalbuminuria. The other 80 participants were assigned to conventional therapy based on the recommendations of the Danish Medical Association. Table 5.2 indicates the threshold of treatment for each of the elements that the study addressed. Since the Danish Medical Association changed their recommendations for the treatment of diabetes in 2000, the treatment criteria were altered for the last year of the study. Elevated levels of glycosylated hemoglobin were treated first with oral hypoglycemics, and if this was unsuccessful, with insulin injections. Patients in the intensive treatment arm of the study were

TABLE 5.2 Steno-2 Study—Treatment Criteria for Conventional and Intensive Therapy Groups

	Conventional Therapy		Intensive Therapy	
	1993–1999	2000–2001	1993–1990	2000–2001
Systolic blood pressure (mm Hg)	<160	<135	<140	<130
Diastolic blood pressure (mm Hg)	<95	<85	<85	<80
Glycosylated hemoglobin (%)	<7.5	<6.5	<6.5	<6.5
Fasting serum total cholesterol (mg/dL)	<250	<190	<190	<175
Fasting serum triglycerides (mg/dL)	<195	<180	<150	<150
Treatment with ACE inhibitor regardless of blood pressure	No	Yes	Yes	Yes
Prophylactic aspirin therapy in patients with known ischemia; or	Yes	Yes	Yes	Yes
peripheral vascular disease;	No	No	Yes	Yes
without coronary artery disease, or peripheral vascular disease	No	No	No	Yes

ACE, angiotensin-converting enzyme.

placed on an ACE inhibitor, or if such a drug was contraindicated, on an angiotensin II receptor agonist, regardless of the blood pressure level. Elevated serum cholesterol levels were treated with statins, and patients with hypertriglyceridemia received fibrates. Aspirin was also prescribed as a secondary preventive measure for macrovascular complications. As expected, the patients in the intensive therapy group had significantly greater declines in glycosylated hemoglobin values, systolic and diastolic blood pressure, fasting serum cholesterol and triglyceride levels, and rate of urinary albumin excretion, but these patients also had significantly lowered risk for cardiovascular complications including stroke, as well as a decreased incidence of nephropathy, retinopathy, and autonomic neuropathy during the 7-year follow-up. There were 20 nonfatal strokes in the conventionally treated group compared to 3 in the intensive treatment group. The authors concluded that a target-driven, long-term intensified intervention aimed at reducing multiple risk factors can reduce the risk of macrovascular complications of diabetes by approximately 50%.

Although no large studies have been performed to evaluate antiplatelet therapy specifically in the diabetic population, no discussion of the prevention of stroke would be complete without a brief review of the use of aspirin or similar medications. A meta-analysis of 142 trials that included >73,000 patients at high risk of vascular complications calculated a 27% reduction in the risk of ischemic stroke, myocardial infarction, and vascular death with the use of antiplatelet drugs.

In summary, although tight control of serum glucose levels is desirable for prevention of microvascular complications of stroke, its role in stroke prevention seems minor. Rigid control of blood pressure appears to be crucial to stroke prevention in the diabetic patient. ACE inhibitors should be considered as first-line treatment for diabetic patients with hypertension, especially in those with additional cardiac risk factors. Initiation of statin drugs should also be contemplated, especially in patients with elevated LDL cholesterol level, and antiplatelet therapy such as aspirin or clopidogrel should be implemented in patients without contraindications. A sleep history should be obtained from all diabetic patients, and evaluation by polysomnography is recommended for all patients with symptoms of sleep apnea.

Hyperglycemia in Acute Stroke

Hyperglycemia is common in the acute stroke setting. There is an approximate 30% increased risk for a poor outcome for patients with immediate poststroke hyperglycemia. Mortality may be increased by as much as three times in these patients as compared to euglycemic patients.

The actual prevalence of immediate poststroke hyperglycemia is unclear and may vary significantly among various demographic subpopulations. Risk factors for the development of poststroke hyperglycemia are also unclear. Given this relative lack of data, the formulation of a treatment paradigm is challenging.

In the Virtual International Stroke Trials Archive (VISTA) study, poststroke hyperglycemia was defined as a glucose level >7.0 mmol per L. In the VISTA population, 36% of nondiabetic patients and 81% of diabetic patients were hyperglycemic on admission, and these numbers increased to 48% of nondiabetic patients and 88% of diabetic patients within 48 hours of presentation. The degree of hyperglycemia was only modestly associated with the severity of the stroke.

TABLE 5.3 Sample Sliding Scale Insulin Orders

Glucose (mg/dL)	Regular Insulin Units SQ (Humulin R)
<200	0
201–250	2
251–300	4
301–350	6
351–400	8
401–450	10
451–500	12
>500, <600	Call MD

The concept that hyperglycemia worsens outcome is an important piece of information. The appropriate management of this hyperglycemia is of paramount importance. Close monitoring of the serum glucose level during the acute stroke phase would seem prudent. Use of sliding scale insulin for the management of the elevated glucose levels also seems appropriate (see Table 5.3 for a sample sliding scale insulin regimen). Further research is needed to define the degree of glucose control that is optimal for neurological outcome.

SELECTED REFERENCES

Air EA, Kissela BM. Diabetes, the metabolic syndrome and ischemic stroke: epidemiology and possible mechanisms. *Diabetes Care* 2007;30: 3131–3140.

Bruno A, Biller J, Adams H, et al. Acute blood glucose level and outcome from ischemic stroke. *Neurology* 1999;52:280–284.

Burroughs V, Weinberger J. Diabetes and stroke: Part 2. Treating diabetes and stress hyperglycemia in hospitalized stroke patients. *Curr Card Reports* 2006;8:29–32.

Capes S, Hunt D, Malmberg K, et al. Stress hyperglycemia and prognosis of stroke in nondiabetic and diabetic patients. A systematic overview. *Stroke* 2001;32:2426–2432.

Combs D, Dempsey R, Kumar S. Focal cerebral infarction in cats in the presence of hyperglycemia and increased insulin. *Metab Brain Dis* 1990;5:169–178.

de Courten-Myers G, Kleinholz M, Holm P, et al. Hemorrhagic infarct conversion in experimental stroke. *Ann Emerg Med* 1992;21:120–126.

de Courten-Myers G, Kleinholz M, Wagner K. Fatal strokes in hyperglycemic cats. *Stroke* 1989;20:1707–1715.

Dietrich W, Alonso O, Busto R. Moderate hyperglycemia worsens acute blood-brain barrier injury after forebrain ischemia in rats. *Stroke* 1993;24:111–116.

Gilmore R, Stead L. The role of hyperglycemia in acute ischemic stroke. *Neurocrit Care* 2006;5:153–158.

Ginsberg M, Prado R, Dietrich W, et al. Hyperglycemia reduces the extent of cerebral infarction in rats. *Stroke* 1987;18:570–574.

Kawai N, Keep R, Betz A. Hyperglycemia and the vascular effects of cerebral ischemia. *Stroke* 1997;28:149–154.

Kissela B, Air E. Diabetes: impact on stroke risk and post-stroke recovery. *Sem Neurol* 2006;26(1):100–107.

Kissela BM, Khoury J, Kleindorfer D, et al. Epidemiology of ischemic stroke in patients with diabetes: the Greater Cincinnati/Northern Kentucky Stroke Study. *Diabetes Care* 2005;28(2):355–359.

Kraft S, Larson C, Shuer L, et al. Effect of hyperglycemia on neuronal changes in a rabbit model of focal cerebral ischemia. *Stroke* 1990;21 :447–450.

Malmberg K. Prospective randomized study of intensive insulin treatment on long term survival after acute myocardial infarction in patients with diabetes mellitus. DIGAMI (Diabetes Mellitus, Insulin-Glucose in Acute Myocardial Infarction) Study Group. *BMJ* 1997;314(7093):1512–1515.

Malmberg K, Ryden L, Hamsten A, et al. Effects of insulin treatment on cause-specific one-year mortality and morbidity in patients with acute myocardial infarction. DIGAMI Study Group (Diabetes Insulin-Glucose in Acute Myocardial Infarction). *Eur Heart J* 1996;17(9): 1337–1344.

Nedergaard M, Diemer N. Focal ischemia of the rat brain, with special reference to the influence of plasma glucose concentration. *Acta Neuropathol*1987;73:131–137.

Nedergaard M, Gjedde A, Diemer N. Hyperglycemia protects against neuronal injury around experimental brain infarcts. *Neurol Res* 1987;9:241–244.

Parsons M, Barber P, Desmond P, et al. Acute hyperglycemia adversely affects stroke outcome: a magnetic resonance imaging and spectroscopy study. *Ann Neurol* 2002;52:20–28.

Prado R, Ginsberg M, Dietrich W, et al. Hyperglycemia increases infarct size in collaterally perfused but not end-arterial vascular territories. *Am J Neurorad* 1991;12:603–609.

Rovlias A, Kotsou S. The influence of hyperglycemia on neurological outcome in patients with severe head injury. *Neurosurgery* 2000; 46(2), 335.

Scott J, Robinson G, French J, et al. Glucose potassium insulin infusions in the treatment of acute stroke patients with mild to moderate hyperglycemia: The Glucose Insulin in Stroke Trial (GIST). *Stroke* 1999;30(4): 793–799.

Van den Berghe G, Wouters P, Weekers F, et al. Intensive insulin therapy in critically ill patients. *N Eng J Med* 2001;345:1359–1367.

Venables G, Miller S, Gibson G, et al. The effects of hyperglycaemia on changes during reperfusion following cerebral ischemia in the cat. *J Neurol Neurosurg Psychiatr* 1985;48:663–669.

Voll C, Auer R. The effect of postischemic blood glucose levels on ischemic brain damage in the rat. *Ann Neurol* 1988;24:638–646.

Weir C, Murray G, Dyker A, et al. Is hyperglycaemia and independent predictor of poor outcome after acute stroke? Results of a long-term follow up study. *BMJ* 1997;314:1303–1306.

Widmer H, Abiko H, Faden A, et al. Effects of hyperglycemia on the time course of change in energy metabolism and pH during cerebral ischemia and reperfusion in rats: correlation of 1H and 31 P NMR spectroscopy with fatty acid and excitatory amino acid levels. *J Cereb Blood Flow Metab* 1992;12:456–468.

Zasslow M, Pearl R, Shuer M, et al. Hyperglycemia decreases acute neuronal ischemic changes after middle cerebral artery occlusion in cats. *Stroke* 1989;20:519–523.

CHAPTER 6

Tobacco and Stroke

ALAN BLUM AND JAMES D. GEYER

OBJECTIVES

- What are the vascular risks of smoking?
- How should a treatment plan be designed?
- What is the role of the physician in smoking cessation?

Tobacco smoking is one of the leading modifiable risk factors for stroke. A truly comprehensive approach to stroke prevention (both primary and secondary) must include an *effective* smoking cessation plan. The approach to the patient is not as easy as handing the patient a prescription. It demands the physician's time and effort. The results of appropriate and aggressive physician counseling cannot be overstated.

CLINICAL APPLICATIONS

Cigarette smoking is the chief avoidable cause of death in our society. Smoking is responsible for 18% of the total deaths in the United States each year. It is one of the primary modifiable risk factors for stroke. An aggressive approach to smoking cessation is an indispensable component of any stroke treatment or prevention strategy.

Tobacco smoking leads to a dependence on nicotine that is distinguishable from other forms of drug dependence. In such a dependency, the drug is needed to maintain an optimal state of well-being. Nicotine, the habituating constituent of tobacco, meets the criteria for addiction because a typical withdrawal syndrome occurs after smoking cessation.

Although cigarette smoking in adults declined from 42% to 27% in the United States between 1964 and 1992, 28% of men and 24% of women continue to use tobacco daily. Approximately 1.3 million persons per year stop smoking. However, each day approximately 3,000 individuals start smoking. Almost half of all smokers start smoking before 18 years of age. Although 80% of those who smoke say that they would like to stop, only 20% of those who try actually succeed in stopping permanently. The likelihood of success increases with the number of attempts, and those with a college education are twice as likely to break the habit as less-educated smokers.

At present, virtually all life insurance companies now offer significant discounts to persons who do not smoke. Actuarial data leave little doubt that the average life expectancy of a 32-year-old man who smokes cigarettes is 72 years versus 79 years for someone who does not smoke. The quality of life for those diminished years is frequently complicated by myriad disorders including stroke and chronic obstructive pulmonary disease (COPD).

HEALTH RISKS ASSOCIATED WITH SMOKING

Cancer

Forty percent of all cancer deaths are attributable to cigarette smoking. Besides lung cancer, smoking is the major cause of cancer of the larynx, oral cavity, and esophagus (see Table 6.1). It is also a contributory factor in cancer of the pancreas, bladder, kidney, stomach, and uterine cervix. Recent studies have implicated smoking in leukemia, colon cancer, Graves disease, depression, and renal disease in persons with diabetes mellitus. A dose–response relationship exists between smoking and all these diseases. As described in Chapter 8, cancers increase the overall risk of stroke.

Cardiovascular Disease

Heart Disease

Nicotine raises systolic blood pressure, heart rate, and cardiac output and causes vasoconstriction. The relationship between cerebral vasoconstriction and anoxia and the intake of carbon monoxide resulting from cigarette smoking could explain the 50% increase in automobile accidents in smokers. The symptoms associated with carbon monoxide intoxication can be a problem, especially for persons with an already compromised coronary or cerebral circulation. Carbon monoxide has an affinity for hemoglobin that is 245 times stronger than that of oxygen. Thus carbon monoxide reduces oxygen delivery to the myocardium and has a decidedly negative inotropic effect. Carboxyhemoglobin also lowers the threshold for ventricular fibrillation and could help explain the higher incidence of sudden death in those who smoke.

TABLE 6.1 Diseases or Conditions Influenced by Cigarette Smoking

Cardiovascular	Cancer	Respiratory	Other
Coronary heart disease	Lung	COPD (emphysema)	Infertility
Stroke	Larynx	Bronchitis	Impotence
Subarachnoid hemorrhage	Esophagus	Pneumonia	Osteoporosis
Aortic aneurysm	Pancreas	Asthma	Premature wrinkling
Hypertension	Uterine	Otitis media	Peptic ulcer
Peripheral vascular disease	Cervix		Alzheimer disease
	Ovary		Graves disease
	Colon		Insomnia
	Bladder		Depression
	Kidney		
	Breast		
	Brain		
	Blood (leukemia)		

COPD, chronic obstructive pulmonary disease.

The risk of myocardial infarction is proportional to the number of cigarettes smoked. The trend toward the use of filtered cigarettes does not appear to have reduced the risk of coronary heart disease. Theoretically, filters on cigarettes reduce the amount of tar (the condensate of tobacco smoke that comprises over 3,000 compounds, including more than 40 carcinogens), but they may increase the amount of carbon monoxide, thus contributing to the increased mortality from coronary heart disease. Persons who smoke cigarettes containing low amounts of nicotine have the same degree of risk of myocardial infarction as those who smoke cigarettes containing larger amounts. Smokers of these low-dose cigarettes still have three times the risk of myocardial infarction as nonsmokers. The good news is that the risk of sudden death decreases immediately on stopping, and within a few years of stopping, the risk of myocardial infarction decreases to a level similar to that in people who have never smoked, even in heavy smokers who have a positive family history of coronary heart disease.

Three-fourths of myocardial infarctions in women younger than 50 years have been attributed to smoking. The risk of myocardial infarction increases progressively to as much as 20-fold in persons smoking 35 or more cigarettes per day. There is no safe level of smoking. Women who smoke and use oral contraceptives have a risk of heart attack that is ten times greater than that of women who do neither.

Silent ischemia probably accounts for most of all cardiac ischemic events. Patients with coronary heart disease who smoke have three times as many episodes of silent ischemia as nonsmokers, and the duration of each is 12 times longer. Frequent episodes of myocardial ischemia, even though asymptomatic, damage the heart. Because smoking also increases platelet adhesiveness and lowers high-density lipoprotein cholesterol, the association with a higher incidence of myocardial infarction is no surprise.

Benefits from stopping smoking can be demonstrated at all ages. No decrease in benefits is seen as one gets older, so it is still worthwhile for someone older than 65 to break the addiction. This benefit can be demonstrated in the cerebral as well as the coronary circulation. Older individuals who stop smoking have significantly higher cerebral perfusion levels than those who continue to smoke. Even those who have smoked for 30 to 40 years have improved cerebral circulation within a relatively short time after stopping smoking.

Stroke

Cigarette smoking is one of the most important modifiable risk factors for stroke. The incidence of stroke in smokers is 50% higher than in nonsmokers (40% higher in men and 60% higher in women). The risk of stroke increases in proportion to the amount of smoking; it is twice as great in those who smoke more than 40 cigarettes per day than in those smoking fewer than 10 cigarettes per day.

When compared with women who have never smoked, the risk of stroke increases 2.2-fold in women smoking 1 to 14 cigarettes per day and 3.7-fold in women smoking 25 or more cigarettes daily. Bonita et al. found a threefold increase in the risk of stroke in smokers in comparison to nonsmokers. Cigarette smokers who are also hypertensive have a 20-fold increased risk of stroke.

Sclerosis of the carotid arteries is directly proportional to the amount of smoke exposure. Smoking increases the risk of ischemic heart disease and cerebrovascular disease regardless of the level of serum cholesterol. Jee et al. found that a low cholesterol level did not protect against smoking-related arteriosclerotic cardiovascular disease in patients in South Korea, where the prevalence of smoking is among the highest in the world at 72% of men.

The risk of stroke declines rapidly after cessation of smoking, and after 5 years, is at the level of nonsmokers, which emphasizes that it is never too late to quit no matter how long one has been smoking.

Subarachnoid Hemorrhage

Habitual smoking also increases the risk of subarachnoid hemorrhage, with an increased relative risk of 3.9 times for men and 3.7 times for women. The risk increases to 22 times that of nonsmokers in women who both smoke and use oral contraceptives.

Other Diseases and Conditions

Diabetes Mellitus

The risk of diabetes increases with the number of cigarettes smoked. People smoking more than one pack per day have 1.5 times the risk for diabetes as those who smoke 1 to 14 cigarettes. Albuminuria as a sign of early renal damage and retinopathy is greater in patients with type 1 diabetes mellitus who smoke and can be shown to improve significantly if the person stops smoking.

Depression

Smokers are more likely to experience major depression than nonsmokers are, and the incidence increases steadily with the number of cigarettes smoked. Conversely, it is estimated that one third of smokers are depressed and self-medicate with tobacco. Kendler et al. suggested that this increased risk could be due to genes that predispose to both conditions.

Insomnia

Smokers are more likely than nonsmokers to have insomnia, and as a consequence, to feel tired in the morning. Smokers will be more restless during sleep and more likely to awaken tired and then smoke during the day for the stimulation. However, smokers also consume more alcohol and caffeine than nonsmokers do, which will contribute to insomnia.

PHYSICIAN INVOLVEMENT IN ENDING THE TOBACCO PANDEMIC

A remarkable grassroots antismoking movement that arose in the 1970s has had a major impact on the goal of achieving a smoke-free society and has impelled traditional health organizations such as the American Cancer Society and the American Medical Association to become more outspoken. The first medical organization to develop proven strategies for the clinic, classroom, and community aimed at counteracting tobacco use and promotion was Doctors Ought to Care (DOC), founded in 1977 by a family physician at the University of Miami. During its 25-year existence, DOC was supported by the American Academy of Family Physicians. Tar Wars, an annual antismoking poster contest for schoolchildren, is a DOC offshoot that has been adopted by numerous state and local family practice organizations.

The *five foci of tobacco control*, the accepted term for this emerging field of public health, included the following: increases in cigarette excise taxes, bans on tobacco advertising and promotion, restrictions on teenagers' access to tobacco products, pharmacologic and behavioral smoking cessation strategies, and legislation to prohibit smoking in public areas and the workplace.

Other tobacco control efforts include regulatory warning labels on cigarette packages, divestment of tobacco stocks, enforcement of laws against cigarette smuggling, an end to tobacco subsidies, and rejection of donations and research grants from the tobacco industry. The American Cancer Society's most visible antismoking effort is an annual day-long event in November, The Great American Smokeout, during which people who smoke are encouraged to quit and use a nicotine-replacement product instead.

SMOKING CESSATION PROGRAMS

Ideally, the validity of the abstinence rate for a method of smoking cessation should depend on the performance of a controlled, double-blind study with follow-up of at least 6 months duration of all subjects who entered the study. Few published outcome evaluations meet such criteria. Before the introduction of nicotine-replacement products in 1984, smoking cessation techniques in the United States consisted of a hodgepodge of unproven but much-touted chemical remedies, diets, aversive stimuli, hypnotherapy, self-help manuals, special filters, acupuncture, and expensive behavior modification clinics or seminars. Many of these methods are quite costly, but having to pay a high price may well be related to the alleged success of a given method.

When the U.S. Food and Drug Administration (FDA) approved the use of nicotine-containing chewing gum (Nicorette) for smoking cessation, the product gained immediate popularity (see Table 6.2 for a listing of pharmacologic therapies for smoking cessation). However, although the gum was approved for the use as an adjunct to a comprehensive program of behavior modification, most physicians offered few instructions and little follow-up. Moreover, some patients became dependent on the gum and perpetuated their

TABLE 6.2 Pharmacologic Therapies Used in Smoking Cessation

Agent	Duration of Therapy	Side Effects	Contraindications
Patch	10 wk	Headache, insomnia, site reactions, jaw pain	Recent MI, arrhythmias, TMJ symptoms
Gum	3 mo		
Lozenge	3 mo		
Nasal spray	3–6 mo		
Inhaler	3 mo		
Bupropion	3–6 m	Headache, dry mouth, tremor, behavioral changes	Eating disorders, seizures, bipolar disorders
Varenicline	3 mo + 3 mo to enhance cessation	Suicide risk, nausea, insomnia, headache	

MI, myocardial infarction; TMJ, temporomandibular joint.

smoking by using the gum at times and in places where they were not permitted to smoke. The high success rates reported in clinical trials may be attributed in part to the fact that the research was conducted in clinics that specialize in the treatment of smoking cessation. This difference may further explain why placebo groups in some studies fared better than the intervention groups of most other methods.

In 1992, all smoking cessation methods began to take a back seat to use of the transdermal nicotine patch. The theory behind the patch is that controlled, continuous release of nicotine provides partial replacement of the nicotine from smoking, thereby reducing the craving and preventing withdrawal. As with users of nicotine gum, relapse is a problem in patients who use the patch. The most significant problem in clinical practice appears to be a combination of the patient's heightened expectations for the patch (based on word-of-mouth testimonials and advertising in the mass media) and the physician's overeager acquiescence in prescribing it.

Pharmaceutical company claims notwithstanding, smoking is not simply an addiction to nicotine. Social and psychological factors also play determining roles. Promotions for various pharmacological agents for smoking cessation wrongly reinforce the notion that smoking is primarily a medical problem with a simple, prescribable, nonindividualized solution. When a patient requests a drug to help stop smoking, the physician, although not wishing to dash expectations, should emphasize that a drug is an adjunct, not the single solution.

The updated clinical practice guideline *Treating Tobacco Use and Dependence*, published by the U.S. Department of Health and Human Services (DHHS), has added bupropion sustained release (SR) (Zyban), nicotine inhaler (Nicotrol), and nicotine nasal spray to its list of first-line medications that patients should be encouraged to use. All three are available exclusively by prescription. Nicotine gum and transdermal nicotine, the only two recommended medications in the original guideline in 1996, remain on the list. The gum is now available exclusively as an over-the-counter medication in either 2 or 4 mg strengths; the latter is recommended for highly dependent smokers. Clonidine, in doses of 0.1 to 0.75 mg per day delivered either transdermally or orally, is recommended as a second-line agent to treat tobacco dependence. Because of a paucity of data, no other pharmacotherapies are recommended as a second-line agent to treat tobacco dependence. Apart from bupropion SR (which is contraindicated in patients who are at risk for seizures or who have had a previous diagnosis of bulimia or anorexia nervosa), no other antidepressant agent has been documented as effective for smoking cessation or approved by the FDA for this use. Neither benzodiazepines nor β-adrenergic blocking agents have been found to have a beneficial effect in smoking cessation.

Two large multicenter studies have found bupropion SR to be efficacious in doubling long-term abstinence rates when compared with placebo. One advantage of this medication is that it can be instituted a week or two before complete cessation is attempted, unlike nicotine-replacement products, which are based on providing gradually reduced amounts of nicotine without the other toxic components of cigarette smoke. A course of treatment with bupropion SR ranges from 7 to 12 weeks. Treatment with nicotine-replacement products ranges from 6 weeks to 6 months.

Combination therapy appears to be a promising, albeit doubly expensive, approach. A 9-week study combining bupropion SR with transdermal nicotine found much greater efficacy than with either medication alone. Overall, the guideline found insufficient evidence to recommend combination therapy as a general treatment strategy.

Varenicline (Chantix) is a selective a_4-β_2 neuronal nicotinic acetylcholine receptor partial agonist that was recently approved for smoking cessation therapy. This drug is felt to help decrease the cravings associated with quitting and the withdrawal from nicotine. While this drug may be of benefit, it must be used in concert with behavior modification. Furthermore, concerns have been raised about potential adverse side effects.

The introduction of bupropion SR and newer forms of nicotine-replacement products, backed by intensive advertising campaigns in both medical journals and the mass media, will doubtless stimulate physicians to take a more informed and personal role in smoking cessation. Such active involvement can be extremely crucial in and of itself. In the 1970s, at a time when efforts by physicians to discourage smoking were much less widespread and accepted, Russell et al. (1979) found that just 1 to 2 minutes of simple but unequivocal advice to the patient to stop smoking resulted in a cessation rate of over 5% measured at 1 year as opposed to only 0.3% in the control group. Moreover, when strong advice is given at the time of recovery from a heart attack or other smoking-related disease (combined with a brochure and a promise of follow-up), over 60% stop smoking and stay off cigarettes (measured at 3 years)—more than twice the rate of those who receive less definitive advice. Although most family physicians routinely ask their patients about smoking and advise them to stop smoking, relatively few provide more than advice and actually counsel patients with state-of-the-art techniques.

OBSTACLES TO CHANGE

Unfortunately, the tobacco pandemic cannot be addressed as though it were a static issue whereby sufficient public health education results in a significant change in societal behavior. Rather, smoking is a dynamic issue, with cigarette advertisers—whose livelihoods depend on maintaining more than 50 million users of tobacco, including 1.25 million teenagers who take up smoking each year—constantly adapting to the challenges brought by the antismoking movement.

Thus, smoking cessation programs for individual patients cannot truly succeed in the long run in the absence of both workplace smoking bans and multimedia counteradvertising strategies that weaken the influence of the tobacco industry and reinforce physician's office-based efforts.

A variety of factors may inhibit physician involvement in smoking cessation, such as a perceived or real lack of time, lack of reimbursement by third-party payers for such counseling, and lack of peer group reinforcement in a technologically oriented, tertiary care-centered, highly intellectualized health care system. Nonetheless, physicians might well find that their increased involvement in efforts to promote smoking cessation among patients, regardless of the minimal enhancement in revenue, becomes a practice-building factor as word spreads about the physicians who care.

OFFICE-BASED STRATEGIES

Physicians can do a great deal to become better teachers about smoking, in lieu of relegating this role to ancillary personnel, a smoking cessation clinic, or a pamphlet. The physician can develop an innovative strategy beginning outside the office. A bus bench, billboard, or sign in the parking lot with a straightforward or humorous health promotion message helps establish a thought-provoking and favorable image. In the waiting area, removal of ashtrays and placement of signs noting that "In the interest of comfort, safety, and health, this is a smoke-free environment" further reinforce the message.

Magazines with cigarette advertisements ought not to appear in the physician's office in the absence of prominent stickers or rubber-stamped messages calling patients' attention to the deceptive, absurd nature of such ads. Although responsibility for the office-based smoking cessation strategy should rest with the physician, it is invaluable to include all office staff as positive reinforcement for patients. Labeling each chart with a small "No Smoking" sticker to indicate the need for such reinforcement may be helpful, although care must be taken to avoid stigmatizing the patient as a smoker. One would do well to reconsider using potentially alienating words such as "smoker" or even "quitter."

The key to successful smoking cessation efforts is a positive approach. A discussion about the diseases caused by smoking and the harmful constituents of tobacco smoke is essential—indeed, the physician must not shrink from imparting, through graphic posters, pamphlets, slides, and other audiovisuals aids, the gruesome consequences of smoking—but the benefits of not smoking must be emphasized at least as strongly. Moreover, solely educating patients about the facts of smoking in a single office visit is unlikely to result in behavioral change.

In contrast, the physician can, through the use of creative analogies related to the patient's occupation, hobbies, or romantic interest, succeed in changing the patient's entire attitude toward smoking. By noting that cyanide is the substance used in the gas chamber in executions, that formaldehyde is used to preserve cadavers, or that ammonia is the predominant smell in urine, however, the physician is likely to cause the patient to think about smoking a bit differently. No one wishes to have "urine breath." Similarly, it does little good to talk about carcinogens in tobacco in an age when the public believes that "everything causes cancer." Sadly, the concept of relative risk is poorly developed in our society because all too many people who smoke choose to think their million-to-one odds of winning the state lottery are better than their one-in-seven chance of actually getting lung cancer.

Metaphors that Motivate

A revocabularization on the part of the physician is essential for making progress in office-based smoking cessation. Instead of "pack-year history," a more relevant measure is the "inhalation count." A pack-a-day smoker will breathe in upward of 1 million doses of cyanide, ammonia, carcinogens, and carbon monoxide in fewer than 15 years, not including the inhalation of other people's smoke (calculated at 10 inhalations per cigarette, 20 cigarettes per pack). Another way to emphasize the enormous amount smoked is to state the financial cost: a pack-a-day cigarette buyer will spend in excess of $1,000 per year (calculated at $3 a pack). That is well over $10,000 in a decade that could be put into a savings account. Patients can look forward to the joyful feeling of finding a $50 bill every 2 weeks—which is what they would indeed find if the money is not spent on cigarettes.

So although patient education in general and smoking cessation in particular depend on the knowledge that both the physician and the patient have about the deleterious aspects of adverse health behavior, the cognitive component alone is insufficient. Both the physician and the patient must be motivated to succeed. Three keys to office-based smoking cessation are to personalize, individualize, and demythologize.

The physician can learn to personalize approaches to smoking cessation by carefully screening the pamphlets and other audiovisual aids available in the office. (Ideally, physicians should consider producing their own.) It is essential to scrutinize all such materials as one would with a new drug or medical device. Personally handing a brochure to the patient while pointing out and underlining certain passages or illustrations will provide an important reinforcing message. The pamphlets, posters, and signs should be changed or otherwise updated every few weeks or months.

In any event, such dialogue must be practiced over and over again like any medical procedure and individualized to the patient. (Remember that no two construction workers, teenagers, or executives are alike.) The counseling should be designed to call attention not only to the inevitable risks of smoking cigarettes but also to the chemically adulterated tobacco product itself, its inflated price, and the ubiquitous and ludicrous way in which the person's brand is promoted. In effect, the physician can shift the focus away from a resistant or guilt-ridden smoker and onto the product.

COMMON MYTHS

The most important myth surrounding smoking is that it relieves stress. This myth can be debunked by pointing out that the stress that is relieved is what resulted from being dependent on cigarettes—the essence of addiction. At the same time, it is important to point out that deep breathing in and of itself has a relaxing effect.

The second and saddest myth is that smoking keeps weight off. Aside from pointing to all the obese women who smoke and attempting to correct the misapprehension that being overweight is a greater health risk than smoking is, one can point out that by damaging the taste buds and other digestive tract cells, smoking does inhibit appetite, but it also results in more sedentary behavior through loss of lung capacity and cardiovascular fitness. One need not gain weight on stopping smoking if one will relearn to enjoy walking and running as much as one relearns the taste of food. By no means will all persons who stop smoking gain weight. Even among those who do, the average weight gain is 6 pounds for men and 8 pounds for women. Although smokers may weigh slightly less than nonsmokers, when they stop smoking they simply return to an average weight. Moreover, the slightly lower weight in many who continue to smoke is associated with a higher-risk body fat distribution.

From the physician's standpoint, perhaps the biggest myth that has been encouraged in the medical literature is that the patient must be "ready to quit." Setting a "quit date," the sine qua non of the smoking cessation literature, may rationalize the continuation of an adverse health practice and may strengthen denial. In other words, it is helpful to remind patients that they can stop now. If they do not stop, it does not mean that you will not treat them next time, but it is important to give encouragement and not reinforce excuses. Most authors do believe that a quit date targeted only 1 week or a few weeks into the future is useful for a motivated patient, for whom denial is less of a problem. Its purpose is to let the individual build up resolve or to permit a gradual reduction in daily cigarette consumption. Giving patients a few written reminders is very helpful (such as lists of the advantages and disadvantages of smoking, the rewards for not smoking and the penalties for lighting up, the situations and environmental influences that encourage one to smoke, and the myths of smoking and smoking cessation). A prescription with a no-smoking symbol signed by the physician and included with the other prescriptions is a thoughtful gesture. The physician should not advise switching to a low-tar cigarette, or changing to a pipe or cigar.

PRACTICAL RECOMMENDATIONS

A tailored approach to smoking cessation must be developed for each patient who smokes. The approach to a teenage woman should be quite different from the approach to an older man. Counseling is the cornerstone of treatment but medication can play an ancillary role as described in this chapter. The patient should be counseled about the role of the medications—helping to begin the transition to a smoke-free life, although drugs are not a magical treatment with immediate and complete results.

An excellent motivational Web site for all patients who use tobacco products is www.whyquit.com. Patients can also obtain self-help materials from the National Quitline, sponsored by the U.S. Department of Health and Human Services, by dialing 1-800-QUITNOW (1-800-332-8615 for hearing impaired) or online at www.smokefree.gov.

SELECTED REFERENCES

Anda RF, Williamson DF, Escobedo LG, et al. Depression and the dynamics of smoking: A national perspective. *JAMA* 1990;264:1541–1545.

Blum A. Preventing tobacco-related cancers. In: DeVita VT, Hellman S, Rosenberg SA, eds. *Cancer: Principles and practices of oncology*. 5th ed. Philadelphia, PA: Lippincott; 1997:545–557.

Blum A. The role of the health professional in ending the tobacco pandemic: clinic, classroom, and community. *J Natl Cancer Inst* 1992;12:37–43.

Blum AM, Solberg EJ. The tobacco pandemic. In: Mengel MB, Holleman WL, Fields SA, eds. *Fundamentals of clinical practice*. 2nd ed. New York: Plenum; 2002:671–687.

Cofta-Woerpel L, Wright KL, Wetter DW. Smoking cessation 3: Multicomponent interventions. *Behav Med* 2007;32:135–149.

Fiore MC, Bailey WC, Cohen SJ, et al. Treating tobacco use and dependence: Clinical practice guideline. Rockville, MD: US Department of Health and Human Services, Public Health Service; 2000.

Klesges RC, Johnson KC, Somes G. Verenicline for smoking cessation: definite promise, but no panacea. *JAMA* 2006;296:94–95.

Rakel RE, Blum A. Nicotine addiction. In: Rakel RE, ed. *Textbook of Family Practice*. 6th ed. Philadelphia, PA: WB Saunders; 2002:1523–1538.

US Department of Health and Human Services, Centers for Disease Control and Prevention, National Center for Chronic Disease Prevention and Health Promotion, Office on Smoking and Health. *The Health Consequences of Smoking: A Report of the Surgeon General*. Washington, DC: US Government Printing Office, 2004.

US Department of Health and Human Services, Centers for Disease Control and Prevention, National Center for Chronic Disease Prevention and Health promotion, Office on Smoking and Health. *The Health Consequences of Involuntary Exposure to Tobacco Smoke. A Report of the Surgeon General*. Washington, DC: US Government Printing Office, 2006.

US Department of Health and Human Services, National Institutes of Health, National Institute on Alcohol Abuse and Alcoholism. Alcohol and tobacco. In: *Alcohol Alert*. 2007; 71.

US Department of Health and Human Services, Public Health Service, Centers for Disease Control, Office on Smoking and Health. *The Health Consequences of Smoking: Cardiovascular Disease. A Report of the Surgeon General*. Washington, DC: US Government Printing Office, 1982; DHHS Publication No. (PHS) 82-50179.

Wannamehee SG, Shaper AG, Whincup PH, et al. Smoking cessation and the risk of stroke in middle-aged men. *JAMA* 1995;274:155–160.

Wolf PA, D'Agostino RB, Kannel WB, et al. Cigarette smoking as a risk factor for stroke: The Framingham Study. *JAMA* 1988;259: 1025–1029.

CHAPTER

7 Management of Cholesterol in Patients with Ischemic Stroke

NADER ANTONIOS AND SCOTT SILLIMAN

OBJECTIVES

- What is the epidemiological evidence that hypercholesterolemia is a risk factor for ischemic stroke?
- What pharmacological agents are used to reduce cholesterol levels?
- What is the practical approach to managing patients with ischemic stroke and hypercholesterolemia?

Over the past few decades, it has been recognized that abnormal levels of certain lipids, particularly cholesterol, are a risk factor for vascular diseases affecting the heart, limbs, and brain. Aggressive management of hypercholesterolemia has become a universal component of risk factor management aimed at preventing coronary heart disease (CHD). Reduction of primary stroke risk, observed in clinical trials of statins published since 1994, has been the impetus for physicians to evaluate the cholesterol levels in patients who are at risk for stroke. Prescribing medications to lower cholesterol levels in these patients is emerging as a common practice.

CLINICAL APPLICATIONS AND METHODOLOGY

Cholesterol as a Risk Factor for Primary Ischemic Stroke

Results of observational studies in different populations indicate that lower blood cholesterol is associated with a reduced risk of CHD for the normal range of cholesterol levels. There is a continuous positive relationship between coronary artery disease and blood cholesterol down to at least 3 to 4 mmol per L (116 to 154 mg per dL), with no threshold below which a lower cholesterol is not associated with a lower risk. Observational studies suggest that a prolonged difference in total cholesterol of about 1 mmol per L (17 mg per dL) is associated with one third fewer CHD deaths in middle age.

In contrast to the epidemiological data supporting a relationship between CHD and total cholesterol level, a link between serum cholesterol concentration and all strokes (hemorrhagic + ischemic) has never been completely established. A meta-analysis of 45 prospective cohorts that included a total of 450,000 people with an average of 16 years of follow-up and 13,000 incident strokes found no association between total cholesterol and stroke. There are several potential explanations for the lack of an association between total cholesterol level and all strokes in this meta-analysis. The cohorts were selected primarily to study the incidence of CHD, and thus recruited mostly middle-aged subjects who may be more at risk of developing myocardial infarction (MI) (mean age of MI was 55 years) than IS, which is seen more frequently in older subjects (>70 years of age). In addition, aggressive management of risk factors in the study patients may have lowered the incidence of stroke in these cohorts. Another potential explanation is that hemorrhagic stroke was not separated from IS in these analyses, thus potentially leading to an undetected association between brain infarction and elevated cholesterol.

Findings from the Multiple Risk Factor Intervention Trial (MRFIT) suggest that there is an association between higher total cholesterol levels and risk of IS. This trial followed 350,977 men for 6 years. At baseline all subjects had no history of MI and their ages ranged from 35 to 57 years. In this study the risk of death from IS increased in proportion to serum cholesterol. There was, however, a negative association between cholesterol <200 mg per dL and the risk of death from hemorrhagic stroke; the lower the cholesterol level the higher the risk of death from hemorrhagic stroke. This relationship between cholesterol and stroke suggested a U-shaped correlation between cholesterol concentration and stroke risk. The findings from this study suggest that the cohorts examined in the Prospective Study Collaboration that counted all strokes and did not differentiate between ischemic and hemorrhagic stroke may have masked the association between low cholesterol and hemorrhagic stroke risk as well as that between high cholesterol concentration and ischemic stroke.

PROTECTIVE EFFECTS OF HIGH-DENSITY LIPOPROTEIN CHOLESTEROL

Low levels of high-density lipoprotein cholesterol (HDL-C) (40 mg per dL) is common and is more prevalent in men (35%) than in women (15%). There is an inverse relationship between HDL-C levels and CHD. Clinical trials that assessed the role of HDL-C and IS were summarized in a recent publication; the adjusted risk of IS in subjects with high HDL-C ranged from 0.34 (95% CI, 0.14 to 0.85) to 0.81 (95% CI, 0.54 to 1.2). One study that demonstrated a consistent decline in the incidence of IS with increasing HDL-C levels was the Honolulu Heart Study. This was a population-based study that enrolled 2,444 men aged 71 to 93 years without stroke, CHD, or cancer at baseline. HDL-C levels were measured at study entry and the subjects were followed prospectively for at least 5 years. The age-adjusted incidence of IS decreased consistently with increasing HDL-C levels ($p = 0.003$). Men with HDL-C <40 mg per dL had a nearly threefold excess of IS compared with those with HDL-C ≥60 mg per dL ($p = 0.001$). The incidence of IS was still lower when adjusted for the presence of elevated total cholesterol, hypertension, and diabetes (p values were 0.509, 0.012, and 0.007, respectively). This study suggested that in older men the risk of IS is inversely related to HDL-C levels. In the Systolic Hypertension in the Elderly Program, in which older Australian patients were recruited, a significant association between lower HDL-C levels and IS was also observed. In summary, elevated HDL-C level (>40 mg per dL) appears to provide protective effect against the risk of IS.

DRUG THERAPY

The four available classes of drugs that are used to treat hyperlipidemia in humans are the 3-hydroxy-3-methyl-glutaryl-CoA (HMG-CoA) reductase inhibitors (statins), nicotinic acid, fibric acid derivatives, and bile acid sequestrants. Ezetimibe, which inhibits intestinal absorption of cholesterol, is a recently approved drug for cholesterol management and represents a fifth alternative to managing lipid disorders.

Statins

Statins, which were first introduced into clinical practice over 20 years ago, interfere with hepatic synthesis of cholesterol. There are currently six statins that have been approved in the United States by the Food and Drug Administration (FDA): lovastatin (Mevacor), simvastatin (Zocor), pravastatin (Pravachol), fluvastatin (Lescol), atorvastatin (Lipitor), and rosuvastatin (Crestor).

The ability of statins to inhibit cholesterol synthesis leads to reduction in the cholesterol content of the liver. This results in increased expression of low density lipoprotein cholesterol (LDL-C) receptors in the liver, consequently leading to reduction of LDL-C in the blood. The increased expression of LDL-C receptors also leads to lowering of intermediate density lipoprotein (IDL) and very low-density lipoprotein (VLDL); the latter effect leads to reduction in triglyceride levels. Statins may also reduce the risk of atherothrombotic disease by a variety of other mechanisms, which include effects on raising HDL-C, lowering triglycerides, promoting plaque stability, decreasing platelet aggregation, decreasing inflammation, improving endothelial function, and decreasing lipoprotein susceptibility to oxidation. Plaque stability may occur via modulation of the activation of macrophages. Reduction in LDL-C varies from 21% to 63% with traditional pharmacological doses. The reduction produced by atorvastatin, fluvastatin, lovastatin, pravastatin, rosuvastatin, and simvastatin is 26% to 60%, 22% to 36%, 21% to 42%, 22% to 34%, 45% to 63%, and 26% to 47%, respectively. Increase in HDL-C varies from 2% to 16%, with all FDA-approved statins having a similar effect on the increase in this cholesterol subtype. Reduction in triglycerides elicited by statins varies from 6% to 53%. Reduction induced by atorvastatin, fluvastatin, lovastatin, pravastatin, rosuvastatin, and simvastatin is 17% to 53%, 12% to 25%, 6% to 27%, 15% to 24%, 10% to 35%, and 12% to 34%, respectively.

The major side effects of concern in statin use are hepatotoxicity and myopathy. The incidence of hepatic transaminase elevation (more than three times the upper limits of normal) is 0.5% to 2%. Transaminase elevation usually reverses with reduction of the statin dose, but it may also occur spontaneously, even with continued use of the same dose. The FDA recommendation is to discontinue a statin if the hepatic transaminase levels exceed three times the upper limit of normal. Liver failure is extremely rare. Statin-induced myopathy is probably related to a disturbance of the myocyte cell membrane stability due to depletion of cholesterol in these membranes. In a population-based follow-up study, in the lipid-lowering group the incidence of myopathy was 2.3 per 10,000 person-years (95% CI, 1.2 to 4.4) versus none in the nontreated group. Death from rhabdomyolysis is extremely rare. The risk of development of side effects appears to increase with escalation of the dose of statin. In particular, the concentration of statin in the plasma is related to the risk of myopathy and rhabdomyolysis. Factors that may increase this risk include high-dose statins, old age, renal or hepatic impairment, diabetes mellitus, postoperative periods, trauma, heavy exercise, excessive alcohol use, hypothyroidism, and myotoxic drugs (e.g., fibrates or niacin). The dose of statin should be reduced to 25% or less of its maximal dose when it is combined with niacin, to reduce the risk of myopathy. The statin–fibrate combination can also increase the risk of myopathy; therefore, when this combination is used the dose of statin should be reduced. The combination of a statin with ezetimibe is associated with an increased incidence of elevation of hepatic transaminases and no increased risk of myopathy. In pregnancy, the safety of statins has not yet been established.

Although the National Cholesterol Education Program (NCEP) guidelines cite active or chronic liver disease as absolute contraindications of statins, the panel also emphasized that the use of statins in chronic liver disease should depend on "clinical judgment that balances proven benefit against risk." Relative contraindications include concomitant use of cyclosporine, macrobide antibiotics, certain antifungal agents, and cytochrome P-450 inhibitors.

In 2006, the final conclusions and recommendations of the National Lipid Association Task Force regarding statin safety and monitoring were published. The task force consisted of four expert panels and assessed the available data from the New Drug Application information, FDA Adverse Event Reporting System, clinical trials, and administrative claims database information. The panel recommended that hepatic transaminases be checked just prior to therapy initiation, 12 weeks after starting therapy, after any dose increase, and "periodically" after that. If there is objective evidence of liver injury, the statin should be discontinued and the patient referred to a hepatologist or gastroenterologist. If there is isolated elevation of transaminases up to three times the upper limits of normal, the statin can be continued with serial monitoring of hepatic transaminases. If the transaminase elevation is persistently greater than three times the upper limits of normal, another cause, other than the statin, should be investigated. If no other cause is found, the statin may be continued, discontinued, or its dose reduced depending on clinical judgment.

The task force defined myopathy as a combination of clinical complaints of muscle pain or soreness, weakness, and/or cramps + elevated creatine kinase (CK) >ten times the upper limit of normal. Rhabdomyolysis was defined as CK level >10,000 or CK >ten times the upper limit of normal + elevation in serum creatinine. If clinical symptoms or elevated CK are found in a patient on statins, other causes should first be ruled out. A baseline CK level should be considered in patients at higher risk of developing myopathy (older patients or those on a combination of statin + medications that may increase risk of myopathy). Routine monitoring of CK in asymptomatic patients while on statins is not necessary; CK should be obtained in symptomatic patients to determine severity of muscle damage and whether statin therapy can be continued. After discontinuation, and once the patient is asymptomatic, the same statin at the same or a lower dose or an alternate statin can be started. If symptoms recur with multiple statins and doses, treatment should be changed to an alternate lipid modifying therapy. In patients with mild muscle complaints or those who are asymptomatic with CK $<$ten times the upper limit of normal, treatment can be continued with the same statin at the same or a lower dose. Statins should be stopped if rhabdomyolysis develops; the patient should be treated with intravenous hydration, and after recovery careful reconsideration for starting statin therapy will depend on the risk versus benefit of the treatment.

Baseline assessment of renal function is recommended before starting statin therapy; however, routine monitoring of creatinine or screening for proteinuria during therapy is not necessary in asymptomatic patients with normal renal function and no rhabdomyolysis. If the serum creatinine becomes elevated or if proteinuria develops during treatment, it is not necessary to discontinue the statin, but depending on the prescribing information of the statin, the dose may be adjusted. Investigation into the underlying cause of renal dysfunction is necessary. Statins can be used in patients with chronic renal disease, with adjustment of the dose in moderate to severe renal insufficiency.

In general, dosage should be started at the lowest end of the recommended range and can be increased gradually as needed to reach the target lipid level. However, it should be kept in mind that most of the efficacy of statins can be demonstrated at the lowest initial dose, and that the higher the dose the greater the risk of side effects. If the dose of statin is doubled, only an additional 6% incremental reduction in the LDL-C can be achieved. For example, if the dose of atorvastatin is increased from 10 to 80 mg daily, only an additional 18% reduction in LDL-C occurs. This concept is referred to by some authors as the "rule of 6."

The dose range varies depending on the statin (see Table 7.1). Usually statins are administered as a single daily dose. To maximize the statin lowering effect on LDL-C, the doses should be taken with dinner or at bedtime. However, if the daily dose of lovastatin is $>$20 mg or if the daily dose of fluvastatin is $>$40 mg, the dose should be divided into two daily doses.

Nicotinic Acid (Niacin)

Niacin is one of the B complex vitamins. This vitamin inhibits lipoprotein synthesis, decreases VLDL production, and inhibits the peripheral mobilization of free fatty acids. At high doses, it can effectively lower triglycerides by 20% to 50%, reduce LDL-C by 5% to 25%, and increase the HDL-C by 15% to 35%. The combination of nicotinic acid with a statin provides a powerful tool to lower the LDL-C (due to the action of the statin), in addition to raising the HDL-C and lowering the triglycerides (owing to the action of nicotinic acid). There is no evidence that combining niacin with a statin increases the risk of myopathy. Side effects of niacin include hyperuricemia, gout, hyperglycemia, flushing, upper gastrointestinal discomfort, retinal edema, nasal stuffiness, conjunctivitis, ichthyosis, acanthosis nigricans, and hepatotoxicity. Hepatotoxicity is more common with the sustained release form of nicotinic acid. Flushing is more common with the use of the crystalline form; the extended release form causes less flushing. Flushing can also be minimized if administered during or after meals. Flushing is thought to be due to prostaglandin D_2 release; this can be decreased by using aspirin, which inhibits prostaglandin D_2, for several days before starting niacin. The daily doses of crystalline and sustained release forms are 1.5 to 4.5 g and 1 to 2 g, respectively, administered in 2 to 3 divided doses per day. The daily dose of the extended release form is 1 to 2 g, administered once daily. Nicotinic acid is contraindicated in severe gout and chronic liver disease. Hyperuricemia, gout, recent peptic ulcer disease, high doses in type II diabetes mellitus, and active liver disease are relative contraindications.

TABLE 7.1 Dose Range of Statins

Statin	Daily Dose Range (mg)
Atorvastatin	10–80
Rosuvastatin	5–40
Fluvastatin	20–80
Lovastatin	10–80
Pravastatin	10–80
Simvastatin	5–80

Fibric Acid Derivatives (Fibrates)

Fibric acid derivatives can reduce LDL-C levels by 5% to 20%, increase HDL-C by 10% to 35%, and decrease triglycerides by 20% to 50%. Their main clinical use is to lower triglyceride levels. The mechanism of action of fibric acid derivatives is complex. Fibrates are agonists for the peroxisome proliferator activated receptor-alpha (PPAR-α), which is a nuclear transcription factor. Through this mechanism, fibrates upregulate genes for fatty acid transport protein and fatty acid oxidation, and consequently lead to the reduction of triglycerides. PPAR-α also increases synthesis of apolipoprotein A-I and A-II; this mechanism, when combined with reduction of triglyceride levels, leads to elevation of HDL-C levels. The available fibrates in the United States include clofibrate, gemfibrozil, and fenofibrate. Dose ranges for these drugs are highlighted in Table 7.2. Potential side effects include upper gastrointestinal discomfort, cholesterol gallstones, and myopathy. Fibric acid derivatives are contraindicated in severe hepatic or renal insufficiency. Fibrates can be used in combination with a statin as an alternative to high doses of statins. This drug combination therapy, however, can be associated with higher risk of myopathy than with statin monotherapy. Several precautions should be considered when this combination is used, which include ensuring that the patient has normal renal function, using a small starting dose of the statin, educating the patient regarding manifestations of myopathy, and checking CK level before therapy and as needed.

TABLE 7.2 Dose Range of Fibrates

Fibrates	Daily Dose Range (mg)
Gemfibrozil	600 (twice daily)
Fenofibrate	200 (daily)
Clofibrate	1,000 (twice daily)

Bile Acid Sequestrants

These agents bind bile acids in the intestine, thus reducing the enterohepatic recirculation of bile acids. Ultimately, reduction of enterohepatic bile acid recirculation leads to reduction in the liver content of cholesterol, enhancement of expression of the LDL-C receptors, and consequently reduction of serum LDL-C. Commercially available bile acid derivatives include cholestyramine, colestipol, and colesevelam. They can reduce LDL-C by 15% to 30% and increase the HDL-C by 3% to 5%. Triglyceride levels are not affected or may potentially be increased by these agents. The daily dosage range for cholestyramine, colestipol, and colesevelam are 4 to 24 g, 5 to 30 g, and 2.6 to 4.4 g, respectively. When used in combination with statins, bile acid sequestrants can decrease LDL-C by up to 70%; low or moderate doses of the sequestrant are sufficient in this case as high doses do not add much. It is best to give the statin at night and the sequestrant in divided doses with each meal; they should not be given concomitantly. However, if colesevelam is used with a statin, separation of the time of administration is not necessary. Nicotinic acid can be added to the sequestrant–statin combination if the LDL-C goal cannot be successfully achieved. Bile acid sequestrants may cause gastrointestinal side effects. All of these agents, except colesevelam, can decrease the absorption of other medications; therefore other drugs should be administered 4 hours after or 1 hour before the dose of the sequestrant. Absolute contraindications to use of bile acid sequestrants include familial dysbetalipoproteinemia and triglyceride level >400 mg per dL.

Ezetimibe

Ezetimibe is approved by the FDA for the treatment of primary hypercholesterolemia, mixed hyperlipidemia, familial homozygous hypercholesterolemia, and familial homozygous sitosterolemia. Ezetimibe selectively inhibits absorption of cholesterol from the intestine by blocking the Niemann-Pick C1 Like 1 (NPC1L1) sterol transporter. At a dose of 10 mg once daily, ezetimibe can lower LDL-C by 17% to 18%. It can be used as monotherapy but its primary usefulness may be in combination with statins in patients who are not able to achieve their target LDL-C level with statin monotherapy. The combination of ezetimibe with a statin achieves reduction of LDL-C level by "dual inhibition,"—that is, inhibition of cholesterol absorption from the intestine by ezetimibe and inhibition of cholesterol synthesis by the statin; ezetimibe can potentially enhance the cholesterol-lowering effect of statins. When combined with a statin, ezetimibe can reduce the LDL-C by 34% to 53%. An additional advantage of combination therapy is that it may achieve the patient's target LDL-C while allowing reduction in dose of statin in patients who have side effects from high-dose statin therapy. Other benefits that can occur with this combination therapy include a small decrease in triglycerides, a small increase in HDL-C, and a decrease in C reactive protein. Contraindications to combination therapy with statins include active liver disease or persistently elevated liver enzymes.

EFFICACY OF CHOLESTEROL-LOWERING DRUGS FOR PREVENTION OF ISCHEMIC STROKE

Large-scale randomized trials that have explored the potential utility of cholesterol-lowering drugs for stroke prevention have primarily focused on statins. In all but one of these trials, stroke was a secondary outcome event since these trials were primarily designed to evaluate the effects of these drugs on cardiac events and mortality. The majority of participants in these trials had no history of stroke; thus the risk reduction of stroke in these studies reflects risk reduction of primary stroke. The Stroke Prevention by Aggressive Reduction in Cholesterol Levels (SPARCL) study is the only multicenter, randomized, placebo-controlled study that has examined the utility of a statin in a population of patients with recent stroke. This study provides information regarding risk reduction of secondary stroke and vascular events produced by a statin. Randomized, double-blind, placebo-controlled studies have demonstrated that bile acid sequestrants decrease the risk of CHD, and other studies showed that nicotinic acid and fibric acid derivatives decrease the risk of MI. These studies were not primarily designed to determine if these agents reduce the risk of stroke. However, in one study, there was a 24% reduction (95% CI, 11% to 36%; $p < 0.001$) of a composite secondary outcome (combined death due to CHD, nonfatal MI, and stroke).

Statins

The Cholesterol Treatment Trialists conduct periodic meta-analyses of all relevant large-scale randomized trials of lipid-modifying treatments. Their first meta-analyses of trials of statins was published in 2005. Randomized trials were eligible for inclusion if (i) the main effect of at least one of the trial interventions was to modify lipid levels; (ii) the trial was unconfounded with respect to this intervention (i.e., no other differences in risk factor modification between the relevant treatment groups was intended); and (iii) the trial aimed to recruit at least 1,000 participants with treatment duration of at least 2 years. The primary meta-analysis was on the effects on clinical outcome in each trial weighted by the absolute LDL-C difference in that trial at the end of the first year of follow-up. The main prespecified outcomes were all-cause mortality, CHD mortality, and non-CHD mortality. Stroke was a prespecified secondary outcome of the analysis. Fourteen trials, which included 90,056 participants, were included in the meta-analysis. All participants had coronary artery disease. At the time of study entry, 42,131 (47%) had pre-existing CHD, 21,575 (24%) were women, 18,686 (21%) had diabetes mellitus, 49,689 (55%) had a history of chronic hypertension, and 13,255 (15%) had other pre-existing vascular disease including history of stroke or transient ischemic attack (TIA). The mean pretreatment LDL-C was 3.79 mmol per L (146.5 mg per dL). In these trials the weighted average difference in LDL-C at 1 year was 1.09 mmol per L (42.1 mg per dL). There were 2,282 strokes among 65,138 participants in nine trials that sought information on stroke type. Hemorrhagic stroke was confirmed in 204 (9%), 1,565 (69%) were ischemic, and 513 (22%) were of unknown type. The incidence of first stroke of any type was proportionally reduced by 17% in favor of statins [1,340 (3.0%) statin vs 1,617 (3.7%) control relative risk (RR) 0.83; 95% CI, 0.78 to 0.88; $p < 0.0001$] per 1 mmol per L LDL-C reduction. This overall reduction in stroke reflected a significant 19% proportional reduction in strokes not attributed to hemorrhage (i.e., presumed IS); RR 0.81; 99% CI, 0.74 to 0.89; $p < 0.0001$ per 1 mmol per L, LDL-C reduction. There was no apparent difference in hemorrhagic stroke. There was a 12% reduction in all-cause mortality for every 1 mmol per L reduction in LDL-C (rate ratio 0.88; 95% CI, 0.84 to 0.91; $p < 0.0001$). The meta-analysis demonstrated that the 5-year incidence of stroke, major coronary events, and coronary revascularization can be safely reduced by one-fifth for each 1 mmol per L reduction of LDL-C with statin therapy. The meta-analysis also supported the concept that patients at high risk for major vascular events should be on long-term statin treatment to achieve and maintain significant reduction in LDL-C levels. Likewise, statin therapy lowers primary IS risk in patients with CHD and/or vascular risk factors.

The only prospective, multicenter, randomized, placebo-controlled trial that has been designed to address the potential benefit of statin therapy in secondary prevention of IS is the SPARCL study. Eligible patients must have had either a stroke (70%) or TIA (30%) 1 to 6 months before randomization, an LDL-C of 100 to 190 mg per dL, no history of symptomatic CHD, and a modified Rankin scale ≤ 3 (functionally independent). Patients with the significant peripheral vascular disease (PVD), atrial fibrillation, prosthetic heart valve, clinically significant mitral stenosis, sinus node dysfunction, uncontrolled hypertension, hepatic dysfunction, renal dysfunction, and stroke caused by revascularization procedure, trauma, or subarachnoid hemorrhage were excluded from study participation. This international study randomized 4,731 patients (60% males and 40% females), in a 1:1 ratio to atorvastatin 80 mg per day or placebo. The patients were instructed to follow the NCEP diet during the study period. The mean age of study subjects was 62.5 years. Seventy percent were enrolled following a stroke. These strokes were primarily ischemic (97%). The mean follow-up period was 4.9 years. In the atorvastatin group, compared to placebo, fatal or nonfatal stroke was reduced over 5 years. The absolute risk reduction (ARR) was 2.2%, the relative risk reduction (RRR) was 16%, and the hazard ratio (HR) was 0.84 (95% CI, 0.71 to 0.99; $p = 0.03$). The number needed to treat with atorvastatin for 5 years to prevent one stroke was 46. There was also a significant reduction of time to stroke or TIA (HR 0.77; 95% CI, 0.6 to 0.91; $p = 0.004$). However, there was a small increase in hemorrhagic strokes (HR 1.66; 95% CI, 1.08 to 2.55; $p = 0.02$). Hemorrhagic stroke occurred in 2% of patients in the placebo group, and in 1.9% of patients in the atorvastatin group. The LDL-C was significantly reduced by 53% in the atorvastatin arm, compared to a 1% rise in the placebo group. Despite the clear benefit of atorvastatin in reducing the risk of recurrent IS in the SPARCL trial, there are some issues that were not clarified by this study. It is still not clear if a lower dose of atorvastatin would be as beneficial as the 80 mg dose. In addition, the correlation between specific LDL-C levels <100 mg per dL and the magnitude of stroke risk reduction is not defined by this study. The study did not explain if the risk of hemorrhage was mostly limited to the patients with hemorrhagic stroke who were enrolled in the study. Further study will be necessary to determine if statins actually contribute to risk of secondary hemorrhagic stroke. In addition, more studies designed to determine the effect of niacin and fibrates on risk of IS are needed.

Fibrates and Niacin

Fibrates and niacin have been less extensively studied than statins in randomized, multicenter trials with respect to their effects on vascular events. Stroke has not been a primary outcome event in any of these trials, and no trial has been designed to evaluate the effectiveness of these agents in a population of stroke survivors. Although the trials demonstrated beneficial effects on the lipid profile, these trials have not conclusively demonstrated that niacin or fibrates produce a significant risk reduction with respect to primary stroke. Despite the benefits of fibric acid derivatives on the lipid profile in these trials, a double-blind placebo-controlled randomized trial did not find benzafibrate 400 mg daily able to reduce the incidence of first stroke (RR 1.34; 95% CI, 0.82 to 2.01). This study included 1,568 men with lower extremity arterial disease; the main outcome measures included a combination of all CHD events and all strokes. Fibrates and niacin alone, or in combination with other antihyperlipidemic agents, are used to raise HDL-C levels. In a randomized double-blind, placebo-controlled study of 2,531 men with CHD, gemfibrozil was reported to significantly reduce the risk of IS; RRR, adjusted for baseline variables, was 31% (95% CI, 2% to 52%; $p = 0.036$). Another randomized clinical trial, however, showed that treatment with benzafibrate was associated with an increase in HDL-C but did not reduce the risk of cerebrovascular events. In one study, in individuals with low HDL-C and CHD, the use of statin therapy combined with extended release niacin stopped the progression of atherosclerosis (evaluated by measuring carotid intima media thickness). Torcetrapib is an inhibitor of cholesteryl ester transfer protein (CETP). In a recent review, significant elevation of HDL-C was achieved in patients who were placed on torcetrapib and atorvastatin combination compared with those placed on atorvastatin alone. In this study the mean HDL-C level in subjects who were placed on atorvastatin alone versus those placed on torceptrapib and atorvastatin combination was 52.4 ± 13.5 mg per dL versus 81.5 ± 22.6 mg per dL, respectively. Mean LDL-C level was 143.2 ± 42.2 mg per dL versus 115.1 ± 48.5 mg per dL, respectively. The increase in HDL-C, however, was not associated with reduction in progression in atherosclerosis; in fact there was even progression of atherosclerosis in the common carotid arteries in those on combination therapy. The average systolic blood pressure increased by 2.8 mm Hg in the subjects who received combination therapy versus those who received atorvastatin alone. The authors suggested that the discrepancy between the improvement in the lipid profile and progression of atherosclerosis in subjects receiving torceptrapib could possibly be due to a "direct vasculotoxic effect" as shown by the rise in systolic blood pressure. A similar discrepancy was noted recently in a study using torceptrapib in patients with coronary artery disease, which showed no significant decrease in progression of coronary atherosclerosis despite a significant increase in HDL-C and decrease in LDL-C. Although some studies have suggested that fibrates can reduce stroke risk via rise in HDL-C, there are other studies that conflict with these results.

PRACTICAL APPROACH TO THE MANAGEMENT OF HYPERCHOLESTEROLEMIA

Patients with IS or TIA are at risk for subsequent cerebrovascular and coronary artery events. Stroke is an important neurological condition that can cause permanent disability and can even be fatal in some cases. In the United States, approximately 700,000 cases of stroke occur every year; 200,000 cases of those are considered recurrent strokes. Stroke is the third leading cause of death after heart disease and cancer; it accounts for 6.5% of all deaths. Among the approximately 5.5 million stroke survivors in the United States, 15% to 30% will have permanent disability. Patients with IS are at increased risk of having MI. Cholesterol reduction is one of the medical interventions that clinicians prescribe to reduce the risk of

TABLE 7.3 CHD Risk Equivalents

1. TIA or stroke of carotid artery origin, and >50% symptomatic carotid stenosis on angiography or ultrasound
2. >50% asymptomatic carotid stenosis on angiography or ultrasound
3. Clinical atherosclerotic disease, for example, renal artery disease and peripheral arterial disease
4. Abdominal aortic aneurysm
5. Diabetes mellitus

TIA, transient ischemic attack.

these secondary vascular events. The American Heart Association/American Stroke Association Council on Stroke recommends that patients with IS or TIA with elevated cholesterol, comorbid heart disease, or evidence of an atherosclerotic origin of the cerebrovascular event should have their cholesterol managed according to the National Cholesterol Education Program Adult Treatment Panel III (NCEP-ATP III) guidelines.

National Cholesterol Education Program Adult Treatment Panel III Guidelines

These treatment guidelines were published in 2002 to provide recommendations for the detection, evaluation, and treatment of high blood cholesterol in adults. The guidelines were developed by a panel of experts from multiple national professional healthcare organizations, and are widely accepted by most health care providers. These guidelines provide evidence-based recommendations on the management of elevated blood cholesterol. Recommendations are primarily based on results of large, randomized controlled clinical trials as well as results of prospective epidemiological studies.

The guidelines delineate certain medical conditions as CHD risk equivalents that carry a risk for major coronary events equal to that of established CHD, that is, greater than 20% over 10 years (i.e., more than 20 of every 100 such individuals will develop CHD or have a recurrent coronary artery event within 10 years). The CHD risk equivalents are summarized in Table 7.3. The following risk factors for CHD were identified: LDL-C >100 mg per dL, HDL-C <40 mg per dL, hypertension (≥140/90 mm Hg, or on antihypertensive medication), current cigarette smoking, and family history of premature CHD (for women ≥ 55 years, and for men ≥ 45 years). It should be noted that the NCEP-ATP III guidelines did not specifically address the management of hyperlipidemia following IS or TIA of noncarotid artery origin since the SPARCL study was published after the NCEP-ATP III guidelines were issued.

NCEP-ATP III Recommendations for Treating Hypercholesterolemia

The NCEP-ATP III identified elevated LDL-C as the primary target of cholesterol-lowering therapy since scientific evidence strongly indicates that elevated LDL-C is a major cause of CHD. The LDL-C target depends on the presence or absence of CHD, CHD risk equivalents, and risk factor for CHD (see Table 7.4). A more recent publication, written by the Coordinating Committee of the NCEP, addressed the implications of recent clinical trials for the NCEP-ATP III guidelines, and suggested that in individuals at very high risk for coronary events it appears to be preferable to have an LDL-C goal of <70 mg per dL. The committee, however, indicated that this treatment goal should be an option until additional trials are completed to confirm this recommendation; until then the LDL-C goal of <100 mg per dL should remain as a strong recommendation. Patients who are at very high risk include individuals with cardiovascular disease with multiple major risk factors (especially diabetes mellitus), severe and poorly controlled risk factors (especially continued cigarette smoking), multiple risk factors of metabolic syndrome (especially triglycerides levels ≥ 200 mg per dL + non-HDL-C ≥ 130 mg per dL with low HDL <40 mg per dL), and patients with acute coronary syndromes. The NCEP-ATP III recommended that the LDL-C goal should be achieved by drug therapy combined with therapeutic life changes (TLCs). The TLC is summarized in Table 7.5. TLC should be tried first for approximately 3 months before initiating drug therapy. LDL-C drug therapy should be started at the same time with TLC in patients with CHD, a CHD risk equivalent, or if the baseline LDL-C ≥130 mg per dL. The NCEP-ATP III guidelines recommend that initial drug therapy should be a statin. After 6 weeks, if the LDL-C goal is not achieved, the statin dose can be increased. Alternatively, physicians can consider adding nicotinic acid, a fibrate, or a bile acid sequestrant. After another 6 weeks, if the LDL-C goal is still not achieved, treatment of other lipid risk factors (including hypertriglyceridemia or low HDL-C) should be initiated by adding nicotinic acid or fibric acid to the statin therapy. Secondary modifiable risk factors of low HDL-C (e.g., cigarette smoking, obesity, or physical inactivity should be eliminated). The response and adherence to treatment should be monitored every 4 to 6 months.

Management of Low HDL-C

The guidelines of the American Diabetes Association and NCEP-ATP III indicate that elevation of HDL-C is considered a secondary target in those individuals with high LDL-C and low HDL-C in an effort to reduce risk of coronary events. Treatment should be aimed primarily at lowering LDL-C. The Expert Group on HDL, however,

TABLE 7.4 Recommended Target LDL-C by the NCEP-ATP III According to CHD and CHD Risk Equivalents

Condition	Recommended LDL-C Goal (mg/dL)
CHD or CHD risk equivalent	<100
Multiple (2+) risk factors for CHD	<130
Multiple risk factors with 10-year risk for MI/CHD death >20%	<100
0–1 risk factor	<160

LDL-C, low density lipoprotein cholesterol; CHD, coronary heart disease.

TABLE 7.5 Therapeutic Life Changes

1. Reducing dietary intake of total fats to 25% to 35% of total calories (saturated fats <7% of calories, polyunsaturated fats ≤10% of calories, and monounsaturated fats ≤20% of total calories)
2. Limiting cholesterol intake to <200 mg/d
3. Including carbohydrate and protein intake of 50% to 60% and 15%, respectively, of total calories
4. Consumption of plant stanols/sterols (2 g/d)
5. Consumption of 20 to 30 g of dietary fiber per day (soluble fiber 10 to 25 g/d)
6. Increasing grain intake (at least 6 servings per day with at least one-third whole grain)
7. Weight reduction (body mass index <25 kg/m^2)
8. Smoking cessation
9. Increasing physical activity of moderate intensity to expend at least 200 kcal/d
10. Limiting alcohol intake to 2 drinks daily for men and ≤1 drink daily for women[a], however, individuals who do not drink alcohol are not encouraged to start alcohol consumption

[a]One alcoholic drink was defined as 5 oz of wine, 12 oz of beer, or 1.5 oz of 80-proof whiskey.

recommends that in patients with diabetes, the metabolic syndrome, or HDL-C levels <40 mg per dL, additional treatment with niacin or fibrate should be considered. Combining niacin with statin therapy can be more effective than either treatment alone in raising HDL-C; combination therapy may increase HDL-C by 18% to 21%. This combination has not been evaluated in a clinical trial that has incorporated IS as an endpoint; thus it is not known if the combination decreases stroke risk. Lifestyle modifications, such as weight reduction, limiting alcohol intake, and increasing physical activity, were reported to have the greatest impact on HDL-C in individuals with high baseline HDL-C levels and the least improvement in those with low HDL-C levels. The most effective strategy to raise HDL-C in patients with IS, who have HDL-C <40 mg per dL, is to use a combination of lifestyle modification, a statin, and extended release niacin; the goal is to increase the HDL-C by 20%.

Practical Recommendations

Elevated cholesterol is a probable risk factor for primary IS, and patients with a history of IS or TIA are at risk for recurrent stroke and CHD. Management of this risk factor is important to help reduce morbidity and mortality following IS. One randomized, placebo-controlled trial (SPARCL) has demonstrated that secondary stroke risk can be reduced if a statin is used in patients with normal and elevated LDL-C.

Lifestyle modifications should be instituted in all patients. In addition, initiation of therapy with a statin is recommended; the target LDL-C in these patients is <100 mg per dL. However, a target of <70 mg per dL is reasonable in patients with multiple risk factors for vascular disease. In patients who cannot tolerate statins, ezetimibe is an option. In patients with HDL-C <40 mg per dL despite treatment with a statin, additional treatment with niacin or fibrate can be considered. Further research will need to be conducted to determine if raising HDL-C alone can reduce secondary stroke risk.

SELECTED REFERENCES

Abbott RD, Wilson PW, Kannel WB, et al. High density lipoprotein cholesterol, total cholesterol screening, and myocardial infarction: the Framingham Study. *Arteriosclerosis* 1988;8:207–211.

Amarence P, Lavallee P, Touboul P-J. Stroke prevention, blood cholesterol, and statins. *Lancet Neurol* 2004;3:271–278.

Assmann G, Schulte H, von Eckardstein A, et al. High density lipoprotein cholesterol as a predictor of coronary heart disease risk: the PROCAM experience and pathophysiological implications for reverse cholesterol transport. *Atherosclerosis* 1996;124(suppl):S11–S20.

Bilheimer DW, Grundy SM, Brown MS, et al. Mevinolin and colestipol stimulate receptor-mediated clearance of low density lipoprotein from plasma in familial hypercholesterolemia heterozygotes. *Proc Natl Acad Sci USA* 1983;80:4124–4128.

Brown BG, Bardsley J, Poulin D, et al. Moderate dose, three-drug therapy with niacin, lovastatin, and colestipol to reduce low-density lipoprotein cholesterol <100 mg/dL in patients with hyperlipidemia and coronary artery disease. *Am J Cardiol* 1997;80:111–115.

Brown BG, Zhao X-Q, Chait A, et al. Simvastatin and niacin, antioxidant vitamins, or the combination for the prevention of coronary disease. *N Engl J Med* 2001;345:1583–1592.

Brown G, Albers JJ, Fisher LD, et al. Regression of coronary artery disease as a result of intensive lipid-lowering therapy in men with high levels of apolipoprotein B. *N Engl J Med* 1990;323:1289–1298.

Cholesterol Treatment Trialists' (CTT) Collaborators. Efficacy and safety of cholesterol-lowering treatment: prospective meta-analysis of data from 90,056 participants in 14 randomised trials of statins. *Lancet* 2005;366: 1267–1278.

Coronary Drug Project Research Group. Clofibrate and niacin in coronary heart disease. *JAMA* 1975;231:360–381.

Curb JD, Abbott RD, Rodriguez BL, et al. High density lipoprotein cholesterol and the risk of stroke in elderly men. *Am J Epidemiol* 2004; 160:150–157.

Davis BR, Vogt T, Frost PH, et al. Risk factors for stroke and type of stroke in persons with isolated systolic hypertension. *Stroke* 1998;29:1333–1340.

Dyslipidemia management in adults with diabetes. *Diabetes Care* 2004;27:68S–71S.

Gotto AM, Brinton EA. Assessing low levels of high-density lipoprotein cholesterol as a risk factor in coronary heart disease: a working group report and update. *J Am Coll Cardiol* 2004;43:717–724.

Gagne C, Bays HE, Weiss SR, et al. Efficacy and safety of ezetimibe added to ongoing statin therapy for treatment of patients with primary hypercholesterolemia. *Am J Cardiol* 2002;90:1084–1091.

Gaist D, Rodriguez LA, Huerta C, et al. Niemann-Pick C1 Like 1 (NCP1L1) is the intestinal phytosterol and cholesterol transporter and a key modulator of whole-body cholesterol homeostasis. *J Biol Chem* 2004; 279:33586–33592.

Gaist D, Rodriguez LA, Huerta C, et al. Lipid lowering drugs and risk of myopathy: a population-based follow up study. *Epidemiology* 2001; 12 (5):565–569.

Gotto AM, Brinton EA. Assessing low levels of high-density lipoprotein cholesterol as a risk factor in coronary heart disease: a working group report and update. *J Am Coll Cardiol* 2004;43:717–724.

Grundy SM, Cleeman JI, Merz CNB, et al. Implications of Recent Clinical Trials for the National Cholesterol Education Program Adult Treatment Panel III Guidelines. *Circulation* 2004;110:227–239.

Hallas J, Sindrup SH. Lipid lowering drugs and risk of myopathy: a population-based follow up study. *Epidemiology* 2001;12(5):565–569.

Helfand M, Carson S, Kelley C. Drug class review on HMG-CoA reductase inhibitors (statins). Final Report. http://www.ohsu.edu/drugeffectiveness/reports/documents/Statins%20Final%20Report%20Update%204%20Unshaded.pdf. Accessed April 2008.

Iso H, Jacobs DR, Wentworth D, et al. Serum cholesterol levels and six-year mortality from stroke in 350,977 men screened for the multiple risk factor intervention trial. *N Engl J Med* 1989;320:904–910.

Kastelin JJP, van Leuven SI, Burgess L, et al. Effect of torcetrapib on carotid atherosclerosis in familial hypercholesterolemia. *N Engl J Med* 2007; 356:1620–1630.

Koren-Morag N, Tanne D, Graff E, et al. Low- and high-density lipoprotein cholesterol and ischemic cerebrovascular disease: the bezafibrate infarction prevention registry. *Arch Intern Med* 2002;162:993–999.

Lipid Research Clinics Program. The lipid research clinics coronary primary prevention trial results. I: Reduction in the incidence of coronary heart disease. *JAMA* 1984;251:351–364.

Lipid Research Clinics Program. The lipid research clinics coronary primary prevention trial results. II: The relationship of reduction in incidence of coronary heart disease to cholesterol lowering. *JAMA* 1984: 251:365–374.

McKenney JM, Davidson MH, Jacobson TA, et al. Final conclusions and recommendations of the national lipid association statin safety assessment task force. *Am J Cardiol* 2006;97(suppl):89C–94C.

Meade T, Zuhrie R, Cook C, et al. Bezafibrate in men with lower extremity arterial disease: randomised controlled trial. *BMJ* 2002;325:1139–1143.

MICROMEDEX Healthcare Series. http://www.thomsonhc.com (accessed on April 20, 2007).

Mikhalidis DP, Wierzbicki AS, Daskalopoulou SS, et al. The use of ezetimibe in achieving low density lipoprotein lowering goals in clinical practice: position statement of a United Kingdom consensus panel. *Curr Med Res Opin* 2005;21(6):959–969.

Nissen SE, Tardif J-C, Nicholis SJ, et al. Effect of torcetrapib on the progression of coronary atherosclerosis. *N Engl J Med* 2007;356: 1304–1316.

Prospective Studies Collaboration. Cholesterol, diastolic blood pressure, and stroke: 13,000 strokes in 450,000 people in 45 prospective cohorts. *Lancet* 1995;346:1647–1653.

Rubins HB, Davenport J, Babikian V, et al. Reduction in stroke with gemfibrozil in men with coronary heart disease and low HDL cholesterol: the Veterans Affairs HDL Intervention Trial (VA-HIT). *Circulation* 2001; 103:2828–2833.

Rubins HB, Robins SJ, Collins D, et al. Gemfibrozil for the secondary prevention of coronary heart disease in men with low levels of high-density lipoprotein cholesterol. Veterans Affairs High-Density Lipoprotein Cholesterol Intervention Trial Study Group. *N Engl J Med* 1999;341(6): 410–418.

Sacco RL, Adams R, Albers G, et al. Guidelines for prevention of stroke in patients with ischemic stroke or transient ischemic attack. *Stroke* 2006; 37:577–617.

Sanossian N, Saver JL, Navab M, et al. High density lipoprotein cholesterol. An emerging target for stroke treatment. *Stroke* 2007;38:1104–1109.

Schoojans K, Staels B, Auwerx J. Role of the peroxisome proliferator-activated receptor (PPAR) in mediating the effects of fibrates and fatty acids on gene expression. *J Lipid Res* 1996;37:907–925.

Simons LA, McCallum J, Friedlander Y, et al. Risk factors for ischemic stroke: Dubbo Study of the Elderly. *Stroke* 1998;29:1341–1346.

Sprecher DL. Raising high density lipoprotein cholesterol with niacin and fibrates: a comparative review. *Am J Cardiol* 2000;86:46L–50L.

Sukhova GK, Williams JK, Libby P. Statins reduce inflammation in atheroma of nonhuman primates independent of effects on serum cholesterol. *Arterioscler Thromb Vasc Biol* 2002:22:1452–1458.

Taylor AF, Sullenberger LE, Lee HJ, et al. Arterial biology for the investigation of the treatment effects of reducing cholesterol (ARBITER) 2. *Circulation* 2004;110:3512–3517.

The Stroke Prevention by Aggressive Reduction in Cholesterol Levels (SPARCL) Investigators. High-dose atorvastatin after stroke or transient ischemic attack. *N Engl J Med* 2006;355:549–559.

American Heart Association. The third report of the national cholesterol education program (NCEP) expert panel on detection, evaluation and treatment of high blood cholesterol in adults (Adult Treatment Panel III). *Circulation* 2002;106:3143.

Vaughan CJ, Gotto AM. Update on statins: 2003. *Circulation* 2004;110: 886–892.

Vu-Dac N, Schoonjans K, Kosykh V, et al. Fibrates increase human apolipoprotein A-II expression through activation of the peroxisome proliferator-activated receptor. *J Clin Invest* 1995;96:741–750.

Williams PT. The relationships of vigorous exercise, alcohol, and adiposity to low and high density lipoprotein-cholesterol levels. *Metabolism* 2004; 53:700–709.

CRITICAL PATHWAY

Management of Hypercholesterolemia in Patients with Ischemic Stroke or TIA

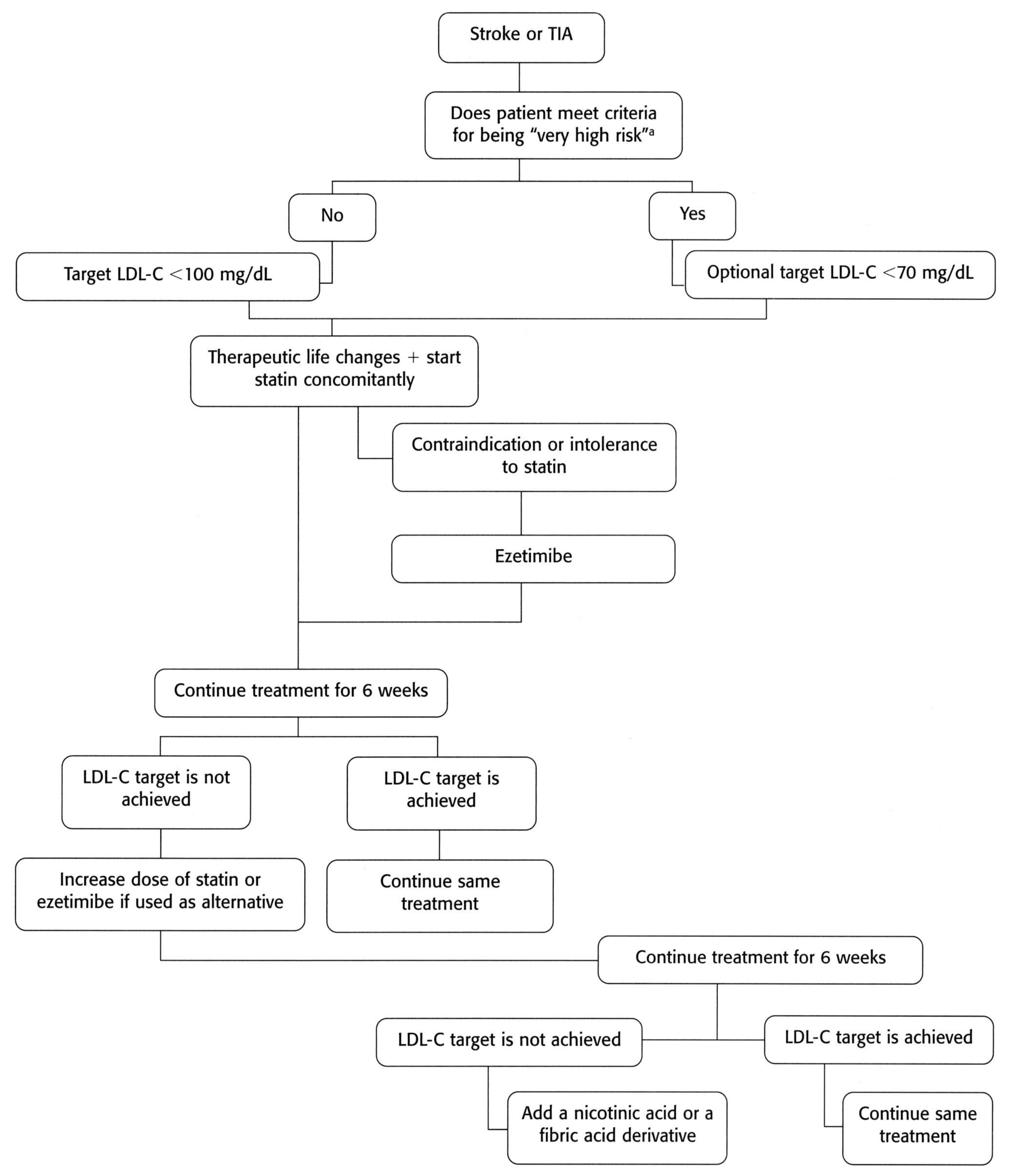

[a]Criteria for "very high risk" patients = presence of any of the following: diabetes mellitus; multiple risk factors for metabolic syndrome (especially triglycerides ≥200 mg/dL, HDL-C <40 mg/dL, and non-HDL-C ≥130 mg/dL); continued cigarette smoking; acute coronary syndrome. TIA, transient ischemic attack.

CHAPTER

8 Cancer and Stroke

BABAK B. NAVI AND ALAN Z. SEGAL

OBJECTIVES

- What is the relationship between cancer and stroke?
- What are the unique mechanisms of stroke in cancer patients?
- Which forms of cancer are most prone to stroke?
- What are the unique treatment considerations in cancer patients with stroke?
- When is anticoagulation indicated in cancer patients with stroke?

Cancer and stroke are the second and third leading causes of death, respectively, in the United States. They are both age-related disorders that increase in incidence and prevalence with advanced age. Given this relationship and the common risk factor of tobacco use, it is not surprising that cerebrovascular disease is common in malignancy. A large autopsy study demonstrated hemorrhagic and ischemic cerebrovascular events to be second only to metastases in frequency of central nervous system (CNS) lesions in cancer patients. These lesions were not always symptomatic, being clinically silent half the time. As with the general population, strokes in patients with cancer are divided into hemorrhagic and ischemic types and frequently occur because of standard mechanisms such as cardiac embolism, small vessel disease, or large vessel disease. However unlike the general population, cancer patients often undergo unique stroke mechanisms that make the diagnosis and management of stroke challenging. These mechanisms are often multifactorial and can be intrinsic to the cancer itself or related to complications of therapy. Cancer-related strokes frequently contain both hemorrhagic and ischemic components and can occur at any point in the duration of the malignancy. In fact, in rare circumstances, strokes have been the first manifestation of an occult malignancy.

BACKGROUND AND RATIONALE

Ischemic Stroke

Ischemic stroke in cancer patients is often caused by unique mechanisms that are not encountered in the general population (see Table 8.1). While atherosclerosis accounts for a subset of strokes in cancer patients, nonbacterial thrombotic endocarditis (NBTE) and cerebral intravascular coagulation account for most symptomatic ischemic strokes in patients with underlying malignancies. Other novel mechanisms of ischemic stroke include septic emboli, tumor emboli, chemotherapy-induced hypercoagulability, microangiopathic hemolytic anemia (MAHA), and radiation therapy (XRT) toxicity (via accelerated atherosclerosis). NBTE, which is the most common cause of stroke in cancer patients, often occurs late in the course of a malignancy and frequently presents with both multifocal strokes and systemic emboli. It is thought to occur via a chronic disseminated intravascular coagulation (DIC) state that predisposes cardiac valves to edema, degeneration, and ultimately deposition of sterile platelet–thrombin vegetations. It is also likely underestimated because of the difficulty of capturing vegetations on echocardiography. Cerebral intravascular coagulation is the second most common mechanism of stroke in cancer patients and is often lethal. It is caused by widespread small vessel occlusions from fibrin thrombi leading to extensive, bilateral infarctions. Given its diffuse nature, it commonly presents as a nonspecific encephalopathy and is only correctly diagnosed at autopsy. As with NBTE, clots are not limited to the brain and are commonly found in other organ systems as well.

Types of cancer differ in their predilection for cerebrovascular disease and some are associated with specific stroke mechanisms (see Table 8.1). Mucinous adenocarcinomas are the most common offenders in ischemic stroke. A large, retrospective study from Memorial Sloan-Kettering Cancer Center demonstrated lung cancer as the most common primary malignancy associated with ischemic stroke, accounting for 30% of cases, followed by primary brain tumors (9%), and prostate cancer (9%). Other authors have cited an increased frequency of ischemic stroke in patients having gastrointestinal tract tumors, genitourinary neoplasms, and lymphoma. In contrast, breast cancer infrequently leads to stroke, and one study showed that it accounted for 18% of hospital admissions but only 4% of strokes. However, in other series, breast cancer patients receiving chemotherapy are reported to have a slightly increased risk of stroke. A large case-controlled study by Geiger et al. found that chemotherapy was associated with an odds ratio of 2.3 in favor of stroke. This was not related to any specific chemotherapy regimen. Tamoxifen, a selective estrogen receptor modulator used commonly in breast cancer treatment, may have

TABLE 8.1 Etiology of Ischemic Infarcts in Cancer Patients

Etiology	Mechanism	Tumors/Associations
NBTE	Cardiac embolism	Mucinous adenocarcinomas, lymphomas, hematologic malignancies: BMT
Cerebral intravascular coagulation	Widespread small arterial thrombosis	Advanced malignancies, leukemia, lymphoma: sepsis
Atherosclerosis	Cardiac embolism, large vessel disease, small vessel disease	Prior radiation
Venous sinus thrombosis	Hypercoagulable state or neoplastic compression	Leukemia, breast cancer and chemotherapy, solid tumors: L-asparaginase
Tumor embolism	Embolism	Sarcoma, cardiac tumors, lung cancer: pneumonectomy
Septic embolism	Cardiac embolism	Hematologic malignancies: sepsis, immunosuppression, indwelling venous catheters
Vasculitis	Infectious and inflammatory invasion of vessel wall	Leukemia: *Aspergillus*, Mucor, Rhizophus, VZV
Leptomeningeal metastasis	Compression and resultant arterial thrombosis	Solid tumors, glioblastoma: advanced metastatic disease
Chemotherapy	Arterial or venous thrombosis from hypercoagulable state	Breast cancer: cisplatin, L-asparaginase, bleomycin, cytarabine, lomustine
Radiation	Accelerated atherosclerosis and subsequent embolism, intracranial vasculopathy	Lymphoma, head and neck cancers, primary brain tumors
Hyperviscosity	Small vessel occlusion	Multiple myeloma, lymphoma, essential thrombocythemia, leukemia-causing hyperleukocytosis
MAHA	Platelet-rich microvascular thrombi	Mucinous adenocarcinomas: chemotherapy, BMT

NBTE, nonbacterial thrombotic endocarditis; BMT, bone marrow transplantation; VZV, varicella zoster virus; MAHA, microangiopathic hemolytic anemia.

prothrombotic tendencies similar to oral contraceptives and hormone replacement therapy. However, in Geiger's study, tamoxifen was not associated with an increased risk of stroke, regardless of cumulative dose, duration, or proximity of use. In addition, a large prospective study, the National Surgical Adjuvant Breast and Bowel Project Protocol 1 (NSABP P-1) Breast Cancer Prevention Trial, also did not show a statistically significant increase in stroke incidence with tamoxifen.

Head and neck cancers and lymphoma are frequently associated with radiation-accelerated atherosclerosis and subsequent ischemic infarctions. The interval from radiotherapy to stroke is usually >6 months but can be quite variable. The arterial stenosis or occlusion will be confined to the prior radiation port and often extends over a longer arterial segment than in standard atherosclerotic disease.

Hemorrhagic Stroke

Hemorrhagic strokes in cancer patients are more often symptomatic than ischemic strokes and are caused by a variety of etiologies (see Table 8.2). Intraparenchymal hemorrhages are the most common type, followed by subdural hematomas, subarachnoid hemorrhages, and epidural hematomas, in the listed order. The most common causes for symptomatic hemorrhages are coagulopathy and tumor-associated hemorrhages. Coagulopathy arises from multiple mechanisms in cancer patients and can be divided into dysfunction of platelets, coagulation factors, or both. Cancer-related platelet dysfunction or deficiency may occur from tumor infiltration of bone marrow, intrinsic bone marrow failure caused by hematologic malignancies (i.e., leukemia, lymphoma, and multiple myeloma), or chemotherapy or XRT toxicity. Causes of coagulation disorders include clotting factor deficiencies from liver disease or vitamin K deficiency, consumptive coagulopathies such as DIC or thrombotic thrombocytopenic purpura (TTP), and therapeutic anticoagulation for systemic thromboses. Tumor-associated hemorrhages most commonly arise from metastatic or primary CNS parenchymal lesions via intratumoral hemorrhage. However, tumors can also cause intracranial hemorrhage via neoplastic aneurysms (specifically cardiac myxoma, lung, and choriocarcinoma have been implicated), skull metastases causing epidural hematomas, and leptomeningeal or subdural metastases leading to subarachnoid or subdural hemorrhages, respectively. Hypertension, which is the leading cause of hemorrhage in the non-neoplastic population, accounted for only 6% of symptomatic intracranial hemorrhages in a large, retrospective study by Graus et al.

Hemorrhagic strokes in cancer patients are more common in hematologic neoplasms than in solid tumors. Leukemic patients in particular are extremely prone to both DIC and thrombocytopenia with subsequent intracranial hemorrhage. In acute promyelocytic leukemia, intrinsic promyelocytic degranulation directly causes the acute DIC state, which can further be exacerbated by tumor lysis syndrome from chemotherapy. Leukemic patients can also rarely have intracerebral hemorrhages via hyperleukocytosis. In the setting of significantly elevated leukocyte count, usually >100,000 cells per mm^3, peripheral blasts can cause leukostasis and eventual rupture of cerebral vessels. Leukostasis-associated bleeds often occur at the initial diagnosis of leukemia and are most common in acute myelogenous leukemia. In addition, hematologic malignancy patients frequently require bone marrow transplantation as a ther-

TABLE 8.2 Etiology of Hemorrhagic Infarcts in Cancer Patients

Etiology	Mechanism	Tumors/Associations
Coagulopathy	Dysfunction or deficiency of clotting factors and/or platelets	Hematologic malignancies (especially APML), bone marrow dysfunction, liver disease, vitamin K deficiency, consumptive coagulopathies, chemotherapy, sepsis, XRT
Tumor associated hemorrhage (intraparenchymal)	Tumor cell necrosis, angiogenesis, blood vessel invasion	Lung cancer, melanoma, glioblastoma, renal cell, thyroid carcinoma, choriocarcinoma, leukemia, hyperleukocytosis
Tumor associated hemorrhage (subdural)	Bridging vein invasion or compression leading to rupture	Meningioma, lung cancer, gastric cancer, prostate adenocarcinoma
Tumor associated hemorrhage (subarachnoid)	Ruptured neoplastic or infectious aneurysms, leptomeningeal compression/rupture of arteries	Choriocarcinoma, cardiac myxoma, bacterial/fungal endocarditis, *Aspergillus*, Mucor/Rhizophus, immunosuppression
Tumor associated hemorrhage (epidural)	Arterial invasion or compression leading to rupture	Hepatocellular carcinoma
Venous sinus thrombosis	Hypercoagulable state or neoplastic compression causing thrombosis and rupture	Leukemia, breast cancer and chemotherapy, solid tumors; L-asparaginase
Hypertension	End arteriole lipohyalinosis and subsequent rupture	No specific cancer predilection though cyclosporine, tacrolimus, and cisplatin are associated with PRES (occasionally hemorrhagic)
MAHA	Platelet-rich microvascular thrombi	Mucinous adenocarcinomas, BMT, chemotherapy
Vasculitis	Infectious and inflammatory invasion of vessel wall	Leukemia; *Aspergillus*, Mucor, Rhizophus, VZV

APML, acute promyelocytic leukemia; XRT, radiation therapy; PRES, posterior reversible leukoencephalopathy; MAHA, microangiopathic hemolytic anemia; BMT, bone marrow transplantation; VZV, varicella zoster virus.

apeutic measure, with subsequent immune compromise producing significant risk of sepsis and DIC.

Tumor-related hemorrhages have been reported with nearly all solid malignancies but are most frequently associated with histologically vascular tumors. Melanoma, choriocarcinoma, renal cell carcinoma, papillary thyroid carcinoma, and lung neoplasms are some common examples. Metastases-associated hemorrhages are postulated to be multifactorial in pathophysiology, with elements of neoangiogenesis, tumor cell necrosis, and parenchymal blood vessel invasion. Of the primary brain tumors, oligodendroglioma and glioblastoma multiforme are most likely to produce parenchymal brain hemorrhage. Subdural hematomas are rare compared to parenchymal hemorrhages in cancer patients but are of obvious import given their potential for rapid neurologic compromise and the need for emergency surgical correction. Meningiomas can occasionally present as subdural hematomas when there is venous sinus invasion. In addition, lung, gastric, and prostate carcinoma have all been reported to cause dural metastases and consequent hematomas.

Combined Ischemic and Hemorrhagic Stroke

Venous sinus thrombosis, which can lead to both ischemic and hemorrhagic stroke, occurs frequently in leukemic patients, particularly those who have received L-asparaginase treatment. This chemotherapeutic agent alters the coagulation cascade by reducing the levels of antithrombin III, protein C, fibrinogen, and plasminogen. However, venous sinus thrombosis can also occur from neoplastic compression of venous structures, particularly in tumors of solid origin.

Patients with cancer are often immunocompromised from chemotherapy, steroid use, or their neoplasm and thus are at risk for opportunistic infections and atypical presentations of common organisms. Infection and sepsis can cause strokes in these patients via a multitude of mechanisms. Cancer patients often have long-term indwelling catheters that predispose them to septicemia followed by bacterial or candidal endocarditis and subsequent septic emboli. They can also suffer from mycotic aneurysms leading to subarachnoid hemorrhage or infectious vasculitis causing potential catastrophic intracranial hemorrhage via the angiophilic species *Aspergillus* and Mucor/Rhizophus.

CLINICAL APPLICATIONS AND METHODOLOGY

The diagnosis and appropriate management of stroke in cancer patients is often complicated by severe systemic illness, numerous toxic medications, and multiple comorbidities. Thus when approaching a stroke in a cancer patient, we recommend following certain guidelines in a stepwise approach to maximize diagnostic accuracy and efficiency. The first guideline is to evaluate the type, duration, and extent of cancer given that many forms of cancer have predilection for specific stroke mechanisms. In addition, the duration between initial cancer diagnosis and presentation may imply a specific pathophysiology. For instance, NBTE is usually a late complication of malignancy, occurring when cancer is widespread and infarction has occurred in other organs. However, there are clearly many exceptions to this as NBTE has been reported as the presenting manifestation of an occult malignancy. This is particularly true in mucin-producing tumors that can result in catastrophic hypercoagulable states. This syndrome has been reported in lung, ovarian, and cervical cancer among others. Similarly, the extent of cancer can be informative in making the diagnosis as established metastatic disease raises the risk of tumor-associated hemorrhage. Cerebral intravascular coagulation is also typically associated with an extensive tumor burden.

The second guideline is to assess the significance of confounding processes.

Immunosuppression and prior bone marrow transplantation are relevant factors in cancer patients with stroke. These patients are at significant risk for developing opportunistic infections and subsequent cerebral infarctions through a variety of mechanisms. In addition, the physician should be attuned to the strong relationship between bone marrow transplantation and NBTE. Patchell et al. demonstrated NBTE in 7.7% of patients who had recently received an allogenic bone marrow transplant. Furthermore, the transplant patient's medication list should be thoroughly evaluated as certain chemotherapeutic agents used in the prevention of graft versus host disease (i.e., cyclosporine and steroids) are known to cause MAHA and resultant stroke.

Patients with previously documented thrombosis in organ systems outside the CNS are likely hypercoagulable and thus more predisposed to ischemic infarctions via NBTE or cerebral intravascular coagulation. In addition, cancer patients will commonly develop DIC, either from sepsis or from their intrinsic malignancy, and in this scenario, they may develop both ischemic and hemorrhagic features of their infarction.

Patients should be assessed for iatrogenic factors that could predispose to stroke. The patient's chemotherapeutic history should be carefully reviewed, as many agents are associated with increased stroke risk. Cisplatin, cytarabine, bleomycin, L-asparaginase, methyl-CCNU, and mitomycin C have all been implicated in stroke. The cancer patient should also be evaluated for prior radiation treatment. Radiation causes premature atherosclerotic plaques via endothelial injury, vessel wall ischemia, and subendothelial fibrosis. Patients with head and neck cancers who have received local XRT are at high risk for carotid atherosclerotic disease and eventual embolic strokes. In addition, radiation also predisposes to vascular malformations in atypical locations that can result in delayed vessel rupture and subarachnoid or intracerebral hemorrhage.

The final guideline in the evaluation of a cancer patient with stroke is to assess the nature of the neurological presentation. Stroke in cancer patients often presents with a diffuse encephalopathy that may lead to incorrect diagnoses. It is paramount that the physician maintains a high clinical suspicion for stroke, even if there is no focus on history or examination. All cancer patients with mental status changes require at least a computerized tomography (CT) scan, and possibly a contrast-enhanced magnetic resonance imaging (MRI), to rule out cerebrovascular disease as the cause of their encephalopathy. In addition, cerebral intravascular coagulation commonly presents as a diffuse encephalopathy with occasional focal signs or seizures and is extremely difficult to diagnose antemortem. Diffusion-weighted imaging (DWI) on MRI may not reveal the infarctions, and often the definitive diagnosis is only made at autopsy. Given these pitfalls in diagnostic evaluation, this condition is likely underdiagnosed.

Once the initial guidelines have been reviewed, the pertinent laboratory and radiologic features of the case need to be evaluated. Complete blood count, coagulation profile, and DIC panel should be ordered on all stroke patients. Patients with platelet values $<50,000\ mm^3$ and particularly less than $10,000\ mm^3$ are at high risk for hemorrhagic stroke. Conversely, patients with certain hematologic malignancies, particularly essential thrombocythemia, will rarely present with ischemic infarctions due to severe thrombocytosis, with platelet counts usually being $>1,000,000\ mm^3$.

Elevated prothrombin and partial thromboplastin time from DIC, liver failure, or vitamin K deficiency (often from poor nutrition) will raise the suspicion for a hemorrhagic stroke. DIC in particular will manifest as elevated D-dimers/fibrin split products levels and reduced fibrinogen level. All patients with suspected DIC should also have a peripheral blood smear to assess for schistocytes. Though chronic DIC is postulated as being the underlying pathophysiology of NBTE, a laboratory confirmation of DIC may be difficult to establish given the numerous confounding factors that are present in cancer patients. This is especially true in patients with systemic metastases who are actively undergoing chemotherapy and radiation, as they will often have coexisting platelet and coagulation factor abnormalities. Kuramoto et al. found 41.9% of their NBTE cohort (217 patients) to have evidence of DIC. Conversely, Cestari et al. found an elevated D-dimer level in 11 of 12 tested patients, but only 3 patients were conclusively diagnosed with NBTE.

Blood cultures, including both bacterial and fungal isolators, should be drawn on all cancer patients with stroke. As mentioned earlier, these patients are often immunocompromised and are at considerable risk for bacteremia and all its potential CNS complications. Patients should be assessed vigilantly for signs of infection. Fever curves should be plotted and patients should be thoroughly examined for stigmata of endocarditis.

Acute stroke imaging should be performed with CT scan. Non–contrast-enhanced CT of the brain is highly sensitive for hemorrhagic stroke. CT has the clear advantage over MRI in terms of speed and ease of completion in critically ill patients. Cancer patients are potential candidates for tissue plasminogen activator (tPA) and other acute stroke treatments, thus necessitating the primary stroke evaluation to be conducted with extreme urgency.

MRI with DWI is highly sensitive for acute ischemic infarction that may not be seen on CT. DWI scans in NBTE patients will usually demonstrate restricted diffusion in several areas of varying size within multiple vascular territories. These patients may also have evidence of old, clinically silent infarctions on T2-fluid attenuated inversion recovery (FLAIR) images. MRI is unfortunately not as helpful in the evaluation of cerebral intravascular coagulation. In fact, MRI is often nondiagnostic in this syndrome with no apparent strokes seen on DWI technique.

MRI imaging should include gadolinium enhancement. Contrast-enhanced imaging is particularly useful in the evaluation of tumor-related hemorrhagic stroke. Precontrast MRI will often be inconclusive in the investigation for underlying metastases and only with contrast administration will the diagnosis be reached. Peri-hematomal enhancement, multiple parenchymal hemorrhages, and the presence of other enhancing masses are highly suspicious for underlying tumor. In addition, excessive or persistent edema, hematoma at the gray–white junction, delayed hematoma evolution, and diminished or absent hemosiderin deposition is also suggestive of cancer. In fact, Tung et al. reported a positive predictive value of 71% for underlying metastases if the ratio of vasogenic edema to mean hematoma diameter was >100%. Contrast-enhanced images are also useful in the evaluation of venous sinus thrombosis, with the thrombosed vein demonstrating a lack of enhancement or the *empty delta sign*. In addition, MRI with contrast is also indicated to rule out leptomeningeal disease as these metastases can rarely invade venous sinuses and cause venous infarction.

Magnetic resonance angiography (MRA) is useful in defining atherosclerotic etiologies of stroke and will assess for potential neoplastic or marantic aneurysms as sources of subarachnoid hemorrhage. It can also be helpful in diagnosing cerebral vasculitis, which is usually caused by angiophilic opportunistic infections. However, cerebral vasculitis often affects only small vessels and may require standard four-vessel angiography for diagnosis. MRA of the neck is helpful in ruling out carotid and vertebral atherosclerotic disease, particularly in patients with prior radiation to these sites. If MRA is not available at an institution or if it is contraindicated, then carotid ultrasound should be performed to assess for carotid atherosclerotic disease.

Cancer patients with stroke require echocardiography to assess for endocarditis. Patients should first be examined via the transthoracic route as it is less invasive. However, transthoracic echocardiography (TTE) has a poor sensitivity for detecting the diminutive vegetations in NBTE, thus frequently requiring follow-up examination via the transesophageal route for diagnosis. Unfortunately, the sensitivity of transesophageal echocardiography (TEE) in marantic endocarditis is also limited. One study reported 55% of their cohort to have a definite or probable cardiac source of embolism but only 18% of patients were found to have vegetations via TEE. Bubble studies assessing for interatrial shunts should also be performed on all patients. These patients are hypercoagulable and at high risk for venous thromboembolism and potential paradoxical embolus.

Cerebral angiography is occasionally indicated in the evaluation of a cancer patient with stroke. Four-vessel angiography is the gold standard for detecting vascular occlusions and is often utilized when noninvasive MRA or CT angiography (CTA) is nondiagnostic. It is also the imaging modality of choice in subarachnoid hemorrhage and cerebral vasculitis. All patients with subarachnoid hemorrhage must undergo angiography to rule out aneurysmal rupture. This is particularly true because neoplastic or marantic aneurysms are often small and peripheral in origin (frequently distal branches of middle cerebral artery) and may be missed on less invasive angiographic modalities.

Patients with suspected NBTE or cerebral intravascular coagulation should be assessed for systemic thromboembolic events. These patients are at high risk for catastrophic and occasionally lethal thromboses in other organ systems, thus mandating the physician to search for systemic signs of coagulapathy. They should be evaluated via electrocardiogram (ECG) and serial cardiac enzymes to rule out myocardial infarction. In addition, limb venous duplex scans and spiral CT may be indicated.

Treatment of the underlying malignancy is essential for optimal stroke management in the cancer patient. Medical therapy aimed solely at cerebrovascular disease is a temporizing measure that will ultimately fail. Only by addressing the underlying malignancy will the patient's risk for recurrent stroke be reduced. In fact, we believe that cerebrovascular disease in cancer patients, particularly ischemic infarctions from NBTE or cerebral intravascular coagulation, may be one of the few indications for emergent chemotherapy. This is particularly applicable in the rare circumstance of NBTE occurring in a patient with a high performance status and localized or occult cancer.

Hemorrhagic stroke treatment should be aimed at correcting the underlying coagulopathy. If thrombocytopenia or qualitative platelet dysfunction (i.e., prior aspirin or clopidogrel use) exists, then platelet transfusions should be administered with a goal platelet value of $>100{,}000\ mm^3$. Patients with elevated prothrombin or partial thromboplastin time should be treated with vitamin K injections and fresh frozen plasma until laboratory values are normalized (i.e., INR <1.2). Treatment of acute DIC should be aimed at suppressing the underlying DIC etiology and replacing coagulation factors. For instance, sepsis should be treated with appropriate antibiotics and acute promyelocytic leukemia should be treated aggressively with chemotherapeutic agents. Some authors advocate the use of heparin in DIC to stop the thrombotic cascade; however, this treatment remains controversial. MAHA carries a poor prognosis and is often refractory to treatment. Therapy consists of red blood cell and platelet transfusions, treatment of the underlying precipitant, and occasionally steroids or plasma exchange. Neurosurgical decompression is rarely indicated in intraparenchymal hemorrhagic stroke and is almost always confined to symptomatic epidural, subdural, or subarachnoid hemorrhages. Three exceptions to this are posterior fossa hematomas at risk for tonsillar herniation or obstructive hydrocephalus, large, superficial, lobar hemorrhages that are causing extensive mass effect and herniation, and acute tumor-associated hemorrhages. Subarachnoid hemorrhages from neoplastic or mycotic aneurysms are difficult to treat and frequently lethal. Aneurysms associated with mass effect from hematoma should be treated with neurosurgical intervention. Those that are multiple, fusiform, or not amenable to surgery are best served with endovascular coiling. Once the aneurysms are secured, medical therapy is required to prevent further aneurysm growth. Neoplastic aneurysms are treated via brain radiation and/or chemotherapy, while mycotic aneurysms are treated with antibiotics. Complications of subarachnoid hemorrhage, such as vasospasm and hydrocephalus, should follow standard therapeutic guidelines.

In tumor-associated hemorrhagic stroke, treatment should be directed at the underlying metastases. Resection is generally indicated if the lesion is solitary and life threatening. Otherwise, radiation or chemotherapy is preferred. Depending on the amount and location of lesions, radiation can be administered via a stereotactic or whole brain approach. The decision between radiation and chemotherapy is often dependent on the histology of the tumor and how sensitive it is to the respective modality. Symptomatic subdural hematomas caused by subdural metastases should be treated via drainage of the hematoma followed by brain radiation to minimize risk of recurrence.

Cancer patients with acute ischemic strokes are candidates for thrombolytic therapy. Though cancer patients may have a theoretically higher risk of intracerebral hemorrhage from occult cerebral metastases undetected on CT, the American Academy of Neurology does not list malignancy as an absolute contraindication to intravenous tPA administration. In addition, there is currently no data evaluating the efficacy or safety of tPA in the cancer population. Despite this lack of data, the authors' recommend that all qualifying cancer patients with acute strokes receive thrombolytic therapy. Intra-arterial tPA and clot retrieval are also options for the cancer patient and may be administered in appropriate cases.

The treatment of ischemic stroke in cancer patients is controversial and non–evidence based. The role of anticoagulation is a particularly contentious issue with little available data to guide practitioners. There have been no prospective trials assessing the role of anticoagulation in malignancy-associated ischemic stroke. The limited data that does exist is flawed by small sample sizes, multiple confounders, and varying results. Regardless of this paucity of information, anecdotal evidence suggests the use of anticoagulation in ischemic strokes of hypercoagulable origin. NBTE and cerebral intravascular coagulation are clearly caused by relentless procoagulant states that pose significant risk for recurrent cerebral and systemic thrombotic events. It is the authors' opinion that the risk of further thrombotic events generally outweighs the risk of bleeding, justifying anticoagulant use.

Anticoagulation is also recommended in venous sinus thromboses with associated infarction or hemorrhage. Though performed in the noncancer population, a study by Fink et al. demonstrated the safety of anticoagulation despite the presence of intraparenchymal hematoma. The treatment of thromboses without associated infarction is more controversial and should be treated on an individual basis. There are no randomized studies comparing anticoagulation to placebo in the cancer patient with venous sinus thromboses, although one study in the non-neoplastic population did show a trend in favor of anticoagulation at 3 weeks and 3 months. Venous sinus thrombosis caused by local venous compression from metastatic disease is best treated via eradication of the underlying tumor.

Anticoagulation should be used as a temporizing measure to treat the hypercoagulable state until the underlying malignancy can be addressed. However, if the malignancy is refractory or untreatable, anticoagulation is likely futile and should not be given. The risks of anticoagulation are also unclear in the cancer population. Treated stroke patients in a study by Rogers et al. demonstrated a reduction in ischemic episodes without an associated rise in brain hemorrhage. This study, however, was flawed by a treated sample size of only 12, indicating the need for large, prospective studies in the future.

Heparin or its derivatives are the preferred anticoagulant in malignancy-associated infarction. There are no prospective trials comparing heparin to coumadin in the prevention or treatment of stroke in cancer patients. There is, however, considerable historic precedence noting the superiority of heparin to coumadin in the treatment of malignancy-related thromboembolic disease. In addition, there is recent data confirming an increased efficacy of low-molecular-weight heparin compared to coumadin for the prevention of deep vein thromboses and pulmonary embolism.

Atherosclerotic strokes in cancer patients should be treated by standard antiplatelet agents. Atherosclerosis is the third most common cause of symptomatic ischemic stroke in cancer patients. Occasionally, a patient's stroke can be linked to his or her extensive atherosclerotic disease, without any traces of a concomitant hypercoagulable state. This scenario commonly arises in vasculopathic patients with remote cancer histories. Anticoagulation is not justified in these settings as the underlying hypercoagulable state does not exist. Chaturvedi et al. supported this premise by demonstrating no difference in recurrent stroke risk among cancer patients with predominantly atherosclerotic-induced stroke treated with aspirin or anticoagulation.

Furthermore, patients with radiation-induced carotid atherosclerotic disease should be treated with either endarterectomy or carotid stenting. Revascularization procedures are safe in these patients; however, symptomatic restenosis may occur. There are no trials at this point comparing the efficacy or safety of surgical versus interventional therapies in cancer patients.

PRACTICAL RECOMMENDATIONS

Cerebrovascular disease is extremely common in cancer patients. It commonly causes severe disability and occasionally death. Strokes in cancer patients frequently arise from unconventional mechanisms that pose significant diagnostic dilemma. These unique mechanisms create extraordinary stroke presentations requiring a high clinical suspicion. Treatment is often unorthodox and ineffective.

We reiterate the following guidelines to maximize chances of a successful outcome. Scrupulous attention should be paid to the type, extent, and duration of cancer. These elements of the history will help form the physician's differential diagnosis. The presence of confounding processes should be investigated and excluded. In addition, the initial presentation should be carefully analyzed for signs of impending deterioration.

Laboratory and radiologic data will assist in accurate diagnosis. Laboratory data should be rigorously assessed for signs of coagulopathy, infection, or systemic disease. After rapidly assessing the history, exam, and laboratory values, CT scan should be urgently performed. Hemorrhage should be suspected until proven otherwise. If acute hemorrhage does not exist and the patient is stable, brain MRI with contrast should then be performed. MRI will generally confirm clinical diagnosis. In the rare circumstance that it does not, cerebral angiography or lumbar puncture may be indicated.

MRA of the head and neck and echocardiography should be performed to investigate the origin of disease. TEE must be performed, as transthoracic views carry a low sensitivity for NBTE. If vegetations are found, the diagnosis of NBTE can only be made after serial blood cultures rule out septicemia. Magnetic resonance venography (MRV) is indicated if suspicion for venous infarction exists. After cerebral infarction is confirmed, evaluation of systemic infarction should also be conducted. ECG, limb duplex scans, and other diagnostic tools may be indicated depending on existing signs and symptoms.

Treatment should target both the underlying malignancy and inciting factors. Bleeding diatheses should be treated with appropriate replacements. If impending herniation is suspected, emergent neurosurgical decompression may be indicated. Thrombolytics should be administered in qualifying cases of acute ischemic stroke. Hypercoagulable states such as NBTE, cerebral intravascular coagulation, and venous sinus thromboses generally require anticoagulation. Anticoagulation with heparin or its derivatives is preferred to coumadin.

Treatment of the underlying cancer is essential. Stroke pathophysiology is often directly related to the background neoplasm. The malignancy should be aggressively treated to eliminate the principal basis of infarction. Cancer treatment should be considered in all circumstances and may be indicated even if severe medical illness or poor performance status exists.

Prognosis is poor in cancer patients with stroke. Despite our vast therapeutic armamentarium, strokes are poorly treated in cancer patients and often herald impending death. Malignancy patients are at high risk for future infarctions despite preventive therapy. Vigilant follow-up is mandatory to assess for recurrent cerebrovascular events.

SELECTED REFERENCES

Al-Mubarak N, Roubin GS, Iyer SS, et al. Carotid stenting for severe radiation-induced extracranial carotid artery occlusive disease. *J Endovasc Ther* 2000;7:36–40.

Atlas SW, Grossman RI, Gomori JM, et al. Hemorrhagic intracranial malignant neoplasms: spin echo MR imaging. *Radiology* 1987;164: 71–77.

Blanchard DG, Ross RS, Dittrich HC. Nonbacterial thrombotic endocarditis. Assessment by transesophageal echocardiography. *Chest* 1992;102: 954–956.

Borowski A, Ghodsizad A, Gams E. Stroke as a first manifestation of ovarian cancer. *J Neuro-Oncol* 2005;71:267–269.

Cestari DM, Weine DM, Panageas KS, et al. Stroke in patients with cancer: incidence and etiology. *Neurology* 2004;62:2025–2030.

Chaturvedi S, Ansell J, Recht L. Should cerebral ischemic events in cancer patients be considered a manifestation of hypercoagulability? *Stroke* 1994;25:1215–1218.

Cornuz J, Bogousslavsky J, Schapira M, et al. Ischemic stroke as the presenting manifestation of localized systemic cancer. *Schweiz Arch Neurol Psychiatr* 1988;139:5–11.

DeBruijn SF, Buddle M, Teunisse S, et al. Long-term outcome of cognition and functional health after cerebral venous sinus thrombosis. *Neurology* 2000;54:1687–1689.

Dignam JJ, Fisher B. Occurrence of stroke with tamoxifen in NSABP B-24. *Lancet* 2000;355:848–849.

Dorresteijn LD, Kappelle AC, Boogerd W, et al. Increased risk of ischemic stroke after radiotherapy on the neck in patients younger than 60 years. *J Clin Oncol* 2002;20:282–288.

Dutta T, Karas MG, Segal AZ, et al. Yield of transesophageal echocardiography for nonbacterial thrombotic endocarditis and other cardiac sources of embolism in cancer patients with cerebral ischemia. *Am J Cardiol* 2006;97:894–898.

El Amrani M, Heinzlef O, Debroucker T, et al. Brain infarction following 5-fluorouracil and cisplatin therapy. *Neurology* 1998;51:899–901.

Fink JN, McAuley DL. Safety of anticoagulation for cerebral venous thrombosis associated with intracerebral hematoma. *Neurology* 2001;57: 1138–1139.

Geiger AM, Fischberg GM, Wansu C, et al. Stroke risk and tamoxifen therapy for breast cancer. *J Natl Cancer Inst* 2004;96:1528–1536.

Gordon LI, Kwaan HC. Thrombotic microangiopathy manifesting as thrombotic thrombocytopenic purpura/hemolytic uremic syndrome in the cancer patient. *Semin Thromb Hemost* 1999;25:217–221.

Graus F, Rogers LR, Posner JB. Cerebrovascular complications in patients with cancer. *Medicine* 1985;64:16–35.

Herrera de Pablo P, Esteban Esteban E, Gimenez Soler JV, et al. Nonbacterial thrombotic endocarditis as initial event of lung cancer. *Am Med Intl* 2004;21:495–497.

Hongo T, Okada S, Ohzeki T, et al. Low plasma levels of hemostatic proteins during the induction phase in children with acute lymphoblastic leukemia: a retrospective study by the Japan Association of Childhood Leukemia. *Pediatr Int* 2002;44:293–299.

Kashyap VS, Moore WS, Quinones-Baldrich WJ. Carotid artery repair for radiation-associated atherosclerosis is a safe and durable procedure. *J Vasc Surg* 1999;29:90–99.

Katz JM, Segal AZ. Incidence and etiology of cerebrovascular disease in patients with malignancy. *Curr Atheroscl Rep* 2005;7:280–288.

Khang-Loon H. Neoplastic aneurysm and intracranial hemorrhage. *Cancer* 1982;50:2935–2940.

Krouwer HG, Wijdickds EF. Neurologic complications of bone marrow transplantation. *Neurol Clin North Am* 2003;21:319–352.

Kuramoto K, Matsushita S, Yamanouchi H. Nonbacterial thrombotic endocarditis as a cause of cerebral and myocardial infarction. *Jpn Circ J* 1984;48:1000–1006.

Kwaan HC, Gordon LI. Thrombotic microangiopathy in the cancer patient. *Acta Haematol* 2001;106:52–56.

Lee AY, Levine MN, Baker RI, et al. Low-molecular-weight heparin versus a coumarin for the prevention of recurrent venous thromboembolism in patients with cancer. *N Engl J Med* 2003;349:146–153.

Lee AY, Rickles FR, Julian JA, et al. Randomized comparison of low molecular weight heparin and coumarin derivatives on the survival of patients with cancer and venous thromboembolism. *J Clin Oncol* 2005; 23:2123–2129.

Lieu AS, Hwang SL, Howng SL, Chai CY. Brain tumors with hemorrhage. *J Formos Med Assoc* 1999;98:365–367.

Little JR, Dial B, Belanger G, et al. Brain hemorrhage from intracranial tumor. *Stroke* 1979;10:283–288.

McKenzie CR, Rengachary SS, McGregor DH, et al. Subdural hematoma associated with metastatic neoplasms. *Neurosurgery* 1990;27: 619–625.

Patchell RA, White CL, Clark AW, et al. Nonbacterial thrombotic endocarditis in bone marrow transplant patients. *Cancer* 1985;55: 631–635.

Peters PJ, Harrison T, Lennox JL. A dangerous dilemma: management of infectious intracranial aneurysms complicating endocarditis. *Lancet Infect Dis* 2006;6:742–748.

Raizer JJ, DeAngelis LM. Cerebral sinus thrombosis diagnosed by MRI and MR venography in cancer patients. *Neurology* 2000;54: 1222–1226.

Rogers LR. Cerebrovascular complications in cancer patients. *Neurol Clin* 2003;21:167–192.

Rogers LR. Cerebrovascular complications in patients with cancer. *Semin Neurol* 2004;24:453–460.

Rogers LR, Cho E, Sanford K, et al. Cerebral infarction from non-bacterial thrombotic endocarditis: clinical and pathologic study including the effects of anticoagulation. *Am J Med* 1987;83:746–756.

Santoro N, Giordano P, Del Vecchio GC, et al. Ischemic stroke in children treated for acute lymphoblastic leukemia. *J Pediatr Hematol Oncol* 2005;27:153–157.

Tung GA, Julius BD, Rogg JM. MRI of intracerebral hematoma: value of vasogenic edema ratio for predicting the cause. *Neuroradiology* 2003;45: 357–362.

Wong AA, Henderson RD, O'Sullivan ID, et al. Ring enhancement after hemorrhagic stroke. *Arch Neurol* 2004;61:1790.

CRITICAL PATHWAY
Approach to a Cancer Patient with Stroke

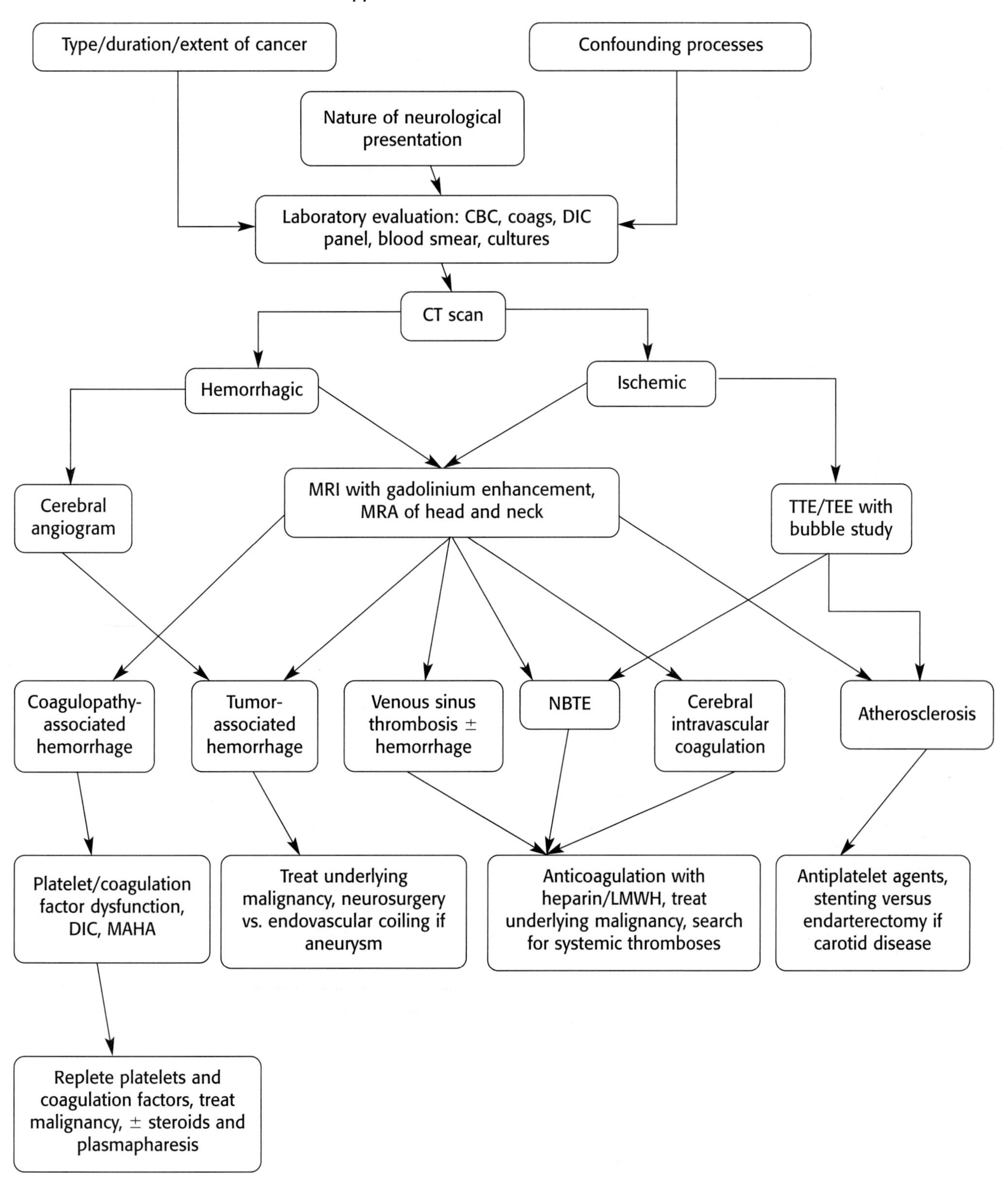

CBC, calcium channel blocker; DIC, disseminated intravascular coagulation; MAHA, microangiopathic hemolytic anemia; CT, computerized tomography; MRI, magnetic resonance imaging; MRA, magnetic resonance angiography;
TTE, transthoracic echocardiography; TEE, transesophageal echocardiography; NBTE, nonbacterial thrombotic endocarditis; LMWH, low molecular weight heparin.

CHAPTER

Management of Atrial Fibrillation

MICHAEL A. SLOAN

OBJECTIVES

- What is the epidemiology and pathophysiology of atrial fibrillation?
- How can stroke risk be predicted?
- How is atrial fibrillation managed?
- What is the evidence supporting antiplatelet and anticoagulation for atrial fibrillation?
- Does rate or rhythm control matter?
- What is the risk of bleeding risk associated with anticoagulant therapy?
- What are the surgical and percutaneous interventional approaches to atrial fibrillation?

Atrial fibrillation (AF) is a supraventricular tachyarrhythmia characterized by uncoordinated atrial activation with consequent deterioration in cardiac mechanical performance. The electrocardiogram (ECG) reveals rapid oscillations, or fibrillatory waves, that vary in amplitude, shape, and timing. These rapid oscillations are accompanied by an irregular ventricular response, which depends upon electrophysiological properties of the atrioventricular (AV) node, other conducting tissues, vagal and sympathetic tone, presence or absence of accessory pathways, and actions of various drugs. The functional refractory period of the AV node correlates inversely with ventricular rate during AF. An irregular, sustained, wide-QRS-complex tachycardia suggests AF with conduction over an accessory pathway or AF with a bundle branch block. AF may occur in association with atrial flutter or atrial tachycardia, and each rhythm may convert into the others.

AF may first be detected in individuals who may or may not be symptomatic. However, there may be uncertainty about the duration of the current episode or whether there have been previous episodes. AF can be classified on the basis of the frequency and duration of its occurrence. If AF occurs after two or more episodes, it is classified as *recurrent*. If AF remits spontaneously within 7 days, it is designated as *paroxysmal*. If AF lasts beyond 7 days, it is termed *persistent*. If AF lasts longer than 1 year, it is considered *permanent*. *Lone AF* applies to individuals younger than 60 years who have no clinical or echocardiographic evidence of cardiopulmonary disease, including hypertension. *Nonvalvular AF* refers to cases without rheumatic mitral valve disease, prosthetic heart valves, or valve repair.

Two major mechanisms are believed to be responsible for AF: a focal triggering mechanism (most frequently present in pulmonary veins) and multiple recurrent wavelets. The focal triggering mechanism is supported by the presence of foci of atrial tissue with shorter refractory periods that can lead to heterogeneity of conduction and reentry located in the pulmonary veins, but may also be present in the superior vena cava, ligament of Marshall, left posterior free wall, crista terminalis, and coronary sinus. The multiple wavelet hypothesis is supported by the observation of a large atrial mass with a short refractory period and delayed conduction that can increase the number of wavelets, thus favoring sustained AF. These mechanisms are not mutually exclusive and may coexist. The most frequent histopathological changes in AF are atrial fibrosis and loss of atrial muscle mass. The degree to which altered atrial architecture contributes to the initiation and maintenance of AF is unknown. However, it is known that the propensity to AF is related to the progressive shortening of the effective refractive period with increasing episode duration, suggesting that "atrial fibrillation begets atrial fibrillation" through the process of electrophysiological remodeling. Inhibition of the renin-angiotensin-aldosterone system, alone or in combination with other therapies, may prevent the onset or maintenance of AF via lower atrial pressure and wall stress, prevention of structural remodeling, inhibition of neurohumoral activation, reduced blood pressure, prevention or amelioration of heart failure, and avoidance of hypokalemia.

Approximately 30% to 45% of paroxysmal AF cases and 20% to 25% of persistent AF cases occur in young patients without demonstrable underlying disease (lone AF). AF may be secondary to a variety of disease states, such as older age with accompanying myocardial stiffness, hypertension (especially with left ventricular hypertrophy), coronary artery disease, acute myocardial infarction, pericarditis, myocardial disease, valvular heart disease (typically mitral valve disease), cardiac arrhythmias (atrial flutter, Wolff-Parkinson-White syndrome, AV nodal re-entrant tachycardia), primary or metastatic disease, obesity with the amount of left atrial dilation related to body mass index, hyperthyroidism, pheochromocytoma, acute pulmonary disease, pulmonary embolism, alcohol intake (holiday heart syndrome) or caffeine ingestion, various metabolic diosorders, postoperative state (cardiac, pulmonary, or esophageal), subarachnoid hemorrhage, and major nonhemorrhagic stroke.

EPIDEMIOLOGY AND PATHOPHYSIOLOGY

AF is the most common arrhythmia in clinical practice, accounting for approximately one third of hospitalizations for cardiac rhythm disorders. In prospective studies, the incidence of AF increases from <0.1% per year in persons younger than 40 years to over 1.5% per year in women and 2.0% per year in men older than 80 years. An estimated 2.3 million people in North America and 4.5 million people in the European Union have paroxysmal or persistent AF, with its prevalence rising rapidly after the age of 60 years to reach nearly 10% in persons aged 80 years and older. The mean age of individuals with AF is 75 years. By the year 2050, the prevalence of AF is expected to increase about 2.5-fold, mostly because of the increasing proportion of individuals living into their 80s and beyond. AF may be paroxysmal (self-limiting), persistent (amenable to cardioversion), or permanent, with paroxysmal AF accounting for 35% to 66% of all cases, peaking at age 50 to 69 years. In a recent cluster randomized trial involving British primary care practices, active screening in interventional practices (with patient education) detected significantly more cases of AF per year than control practices [1.63% versus 1.04%; absolute difference 0.58%; 95% confidence interval (CI), 0.20–0.98], However, systematic (entire population screened by ECG) and opportunistic (irregular pulse confirmed by ECG) screening detected similar numbers of new AF cases (1.62% versus 1.64%). There are three objectives in the management of patients with AF: rate control, prevention of thromboembolism, and correction of the rhythm disturbance. In general, for complex or high-risk situations and long-term management, consultation with internal medicine or cardiology is recommended.

The pathophysiology of thromboembolism in AF is complex. Ischemic stroke in AF is generally attributed to embolism of left atrial thrombus due to stasis. Decreased flow in the left atrium or left atrial appendage has been associated with spontaneous echo contrast, thrombus formation, and embolic events. However, the presence of spontaneous echo contrast, a marker of left atrial or left atrial appendage stasis, has not been shown to be useful for risk stratification. After successful cardioversion by spontaneous, pharmacological or electrical means, stunning of the left atrial appendage with resultant decrease of atrial transport function may account for an increased risk of thromboembolic events (1% to 5%) for up to 3 to 4 weeks. In this setting, >80% of thromboembolic events occur within the first 3 days and almost 100% within 10 days. Left ventricular systolic dysfunction has been associated with left atrial thrombus formation and noncardioembolic strokes in AF patients. In addition, up to 25% of strokes in AF patients may be associated with intrinsic cerebrovascular diseases, such as internal carotid artery stenosis, aortic atherosclerosis, or other sources of embolism.

STROKE OCCURRENCE AND STROKE RISK PREDICTION

AF increases the risk of stroke four- to sixfold across all age groups. In Olmstead County, Minnesota, the 15-year cumulative stroke rate in individuals younger than 60 years with lone AF was 1.3%. The rate of ischemic stroke among patients with nonvalvular AF averages 5% (range 3% to 8%) per year or two- to sevenfold higher than patients without nonvalvular AF. If one includes patients with transient ischemic attacks or silent strokes detected by brain imaging, the stroke risk exceeds 7% per year. It is believed that AF accounts for approximately 15% of strokes, with the population attributable risk rising from 1.5% for persons in their 50s to 23.5% for those in their 80s. In the Stroke Prevention in Atrial Fibrillation I-III (SPAF) studies, the annualized risk of ischemic stroke during aspirin treatment was similar in patients with paroxysmal (3.2%) and permanent (3.3%) AF. In the Framingham Heart Study (FHS), the stroke risk of patients with rheumatic AF increased 17-fold over age-matched controls, with attributable risk being fivefold higher than that in nonrheumatic AF. In the Japan Multicentre Stroke Investigators' Collaboration, AF was an independent predictor of severe stroke and early death. The risk of thromboembolism in patients with atrial flutter is not as well established as it is for AF but is believed to be higher than that for patients in normal sinus rhythm and less than that for persistent or permanent AF.

In patients with nonvalvular AF enrolled in randomized clinical trials, independent risk factors for stroke include previous stroke or transient ischemic attack [relative risk (RR) = 2.5], diabetes mellitus (RR = 1.7), history of hypertension (RR = 1.6), heart failure (RR = 1.4), and advanced age (per decade) (RR = 1.4). A number of epidemiological studies and other secondary analyses of clinical trials have also been conducted, and consideration of issues relating to stroke prediction, optimal treatment, complications of therapy, and cost effectiveness has recently been published and reviewed. The risk of stroke with nonvalvular AF is now recognized to be heterogeneous. Risk factors for stroke include increasing age (per decade >65 years), history of hypertension, diabetes mellitus, previous transient ischemic attack or stroke, moderate to severe reduced left ventricular function, and congestive heart failure. In a recent meta-analysis of studies, observed absolute annual stroke rates for non-anticoagulated patients with single independent risk factors were 6% to 9% for prior stroke/transient ischemic attack (TIA), 1.5% to 3.0% for history of hypertension, 1.5% to 3.0% for age >75 years, and 2.0% to 3.5% for diabetes. Among high-risk AF patients, impaired left ventricular systolic function on transthoracic echocardiography, thrombus, dense spontaneous echo contrast or smoke, reduced left atrial appendage flow velocity, and complex atheromatous plaque in the thoracic aorta on transesophagral echocardiography have been associated with thromboembolism. However, absence of left atrial clot or smoke on transesophageal echocardiography (TEE) does not necessarily confer a low stroke risk.

Three risk scores have been developed for predicting stroke in nonvalvular AF on the basis of clinical trial data or administrative databases in patients not receiving antithrombotic therapy. Based on nonrheumatic atrial fibrillation (NRAF) data, the Cardiac Failure, Hypertension, Age, Diabetes, Stroke (Doubled) (CHADS2) score (see Table 9.1) assigns two points for stroke or TIA and one point for the other factors. The discriminative power (c-index) [proportion (%) of predictive power of the risk factors contained in the risk score] of these risk scores are as follows: AFI – c-index = 0.68 (95% CI, 0.65 to 0.71), SPAF – c-index = 0.74 (95% CI, 0.71 to 0.76), and CHADS2 (NRAF) – c-index = 0.82 (95% CI, 0.80 to 0.84). In the CHADS2 score, the stroke rate per 100 patient-years increased 1.5-fold for every one point increase in the CHADS2 score. A new risk score for stroke using the FHS dataset shows similar results between FHS (c-index = 0.66) and the other three

TABLE 9.1 Stroke Risk in Nonvalvular Atrial Fibrillation According to the CHADS2 Index

CHADS2 Risk Criteria	Score
Prior stroke or TIA	2
Age >75 years	1
Hypertension	1
Diabetes mellitus	1
Heart failure	1

CHADS2, Cardiac failure, Hypertension, Age, Diabetes, Stroke (doubled).

Patients (n = 1,733)	Adjusted Stroke Rate (%/yr, 95% CI)	CHADS2 Score
120	1.9 (1.2–3.0)	0
463	2.8 (2.0–3.8)	1
523	4.0 (3.1–5.1)	2
337	5.9 (4.6–7.3)	3
220	8.5 (6.3–11.1)	4
65	12.5 (8.2–17.5)	5
5	18.2 (10.5–27.4)	6

CHADS2, Cardiac Failure, Hypertension, Age, Diabetes, Stroke (Doubled); TIA, transient ischemic attack.
From Gage BF, Waterman AD, Shannon W, et al. Validation of clinical classification schemes for predicting stroke: results from the National Registry of Atrial Fibrillation. *JAMA* 2001;285:2864–2870 and van Walraven WC, Hart RG, Wells GA, et al. A clinical prediction rule to identify patients with atrial fibrillation and a low risk for stroke while taking aspirin. *Arch Intern Med* 2003;163:936–943, with permission.

(AFI – c-index = 0.61, SPAF – c-index = 0.62, CHADS2 – c-index = 0.62), while the risk score for stroke and death was slightly better (c-index = 0.70). Application of these risk scores may be useful to guide the choice of antithrombotic therapy in AF patients.

Systemic (especially cerebral) embolism is an important complication of valvular heart disease. For rheumatic mitral valvular disease, the incidence of emboli varies from 1.5% to 4.7% per year and is increased in case of older patients, lower cardiac indices, presence of left atrial clot, and significant aortic regurgitation; atrial fibrillation increases the risk by approximately sevenfold. Maintenance of normal sinus rhythm with an enlarged left atrium and mitral valvuloplasty do not appear to reduce the risk of thromboembolism. Observational studies have shown reduction in annual stroke risk (10% to 0.8% to 3%) and death from embolism with oral anticoagulation therapy. Mitral annular calcification (MAC) is associated with a 2.1-fold increase in stroke risk and can be associated with AF (12-fold increase), aortic atheroma, and carotid atheroma. In the absence of associated mitral valve disease or AF, systemic embolism in patients with aortic valve disease is uncommon.

Thromboembolic complications of the various types of prosthetic valves are common and have recently been reviewed. The rate of embolism in patients with mechanical prosthetic valves is estimated to be 2% to 4% per year, even with proper anticoagulant therapy. Factors associated with thrombus formation include left atrial enlargement, atrial stasis, coexistent AF, valve type and position, and the presence of ventricular pacemakers. In patients who experience additional thromboembolic events despite adequate anticoagulation, TEE should be performed to look for atrial, ventricular, or valve thrombi, infective vegetations, and spontaneous echodensities. In selected cases, the dose of vitamin K antagonists (VKA) can be increased or an antiplatelet agent can be added, albeit with an increased risk of bleeding.

With combined antiplatelet and oral anticoagulant therapy, the risk of major hemorrhage varies from 1.3% to 24.7% . The observation in some studies that the risk of thromboembolism is reduced with the addition of aspirin is tempered by the observation of poor international normalized ratio (INR) control. Anticoagulation may be continued in the setting of infective prosthetic valve endocarditis, although the opinion is divided on the effectiveness of anticoagulation in reducing thromboembolic events in this setting.

ACUTE MANAGEMENT OF ATRIAL FIBRILLATION

Acute stroke patients may have AF with rapid ventricular response (RVR) on presenting at the hospital or they develop it during the acute hospitalization. The three major issues in this setting are determination of the type of AF (paroxysmal, persistent, recurrent or permanent), rate control, and cardioversion. Drugs that prolong the refractory period of the AV node are generally effective for rate control, resulting in rate reduction and improved cardiovascular hemodynamics. Criteria for rate control vary with age, but usually involve achieving ventricular rates of 60 to 80 per minute at rest and between 90 and 115 per minute during moderate exercise. Intravenous therapy is indicated if rapid rate control is necessary or if oral therapy is not feasible, while oral therapy may be used in hemodynamically stable patients. If pharmacological rate control therapy offers inadequate symptom relief or if the patient develops symptomatic hypotension, angina, or heart failure, then pacing, AV node ablation in conjunction with permanent pacing, or cardioversion are indicated. If cardioversion is considered, it should not be delayed to deliver therapeutic anticoagulation. In this setting, intravenous unfractionated heparin (UFH) or subcutaneous low-molecular-weight (LMW) heparin should be initiated before cardioversion or intravenous antiarrhythmic therapy. Treatment must be tailored to each individual, depending on the nature, severity, and frequency of symptoms; patient preferences; comorbid conditions; and the ongoing response to treatment.

If the patient has newly discovered paroxysmal AF, the only therapy needed is anticoagulation, unless there are significant symptoms. For the patient who has recurrent paroxysmal AF, anticoagulation and rate control are needed; if there are significant symptoms, then antiarrhythmic drugs or AV nodal ablation for antiarrhythmic drug–resistant cases may be necessary. If the patient has newly discovered persistent AF or has symptomatic AF lasting many weeks, initial therapy may be anticoagulation and rate control, while the long-term goal is to restore sinus rhythm with antiarrhythmic drugs or cardioversion. For the patient who has recurrent persistent AF, anticoagulation and rate control are needed; if there are significant symptoms, then antiarrhythmic drugs or electrical cardioversion may be necessary. In cardioversion-resistant cases, AV nodal ablation should be considered. Depending on symptoms, rate control may be a reasonable initial therapy in older patients with persistent AF who have hypertension or heart disease. For younger individuals, especially those with paroxysmal or lone AF, rhythm control may be a better initial approach. Table 9.2 shows

TABLE 9.2 Pharmacological Agents for Heart Rate Control in Atrial Fibrillation

Drug	Recommendation	Loading Dose	Onset	Maintenance Dose
Acute Setting				
No accessory pathway				
Esmolol	1C	500 μg/kg IV, 1 min	5 min	60–200 μg/kg/min IV
Metoprolol	1C	2.5–5.0 mg IV, 2 min X 3	5 min	—
Propanolol	1C	0.15 mg/kg IV	5 min	—
Diltiazem	1B	0.25 mg/kg IV, 2 min	2–7 min	5–15 mg/h IV
Verapamil	1B	0.075–0.15 mg/kg IV, 2 min	3–5 min	—
Accessory pathway				
Amiodarone	2aC	150 mg, 10 min	Days	0.5–1.0 mg/min IV
Heart failure, no accessory pathway				
Digoxin	1B	0.25 mg IV q2h to 1.5 mg	60+ min	0.125–0.375 mg/d
Amiodarone	2aC	150 mg, 10 min	Days	0.5–1.0 mg/min IV
Nonacute Setting, Chronic Maintenance				
Heart rate control				
Metoprolol	1C	—	4–6 h	25–100 mg BID
Propanolol	1C	— —	60–90 min	80–240 mg daily
Diltiazem	1B		2–4 h	120–360 mg daily
Verapamil	1B	—	1–2 h	120–360 mg daily
Heart failure, no accessory pathway				
Digoxin	1C	0.5 mg PO	2 ds	0.125–0.375 mg daily
Amiodarone	2bC	800 mg daily 1 wk, 1–3 wk	200 mg daily	
		600 mg daily 1 wk	400 mg daily 4–6 wk	

IV, intravenous; PO, orally; BID, twice daily.

From Fuster V, Ryden LE, Cannom DS, et al. ACC/AHA/ESC 2006 guidelines for the management of patients with atrial fibrillation. A report of the American College of Cardiology/American Heart Association Task Force on Practice Guidelines and the European Society of Cardiology Committee for Practice Guidelines. *J Am Coll Cardiol* 2006;48:854–906, with permission.

the pharmacological agents used to control heart rate, whether or not the patient has an accessory pathway or heart failure. Side effects of β-blockers include bradycardia, heart block, hypotension, and precipitation of heart failure or asthma. Side effects of calcium channel blockers include bradycardia, heart block, and heart failure; verapamil interacts with digoxin. Side effects of amiodarone include bradycardia, heart block, hypotension, pulmonary toxicity, skin discoloration, thyroid dysfunction, corneal deposits, optic neuropathy, and warfarin interaction.

For patients with Wolff-Parkinson-White syndrome or ventricular preexcitation, agents that slow AV node conduction will facilitate conduction across the accessory pathway, leading to ventricular tachycardia or ventricular fibrillation. In these patients, type 1 antiarrhythmic agents (disopyramide, procainamide, quinidine, mexiletine, flecainide) or amiodarone may be used acutely, while β-blockers and calcium channel blockers may be used for long-term therapy.

Cardioversion may be accomplished with pharmacological agents (simpler) or direct current electrical means (more efficacious). Conversion of AF to sinus rhythm results in transient stunning of mechanical function, with resultant stasis and potential for thrombus formation. It is common practice to administer anticoagulants for 3 weeks before and 4 weeks after electrical cardioversion for patients with AF of unknown duration or with AF for >48 hours.

The quality of evidence for evaluation of pharmacological cardioversion is limited by studies with small sample sizes, lack of standard inclusion criteria, variable intervals from drug administration to outcome assessment, and arbitrary dose selection. Pharmacologicalal cardioversion seems most effective for AF episodes >7 days in duration. Most of these patients have first-documented AF or AF with an unknown pattern, with many undergoing spontaneous conversion within 24 to 48 hours. For patients with AF episodes lasting >7 days, drug therapy is much less effective.

Table 9.3 summarizes the antiarrhythmic drugs used for pharmacological conversion and for maintaining normal sinus rhythm. Side effects of these drugs include QT-prolongation and torsade de pointes. Flecainide and propafenone may produce hypotension or atrial flutter with high ventricular rates, which may be

TABLE 9.3 Recommendations for Pharmacological Cardioversion of Atrial Fibrillation

Drug	Route of Administration	AF Duration[a]		Dosage
		<7 d	≥7 d	
Agents with proven efficacy				
Dofetilide	PO	1A	1A	Ccr: >60: 500 μg BID 40–60: 250 μg BID 20–40: 125 μg BID <20: –
Flecainide	PO, IV	1A	–	PO: 200–300 mg IV: 1.5–3.0 mg/kg, 10–20 min
Ibutilide	IV	1A	2aA	1 mg, 10 min (1–2×)
Propafenone	PO, IV	1A	–	PO: 600 mg IV: 1.5–2.0 mg/kg, 10–20 min
Amiodarone	PO, IV	2aA	2aA	IV/PO: 5–7 mg/kg, 30–60 min; then 1.2–1.8 g/d IV/PO until 10 g; then 200–400 mg/d maintenance
Less effective or incompletely studied agents				
Disopyramide	IV	2bB	2bB	
Procainamide	IV	2bB	2bC	
Quinidine	PO	2bB	2bB	
Propafenone	PO, IV	–	2bB	
Flecainide	PO, IV	–	2bB	
Should not be administered				
Digoxin	PO, IV	3A	3B	
Sotalol	PO, IV	3A	3B	

d = number of days in atrial fibrillation; PO, oral; BID, twice daily; IV, intravenous.

[a]AF duration indicates the number of days in atrial fibrillation, with numbers and letters in each column referring to the class and level of evidence of the recommendation.

From Fuster V, Ryden LE, Cannom DS, et al. ACC/AHA/ESC 2006 guidelines for the management of patients with atrial fibrillation. A report of the American College of Cardiology/American Heart Association Task Force on Practice Guidelines and the European Society of Cardiology Committee for Practice Guidelines. *J Am Coll Cardiol* 2006;48:854–906, with permission.

reduced with concomitant nondihydropyridine calcium channel antagonist therapy. The doses of digoxin and warfarin should usually be reduced on initiation of amiodarone therapy. In addition, antiarrhythmic drugs may interact with warfarin, leading to over- or under-anticoagulation and bleeding or thromboembolic complications, respectively.

Direct-current cardioversion involves delivery of a synchronized electrical shock to ensure that electrical stimulation does not occur during a vulnerable phase of the cardiac cycle. The procedure may be done under conscious sedation or general anesthesia. An initial energy of 200 J is recommended. Successful cardioversion of AF depends on the underlying heart disease and presence of therapeutic concentrations of antiarrhythmic agents. Complete shock failure and immediate recurrence occur in approximately 25%, while subacute recurrences within 2 weeks occur in approximately 25%.

Most AF patients will likely experience recurrent AF and may eventually need prophylactic antiarrhythmic drug therapy. Risk factors for AF recurrence are similar to risk factors for stroke and include advanced age, female gender, heart failure, hypertension, left atrial enlargement, and left ventricular dysfunction. The duration of anticoagulation after cardioversion depends on the likelihood that AF will recur and the patient's intrinsic risk of thromboembolism. There is no evidence that the risk of thromboembolism or stroke differs between pharmacological and electrical methods of cardioversion. There is also no evidence that cardioversion followed by prolonged maintenance of sinus rhythm effectively reduces thromboembolism in AF patients.

ANTIPLATELET AND ANTICOAGULANT THERAPY FOR ATRIAL FIBRILLATION

The coagulation cascade, pharmacology, mechanisms, sites of action, dosing, methods of administration, and monitoring of and indications for the various antiplatelet agents and old and new anticoagulant agents have recently been reviewed. A brief discussion of the anticoagulant agents is warranted.

UFH is composed of a heterogeneous group of branched glycosaminoglycans that inactivate thrombin via three dose-related mechanisms: interaction with antithrombin III, a charge-dependent interaction, and modulation of factor Xa generation. The relatively low affinity of heparin for antithrombin III leads to a relatively greater effect on platelet function when heparin binds to platelet factor 4 (PF4).

VKA or coumarins interfere with the cyclic interconversion of vitamin K and its 2, 3-epoxide via the enzyme vitamin K epoxide reductase complex 1 (VKORC1), thereby modulating the γ-carboxylation of glutamate residues on the *N*-terminal regions of vitamin K–dependent proteins (factors II, VII, IX, and X; proteins C and S). The relationship between dose and response to VKAs is modified by genetic (*CYP2C9* polymorphism of cytochrome P-450 system) and environmental (drugs, diet, disease states) factors. The VKAs in clinical use include warfarin in the United States and acenocoumarol or phenprocoumon in European and other countries. Drugs such as aspirin, nonsteroidal anti-inflammatory agents, high-dose penicillin, and moxalactam may increase VKA-related bleeding by inhibiting platelet function, while acetaminophen may interfere with cytochrome P-450 enzymes. However, in one study, acetaminophen was not shown to produce excessive anticoagulation or bleeding in a multivariate analysis. A recent study identified 10 common noncoding single-nucleotide polymorphisms and five haplotypes of VKORC1, thus permitting stratification of warfarin dose groups by VKORC1 haplotypes across race/ethnic groups. The role of genetic screening for evaluating responsiveness to warfarin therapy remains to be determined.

Direct thrombin inhibitors bind directly to both fibrin-bound and fluid-phase thrombin and block its interaction with various clotting factors and endothelial cell receptors. There are two potential advantages of these agents. First, the lack of binding to plasma proteins produces a more predictable anticoagulant response. Second, the lack of binding to PF4 means that drug action is not affected by the large amounts of PFD4 present in the vicinity of platelet-rich thrombi. Ximelagatran has several advantages over warfarin therapy: use of a fixed dose, no need to monitor anticoagulation levels, and almost no food or drug interactions.

Nonvalvular Atrial Fibrillation

Details of the randomized clinical trials comparing oral anticoagulants with placebo and aspirin/triflusal (nonaspirin salicylate) in varying doses for primary or secondary stroke prevention have recently been reviewed and are briefly summarized in Table 9.4. For example, the doses of salicylates include 75 mg of aspirin in the AFASAK study, 325 mg of aspirin in the SPAF studies, and 600 mg of triflusal in the National Study for Prevention of Embolism in Atrial Fibrillation (NASPEAF). The type of oral anticoagulant was acenocoumarol or phenprocoumon in European Atrial Fibrillation Trial (EAFT, 1993), acenocoumarol in NASPEAF, ximelagatran in SPORTIF III and V, and warfarin in the others. The intention-to-treat analysis of pooled data from the primary prevention trials revealed an annual stroke rate of 6.0% in the control group and 2.2% in the adjusted-dose warfarin group, for a relative risk reduction (RRR) of 64% (95% CI, 49% to 74%) and a number needed to treat for 1 year of 26. In a pooled analysis of the first five primary prevention trials, the effect was more significant in women (RRR = 84%; 95% CI, 55% to 95%) than men (RRR = 60%; 95% CI, 35% to 76%). In addition, anticoagulant therapy was associated with a 33% RRR (95% CI, 9% to 51%) in all cause mortality and a 48% RRR (95% CI, 34% to 90%) in the composite outcome of stroke, systemic embolism, and death. In a meta-analysis of seven trials comparing aspirin with placebo, aspirin therapy was associated with an RRR of 19% (95% CI, −1% to 35%). Among patients who received aspirin in the SPAF I to III trials, the risk of stroke was similar in patients with persistent and paroxysmal AF. In SPAF I, aspirin appeared to be more effective in preventing noncardioembolic strokes than cardioembolic strokes. One meta-analysis showed that aspirin is more effective in preventing nondisabling strokes than disabling strokes. In the secondary prevention trial, the annual stroke rate was 12% in the aspirin group and 4% in the oral anticoagulant group, for an RRR of 66% (95% CI, 43% to 80%). In a meta-analysis of 11 randomized trials comparing various antiplatelet regimens with oral anticoagulants in patients with chronic or paroxysmal AF, oral anticoagulant therapy was associated with an RRR of 37% (95% CI, 23% to 48%). Finally, reduction in all-cause mortality was greatest with warfarin-containing regimens—adjusted-dose warfarin versus control or placebo: RRR = 26% (95% CI, 3% to 43%); aspirin versus control or placebo: RRR = 14% (95% CI, −7% to 31%); adjusted-dose warfarin versus aspirin: RRR = 9% (95% CI, −19% to 30%). The

TABLE 9.4 Summary of Major Antithrombotic Trials for Stroke Prevention in Nonvalvular Atrial Fibrillation

Trial Type	Number of Trials	Secondary Prevention (%)	INR Range or Antiplatelet Dose	Strokes/ Patient- Years	RRR (95% CI)	Prevention ARR (%/y)
ADW vs. P	6	20	1.0–4.5	53/2,396 vs. 133/2,207	64 (49–74)	Primary: 2.7 Secondary: 8.4
ASA vs. P	7	30	75–1,200 mg	179/3,432 vs. 209/3,302	19 (−1–35)	Primary: 0.8 Secondary: 2.5
ADW vs. ASA	8	21	1.6-4.5	91/3,740 vs. 142/3,730	38 (18–52)	Primary: 0.7 Secondary: 7.0
ADW vs. nASA	3	22	2.0–3.5	89/5,206 vs. 140/5,216	36 (25–46)	Primary: 1.0 Secondary: NC
ADW vs. W + A	2	24	2.0–3.0	25/936 vs. 59/935	39 (22–52)	Primary: 0.9 Secondary: NC
X vs. W	2	21	2.0–3.0	77/5,606 vs. 82/5,627	8 (−38–38)	Primary: NC Secondary: NC

INR, international normalized ratio; RRR, relative risk reduction; ARR, absolute risk reduction; ADW, oral anticoagulant drug (coumarins); P, placebo or no treatment; ASA, aspirin; nASA, nonaspirin antiplatelet regimens, especially aspirin and clopidogrel; W + A, warfarin (varying doses) plus aspirin; NC, not computed; X, ximelagatran.

From Hart RG, Pearce LA, Aguilar MI. Meta-analysis: antithrombotic therapy to prevent stroke in patients who have nonvalvular atrial fibrillation. *Ann Intern Med* 2007;146:857–867, with permission.

ACTIVE-W trial (ACTIVE Writing Group, 2006) studied 6,706 patients and showed that in previously anticoagulated patients, anticoagulation therapy was superior to aspirin plus clopidogrel (RRR = 40%; 95% CI, 18% to 56%). Most recently, the Birmingham Atrial Fibrillation Treatment of the Aged (BAFTA) trial randomized 973 patients aged 75 years and older to warfarin (INR 2 to 3) versus aspirin 75 mg per day and showed that warfarin use was superior to aspirin for preventing stroke, systemic embolism, and intracranial hemorrhage (RR = 0.48; 95% CI, 0.28 to 0.80). The SPORTIF III and V trials included 7,329 patients and showed that ximelagatran is equivalent to warfarin in terms of preventing stroke (RRR = 8%, 95% CI, −38% to 38%) and systemic embolism. However, the addition of aspirin to either warfarin or ximelagatran did not reduce the occurrence of stroke, myocardial infarction, or systemic embolism. In addition, the use of ximelagatran was associated with a transient >3-fold increase in liver function tests in 6% of treated patients. As a result, ximelagatran was not approved by the Food and Drug Administration. In the NAS-PEAF study, the primary endpoint was lower in the combined treatment group of triflusal 600 mg and acenocoumarol (INR 1.4 to 2.4) than in the acenocoumarol group (INR 2.0 to 3.0) in both the intermediate-risk group (hazard ratio (HR) = 0.33; 95% CI, 0.12 to 0.91) and high-risk group (HR = 0.51; 95% CI, 0.27 to 0.96). Results were similar in patients with or without mitral stenosis and for primary or secondary stroke prevention.

DOES RATE CONTROL OR RHYTHM CONTROL MATTER?

It is logical to presume that eliminating AF and restoring sinus rhythm would abolish the perturbed physiology generating the arial thrombi, improve cardiac hemodynamics, improve exercise tolerance and quality of life and reduce mortality. Table 9.5 summarizes the five randomized clinical trials that have tested this

TABLE 9.5 Trials Comparing Rate Control and Rhythm Control in Atrial Fibrillation

Trial	Number of Patients	Age (Mean ± SD)	Percentage in SR	Stroke/ Thromboembolism(%)		Death (%)	
				Rate	Rhythm	Rate	Rhythm
AFFIRM	4060	70 ± 9 y	35% vs 63%	4.3	4.5	15.3	17.5
RACE	522	68 ± 9 y	10% vs 39%	2.7	6.0	7.0	6.8
PIAF	252	61 ± 10 y	10% vs 56%	0	1.6	1.6	1.6
STAF	200	66 ± 8 y	11% vs 26%	2.0	5.0	8.0	4.0
HOT CAFÉ	205	61 ± 11 y	NR vs 64%	1.0	2.9	1.0	2.9

SD, standard deviation; SR, sinus rhythm; AFFIRM, Atrial Fibrillation Follow-up Investigation of Rhythm Management; RACE, Rate Control Versus Electrical Cardioversion for Persistent Atrial Fibrillation; PIAF, Pharmacologic Intervention in Atrial Fibrillation; STAF, Strategies of Treatment of Atrial Fibrillation; HOT CAFÉ, How To Treat Chronic Atrial Fibrillation .

From Fuster V, Ryden LE, Cannom DS, et al. ACC/AHA/ESC 2006 guidelines for the management of patients with atrial fibrillation. A report of the American College of Cardiology/American Heart Association Task Force on Practice Guidelines and the European Society of Cardiology Committee for Practice Guidelines. *J Am Coll Cardiol* 2006;48:854–906, with permission.

hypothesis. The largest trial, the Atrial Fibrillation Follow-up Investigation of Rhythm Management (AFFIRM) trial, showed that there was no difference in all strokes, individual stroke subtypes, and mortality between the rate- and rhythm-management groups but that warfarin use reduced stroke risk regardless of assigned treatment strategy. When one considers all five trials, the rates of thromboembolism were 1.6% to 6.0% in the rhythm-control group and 0% to 4.3% in the rate-control group. The rates of mortality were 1.6% to 17.5% in the rhythm-control group and 1.0% to 15.3% in the rate-control group. There are two likely explanations for these results. First, many patients were likely to not be in sustained normal sinus rhythm. In another study of intensive monitoring of paroxysmal AF patients, there were 12 asymptomatic episodes of asymptomatic AF for every sympto-matic episode. Second, anticoagulation was more commonly discontinued in the rhythm-control group in the two largest studies. While it appears that rate control and rhythm control have similar outcomes, optimal management may require both, as well as anticoagulation.

BLEEDING RISK ASSOCIATED WITH ANTICOAGULANT THERAPY

Hemorrhage is the most important complication of anticoagulant therapy. For purposes of comparison, Table 9.6 summarizes data on systemic and intracranial hemorrhage complicating anticoagulant therapy in diverse disease states.

In an early pooled analysis, the annual rate of major hemorrhage was 1.0% in control patients and 1.3% in warfarin-treated patients. The most recent meta-analysis showed that the risk of major extracranial hemorrhage was higher in warfarin-containing regimens—adjusted-dose warfarin versus aspirin: RRR = −70% (95% CI, −234% to 14%); adjusted-dose warfarin versus control or placebo: RRR = −66% (95% CI, −235% to 18%); and aspirin versus placebo or no treatment: RRR = 2% (95% CI, −98% to 52%). In the SPORTIF III and SPORTIF V trials, the annual rates of major bleeding were: warfarin = 1.5%; warfarin + aspirin = 4.95% ($p = 0.004$); ximelagatran = 2.35%; ximelagatran + aspirin = 56.09% ($p = 0.046$). Although the number of observations in NASPEAF was small, the risk of severe bleeding was 0.92% to 2.09% in the combined treatment group and 1.80% to 2.13% in the anticoagulant therapy group. In general, factors associated with systemic bleeding include increasing age, hypertension, history of cerebrovascular disease, ischemic stroke, serious heart disease, renal insufficiency, history of gastrointestinal bleeding, history of malignancy, concomitant medications (such as aspirin), intensity of anticoagulation, and increased variation in INR values independent of the mean INR. Models for prediction of hemorrhage risk have been generated, but they should be used in conjunction with the

TABLE 9.6 Hemorrhagic Complications of Anticoagulant Therapy According to Disease State

Disease State	INR Range	Frequency of Hemorrhage (%)		
		Major	Fatal	Intracranial
Atrial fibrillation	1.5–4.5	0–6.6	0–1.1	0.2–0.5
Coronary artery disease				
UFH	–	1.0–6.8	0–0.2	–
LMWH	–	0–6.5	0–0.2	–
VKA	1.3–5.0	0–19.3	0–2.9	up to 0.4
Prosthetic heart valves	2.0–9.0	1.0–19.2	0-0.7	0–1.5
Venous thromboembolism	2.0–4.4	0–16.7	0–0.9	–
Acute ischemic stroke				
Control	–	0.3	0.1	0.3
Aspirin	–	0–1.8	0.2–1.9	0.5
UFH-SC	–	0–1.4	0.4–0.5	0.7–9.6
LMWH-SC	–	0–5.9		0–6.1
Stroke prevention				
Noncardioembolic	1.4–4.5	3.4–8.1	0.6–2.6	4.1
Intracranial stenosis	2.0–3.0	8.3	0.7	0.7

Note: Intracranial hemorrhage in atrial fibrillation or stroke prevention trials primarily refers to parenchymal or subdural hematoma, and hemorrhagic transformation in acute ischemic stroke trials.

INR, international normalized ratio; UFH, unfractionated heparin; LMWH, low-molecular-weight heparin; VKA, vitamin K antagonist; SC, subcutaneous.

From Adams HP, Davis PH. Antithrombotic therapy for acute ischemic stroke. In: Mohr JP, Choi DW, Grotta JC, Weir B, Wolf PA, eds. *Stroke: Pathophysiology, Diagnosis and Management.* 4th ed. Philadelphia, PA: Churchill Livingstone; 2004:953–969; Benavente O, Sherman D. Secondary prevention of cardioembolic stroke. In: Mohr JP, Choi DW, Grotta JC, Weir B, Wolf PA, eds. *Stroke: Pathophysiology, Diagnosis, and Management.* 4th ed. Philadelphia, PA: Churchill Livingstone; 2004:1171–1186; and Hart RG, Pearce LA, Aguilar MI. Meta-analysis: antithrombotic therapy to prevent stroke in patients who have nonvalvular atrial fibrillation. *Ann Intern Med* 2007;146:857–867; and Sloan MA. Use of anticoagulant agents for stroke prevention. *Continuum* 2005;11:97–127, with permission.

patient's functional and cognitive status, likelihood of compliance, risk of thrombosis, and patient preference. The relative value of anticoagulation clinics or services, point-of-care INR testing, or patient self-testing in minimizing anticoagulant-related bleeding complications remains to be determined.

Intracranial hemorrhage is the most common, most feared, and least treatable complication of oral anticoagulant therapy in the elderly. In an early pooled analysis, the annual rate of intracranial hemorrhage (ICH) was 0.1% in control patients and 0.3% in warfarin-treated patients. The most recent meta-analysis showed that the risk of ICH was greatest in the adjusted-dose warfarin versus aspirin trials (RRR = −128%; 95% CI, −399% to 14%). In SPAF II, the risk of ICH appeared highest in patients aged 75 years and older. However, in BAFTA, the annual risk of ICH was 1.4% in the warfarin group and 1.6% in the aspirin group. In the SPAF trials, virtually all intracranial hemorrhages were associated with an INR >3.0. Although the number of observations in NASPEAF was small, the risk of severe bleeding and ICH was 0.92% to 2.09% and 0% to 1%, respectively, in the combined treatment group and 1.80% to 2.13% and 1% to 3%, respectively, in the anticoagulant therapy group. The types of hemorrhages in long-term AF trials include parenchymal hemorrhage and subdural hematoma.

In general, oral anticoagulants increase the risk of parenchymal hemorrhage by 7- to 10-fold, with a mortality of 46% to 68%. In patients older than 60 years, the absolute risk of intraparenchymal hemorrhage is 0.3% to 1.0% per year. Factors associated with an increased risk of parenchymal hemorrhage include increasing age, intensity of anticoagulation, prior ischemic stroke, and hypertension, although precise prediction in specific patient groups is difficult. In a combined analysis of the SPIRIT and EAFT trials, patients with cerebral ischemia of presumed arterial origin had a 19-fold (95% CI, 2.4) increased risk of intracranial (89% parenchymal) hemorrhage than patients with AF after correcting for baseline differences. Independent predictors for all anticoagulant-related and intracranial hemorrhage were the intensity of INR (1.37 for each 0.5 unit increase in INR), age ≥65 years (HR = 1.9; 95% CI, 3.4) and the presence of leukoaraiosis on computed tomography (CT) scan (HR = 2.7; 95% CI, 1.4 to 5.3). Similar findings were reported in another study.

The role of neuroimaging studies in clarifying the risk of ICH with oral anticoagulant therapy is increasingly being recognized. In one study of patients with ischemic stroke, myocardial infarction, and peripheral vascular disease, the presence of white matter lesions, lacunes, cortical infarcts, and cerebral atrophy was each significantly more common in the patients with ischemic stroke. In addition, the presence of local hemosiderin deposits indicative of old microhemorrhage on magnetic resonance imaging (MRI) scans was 26% in stroke patients, 4% in myocardial infarction patients, and 13% in peripheral vascular disease patients ($p = 0.002$), with a stronger association in patients with white matter lesions. One recent study showed that the burden of cerebral microhemorrhage relates to the chronicity and severity of hypertension. Another study in patients with lobar intracerebral hemorrhage showed a correlation between white matter damage and number of microhemorrhages on gradient echo MRI, cognitive impairment before lobar hemorrhage, and cognitive decline. Small hemosiderin deposits (asymptomatic microhemorrhages) are frequently detected by gradient-echo MRI scans in patients with small vessel and white matter disease, although an association between these microvascular lesions and parenchymal hemorrhage has to date been shown for aspirin. However, accumulating data indicate that it is reasonable and prudent to be concerned that both leukoaraiosis and microhemorrhages may predispose to parenchymal bleeding during warfarin therapy.

Oral anticoagulants increase the risk of subdural hematoma by 4- to 15-fold, with a mortality of approximately 20%. The absolute rate of subdural hematoma is approximately 0.2% per year in elderly patients on oral anticoagulants. Factors associated with subdural hematoma include advanced age of the patient, intensity of anticoagulation, and perhaps cerebral atrophy.

SURGICAL AND PERCUTANEOUS INTERVENTIONAL TECHNIQUES FOR ATRIAL FIBRILLATION

Interventional approaches are based on the reentrant mechanism of AF development and maintenance and the concept that atrial incisions at critical locations would create barriers to conduction and sustained AF. The three main categories of intervention include surgical procedures, catheter ablation, and obliteration of the left atrial appendage.

Surgical techniques include the Maze procedure, which uses cut-and-sew techniques that ensure transmural lesions to isolate the pulmonary veins, connect these dividing lines to the mitral valve annulus, and thereby prevent macroentrant rhythms, such as AF and atrial flutter. The Maze procedure can be performed as an isolated procedure or be added to another cardiac operation. This procedure can be performed with a minimally invasive small chest wall incision, although the operation typically requires cardiopulmonary bypass. Atrial transport function is preserved in over 90% of cases. Rates for restoration of sinus rhythm have varied from 70% to 99%, with an operative mortality of <1% to 2% and the need for permanent pacemaker in 5% to 10%. When combined with obliteration of the left atrial appendage, there is a substantial reduction in postoperative thromboembolic events, such as stroke. Other risks of the procedure include bleeding necessitating reoperation, impaired atrial transport, transient postoperative AF in up to 38%, delayed atrial arrhythmias such as atrial flutter, and atrioesophageal fistula.

The technique of radiofrequency catheter ablation has evolved from the targeting of individual foci to the circumferential electrical isolation of the entire pulmonary vein musculature. Variations of this latter technique have been associated with approximately 90% success for paroxysmal AF and 80% success for persistent AF. In select patients, ablation has led to improved quality of life and reduced morbidity and mortality due to heart failure and thromboembolism. Complications occur in up to 6% and include pulmonary vein stenosis, thromboembolism, stroke (0% to 5%), atrioesophageal fistula, and left atrial flutter. However, the long-term efficacy of this procedure has not been firmly established. In addition, there is a need for randomized trials in which there is blinded evaluation of outcomes.

Obliteration of the left atrial appendage is based on the observations that left atrial appendage thrombus occurs in 57% of valvular AF patients and 90% of nonvalvular AF patients and the concept that such obliteration may reduce stroke risk. Techniques include left atrial obliteration (typically at the time of open mitral valve surgery), thoracoscopic left atrial appendectomy, or percutaneous transcatheter occlusion. Surgical occlusion is associated with complete occlusion rates of 45% to 72%. Current research involves use of the PLAATO and WATCHMAN percutaneous systems, which often require general anesthesia. Preliminary data report incomplete occlusion in 0% to 2% and stroke in 0% to 3%. Complications of percutaneous techniques include over- or undersizing of the device, migration of the device, dislodgement, embolization, cardiac perforation, hemopericardium (6%), and water retention due to reduced release of atrial natriuretic factor.

SPECIAL PRACTICE SITUATIONS

Warfarin effectively reduces the annual risk of stroke from nonvalvular AF. Recent data confirm its benefit in patients older than 75 years. Warfarin therapy has been shown to be highly cost effective. The choice of optimal antithrombotic therapy varies according to individual patient characteristics and clinical settings. There are several common or serious scenarios that require special consideration.

Table 9.7 summarizes current guidelines on antithrombotic therapy for AF. Patients younger than 65 years and with no stroke risk factors or those with lone AF have a low stroke risk (<1% per year); aspirin therapy (81 to 325 mg) seems adequate in these populations. The threshold for use of anticoagulation may be an annual stroke risk of 3% to 5%. All patients with a history of prior stroke or TIA require anticoagulation unless contraindications exist. One early observational study showed that anticoagulation resulting in an INR of ≥2.0 reduces the frequency, severity, and risk of death from AF-related stroke. More recent studies demonstrate up to 53% reduction in poststroke mortality with warfarin therapy, even in patients aged 75 years and older. Table 9.8 summarizes the treatment recommendations for antithrombotic therapy for AF in diverse settings. The combination of aspirin and warfarin is associated with an increased risk of major hemorrhage and should be avoided unless there is a compelling indication. In patients who have atrial flutter, it is reasonable and prudent to estimate stroke risk using similar stratification criteria until more robust data become known.

The question frequently arises as to whether patients with an acute AF-related ischemic stroke should receive intravenous heparin. Data summarized from three recent clinical trials indicate an early recurrent ischemic stroke rate of approximately 5% within 2 weeks of onset of an AF-associated ischemic stroke. As such, urgent anticoagulation with UFH or LMW heparin is not recommended to prevent early recurrent ischemic stroke. Aspirin and warfarin may be begun within 48 hours of stroke onset and the aspirin can be discontinued when the INR reaches target value.

An acute stroke patient with AF or atrial flutter and rapid ventricular response may experience angina, heart failure, or hypotension that does not respond to medical management. However, formal data to systematically address this issue are not available. In the nonacute stroke setting, TEE may be used to detect left atrial or left atrial appendage thrombus. If clot is detected, a high risk of thromboembolism is identified and several weeks of anticoagulation is recommended before attempted cardioversion. If TEE does not show clot, then intravenous anticoagulation is initiated followed by cardioversion. In the setting of AF-related acute stroke with the aforementioned significant cardiovascular symptoms and signs, the following approach might be considered. If

TABLE 9.7 2006 AHA/ACC/ESC Recommendations: Antiplatelet/Anticoagulant Therapy for Stroke Prevention in Nonvalvular Atrial Fibrillation

Risk Category	Recommended Therapy
No risk factors	Aspirin, 81–325 mg daily
One moderate risk factor	Aspirin, 81–325 mg daily, or warfarin (INR 2.0–3.0, target 2.5)
Any high risk factor or .1 moderate risk factor	Warfarin (INR 2.0–3.0, target 2.5)

Risk Factors

Less validated/weaker	*Moderate*	*High*
Female gender	Age ≥75 y	Prior stroke, TIA, or embolism
Age 65–74 y	Hypertension	Mitral stenosis
Coronary artery disease	Heart failure	Prosthetic heart valve[a]
Thyrotoxicosis	LV EF ≤ 35%	
	Diabetes mellitus	

AHA, American Heart Association; ACC, American College of Cardiology; ESC, European Society of Cardiology; INR, international normalized ratio; TIA, transient ischemic attack; LV, left ventricular; EF, ejection fraction.

[a] If mechanical valve, target INR >2.5.

From Guyatt G, Schunemann HJ, Cook D, et al. Applying the grades of recommendation for antithrombotic and thrombolytic therapy. *Chest* 2004;126:179S–187S.; Salem DN, Stein PD, Al-Ahmad A, et al. Antithrombotic therapy in valvular heart disease—native and prosthetic. *Chest* 2004;126:457S–482S.; Singer DE, Albers GW, Dalen JE, et al. Antithrombotic therapy in atrial fibrillation. *Chest* 2004;126: 429S–456S and Sloan MA. Use of anticoagulant agents for stroke prevention. *Continuum* 2005;11: 97–127, with permission.

TABLE 9.8 2004 ACCP Recommendations: Antiplatelet/Anticoagulant Therapy for Stroke Prevention in Atrial Fibrillation

Indication	Agent	aPTT/INR Range	Grade
Nonvalvular AF			
Age <65 y, no stroke risk factors	Aspirin 325 mg	—	1B
Age 65–75 y, no stroke risk factors	Aspirin 325 mg or VKA	2.5 (2.0–3.0)	1A
Any age, ≥1 stroke risk factor	VKA	2.5 (2.0–3.0)	1A
After cardiac surgery, >48 h duration	VKA	2.5 (2.0–3.0)	2C
Cardioversion			
Elective CV planned, AF duration >48 h or unknown	VKA3 wk pre, 4 wk post	2.5 (2.0–3.0)	1C+
CV urgent/emergent, AF duration <48 h	UFH	50-70 s	
	VKA 4 wk post	2.5 (2.0–3.0)	2C
TEE shows clot, CV cancelled	VKA	2.5 (2.0–3.0)	1B
Contraindication to anticoagulant therapy	Aspirin	—	1A
Valvular AF	VKA	2.5 (2.0–3.0)	1C+
Rheumatic mitral valve disease	VKA	2.5 (2.0–3.0)	1C+
Prosthetic heart valves (mechanical, tissue)	VKA	2.5 (2.0–3.0)	2C
Atrial Flutter, with or without CV			

aPTT, activated partial thromboplastin time; INR, international normalized ratio; AF, atrial fibrillation; VKA, vitamin K antagonist; UFH, unfractionated heparin; TEE, transesophageal echocardiography.

From Guyatt G, Schunemann HJ, Cook D, et al. Applying the grades of recommendation for antithrombotic and thrombolytic therapy. *Chest* 2004;126:179S–187S; Salem DN, Stein PD, Al-Ahmad A, et al. Antithrombotic therapy in valvular heart disease—native and prosthetic. *Chest* 2004;126:457S–482S; Singer DE, Albers GW, Dalen JE, et al. Antithrombotic therapy in atrial fibrillation. *Chest* 2004;126:429S–456S. and Sloan MA. Use of anticoagulant agents for stroke prevention. *Continuum* 2005;11:97–127, with permission.

antiarrhythmic therapy has not been administered, it should be given following anticoagulation and before cardioversion. If TEE shows no clot, then anticoagulation followed by cardioversion may be performed at unknown but likely higher stroke risk. If TEE shows clot, anticoagulation followed by cardioversion may be performed at high risk. In a life-threatening situation, the benefits of this approach may outweigh the risks.

The results of clinical trials translate well into clinical practice, with similar rates of stroke and major bleeding and an increased risk of minor bleeding. Despite these findings, warfarin therapy for stroke prevention in nonvalvular AF in fee-for-service Medicare beneficiaries is either underutilized or inappropriately utilized, with little incremental change from 1998 to 2001. It is possible that clinicians may fear selection of warfarin therapy because of the risk of falls. Interestingly, a recent Markov decision analytic model determined that for patients with average risk of stroke and falling, warfarin therapy was associated with 12.90 quality-adjusted life-years per patient, aspirin therapy was associated with 11.17 quality-adjusted life-years per patient, and no antithrombotic therapy was associated with 10.15 quality-adjusted life-years per patient. Sensitivity analyses demonstrated that regardless of age or baseline stroke risk, the risk of falling was not an important factor in determining the choice of antithrombotic therapy. However, in practice, the nature and severity of the stroke-related neurological deficit and any preexisting neurological findings (such as loss of proprioception due to peripheral neuropathy or a gait disorder) are important factors in choosing antithrombotic therapy. The greater the degree of gait instability of any cause, the less likely a patient will be placed on oral anticoagulation.

Fortunately, patients may only infrequently experience intracerebral, subdural, or subarachnoid hemorrhage while on anticoagulant therapy. Data from CT and MRI scans have assumed more importance in the resumption of antithrombotic therapies in this setting. The presence of microhemorrhages on the gradient echo sequence of MRI studies may indicate the presence of an underlying cerebral microangiopathy or cerebral amyloid angiopathy. In one study, the risk of anticoagulant-related intracranial hemorrhage was 9.3% in patients with microhemorrhages and 1.3% in patients without microhemorrhages. A recent decision analysis recommended against restarting anticoagulation in patients with lobar hemorrhage (possibly secondary to cerebral amyloid angiopathy) and AF. Such findings would increase the likelihood that an otherwise appropriate patient may not receive warfarin therapy. However, if the CHADS2 score indicates high stroke risk, then under certain circumstances one might favor more tightly controlled warfarin therapy, such as INR 2.0 to 2.5, unless a contraindication exists. In general, anticoagulation may be resumed 3 to 4 weeks after intracerebral or subdural hemorrhage. Patients with aneurysmal subarachnoid hemorrhage must have the aneurysm secured before anticoagulation can be resumed. However, recent data suggest that the risk of oral anticoagulant-related intracerebral hemorrhage appears to be increasing; stringent control of the INR assumes even greater importance.

On occasion, patients may require interruption of long-term oral anticoagulation for diagnostic or therapeutic procedures. In patients with mechanical prosthetic heart valves, it is generally appropriate to substitute UFH or LMW heparin to prevent thrombosis. In patients with AF who do not have mechanical prosthetic valves, anticoagulation may be interrupted for up to 1 week for diagnostic or surgical procedures that carry a high risk of bleeding without substituting heparin. In high-risk patients (prior stroke, TIA, systemic embolism), or when a series of procedures requires interruption of oral anticoagulant therapy for longer periods, UFH or LMW heparin may be administered intravenously or subcutaneously.

The role of interventional techniques in the management of AF is evolving. In patients with recurrent paroxysmal or recurrent persistent AF where antiarrhythmic treatment does not result in maintenance of sinus rhythm, ablation may be considered. For prevention of stroke, data are too limited to recommend use of the PLAATO and WATCHMAN systems outside of randomized clinical trials.

CONCLUSION

The benefit of careful oral anticoagulant therapy for stroke prevention is clearly established in patients with nonvalvular AF. At this time, careful patient selection and strict attention to maintaining the INR within the therapeutic range are the best ways to minimize both ischemic and hemorrhagic complications of therapy. On the basis of their properties, the direct thrombin inhibitors appear to be the most promising pharmacological agents to be studied in future clinical trials of stroke prevention in AF. The role of left atrial appendage obliteration is undefined.

SELECTED REFERENCES

ACTIVE Writing Group on behalf of the ACTIVE Investigators. Clopidogrel plus aspirin versus oral anticoagulation for atrial fibrillation in the Atrial fibrillation Clopidogrel Trial with Irbesatan for prevention of Vascular Events (ACTIVE-W): a randomised controlled trial. *Lancet* 2006; 367:1903–1912.

Adams HP, Davis PH. Antithrombotic therapy for acute ischemic stroke. In: Mohr JP, Choi DW, Grotta JC, Weir B, Wolf PA, eds. *Stroke: Pathophysiology, Diagnosis and Management.* 4th ed. Philadelphia, PA: Churchill Livingstone; 2004:953–969.

Albers GW, Amarenco P, Easton JD, et al. Antithrombotic and thrombolytic therapy for ischemic stroke. *Chest* 2004;126:483S–512S.

Albers GW, Diener HC, Frison L, et al. Ximelagatran versus warfarin for stroke prevention in patients with nonvalvular atrial fibrillation: a randomized trial. *JAMA* 2005;293:690–698.

Akins PT, Feldman HA, Zoble R, et al. Secondary stroke prevention with ximelagatran versus warfarin in patients with atrial fibrillation. *Stroke* 2007;38:874–880.

Andersen KK, Olsen TS. Reduced poststroke mortality in patients with stroke and atrial fibrillation treated with anticoagulants. Results from a Danish quality-control registry of 22,179 patients with ischemic stroke. *Stroke* 2007;38:259–263.

Ansell J, Hirsh J, Poller L, et al. The pharmacology and management of the vitamin K antagonists. *Chest* 2004;126:204S–233S.

Atrial Fibrillation Investigators. Risk factors for stroke and efficacy of antithrombotic therapy in atrial fibrillation. *Arch Intern Med* 1994;154: 1449–1457.

Atrial Fibrillation Investigators. Echocardiographic predictors of stroke in patients with atrial fibrillation: a prospective study of 1066 patients from 3 clinical trials. *Arch Intern Med* 1998;158:1316–1320.

Atrial Fibrillation Investigators. The efficacy of aspirin in patients with atrial fibrillation: analysis of pooled data from 3 randomized trials. *Arch Intern Med* 1997;157:1237–1240.

Benavente O, Sherman D. Secondary prevention of cardioembolic stroke. In: Mohr JP, Choi DW, Grotta JC, Weir B, Wolf PA, eds. *Stroke: Pathophysiology, Diagnosis, and Management.* 4th ed. Philadelphia, PA: Churchill Livingstone; 2004:1171–1186.

Berge E, Abdelnoor M, Nakstad PH, et al. Low-molecular-weight heparin versus aspirin in patients with acute ischaemic stroke and atrial fibrillation: a double-blind randomized study. HAEST Study Group. *Lancet* 2000;355:1205–1210.

Beyth RJ, Quinn LM, Landefeld CS. Prospective evaluation of an index for predicting risk of major bleeding in outpatients treated with warfarin. *Am J Med* 1998;105:91–99.

Boston Area Anticoagulation Trial for Atrial Fibrillation Investigators. The effect of low-dose warfarin on the risk of stroke in patients with nonrheumatic atrial fibrillation. *New Engl J Med* 1990;323:1505–1511.

Cappato R, Calkins H, Chen SA, et al. Worldwide survey on the methods, efficacy, and safety of catheter ablation for human atrial fibrillation. *Circulation* 2005;111:1100–1105.

Carlsson J, Miketic S, Windeler J, et al. STAF Investigators.: Randomized trial of rate-control versus rhythm-control in persistent atrial fibrillation: the Strategies of Treatment of Atrial Fibrillation (STAF) study. *J Am Coll Cardiol* 2003;41:1690–1696.

Connolly SJ, Laupacis A, Gent M, et al. Canadian Atrial Fibrillation Anticoagulation (CAFA) study. *J Am Coll Cardiol* 1991;18:349–355.

Cox JL, Ad N, Palazzo T, et al. Current status of the Maze procedure for the treatment of atrial fibrillation. *Semin Thorac Cardiovasc Surg* 2000; 12:15–19.

Eckman MH, Rosand J, Knudsen KA, et al. Can patients be anticoagulated after intracerebral hemorrhage? A decision analysis. *Stroke* 2003; 34:1710–1716.

European Atrial Fibrillation Trial Study Group. Secondary prevention in non-rheumatic atrial fibrillation after transient ischaemic attack or minor stroke. *Lancet* 1993;342:1255–1262.

Evans A, Kalra L. Are the results of randomized controlled trials on anticoagulation in patients with atrial fibrillation generalizable to clinical practice? *Arch Intern Med* 2001;161:1443–1447.

Executive Steering Committee on behalf of the SPORTIF III Investigators. Stroke prevention with the oral direct thrombin inhibitor ximelagatran compared with warfarin in patients with non-valvular atrial fibrillation (SPORTIF III): randomised controlled trial. *Lancet* 2003;362:1691–1698.

Ezekowitz MD, Bridgers SL, James KE, et al. Warfarin in the prevention of stroke associated with nonrheumatic atrial fibrillation. *New Engl J Med* 1992;327:1406–1412.

Ezekowitz MD, Levine JA. Preventing stroke in patients with atrial fibrillation. *JAMA* 1999;281:1830–1835.

Fan YH, Zhang L, Lam WW, et al. Cerebral microbleeds as a risk factor for subsequent intracerebral hemorrhages among patients with acute ischemic stroke. *Stroke* 2003;34:2459–2462.

Fitzmaurice DA, Hobbs FDR, Jowett S, et al. Screening versus routine practice in detection of atrial fibrillation in patients aged 65 years and older: cluster randomized controlled trial. *BMJ* 2007;ONLINE FIRST:1–6.

Flaherty ML, Kissela B, Woo D, et al. The increasing incidence of anticoagulant-associated intracerebral hemorrhage. *Neurology* 2007;68: 116–121.

Fuster V, Ryden LE, Cannom DS, et al. ACC/AHA/ESC 2006 guidelines for the management of patients with atrial fibrillation. A report of the American College of Cardiology/American Heart Association Task Force on Practice Guidelines and the European Society of Cardiology Committee for Practice Guidelines. *J Am Coll Cardiol* 2006;48:854–906.

Gage BF, Cardinalli AB, Albers GW, et al. Cost effectiveness of warfarin and aspirin for prophylaxis of stroke in patients with nonvalvular atrial fibrillation. *JAMA* 1995;274:1839–1845.

Gage BF, Waterman AD, Shannon W, et al. Validation of clinical classification schemes for predicting stroke: results from the National Registry of Atrial Fibrillation. *JAMA* 2001;285:2864–2870.

Gillinov AM, McCarhy PM. Advances in the surgical treatment of atrial fibrillation. *Cardiol Clin* 2004;22:147–157.

Gillinov AM. Advances in surgical treatment of atrial fibrillation. *Stroke* 2007;38(Part 2):618–623.

Go AS, Hylek EM, Phillips KA, et al., for the AnTicoagulation and Risk Factors in Atrial Fibrillation (ATRIA) Study. Prevalence of diagnosed atrial fibrillation in adults: national implications for rhythm management and stroke prevention. *JAMA* 2001;285:2370–2375.

Go AS, Hylek EM, Chang Y, et al. Anticoagulation therapy for stroke prevention in atrial fibrillation: How well do randomized trials translate into clinical practice? *JAMA* 2003;290:2685–2692.

Gorelick PB. Combining aspirin with oral anticoagulant therapy: Is this a safe and effective practice in patients with atrial fibrillation? *Stroke* 2007;38:1652–1654.

Gorter JW. Major bleeding during anticoagulation after cerebral ischemia: patterns and risk factors. Stroke Prevention in Reversible Ischemia Trial (SPIRIT) and European Atrial Fibrillation Trial (EAFT) study groups. *Neurology* 1999;53:1319–1327.

Gullov AL, Koefoed BG, Petersen P, et al. Fixed mini-dose warfarin and aspirin alone and in combination versus adjusted-dose warfarin for stroke prevention in atrial fibrillation: Second Copenhagen Atrial Fibrillation, Aspirin, and Anticoagulation Study. *Arch Intern Med* 1998;158: 1513–1521.

Guyatt G, Schunemann HJ, Cook D, et al. Applying the grades of recommendation for antithrombotic and thrombolytic therapy. *Chest* 2004;126:179S–187S.

Halperin JL, Ximelagatran: direct thrombin inhibition as anticoagulant therapy in atrial fibrillation. *J Am Coll Cardiol* 2005;45:1–9.

Hart RG. What causes intracerebral hemorrhage during warfarin therapy? *Neurology* 2000;55:907–908.

Hart RG, Boop BS, Anderson DC. Oral anticoagulants and intracranial hemorrhage: facts and hypotheses. *Stroke* 1995;26:1471–1477.

Hart RG, Halperin JL. Atrial fibrillation and thromboembolism: a decade of progress in stroke prevention. *Ann Intern Med* 1999;131:688–695.

Hart RG, Pearce LA, McBride R, et al. Factors associated with ischemic stroke during aspirin therapy in atrial fibrillation: analysis of 2012 participants in the SPAF I-III clinical trials. *Stroke* 1999;30:1223–1229.

Hart RG, Palacio S, Pearce LA. Atrial fibrillation, stroke, and acute antithrombotic therapy: analysis of randomized clinical trials. *Stroke* 2002;33:2722–2727.

Hart RG, Pearce LA, Rothbart RM, et al. Stroke with intermittent atrial fibrillation: incidence and predictors during aspirin therapy. *J Am Coll Cardiol* 2000;35:183–187.

Hart RG, Pearce LA, Aguilar MI. Meta-analysis: antithrombotic therapy to prevent stroke in patients who have nonvalvular atrial fibrillation. *Ann Intern Med* 2007;146:857–867.

Healey JS, Crystal E, Lamy A, et al. Left atrial appendage occlusion study (LAAOS): results of randomized controlled pilot study of left atrial appendage occlusion during coronary artery bypass surgery in patients at risk for stroke. *Am Heart J* 2005;150:288–293.

Hellemons BS, Langenberg M, Lodder J, et al. Primary prevention of arterial thromboembolism in non-rheumatic atrial fibrillation in primary care: randomised controlled trial comparing two intensities of coumarin with aspirin. *BMJ* 1999;319:958–964.

Healy JS, Baranchuk A, Crystal E, et al. Prevention of atrial fibrillation with angiotensin-converting enzyme inhibitors and angiotensin receptor blockers: a meta-analysis. *J Am Coll Cardiol* 2005;45:1832–1839.

Hirsh J, Raschke R. Heparin and low-molecular-weight heparin. *Chest* 2004;126:188S–203S.

Hohnloser SH, Kuck KH, Lilienthal J. Rhythm or rate control in atrial fibrillation—Pharmacologic Intervention in Atrial Fibrillation (PIAF): a randomized trial. *Lancet* 2000;356:1789–1794.

Hsu LF, Jais P, Sanders P, et al. Catheter ablation for atrial fibrillation in congestive heart failure. *New Engl J Med* 2004;351:2373–2383.

Hylek EM, Singer DE. Risk factors for intracranial hemorrhage in outpatients taking warfarin. *Ann Intern Med* 1994;120:897–902.

Hylek EM, Heiman H, Skates SJ, et al. Acetominophen and other risk factors for excessive warfarin anticoagulation. *JAMA* 1998;279:657–662.

Hylek EM, Go AS, Chang Y, et al. Effect of intensity of oral anticoagulation on stroke severity and mortality in atrial fibrillation. *New Engl J Med* 2003;349:1019–1026.

Jencks SF, Cuerdon T, Burwen DR, et al. Quality of medical care delivered to Medicare beneficiaries: a profile at state and national levels. *JAMA* 2000;284:1670–1676.

Jencks SF, Huff ED, Cuerdon T. Change in the quality of care delivered to Medicare beneficiaries, 1998–1999 to 2000–2001. *JAMA* 2003;289: 305–312.

Kato H, Izumiyama M, Izumiyama K, et al. Silent cerebral microbleeds on T2-weighted MRI: correlation with stroke subtype, stroke recurrence, and leukoaraiosis. *Stroke* 2002;33:1536–1540.

Kim DE, Bae HJ, Lee SH, et al. Gradient echo magnetic resonance imaging in the prediction of hemorrhagic vs. ischemic stroke: a need for the consideration of the extent of leukoaraiosis. *Arch Neurol* 2002;59: 425–429.

Kimura K, Minematsu K, Yamaguchi T, for the Japan Multicenter Stroke Investigator's Collaboration (J-MUSIC). Atrial fibrillation as a predictive factor for severe stroke and early death in 15,831 patients with acute ischaemic stroke. *J Neurol Neurosurg Psych* 2005;76:679–683.

Kopecky SL, Gersh BJ, McGoon MD, et al. The natural history of lone atrial fibrillation. A population-based study over three decades. *New Engl J Med* 1987;317:669–674.

Kwa VIH, Franke CL, Verbeeten B, et al., for the Amsterdam Vascular Medicine Group. Silent intracerebral microhemorrhages in patients with ischemic stroke. *Ann Neurol* 1998;44:372–377.

Levine MN, Raskob G, Beyth RJ, et al. Hemorrhagic complications of anticoagulant treatment. *Chest* 2004;126:287S–310S. *Mayo Clin Proc* 1999;74:862–869.

Levy S, Maarek M, Coumel P, et al. Characteristics of different subsets of atrial fibrillation in general practice in France: the AIFLA study. The College of French Cardiologists. *Circulation* 1999;99:3028–3035.

Mant J, Hobbs R, Fletcher K, et al., on behalf of the BAFTA Investigators and the Midland Research Practices Network (MidReC). Warfarin versus aspirin for stroke prevention in an elderly community population with atrial fibrillation (the Birmingham Atrial Fibrillation Treatment of the Aged Study, BAFTA): a randomized controlled trial. *Lancet* 2007;370:493–503.

Meier B, Palacios I, Windecker S, et al. Transcatheter left atrial appendage occlusion with Amplatzer devices to obviate anticoagulation in patients with atrial fibrillation. *Catheter Cardiovasc Interv* 2003;60:417–422.

Miller VT, Rothrock JF, Pearce LA, et al., on behalf of the Stroke Prevention in Atrial Fibrillation Investigators. Ischemic stroke in patients with atrial fibrillation: effect of aspirin according to stroke mechanism. *Neurology* 1993;43:32–36.

Onalan O, Crystal E. Left atrial appendage exclusion for stroke prevention in patients with nonrheumatic atrial fibrillation. *Stroke* 2007;38(Pt 2):624–630.

Opolski G, Torbicki A, Kosior DA, et al. Investigators of the Polish How to Treat Chronic Atrial Fibrillation Study. Rate control vs rhythm control in patients with nonvalvular atrial fibrillation: the results of the Polish How to Treat Chronic Atrial Fibrillation (HOT CAFÉ) Study. *Chest* 2004; 126:476–486.

Oral H, Scharf C, Chugh A, et al. Catheter ablation for paroxysmal atrial ablation. *Circulation* 2003;108:2355–2360.

Ostermayer SH, Reisman M, Kramer PH, et al. Percutaneous left atrial appendage occlusion (PLAATO System) to prevent stroke in high-risk patients with non-rheumatic atrial fibrillation: results from the international multicenter feasibility trials. *J Am Coll Cardiol* 2005;46:9–14.

Page RL, Wilkinson WE, Clair WK, et al. Asymptomatic arrhythmias in patients with symptomatic paroxysmal atrial fibrillation and paroxysmal supraventricular tachycardia. *Circulation* 1994;89:224–227.

Pappone C, Rosanio S, Augello G, et al. Mortality, morbidity, and quality of life after circumferential pulmonary vein ablation for atrial fibrillation: outcomes from a controlled nonrandomized long-term study. *J Am Coll Cardiol* 2003;42:185–197.

Perez-Gomez F, Alegria E, Berjon J, et al., for the NASPEAF Investigators. Comparative effects of antiplatelet, anticoagulant, or combined therapy in patients with valvular or nonvalvular atrial fibrillation. *J Am Coll Cardiol* 2004;44:1557–1566.

Peters NS, Schilling RJ, Kanagaratnam P, et al. Atrial fibrillation: strategies to control, combat, and cure. *Lancet* 2002;359:593–603.

Petersen P, Boysen G, Godtfredsen J, et al. Placebo-controlled, randomized trial of warfarin and aspirin for prevention of thromboembolic complications in chronic atrial fibrillation. *Lancet* 1989;1:175–179.

Powers WJ. Oral anticoagulant therapy for the prevention of stroke. *New Engl J Med* 2001;345:1493–1495.

Psaty BM, Manolio TA, Kuller LH, et al. Incidence of and risk factors for atrial fibrillation in older adults. *Circulation* 1997;96:2455–2461.

Reider MJ, Reiner AJ, Gage BF, et al. Effect of VKORC1 haplotypes on transcriptional regulation and warfarin dose. *New Engl J Med* 2005;352:2285–2293.

Salem DN, Stein PD, Al-Ahmad A, et al. Antithrombotic therapy in valvular heart disease—native and prosthetic. *Chest* 2004;126:457S–482S.

Saxena R, Lewis S, Berge E, et al., for the International Stroke Trial Collaborative Group. Risk of early death and recurrent stroke and effect of heparin in 3169 patients with acute ischemic stroke and atrial fibrillation in the International Stroke Trial. *Stroke* 2001;32:2333–2337.

Sherman DG. Stroke prevention in atrial fibrillation. Pharmacological rate versus rhythm control. *Stroke* 2007;38(Pt 2):615–617.

Singer DE, Albers GW, Dalen JE, et al. Antithrombotic therapy in atrial fibrillation. *Chest* 2004;126:429S–456S.

Sloan MA. Use of anticoagulant agents for stroke prevention. *Continuum* 2005;11:97–127.

Smith EE, Rosand J, Knudsen KA, et al. Leukoaraiosis is associated with warfarin-related hemorrhage following ischemic stroke. *Neurology* 2002;59:193–197.

Smith EE, Gurol ME, Eng JA, et al. White matter lesions, cognition, and recurrent hemorrhage in patients with lobar intracerebral hemorrhage. *Neurology* 2004;63:1606–1612.

Stroke Prevention in Atrial Fibrillation Investigators. Stroke Prevention in Atrial Fibrillation Study: Final results. *Circulation* 1991;84:527–539.

Stroke Prevention in Atrial Fibrillation Investigators. Warfarin versus aspirin for prevention of thromboembolism in atrial fibrillation: Stroke Prevention in Atrial Fibrillation II Study. *Lancet* 1994;343:687–691.

Stroke Prevention in Atrial Fibrillation Investigators. Bleeding during antithrombotic therapy in patients with atrial fibrillation. *Arch Intern Med* 1996;156:409–416.

Stroke Prevention in Atrial Fibrillation Investigators. Risk factors for thromboembolism during aspirin therapy in patients with atrial fibrillation: the Stroke Prevention in Atrial Fibrillation Study. *J Stroke Cerebrovasc Ds*_1995;5:147–157.

Stroke Prevention in Atrial Fibrillation Investigators. Adjusted-dose warfarin versus low-intensity, fixed-dose warfarin plus aspirin for high risk patients with atrial fibrillation: Stroke Prevention in Atrial Fibrillation III randomised clinical trial. *Lancet* 1996a;348:633–638.

The Stroke Risk in Atrial Fibrillation Working Group. Independent predictors of stroke in patients with atrial fibrillation. *Neurology* 2007;69:546–554.

Tsivgoulis G, Spengos K, Zakopoulos N, et al. Efficacy of anticoagulation for secondary stroke prevention in older people with non-valvular atrial fibrillation: a prospective case series study. *Age Ageing* 2005;34:35–40.

Van Gelder IC, Hagens VE, Bosker HA, et al. Rate Control versus Electrical Cardioversion for Persistent Atrial Fibrillation Study Group: a comparison of rate control and rhythm control in patients with recurrent persistent atrial fibrillation. *New Engl J Med* 2002;347:1834–1840.

van der Meer FJ, Rosendaal FR, Van Den Broucke JP, et al. Bleeding complications in oral anticoagulant therapy: an analysis of risk factors. *Arch Intern Med* 1993;153:1557–1562.

van Walraven C, Hart RG, Singer DE, et al. Oral anticoagulants vs aspirin in nonvalvular atrial fibrillation: an individual patient meta-analysis. *JAMA* 2002;288:2441–2448.

van Walraven WC, Hart RG, Wells GA, et al. A clinical prediction rule to identify patients with atrial fibrillation and a low risk for stroke while taking aspirin. *Arch Intern Med* 2003;163:936–943.

Vemmos KN, Tsivgoulis T, Spengos K, et al. Anticoagulation influences long-term outcome in patients with non-valvular atrial fibrillation and severe ischemic stroke. *Am J Geriatr Pharmacother* 2004;2:265–273.

Wang TJ, Massaro JM, Levy D, et al. A risk score for predicting stroke or death in individuals with new-onset atrial fibrillation in the community: The Framingham Heart Study. *JAMA* 2003;290:1049–1056.

Wang TJ, Parise H, Levy D, et al.. Obesity and the risk of new-onset atrial fibrillation. *JAMA* 2004;292:2471–2477.

Wazni OM, Marrouche NF, Martin DO, et al. Radiofrequency ablation vs. antiarrhythmic drugs as first-line treatment of symptomatic atrial fibrillation: a randomized trial. *JAMA* 2005;293:2634–2640.

Weitz JI, Hirsh J, Samama MM. New anticoagulant drugs. *Chest* 2004;126:265S–286S.

Wintzen AR, Tijssen JGP. Subdural hematoma and oral anticoagulant therapy. *Arch Neurol* 1982;39:69–72.

Wolf PA, Abbott RD, Kannel WB. Atrial fibrillation as an independent risk factor for stroke: the Framingham Study. *Stroke* 1991;22:983–988.

Wong KS, Chan YL, Liu JY, et al. Asymptomatic microbleeds as a risk factor for aspirin-associated intracerebral hemorrhages. *Neurology* 2003;60:511–513.

Wyse DG, Waldo AL, DiMarco JP, et al. Atrial Fibrillation Follow-up Investigation of Rhythm Management (AFFIRM) Investigators: a comparison of rate control and rhythm control in patients with atrial fibrillation. *New Engl J Med* 2002;347:1825–1833.

CHAPTER 10

Management of Extracranial Carotid Artery Pathology

CAMILO R. GOMEZ AND JAMES D. GEYER

OBJECTIVES

- What are the goals of therapy in patients with extracranial carotid artery pathology?
- What criteria need to be used to decide how to treat patients with extracranial carotid artery pathology?
- When is endovascular therapy of the extracranial carotid artery indicated?
- When is surgical therapy indicated?
- Which patients should be considered for each form of revascularization?
- What is the best approach to the asymptomatic patient?

Carotid artery pathology is one of the most important risk factors for ischemic stroke. Therefore, stroke prevention by appropriate management of carotid artery pathology is a very important aspect of every day neurological practice. The primary goals are to identify patients at risk for stroke from carotid artery pathology and to allocate each of them to the best therapeutic strategy available. Such an approach requires fundamental knowledge about the multiple dimensions of carotid artery pathology and a clear understanding of the various treatment modalities, including their shortcomings.

BACKGROUND AND RATIONALE

General Considerations

In general, carotid artery pathology is loosely understood to refer to atherosclerotic plaques that affect the common carotid bifurcation, often extending into the origin of the internal carotid artery. However, it is imperative to have a broader view of carotid artery pathology and to consider other types of lesions that may also result in increased stroke risk. These lesions may differ from the lesions more commonly diagnosed as carotid stenosis by virtue of their location (e.g., common carotid ostial stenoses) or the underlying pathological process [e.g., dissection or fibromuscular dysplasia (FMD)]. These two dimensions of carotid pathology must therefore be considered to optimize the patient's treatment. It follows that not all patients, and certainly not all lesions, can be readily managed by following a single-minded approach to either medical therapy or revascularization.

The literature on how carotid artery pathology leads to an increase risk of stroke has fluctuated over the years between two primary theories: flow reduction and emboligenicity. The former relates the production of ischemia to the severity of flow compromise caused by the lesion as it narrows the carotid artery. The latter is based on the tendency of the embolism to produce ischemic strokes distal to the carotid artery pathology. Extensive and critical review of the existing literature should convince the reader that both mechanisms operate concurrently. Indeed, downstream ischemic events are most frequently the result of artery-to-artery embolism. However, the importance of hemodynamic compromise is evidenced by the fact that the effect of revascularization (measured by stroke risk reduction) is proportional to the preoperative degree of vascular narrowing, at least in symptomatic patients.

The present chapter examines the various manifestations of carotid artery pathology, with an emphasis on how to strategically plan the best course of therapeutic action, and its implementation.

Variability of Extracranial Carotid Pathology

Atherosclerotic plaques represent the most common and best studied lesions affecting the extracranial carotid arteries, but not the only ones. Indeed, dissection, FMD, and radiation angiitis, among others (see Table 10.1), are also capable of causing narrowing of the carotid artery and carry their own inherent risk for stroke. It must also be pointed out that atherosclerotic plaques comprise the only type of carotid pathology that, when located in a surgically accessible site, has been the subject of randomized prospective controlled studies of the effect of revascularization. In contrast, nonatherosclerotic lesions have not been as widely studied, largely because the populations affected are so small that it becomes difficult to organize valid prospective studies. In many of these patients, surgical intervention is not as simple, effective, or even available, while the efficacy of medical treatment is often unpredictable. From this point of view, in fact, the only form of carotid pathology for which specific surgical intervention has been convincingly shown to

TABLE 10.1 Nonatherosclerotic Types of Extracranial Carotid Pathology

Dissection
Fibromuscular dysplasia
Inflammatory conditions
  Infectious
  Necrotizing (e.g., polyarteritis nodosa)
  Collagen vascular disease (e.g., scleroderma)
  Giant cell arteritis (e.g., Takayasu's arteritis)
Radiation angiitis

benefit patients is atherosclerotic narrowing of the bifurcation of the common carotid artery. However, even in this subpopulation, there are circumstances that make the application of surgical intervention unwarranted, underlying the importance of alternative approaches.

Benefits and Shortcomings of Available Treatment Methods

The treatment of patients at risk for stroke from carotid pathology can be categorized as *medical*, *surgical*, or *endovascular*. The first and second treatments have been the only ones traditionally available, and their effectiveness (and limitations) provides perspective to our discussion of the latter treatment. From the point of view of *medical* therapy, the utilization of antithrombotic agents (i.e., antiplatelets and anticoagulants) has been the subject of considerable study in recent years. An indepth discussion and comparison of the differential efficacy of the various drugs available is beyond the scope of the present chapter and is covered elsewhere in the book (see Chapter 24). The same is true for the medical management of lipid disorders, an important dimension to the management of patients with carotid atherosclerosis. In this context, we must emphasize that nearly every patient with carotid artery pathology is likely to benefit from aggressive medical management, alone or as a complement to revascularization.

In case of *surgical* therapy, the benefit of carotid endarterectomy (CEA) over medical therapy alone has been demonstrated in several randomized, prospective, controlled trials encompassing both symptomatic and asymptomatic patients (see Table 10.2). This benefit holds true only if the procedural risk of stroke and death is kept at <6% in symptomatic patients and <3% in asymptomatic patients. Both these numbers are widely quoted as somewhat dogmatic benchmarks that clinicians should demand of their surgeons before referring patients for CEA. In addition, these numbers have been used as a point of comparison to judge the potential viability of newer, alternative therapeutic procedures. However, the absolute numbers quoted do not convey the entire experience with CEA, as well as some of its limitations. For example, in the North American Symptomatic Carotid Endarterectomy Trial (NASCET), the incidence of cranial nerve injuries resulting from CEA approximated 7%, creating another subgroup of patients with neurological deficits related to surgery. Furthermore, the results of the European Carotid Surgery Trial (ECST) are somewhat different from those of NASCET. Despite having a slightly different methodology, the procedural major stroke and death rates in ECST approximated 7%, three times the 2.1% major stroke and death rates of NASCET.

Another shortcoming of the CEA data is related to one of the fundamental principle of statistics: The sample population must be representative of the overall population to which the results of a study will be applied. The patients in the NASCET comprised an extremely healthy, low-risk group, somewhat different from those we find on a daily basis in our practice. The overwhelming majority of them were younger than 80 years, and their clinical profiles lacked clinically significant coronary artery disease, as evidenced by only 19% of them having had a previous myocardial infarction and 23% having preexisting angina. In addition, only 2.6% of them had congestive heart failure, 5% had cardiac arrhythmias, 2% had valvular heart disease, and by exclusion, none suffered renal failure, hepatic insufficiency, or cancer. Other demographic characteristics of these patients included the fact that less than two third were hypertensive, less than one fifth were diabetic and dyslipidemic, and only one third were smokers. In fact, in NASCET, the existence of certain comorbidities significantly increased the stroke and death risk of CEA, particularly contralateral carotid occlusion (14%) and tandem siphon lesions (9%). In parallel, the Asymptomatic Carotid Artery Study (ACAS) showed that CEA is effective so long as the procedural risk for stroke and death is <3%. However, the ACAS patients also comprised an extremely healthy, handpicked, low-risk population.

Therefore, it has been fair to question whether the benefit of CEA holds true to the same degree in other higher risk patient populations, particularly as endovascular techniques have become available. Along these lines, a review of the utilization of CEA to treat Medicare patients (i.e., real life individuals) showed that the mortality from CEA across the country varied from 1.7% to 2.5% (more than twice the 0.6% seen in NASCET), with the highest rate being related to the lesser volume of procedures carried out by the surgeons. These results underscore the operator dependency of CEA, not different from any other aspect of the practice of medicine (see following text). There is also evidence that the rate of

TABLE 10.2 The Most Important Prospective Randomized Studies of Carotid Endarterectomy versus Medical Therapy Alone

Study (y)	Number of Patients (Type)	Endpoints	CEA Risk (%)	Absolute Risk Reduction (%)
ECST (1991)	778 (Sx)	Stroke and death	7.5	6.5
NASCET (1991)	659 (Sx)	Stroke and death	5.8	17
ACAS (1995)	1662 (Asx)	Stroke and death	2.3	8 (for men) 1.4 (for women)

CEA, carotid endarterectomy; ECST, European Carotid Surgery Trial; Sx, symptomatic; NASCET, North American Symptomatic Carotid Endarterectomy Trial; ACAS, Asymptomatic Carotid Artery Study; Asx, asymptomatic.

TABLE 10.3 Studies and Registries Showing Competitive Complication Rates for Carotid Artery Stenting

Study (y)	Patients (Type)	Primary Endpoints (30 d)	CAS Risk (vs. CEA)
SAPPHIRE (2004)	334 (Sx and Asx)	Death, stroke, and MI	4.8% (9.8%)
SPACE (2006)	1,200 (Sx)	Stroke and death	6.84% (6.34%)
CAPTURE (2007)	3,500	Death, stroke, and MI	6.3%

CAS, carotid artery stenting; CEA, carotid endarterectomy; SAPPHIRE, Stenting and Angioplasty with Protection in Patients at High Risk for Endarterectomy; Sx, symptomatic; Asx, asymptomatic; MI, myocardial infarction; SPACE, Stent-Supported Percutaneous Angioplasty of the Carotid Artery vs Endarterectomy; CAPTURE, Carotid Acculink/Accunet Post-Approval Trial to Uncover Unanticipated or Rare Events.

CEA complications reported in the literature depends in part on the specialty of the authors of the study being published. As such, studies in which a neurologist was one of the investigators have reported a higher rate of complications. This may result from the inherent ability of neurologists to recognize neurological complications, and this suggests that the involvement of a neurologist in the decision-making process about CEA is of significant value.

At present, the *endovascular* treatment of carotid pathology largely includes carotid artery stenting (CAS) because balloon angioplasty alone has been widely abandoned. Its application is based on the results of various randomized prospective studies, as well as several registries (see Table 10.3). Among these, we must discuss the ones we consider most important from the perspective of their effect on the acceptance of CAS by the medical community, insurance carriers, and government regulatory agencies are discussed. In 2004, Medicare announced its intention to cover payments for CAS performed under specific circumstances, largely derived from the inclusion criteria in the Stenting and Angioplasty with Protection in Patients at High Risk for Endarterectomy (SAPPHIRE) report. This was a randomized study of CAS versus CEA in *surgical high-risk* patients. The surgical high risk patient was determined by either medical comorbidities or lesion characteristics (see Table 10.4), and a CEA expert surgeon was required to declare a patient as being at surgical high risk. The results, as displayed in Table 10.3, showed rates of stroke, death, and myocardial infarction as 4.8% versus 9.8% in favor of CAS versus CEA at 30 days. Moreover, the superiority of CAS over CEA in this patient population has remained even 1 year after the procedure (see Fig. 10.1).

TABLE 10.4 Criteria Used in SAPPHIRE and Other Studies to Define High Surgical Risk for CEA

- Clinically significant cardiac disease (i.e., Ejection Fraction <30% or NYHA ≥III)
- Severe pulmonary disease (FEV_1<30%)
- Contralateral carotid occlusion
- Contralateral laryngeal nerve palsy
- Previous radical neck surgery
- Previous radiation to the neck
- Recurrent stenosis after CEA
- Age >80 y
- Surgically inaccessible lesion
- Tracheostomy stoma

SAPPHIRE, Stenting and Angioplasty with Protection in Patients at High Risk for Endarterectomy; CEA, carotid endarterectomy; NYHA, New York Heart Association; Forced Exploratory Volume; FEV_1, forced expiratory volume in 1 second.

Along the same lines, other studies have confirmed that the complication rate of CAS is sufficiently competitive to warrant its application in high-risk patients (Table 10.3). Nevertheless, we would be remiss if we did not examine other studies are not examined whose results have not been as favorable to CAS as those listed earlier have. Such studies, shown in Table 10.5, generally underscore the importance of operator's experience and expertise as a requirement for CAS to be of any benefit to patients. In fact, the common denominator of the studies cited is the relative inexperience of the interventionists, evidenced not only in procedural technique but also in the patients' care (e.g., inadequate antiplatelet therapy perioperatively). In fact, to illustrate the importance of this issue, we steer the reader to look at our own experience of over a decade of performing this procedure (see Fig. 10.2). The graph illustrates the effect of experience, as well as that of the introduction of technological advances (i.e., distal protection devices). Furthermore, we must emphasize the fact that all credible studies of CAS have systematically required for neurologists to be involved in the assessment, selection, and postoperative monitoring of the patients, enhancing the accuracy of the identification of neurological complications.

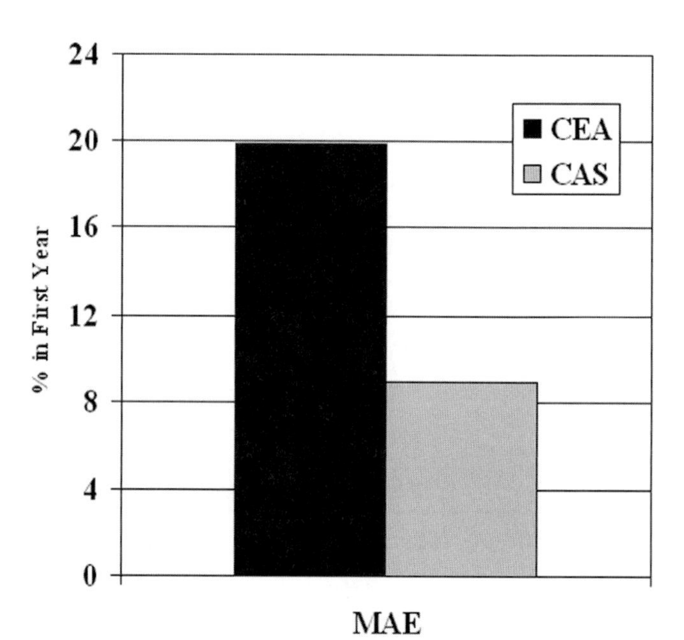

FIGURE 10.1. Comparison of the number of major adverse events (MAEs) occurring in the Stenting and Angioplasty with Protection in Patients at High Risk for Endarterectomy (SAPPHIRE) patients within the first 365 days of follow-up, showing the superiority of stenting. CAS, carotid artery stenting; CEA, carotid endarterectomy.

TABLE 10.5 Principal Studies Showing Unfavorable Results about Carotid Stenting, with Comments Regarding Limitations

Study	Patients	Endpoints	CAS Risk	Commentary
Wallstent (2001)	219 (Sx)	Stroke and death	12%	Inexperienced interventionists, suboptimal technique
ARCHeR 3 (2006)	145 (Sx and Asx)	Stroke, death, and MI	8.3%	Extremely high-risk patients
EVA-3S (2005)	527 (Sx)	Stroke, death, and MI	10%	Inexperienced interventionists, inadequate antiplatelet therapy

CAS, carotid artery stenting; Sx, symptomatic; ARCHeR, ACCULINK for revascularization of carotids in high-risk patients; EVA-3S, endarterectomy versus stenting in patients with symptomatic severe carotid stenosis.

The currently available follow-up data on the durability of CAS from the international CAS registry shows stroke occurrence of 3% over a follow-up period of 24 to 36 months and a restenosis (i.e., >50% stenosis of the treated vessel) rate of approximately 4% over the same period. These results are also quite competitive when one considers that the stroke rate in the surgical arm of the NASCET was 14% over 3 years, and that of the ACAS was 10% over 5 years.

CLINICAL APPLICATIONS AND METHODOLOGY

General Considerations

The application of revascularization techniques to the treatment of carotid artery pathology involves two different issues: feasibility versus reasonableness. The former relates to whether a procedure *can be* performed as the treatment of a specific lesion, while the latter relates to whether such a procedure *should be* performed, even if feasible. It is important to differentiate these two aspects when assessing patients with extracranial carotid pathology. We adhere to the notion that the ability to revascularize a lesion (by any method) should not automatically translate into a procedure that may or may not be needed.

Candidacy for Surgical or Endovascular Intervention

In general, to discuss patients' eligibility for treatment with one or another strategy, we must begin by dividing the patient populations into more or less homogeneous groups. This approach facilitates the assessment of the applicability of the existing data. For example, one major categorization of patients with carotid artery pathology is that of labeling them as symptomatic (i.e., the carotid pathology has already resulted in brain ischemia) or asymptomatic (i.e., the carotid lesion is found incidentally or as part of a surveillance protocol). Furthermore, patient definition would require the subdivision each of these according to their surgical risk (i.e., low versus high) (see Fig. 10.3). In parallel, lesions can be categorized using various dichotomies, such as their severity (i.e., hemodynamically significant or not), their location (i.e., surgically accessible or not), and their morphology (i.e., atheromatous or not). On the basis of these criteria, it is possible to allocate every patient to a specific group, each with a relatively predictable risk-to-benefit ratio, and to decide what therapeutic course is most advantageous and valuable for the patient.

The decisions about symptomatic patients must consider the significantly increased risk of stroke caused by a lesion that has

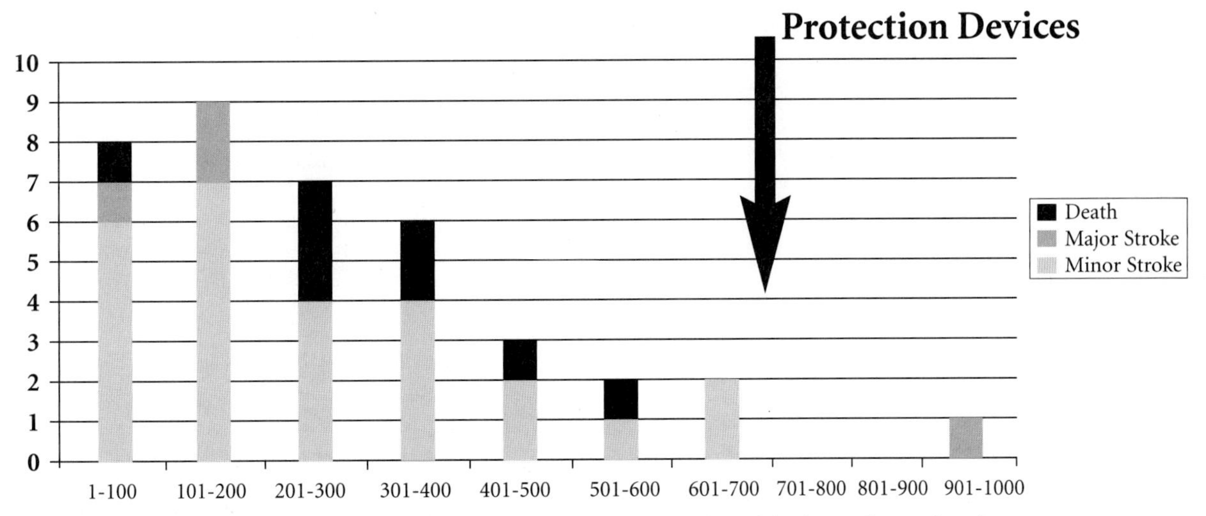

FIGURE 10.2. Bar graph showing practitioners' experience in terms of stroke and death rates by centiles of vessels treated over the course of time. Note the point of introduction of distal protection devices and its effect.

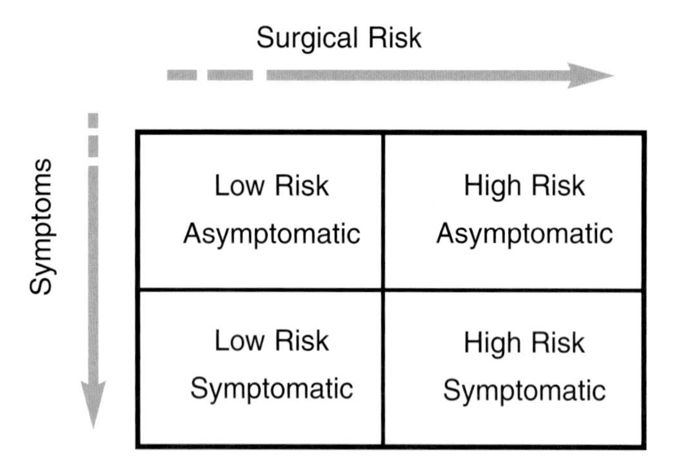

FIGURE 10.3. Contingency table displaying the four major patient subgroups based on whether they have had symptoms of brain ischemia, and their surgical risk.

already been found to be capable of producing brain ischemia (transient or not). From this perspective, and drawing from the existing literature, the sense of urgency and need to revascularize hemodynamically significant lesions (i.e., causing >50% stenosis by NASCET criteria) overwhelms the benefit of any strategy that does not include correction of the hemodynamic compromise. Clearly, in low-surgical-risk patients, CEA has been shown to be extremely effective when performed by expert surgical teams that maintain a high volume practice. The benefit of CAS in these patients, although intuitively expected, awaits the results of ongoing prospective randomized trials. On the basis of current information, high-surgical-risk patients may be better off treated by CAS, provided the operator is an experienced interventionist with ample understanding of the cerebral circulation, both anatomically and physiologically. Finally, surgically inaccessible or nonatherosclerotic lesions should be considered for endovascular therapy only, provided the operator meets the criteria noted earlier in this section. Under these circumstances, we cannot overemphasize the importance of having neurological expertise during the decision-making process, particularly as the literature available to conduct a risk-to-benefit assessment is scant.

Asymptomatic patients, on the other hand, represent a very different problem. Their risk for stroke is relatively small, and the benefits of revascularization may be marginal. In these patients, only lesions that cause severe hemodynamic compromises (i.e., >80% stenosis by NASCET criteria) should be considered for revascularization. Even in these cases, the presence of a high surgical risk should be a major warning about the pitfalls involved in blindly applying data from the literature without considering the individual characteristics of the patient. Considering the existing evidence that both CEA and CAS carry a higher procedural risk in patients such as those described in Table 10.4 than that in low-risk patients, clinicians must find compelling reasons to suggest revascularization by any method. In such circumstances, it is even more important that the operator's expertise is equivalent to "best in class" to minimize the chances of catastrophic complications.

Procedural Safety

The safety of both CEA and CAS has been a subject of concern spanning the last two decades. To arrive at a positive risk-to-benefit assessment, the risk imposed by the procedure must be smaller (for that patient) than the risk of stroke from the carotid artery pathology if only medical treatment is applied. Safety data now exist for both CEA and CAS, although the former is an older and more mature procedure. In fact, the relative immaturity of CAS must be taken into consideration when reviewing the literature to put each of the studies published in the context of the evolution of a technique that has only recently been considered fully developed.

A major advance in the evolution of CAS and its safety record was the introduction of distal embolic protection devices (see Fig. 10.4). The early experience of CAS invariably showed that a few patients (approximately 6% to 7%) had small nondisabling stroke during the intervention (Fig. 10.2). These largely resulted in subtle neurological deficits from which the patients usually recovered within a few days. Nevertheless, such an unpredictable occurrence led to the development of devices that, when deployed distally in the internal carotid artery, would essentially capture the embolic debris and limit the chances of complicating stroke during the procedure (Fig. 10.4). The introduction of distal embolic protection devices resulted in an immediate decrease in the rates of procedural strokes complicating CAS (Figs. 10.2 and 10.5).

Operator's Expertise

Operator's expertise is perhaps the single most important variable that affects the outcome of both CEA and CAS. From the surgical perspective, it is important to point out that large randomized CEA trials (e.g., NASCET, ACAS, and ECST) owe their success to the technical expertise of their surgeons. All operators in these studies were handpicked, screened for a number of months before the study, and closely monitored. In daily practice, on the other hand, this may or may not be the case. The same cannot be said about all the CAS studies. In fact, a close scrutiny of those studies with unusually high procedural complication rates reveals a lack of systematic credentialing of the operators (e.g., Wallstent study) or the inclusion of inexperienced operators [e.g., Stent-Supported Percutaneous Angioplasty of the Carotid Artery vs. Endarterectomy (SPACE)].

Three major features characterize expert operators: (a) patient selection skills, (b) phenotypic and genotypic interventional attributes, and (c) high volume of cases (i.e., experience). The best operators spend considerable amount of time making sure that the patient in question is as close an ideal candidate for the procedure as possible. They do not take chances by operating on patients who may not benefit from the procedure or whose circumstances are such that they pose an unusually high procedural risk. To be able to select patients properly, operators must have fundamental knowledge of neuroanatomy, neurophysiology, clinical neurology, neuroimaging, neuropathology, and neuropharmacology.

The phenotypic characteristics of an operator derive from his or her procedural education; that is, having performed a large number of procedures under the supervision of a qualified mentor, affording him the ability to learn all aspects of the

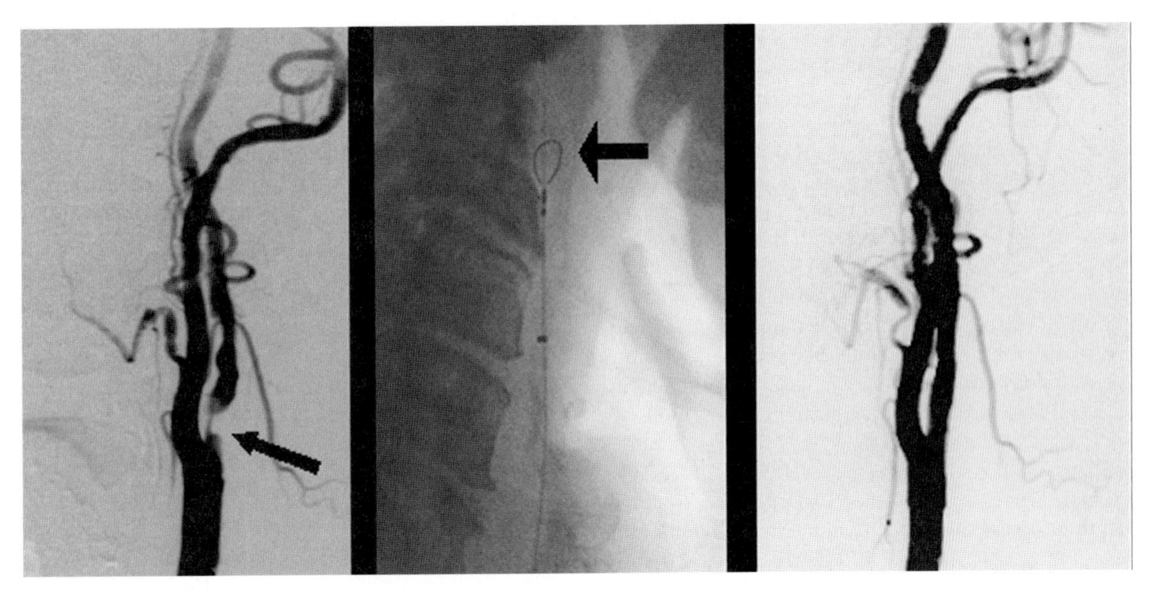

FIGURE 10.4. Basic images of a carotid stenting procedure. *Left to right:* The preprocedural image demonstrates a severe stenosis of the origin of the internal carotid artery. Deployment of a distal protection device is standard practice and reduces the risk of complications. The final image demonstrates effective treatment of the target vessel.

procedure. More important, procedural education must be then translated into learning the principles that would allow the operator to troubleshoot when confronted with a situation not previously encountered. The supervised experience must be sufficient to facilitate the learning curve, while conferring the operator's fundamental knowledge about cerebral catheterization, neuroangiography, and specific competence with the devices to be used. The other set of characteristics, genotypic, constitute a subject that is not often addressed: Not everyone who wants to operate should! In addition to clinical judgment (i.e., for patient selection) and procedural knowledge (i.e., phenotypic skills), the operator must possess the hand–eye coordination, which is inborn and cannot be taught. Just as Michael Jordan was born to play basketball, everyone is born with inherent skills that separate excellence from mediocrity. In our opinion, it is incumbent upon postgraduate program directors to see that individuals without natural aptitudes do not advance the thinking that they can operate just as their mentors do.

The final aspect of the operator's expertise is related to the volume of procedures performed. There is absolutely no substitute for experience, and the literature shows that both for CEA and CAS, the larger the experience and practice volume of the operator, the better the outcomes. Our own experience reflects the importance of this point (Fig. 10.2).

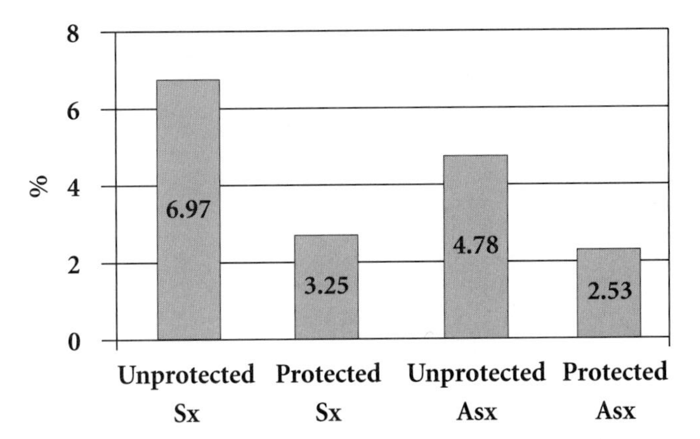

FIGURE 10.5. Effect of the introduction of distal protection devices for carotid stenting in the incidence of stroke and death resulting from the procedure. The graph is derived from the experience of more than10,000 patients treated internationally. Sx, symptomatic; Asx, asymptomatic.

PRACTICAL RECOMMENDATIONS

In our experience, patients with carotid artery pathology present via one of two routes. The first is the patient who has had a focal nondisabling neurological deficit presumably resulting from ischemia (transient or not) and the other is the patient referred because of a carotid lesion found in the course of his or her treatment (typically following an ultrasound done for surveillance or to evaluate an asymptomatic bruit). Although our approach to either of these patients is fundamentally similar, the weight of the choices at each node of the decision tree varies somewhat.

Symptomatic Patient

A patient who has developed a nondisabling deficit from a carotid artery lesion must be taken seriously, with a sense of urgency that cannot be overemphasized. The reason is simple—the symptoms constitute our only opportunity to preempt what could be a catastrophic cerebral infarction. Our first step is to examine the evidence for the presence of carotid artery pathology and to decide whether the lesion is atherosclerotic. Once this decision is made, different issues will have to be addressed, the first one being the degree of hemodynamic compromise. Irrespective of the nature of the lesion (i.e., atherosclerotic or not), if no significant hemodynamic compromise is evident, medical therapy alone is our recommended strategy. As noted earlier, details about the various components of medical therapy are discussed in other chapters of the book. Nevertheless, we recommend the use of double antiplatelet therapy as the primary pharmacological intervention. In patients with atherosclerotic lesions, the combination of statins (e.g., Atorvastatin) and renin–angiotensin system modulators (i.e., angiotensin-converting enzyme inhibitors or angiotensin receptor blockers) for patients with dyslipidemia and hypertension, respectively, is reasonable. The decision to use these medications in patients who lack these diagnoses is more controversial and a matter of personal preference. In any case, patients with carotid artery lesions and no evidence of significant hemodynamic compromise must be placed in an imaging surveillance program to ensure early detection of progression of the underlying process. An important practical point about the aforementioned recommendation refers to the definition of significant hemodynamic compromise. We have covered this subject extensively in Chapter 22 in the book, but suffice to say, it is imperative that we understand the limitations of every imaging technique, as well as the inherent inadequacy of using diameter stenosis as a surrogate for flow compromise (the actual variable to consider). In addition, we must recognize that the benefit of CEA in symptomatic patients, as demonstrated in NASCET, requires diameter measurements using selective digital angiography. If there is a suggestion of significant hemodynamic compromise (equivalent to >50% diameter stenosis by angiography using the NASCET method), further assessment of the patient will depend on the type of lesion suspected.

Atherosclerotic lesions, the only ones for which there is significant evidence of the benefit of CEA, must then be examined for their surgical accessibility and the surgical risk level of the patient. If (and only if) the lesion is surgically accessible AND the surgical risk is low, CEA can be promptly considered and carried out by an experienced surgeon without any delay in most situations. In general, the literature supports the concept of not waiting for the traditional 6 weeks, which was a common practice in the past. However, as with any other rule, we feel there are exceptional circumstances that warrant delaying revascularization, notably when the carotid lesion is upstream from a recent hemorrhagic infarction and the degree of flow compromise is severe. Under certain circumstances, a low-risk patient with a surgically accessible lesion may be considered for CAS, but it must be clearly understood that data to support such a decision are, at the moment of this writing, preliminary and incomplete. Patients who have surgically inaccessible lesions, or a high-surgical-risk profile, should be considered for CAS. It is important to note that the former includes lesions that *could* be accessed surgically but that should not. For example, it is possible to perform a CEA in an internal carotid lesion above the angle of the mandible. However, this requires mandibular disarticulation and constitutes a procedure substantially different from the CEA techniques tested in the randomized prospective trials. Treatment of these lesions by CAS must be found to be feasible and reasonable before they are undertaken.

The management of symptomatic nonatherosclerotic lesions that cause significant hemodynamic compromise should not include a consideration for surgery, but solely a consideration for CAS. The first step in recognizing such a lesion is to decide whether CAS is feasible, a step that often requires digital angiography. Then, we must ascertain whether it is reasonable to use CAS to treat the specific patient. The answers to these questions greatly depend on the underlying pathology and we must consider them separately.

Radiation Angiitis

The decision to treat these patients with CAS rests on the balance between the low emboligenicity of these lesions when compared to atherosclerotic lesions and the significant hemodynamic compromise they are capable of causing. The same criteria used for atherosclerotic lesions can be applied to decide whether to proceed with CAS. In general, the procedure is safer and the results seem to be durable.

Dissection

The decision to treat traumatic injuries of the carotid artery depends on how symptomatic the lesion is and whether it has responded to antithrombotic therapy. In general, flow-reducing dissections should be treated with anticoagulation despite the lack of prospective data. Since the overwhelming majority of dissections heal spontaneously, our approach has been to treat them with warfarin for a period of no more than 6 months, then reassess them. We reserve CAS for patients who have recurrent or progressive symptoms despite anticoagulation or for those who after 6 month continue to have significant hemodynamic compromise from a poorly healed dissection. The exciting prospect of performing CAS in a patient with dissection must be tempered by the understanding of the technical complexities of treating a vessel with a damaged vascular wall, as well as the pitfalls of instrumenting the false lumen.

Fibromuscular Dysplasia

The treatment of FMD also requires moderation in the interventional strategy. The lesions respond well to CAS but the difficulty is in deciding whether revascularization is needed or not. Characteristically, angiography has a limited view of the vascular lesion and measurements of stenosis are not easy. Furthermore, the operator must understand that the vascular wall is abnormal and that there is a risk of creating a dissection during instrumentation.

Inflammatory Vasculopathies

These processes must be treated medically before any attempt at CAS. High-dose steroids must be used to ensure that the angiographic picture is not simply caused by inflammation that can be medically corrected, obviating the need for intervention. CAS has been successfully applied to conditions where intervention is needed.

A final word about medical therapy for all patients undergoing CAS. It is imperative for these individuals to be treated with aspirin and clopidogrel before the procedure to remove the risk of acute stent thrombosis. Once the CAS is completed, both antiplatelet agents must be continued for at least 4 weeks, but preferably indefinitely.

Asymptomatic Patient

The approach to the asymptomatic patient with a carotid artery lesion, although following a similar path to that described for symptomatic patients, requires considerably more thought and a different threshold within the decision tree. For instance, we do not consider any form of revascularization in an asymptomatic patient unless the flow compromise is severe (i.e., equivalent to >80% diameter stenosis angiographically by the NASCET method). Furthermore, we give a slightly higher weight to the characteristics that make the patient a high-risk surgical candidate, since they are quickly imbalanced by the marginal stroke risk reduction from revascularization. A particular problem in this population involves the surgeons who insist in performing CEA without angiographic imaging and based solely on ultrasound results. This practice, although widely accepted, does not have a logical basis and currently results in numerous CEA procedures that may not be needed. Conversely, the popularity of CAS has resulted in frequent drive-by carotid angiograms following coronary angiography. These procedures are not only technically suboptimal but also commonly followed by stenoses measurements not based on accepted standards (i.e., NASCET method), with overestimation of the degree of narrowing and often the performance of a CAS that may also not be needed.

SELECTED REFERENCES

Chang YJ, Golby AJ, Albers GW. Detection of carotid stenosis. From NASCET results to clinical practice. *Stroke* 1995;26(8):1325–1328.

Clinical alert: benefit of carotid endarterectomy for patients with high-grade stenosis of the internal carotid artery. National Institute of Neurological Disorders and Stroke Stroke and Trauma Division. North American Symptomatic Carotid Endarterectomy Trial (NASCET) investigators. *Stroke* 1991;22(6):816–817.

Gray WA, Yadav JS, Verta P, et al. The CAPTURE registry: Results of carotid stenting with embolic protection in the post approval setting. *Catheter Cardiovasc Interv* 2007;69(3):341–348.

Hennerici M, Daffertshofer M, Meairs S. Concerns about generalisation of premature ACAS recommendations for carotid endarterectomy. *Lancet* 1995;346(8981):1041.

Hobson RW, II, Brott T, Ferguson R, et al. CREST: carotid revascularization endarterectomy versus stent trial. *Cardiovasc Surg* 1997;5(5):457–458.

Hobson RW, II. CREST (Carotid Revascularization Endarterectomy versus Stent Trial): background, design, and current status. *Semin Vasc Surg* 2000;13(2):139–143.

Houdart E, Mounayer C, René Chapot R, et al. Carotid stenting for radiation-induced stenoses: a report of 7 cases. *Stroke* 2001;32(1): 118–121.

Moore WS. Efficacy of carotid endarterectomy in randomized trials. *West J Med* 1991;155(4):407.

Myers, K.A. Selection process for surgeons in ACAS. *Stroke* 1992; 23(5):781.

Roubin GS, Hobson RW, White R, et al. CREST and CARESS to evaluate carotid stenting: time to get to work! *J Endovasc Ther* 2001;8(2):107–110.

Setacci C, Cremonesi A, SPACE and EVA-3S trials: the need of standards for carotid stenting. *Eur J Vasc Endovasc Surg* 2007;33(1):48–49.

Wholey MH, Wholey M, Bergeron P, et al. Current global status of carotid artery stent placement. *Cathet Cardiovasc Diagn* 1998;44(1): 1–6.

Yadav JS, Wholey MH, Kuntz RE, et al. Protected carotid-artery stenting versus endarterectomy in high-risk patients. *N Engl J Med* 2004;351(15): 1493–1501.

CRITICAL PATHWAY
Management of Extracranial Carotid Artery Pathology

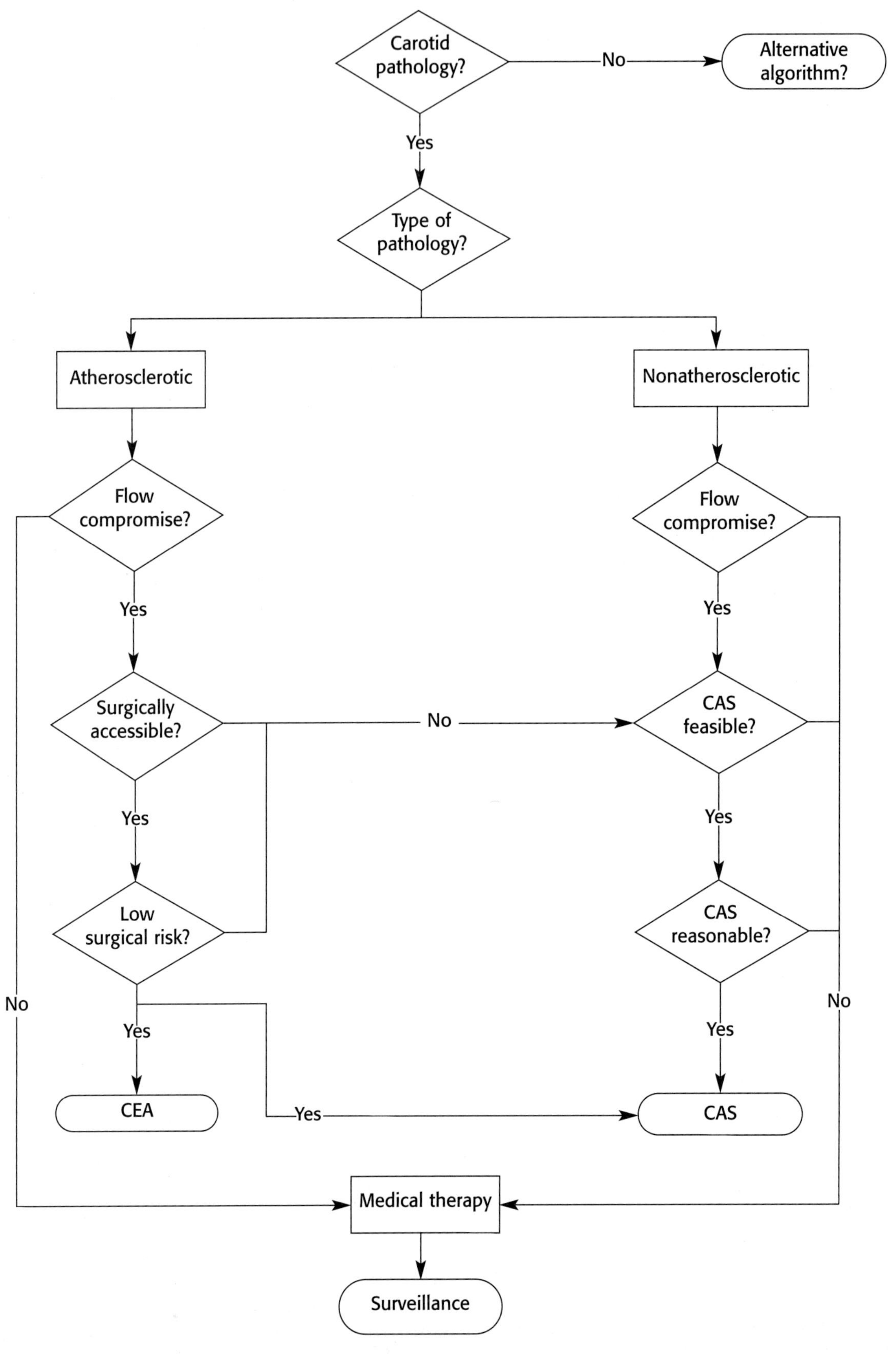

CEA, Carotid endar terectomy; CAS, Carotid artery stenting.

CHAPTER

Management of Extracranial Vertebral Artery Pathology

CAMILO R. GOMEZ AND JAMES D. GEYER

OBJECTIVES

- What are the goals of therapy in patients with extracranial vertebral artery pathology?
- What criteria need to be used to decide how to treat patients with vertebral artery pathology?
- When is endovascular therapy of the extracranial vertebral artery indicated?
- Which patients should be considered for revascularization?
- What is the best approach to the asymptomatic patient?

When compared to the pathology of the carotid artery, the incidence of extracranial vertebral artery stenosis is not widely appreciated, making vertebrobasilar insufficiency an underdiagnosed condition. Medical therapy has traditionally been the mainstay of treatment of patients with extracranial vertebral artery pathology, primarily because of the complexity and high morbidity of surgical intervention. During the 1980s, various authors reported moderately acceptable results using percutaneous transluminal angioplasty to correct extracranial vertebral artery stenoses. However, this technique has significant limitations, including the common elastic recoil of vertebral ostial lesions and the inherent challenges associated with the treatment of vertebral artery dissections. More recently, several groups (including ours) have shown that vertebral artery stenting is feasible in patients who have significant vertebral artery stenosis, with a predictably good angiographic and clinical result. This chapter is a review of the existing experience in the management of extracranial vertebral artery pathology, with an emphasis on the different available approaches, and the selection of the most appropriate technique for each clinical scenario.

BACKGROUND AND RATIONALE

Variability of Extracranial Vertebral Pathology

Atherosclerosis of the extracranial vertebral artery is relatively common, having been found in approximately 25% to 40% of the population in some series. Its true association with brainstem ischemia and disabling stroke is uncertain, since this vessel is harder to study than the extracranial portion of the carotid artery. However, recent advances in imaging technology (e.g., magnetic resonance angiography) have made this task significantly easier. In this context, more recent data suggest that extracranial vertebral artery pathology is common in patients with vertebrobasilar ischemia and that it is found to be the sole cause of the symptoms in almost 10% of the patients. Atherosclerotic plaques are most frequently found in the origin of the vertebral artery, as well as in its most distal segments (i.e., V3 and V4). The latter will be addressed in the context of managing intracranial arterial lesions.

In addition to atherosclerotic plaques, the vertebral artery can be the target of other pathologic processes, such as dissection, fibromuscular dysplasia, radiation angiitis, and giant cell arteritis. These conditions, all risk factors for stroke to one degree or another, require identification and appropriate treatment. Vertebral artery dissection results from trauma (even if trivial) to the arterial wall, with resulting separation of its layers and creation of a false lumen. The latter becomes the nidus of thrombus formation and often progresses to vascular occlusion. Dissection of the vertebral artery is more frequent in the intracanalicular (i.e., V2) segment of the vessel, largely because of the mechanical interaction between the artery and the bony canal. In fact, it is this interaction that predisposes individuals to vascular injury following certain movements or trauma. Fibromuscular dysplasia is an anomalous development of the arterial wall, leading to segmental tandem points of narrowing and trabeculation. Its importance is compounded by the fact that its presence increases the patient's predisposition to arterial dissection. Other types of vertebral pathology, although less common, also demand diagnostic attention because of the various therapeutic implications.

Benefits and Shortcomings of Available Treatment Methods

The treatment of patients at risk for stroke from vertebral pathology involves *medical*, *surgical*, or *endovascular* strategies. *Medical* therapy largely encompasses the utilization of antithrombotic agents (i.e., antiplatelets and anticoagulants) and the management of other stroke risk factors (e.g., hypertension, diabetes, and dyslipidemia). Indepth discussions of each of these aspects of medical treatment can be found elsewhere in this book (e.g., see Chapter 24). Suffice it to say, nearly every patient with vertebral artery pathology is likely to benefit from aggressive medical management, either alone or as a complement to revascularization techniques.

The *surgical* treatment of patients with extracranial vertebral artery atherosclerotic pathology has been the subject of some study, although not as rigorous as that of extracranial carotid pathology. The techniques used in the past vary widely, ranging from endarterectomy to transection of the vertebral artery above the stenosis and reimplantation in either the ipsilateral carotid or subclavian arteries. In addition to the risk of stroke, these procedures have significant limitations, including an overall 10% to 20% risk of injury to the sympathetic fibers—the phrenic, the recurrent laryngeal, or the vagus nerves—as well as the potential for pulmonary complications from thoracotomy. In the largest reported series of vertebral artery operations, the Joint Study of Extracranial Arterial Occlusion, 165 vertebral arteries were treated with a mortality of 4.2% and an incidence of perioperative vertebral artery occlusion of 6%. In another large series, 109 vertebral operations were performed with a 3% mortality rate and a 2% rate of immediate thrombosis. These facts underscore the advantage of a minimally invasive, low morbidity revascularization technique for the vertebral artery, with better long-term patency rates. There is essentially no information about the surgical treatment of nonatherosclerotic vertebral artery pathology.

In regards to *endovascular* treatment of extracranial vertebral atherosclerotic lesions, balloon angioplasty alone has been performed safely and widely since the early 1980s. The procedure is, however, not without complications, with one of the largest series of extracranial vertebral artery angioplasties reporting 34 patients who, as a result of the procedure, were noted to have an 8.8% incidence of transient neurologic complications with no permanent neurologic deficits. Interestingly, a review of the illustrations in previous vertebral angioplasty reports demonstrates significant residual postprocedure stenoses, probably underscoring the problem of elastic recoil. In the past, the use of larger balloons in an attempt to overcome recoil has often resulted in dissection, as seen in similarly proportioned coronary arteries. These limitations fueled the interest in treating vertebral lesions using stents, a procedure that has been used for >10 years. We previously reported the feasibility, safety, and outcome of elective extracranial vertebral artery stenting in 50 patients (55 vessels)—at that time the largest series available. Technical success was achieved in 54 of 55 vessels (98%) with no procedure-related complications. However, one patient died of non-neurologic causes (2%) and one patient had a stroke (2%) during a subsequent complicated coronary intervention performed within the 30-day period following vertebral artery stenting. Clinical follow-up at a mean of 25 ± 10 months revealed two patients with recurrence of vertebrobasilar symptoms (4%). Six-month angiographic follow-up was carried out in 90% of eligible patients with a 10% incidence of restenosis as defined by >50% luminal narrowing. The 30-day morbidity and mortality of 4% in our series compared well with previously published data, particularly when we consider that the two perioperative events did not occur as a direct result of the vertebral revascularization. The rate of restenosis also appeared rather low, even if one considers the inherent limitations to a short-term (6-month) follow-up. Since then, our series has expanded to >150 vessels treated, and no additional procedural complications have been recorded. This means that our stroke and death procedural rate (i.e., within 30 days) presently approximates 1.5%. Other groups, some with comparable number of vessels treated, have confirmed this very competitive statistic. In fact, from an interventional point of view, elective stenting of extracranial vertebral atherosclerotic lesions is the safest and technically simplest procedure. It is fair to say, however, that everyone's experience of treating larger number of vessels has shown the rate of restenosis to approximate 25% to 30%, comparable to that in coronary arteries. This finding has led many, our group included, to shift to the use of drug-eluding stents almost exclusively. In addition, it underscores the need for aggressive medical management of atherogenic risk factors.

The endovascular treatment of nonatherosclerotic lesions deserves particular attention. Some of these conditions, specifically dissection, are perfectly suitable for stenting. Indeed, tacking up the separated arterial wall layers with a stent seems intuitively to be the best method for correcting the vascular pathology and preventing stroke. As we will see in the following section, however, many of these patients fare well without need for any intervention, and deciding who is to be treated requires an expert view of all the factors in the therapeutic equation. To compound the problem, nonatherosclerotic lesions are often not confined to a focal segment of the vessel, requiring a more reconstructive stenting procedure. This is a more complex intervention, for which there is less experience and a list of additional potential complications.

CLINICAL APPLICATIONS AND METHODOLOGY

General Considerations

The application of endovascular techniques to the treatment of vertebral artery pathology involves two different issues: feasibility versus reasonableness. The former relates to whether a procedure *can be performed* as the treatment of a specific lesion, while the latter relates to whether such a procedure *should be performed*, even if feasible. As noted elsewhere in the book, the ability to revascularize a lesion should not automatically translate into a procedure that may or may not be needed. With regards to the treatment of extracranial vertebral atherosclerotic lesions, the experience described earlier is such that issues of feasibility should not be a major concern. The difficulty lies with the decision of whether or not the patient *needs* the intervention.

Candidacy for Endovascular Intervention

In general, to discuss patients' eligibility for endovascular vertebral artery treatment we must begin by considering the different patient populations individually. Let us begin by dividing patients into those with vertebrobasilar symptoms and those without. Each one of these populations must then be considered in the light of (a) vertebral arteries anatomy, (b) location of the vertebral artery lesion, and (c) nature and severity of the lesion. On the basis of these criteria, the ideal patient for endovascular treatment is one who has recurrent vertebrobasilar symptoms directly attributable to a severely stenotic atherosclerotic ostial lesion in a solitary vertebral artery (i.e., the contralateral being occluded or congenitally nonfunctional). The more the patient deviates from these characteristics, the greater the uncertainty about the procedure's beneficial effect.

There are several aspects of the anatomy of the vertebral arteries that must be taken into consideration. The most important is whether the patient has two vertebral arteries. It is relatively common to encounter patients who display either a dominant or a single vertebral artery. In the former situation, the contralateral vertebral artery is hypoplastic and often terminates in the posterior inferior cerebellar artery (PICA), without communicating with the basilar artery at all. A single vertebral artery is sometimes seen in patients whose contralateral vessel is absent, congenitally or as a result of atherosclerotic occlusion. Clearly, a patient with a single (or isolated) dominant vertebral artery is at a potentially greater disadvantage from acute occlusion and must be considered to be at higher risk from a stenotic lesion.

The effect of the location, nature, and severity of the lesion on the decision making process is self-evident. Ostial atherosclerotic lesions that cause severe hemodynamic compromise are readily accessible and represent an easy interventional target in experienced hands (see Fig. 11.1). On the other hand, extensive intracannalicular (i.e., in the V2 segment) dissections with difficult identification of the true lumen are considerably riskier to treat. Furthermore, lesions in the V2 segment in general require great care during the angioplasty process because of their tendency to dissect when the balloon expands the arterial wall against the bony elements that comprise the vertebral canal.

A particularly challenging situation arises when the patient has a lesion such as that described to be ideal, except that he has no symptoms. The treatment of the asymptomatic patient with a potentially ominous vertebral artery lesion must take into account the likelihood of it becoming symptomatic, the incidence of unheralded stroke resulting from such lesions, and the fact that interventional treatment of these lesions is technically feasible. Our bias has been to treat these patients, particularly because the incidence of unheralded stroke is so high, while urgent treatment of an acutely occluded vertebrobasilar system is comparably more difficult and less successful. We have also learned over the years to further explore the presence of symptoms, which may be unrecognized or ill defined. Anecdotally, it is not uncommon for patients who have been asymptomatic to feel significantly improved by vertebral artery stenting of lesions otherwise ideal. This underscores the fact that many symptoms from vertebrobasilar insufficiency may not be easily recognizable or are not those that are traditionally considered as such (e.g., hemiparesis).

Procedural Safety

The safety of vertebral artery stenting has been described earlier in this chapter. The existing data are summarized in Table 11.1. As noted, this is a relatively simple, safe, and effective procedure. An interesting point to consider is that of using distal protection devices (e.g., filters) during vertebral stenting. Although this has been introduced recently by various groups, we fail to see the necessity of routinely deploying distal protection devices based on the enormous success of the unprotected procedure (Table 11.1). However, we have occasionally encountered lesions that seem to have intraluminal thrombus that does not disappear even after a period of anticoagulation. In these instances, we have successfully performed the procedure with a distal protection device (see Fig. 11.2). The reader must understand that the addition of a distal protection device, if not of significant clinical benefit, would only increase the complexity and cost of the procedure.

Operator's Expertise

Just as with any other endovascular procedure, the operator's expertise is perhaps the single most important variable that affects the outcome of vertebral artery stenting (just as with any other endovascular procedure). Three major features characterize expert operators: (a) patient selection skills, (b) phenotypic and genotypic interventional attributes, and (c) high volume of cases (i.e., experience). The best operators spend considerable amount of time

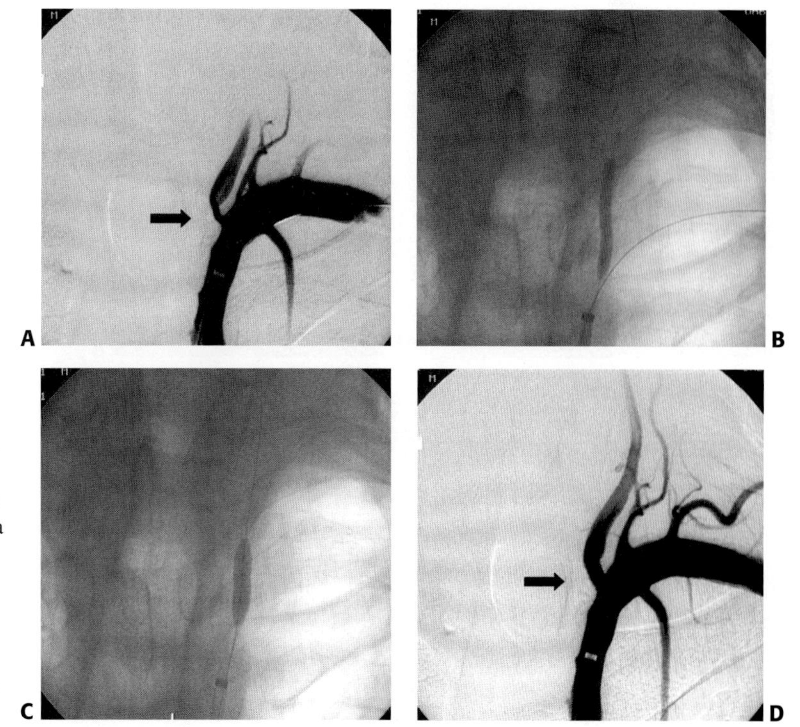

FIGURE 11.1. The basic technique for stenting of atherosclerotic plaques of the ostium of the vertebral artery. **A:** The lesion is imaged and defined before treatment. The arrow indicates the point of stenosis. **B:** After positioning a guide catheter and securing it in place with a 0.014″ wire advanced into the subclavian. The lesion was crossed with a second 0.014″ wire and predilated with a moderately compliant coronary balloon. **C:** Following predilation, deployment of a balloon expandable coronary stent provides definitive treatment. **D:** The result is a complete correction of the stenosis.

TABLE 11.1 Published Series that Address the Topic of Stenting Atherosclerotic Lesions of the Extracranial Vertebral Artery

Author (y)	Patients (Vessels)	Stroke and Deaths	Comments
Fessler (1998)	6 (6)	None	Some perioperative complications
Chastain (1999)[a]	50 (55)	2 (4%)	Stroke and death were delayed
Jenkins (2001)	32 (38)	None	One TIA
Weber (2005)	38 (38)	None	One TIA; restenosis = 36%
Qureshi (2006)	12 (12)	None	Using distal protection
Du (2007)	41 (48)	1 (2%)	Restenosis = 34.6%
Authors' present results[b]	150 (158)	3 (1.5%)	Without distal protection

TIA, transient ischemic attack.
[a]This is the authors' original series.
[b]Unpublished data.

making sure that the patient in question is as close to the ideal candidate described in the earlier section as possible. They do not take chances by operating on patients who may not benefit from the procedure, or whose circumstances are such that they pose a procedural risk that is unusually high. To be able to select patients properly, operators must have fundamental knowledge of neuroanatomy, neurophysiology, clinical neurology, neuroimaging, neuropathology, and neuropharmacology.

The phenotypic characteristics of an operator derive from having performed a large number of procedures under the supervision of a qualified mentor, affording an opportunity to learn all aspects of the procedure. More important, procedural education must be then translated in learning the principles that would allow the operator to troubleshoot when confronted with a situation not previously encountered. The supervised experience must be sufficient to facilitate the learning curve, while conferring to the operator fundamental knowledge about cerebral catheterization, neuroangiography, and specific competence with the devices to be used. The genotypic characteristics constitute a subject that is not often addressed: Not everyone who wants to operate should! In addition to clinical judgment (i.e., for patient selection) and procedural knowledge (i.e., phenotypic skills), the operator must possess inherent hand–eye coordination, which is inborn and cannot be taught. Just as Michael Jordan was born to play basketball, everyone is born with inherent abilities that separate excellence from mediocrity. In our opinion, it is incumbent on postgraduate program directors to see that individuals without natural aptitudes do not advance the thinking that they can operate just as their mentors do.

The final aspect of the operator's expertise relates to the volume of procedures performed. There is absolutely no substitute for experience, and this is supported by the literature relative to any interventional procedure, and vertebral artery stenting is no exception.

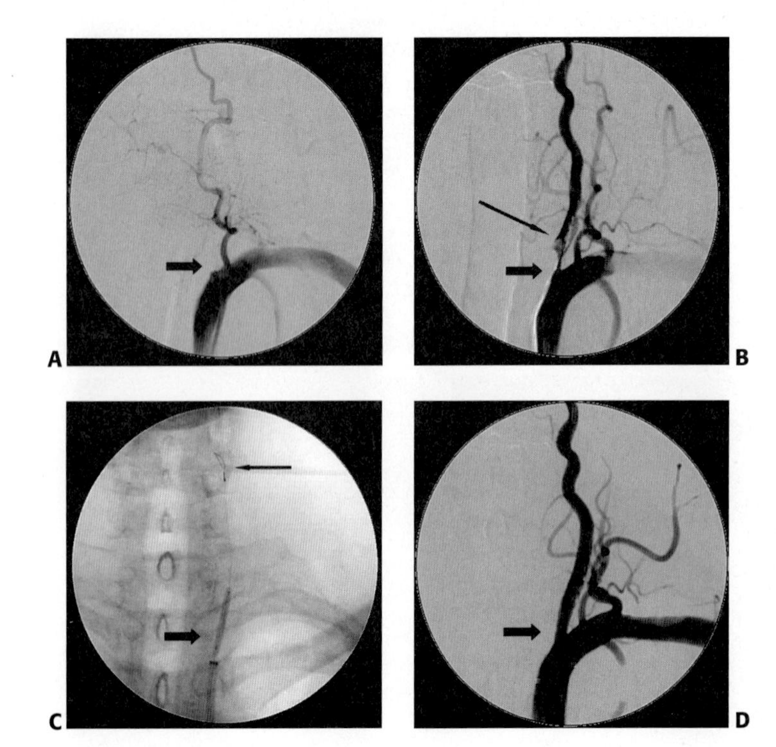

FIGURE 11.2. A complex case is represented by this functional occlusion of the left vertebral artery **(A,** *arrow*). Once the point of occlusion was crossed with a 0.014-inch wire (**B**), there was a suggestion of the presence of intraluminal thrombus **(B,** *long arrow*). This resulted in a decision to use a distal protection device, which was deployed successfully in the V2 segment **(C,** *long arrow*). Once this was accomplished, treatment of the proximal stenosis was carried out with optimal results **(D,** *arrow*).

PRACTICAL RECOMMENDATIONS

Patients with extracranial vertebral artery pathology usually present via one of two routes. The first is the patient who has had neurologic symptoms suggestive of vertebrobasilar ischemia (transient or not) secondary to an identified vertebral artery lesion in the V1, V2, or proximal V3 segments. The second is the patient found to have a vertebral artery lesion that is considered incidental. This scenario typically follows the acquisition of noninvasive images for other reasons (e.g., carotid artery pathology). Although our approach to either of these patients is fundamentally similar, the weight of the choices at each node of the decision tree varies to a certain extent.

Symptomatic Patient

It cannot be overemphasized that a patient who has developed a nondisabling deficit from a vertebral artery lesion must be treated with a sense of urgency. The reason is simple, the symptoms constitute our only opportunity to pre-empt what could be a catastrophic brainstem or cerebellar infarction. Once we confirm the presence and character of a lesion (i.e., atherosclerotic or not), we must consider its degree of hemodynamic compromise. Irrespective of the nature of the lesion, if no significant hemodynamic compromise is evident, medical therapy alone is our recommended strategy. Details about the various components of medical therapy are discussed in other chapters of the book. We recommend the use of double antiplatelet therapy as the primary pharmacologic intervention. In patients with atherosclerotic lesions, the combination of statins (e.g., atorvastatin) and renin–angiotensin system modulators (i.e., angiotensin-converting enzyme inhibitors or angiotensin receptor blockers) for patients with dyslipidemia and hypertension, respectively, is very reasonable. Whether to use these medications in patients who lack these diagnoses is more controversial and a matter of personal preference. In any case, patients with vertebral artery lesions that do not cause significant hemodynamic compromise must be placed in an imaging surveillance program to assure early detection of progression of the underlying process. An important practical point regarding the aforementioned recommendation refers to the definition of significant hemodynamic compromise. We have covered this subject extensively in Chapter 22 later in the book, but suffice to say, it is imperative that we understand the limitations of every imaging technique, as well as the inherent inadequacy of using diameter stenosis as a surrogate for flow compromise (the actual variable to consider). If there is a suggestion of significant hemodynamic compromise (equivalent to >50% diameter stenosis by angiography), further management of the patient will depend on the type of lesion suspected.

Atherosclerotic lesions, particularly those readily accessible (e.g., ostial), can be treated immediately by stenting (see Fig. 11.3). In general, we do not wait to treat these lesions unless an intraluminal thrombus is suspected. When an intraluminal thrombus is suspected, we anticoagulate the patients for a finite period (i.e., 6 to 12 weeks) and then bring them back for intervention. This approach is based on our conviction that most clots produced by flow stagnation will disappear after a few weeks in the presence of adequate anticoagulation (international normalized ratio = 2 to 3), as they do in other clinical scenarios.

Nonatherosclerotic lesions are handled somewhat differently. Patients with acute dissections who show stable symptoms while receiving intravenous heparin should probably be anticoagulated with warfarin for finite period (i.e., up to 6 months). The reason is that the overwhelming majority of them will heal over time, making intervention not necessary. After the conclusion of anticoagulant treatment, the vessel should be reimaged, and if the dissection is completely healed, the patient may be switched from

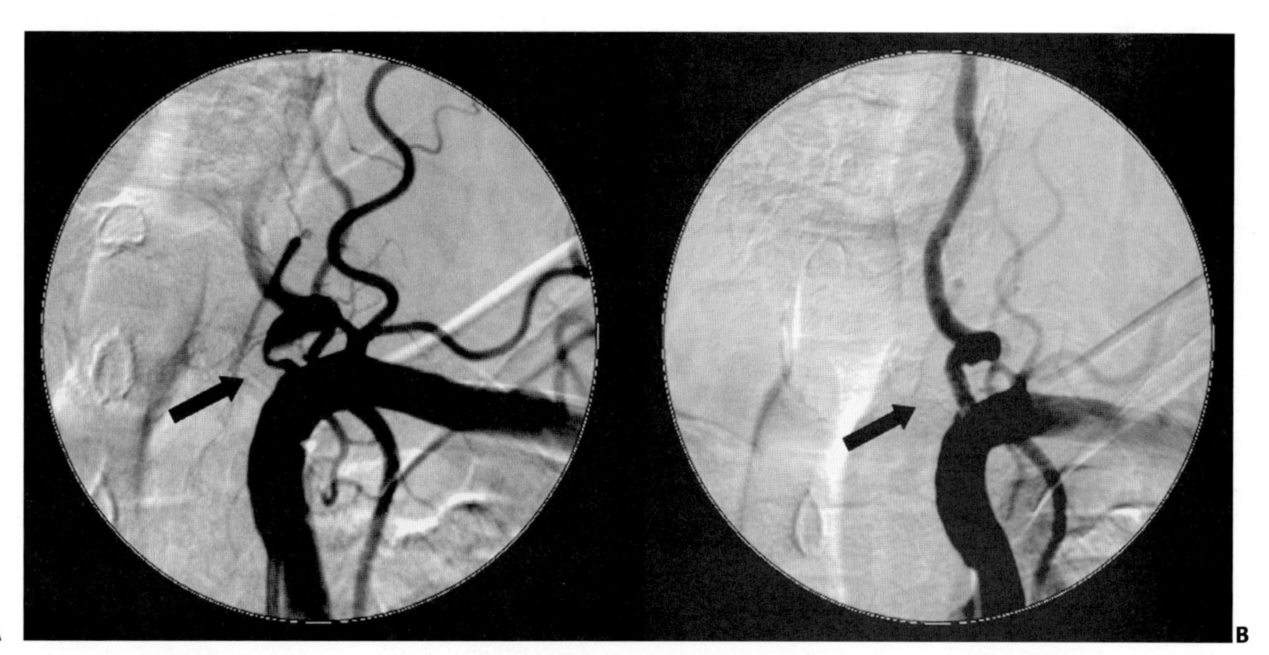

FIGURE 11.3. One potential level of complexity that should be avoided by inexperienced operators is the vertebral artery with significant tortuosity **(A,** *arrow***)**. The tortuosity creates a significant technical challenge for stenting of such lesion. However, in experienced hands, this can be accomplished successfully and without complications **(B,** *arrow***)**.

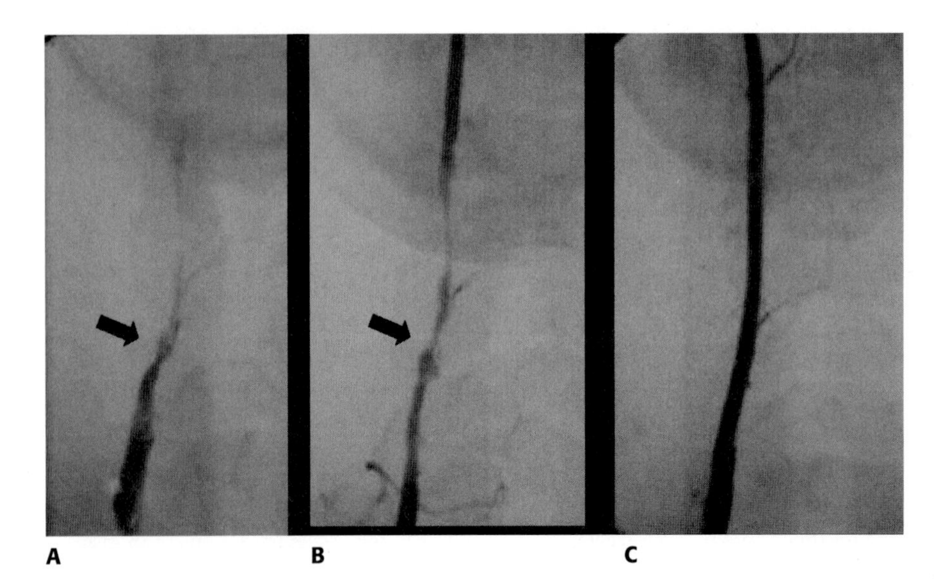

FIGURE 11.4. Treatment of vertebral artery dissections is somewhat more complex. In this case, dissection of the V2 segment of the right vertebral artery results in multiple channels [*arrows* in **(A)** and **(B)**], only one of which is the true lumen. However, after careful instrumentation, and using self-expandable coronary stents, the true lumen is restored **(C)**.

warfarin to double antiplatelet therapy. If, on the other hand, the vessel remains dissected, endovascular repair (i.e., reconstruction) may be carried out. A particular problem is reflected by partially healed dissections, whose endovascular treatment must be balanced against the likelihood of additional healing over a second period of finite anticoagulation. In our experience, it becomes a matter of judgment when to repair these vessels. Finally, there is one more point of view to discuss relative to the treatment of dissections: How to handle the patient who has an underlying condition that predisposes to recurrent future dissections (e.g., fibromuscular dysplasia). These are instances in which, despite complete healing, we may consider endovascular preventive stenting to reinforce the vascular wall for the future and curtail future dissections.

Following the same lines of thought, *ceteris paribus*, the treatment of other nonatherosclerotic lesions, depends on the potential benefit of stenting versus their expected natural history. Certainly, the emboligenic potential of radiation angiitis seems to be lower than that of atherosclerotic lesions, yet for severely stenotic lesions, stenting is a reasonable approach to preserve flow. We have already discussed certain aspects of fibromuscular dysplasia but another aspect to consider is that the weblike intraluminal architecture of many of these lesions is very difficult to demonstrate angiographically. Thus, the possibility of underestimating the hemodynamic effect of these lesions must be balanced against the small yet definite risk of dissecting the vessel during the endovascular procedure. One solution to minimize this risk is the use of small coronary self-expandable (rather than balloon-expandable) stents (Fig. 11.4).

A final word about medical therapy for all patients undergoing vertebral artery stenting: It is imperative that patients are treated with aspirin and clopidogrel before the procedure, to remove the risk of acute stent thrombosis. Once the intervention has been completed, both antiplatelet agents must be continued for at least 4 weeks, and in our opinion, indefinitely.

Asymptomatic Patient

The approach to the asymptomatic patient with a vertebral artery lesion, although following a similar path to that described for symptomatic patients, requires considerably more thought and a different threshold within the decision tree. For instance, we do not consider any form of revascularization in an asymptomatic patient unless the flow compromise is severe (i.e., equivalent to more than 80% diameter stenosis angiographically).

SELECTED REFERENCES

Caplan LR. Lateral medullary ischemic events in young adults with hypoplastic vertebral artery and Arterial occlusions-does size matter? Hypoplastic Vertebral Artery; Frequency and Associations with Ischemic Stroke Territory. *J Neurol Neurosurg Psychiatr* 2007: 78:916.

Chastain HD, II, Campbell MS, Iyer S, et al. *Extracranial vertebral artery stent placement: in-hospital and follow-up results. J Neurosurg* 1999;91(4): 547–552.

Chiaradio JC, Guzman L, Padilla L, et al. Intravascular graft stent treatment of a ruptured fusiform dissecting aneurysm of the intracranial vertebral artery: technical case report. *Neurosurgery* 2002;50(1):213–216; discussion 216–217.

Chuang Y-M, Huang Y-C, Hu H-H, et al. Toward a further elucidation: role of vertebral artery hypoplasia in acute ischemic stroke. *Eur Neurol* 2006;55(4):193–197.

Cohen JE, Gomori JM, Umansky F. Endovascular management of symptomatic vertebral artery dissection achieved using stent angioplasty and emboli protection device. *Neurol Res* 2003;25(4): 418–422.

Du B, Dong KH, Xu XT, et al. Stent-assisted angioplasty and long-term results in atherosclerotic vertebral artery ostial stenosis. *Zhonghua Nei Ke Za Zhi* 2007;46(3):204–207.

Fessler RD, Wakhloo AK, Lanzino G, et al. Stent placement for vertebral artery occlusive disease: preliminary clinical experience. *Neurosurg Focus* 1998;5(4):e15.

Giannopoulos S, Kosmidou M, Pelidou SH, et al. Vertebral artery hypoplasia: a predisposing factor for posterior circulation stroke? *Neurology* 2007;68(22):1956–1957.

Gonzalez A, Mayol A, Gil-Peralta A, et al. Endovascular stent-graft treatment of an iatrogenic vertebral arteriovenous fistula. *Neuroradiology* 2001;43(9):784–786.

Hüttl K, Sebestyén M, Entz L, et al. Covered stent placement in a traumatically injured vertebral artery. *J Vasc Interv Radiol* 2004;15 (2 Pt 1):201–202.

Jenkins JS, White CJ, Ramee SR, et al. Vertebral artery stenting. *Catheter Cardiovasc Interv* 2001;54(1):1–5.

Katsaridis V, Papagiannaki C, Violaris C. Treatment of an iatrogenic vertebral artery laceration with the Symbiot self expandable covered stent. *Clin Neurol Neurosurg* 2007;109(6):512–515.

Kim SR, Baik MW, Yoo SH, et al. Stent fracture and restenosis after placement of a drug-eluting device in the vertebral artery origin and treatment with the stent-in-stent technique. Report of two cases. *J Neurosurg* 2007;106(5):907–911.

Mehta B, Burke T, Kole M, et al. Stent-within-a-stent technique for the treatment of dissecting vertebral artery aneurysms. *AJNR Am J Neuroradiol* 2003;24(9):1814–1818.

Nazir FS, Muir KW. Prolonged interval between vertebral artery dissection and ischemic stroke. *Neurology* 2004;62(9):1646–1647.

Park JH, Kim JM, Roh JK. Hypoplastic vertebral artery; frequency and associations with ischemic stroke territory. *J Neurol Neurosurg Psychiatr* 2007;78:954–958.

Qureshi AI, Kirmani JF, Harris-Lane P, et al. Vertebral artery origin stent placement with distal protection: technical and clinical results. *AJNR Am J Neuroradiol* 2006;27(5):1140–1145.

Saket RR, Razavi MK, Sze DY, et al. Stent-graft treatment of extracranial carotid and vertebral arterial lesions. *J Vasc Interv Radiol* 2004;15(10): 1151–1156.

Sharma S, Bhambi B. Vertebral artery stenting utilizing distal embolic protection with filter wire and a drug-eluting Taxus stent. *Acute Card Care* 2006;8(4):235–237.

Waldman DL, Barquist E, Poynton FG, et al. Stent graft of a traumatic vertebral artery injury: case report. *J Trauma* 1998;44(6): 1094–1097.

Weber W, Mayer TE, Henkes H, et al. Efficacy of stent angioplasty for symptomatic stenoses of the proximal vertebral artery. *Eur J Radiol* 2005; 56(2):240–247.

CRITICAL PATHWAY
Management of Vertebral Artery Atherosclerotic Lesions

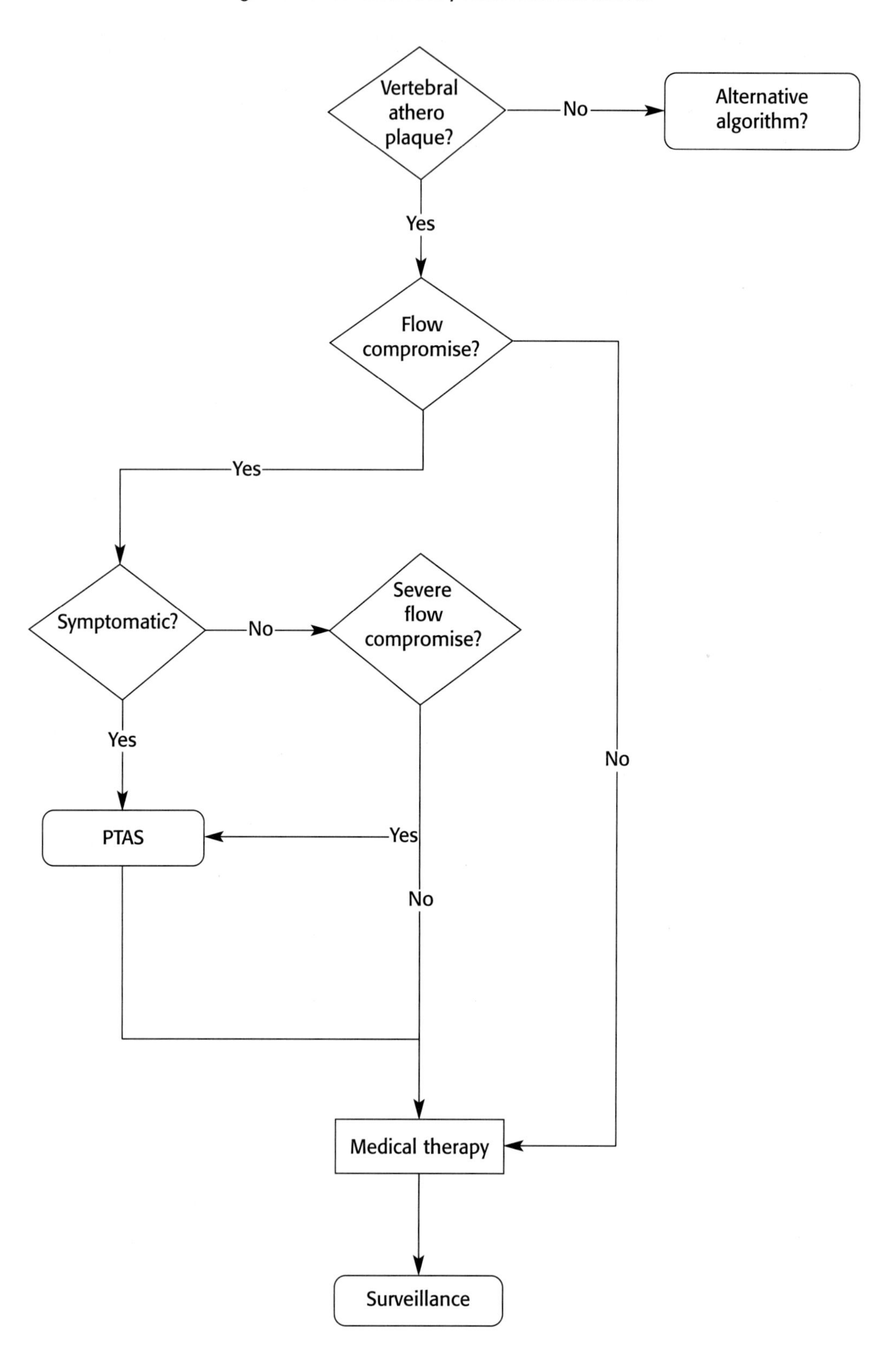

PTAS, percutaneous transluminal angioscopy.

CRITICAL PATHWAY
Management of Vertebral Artery Dissections

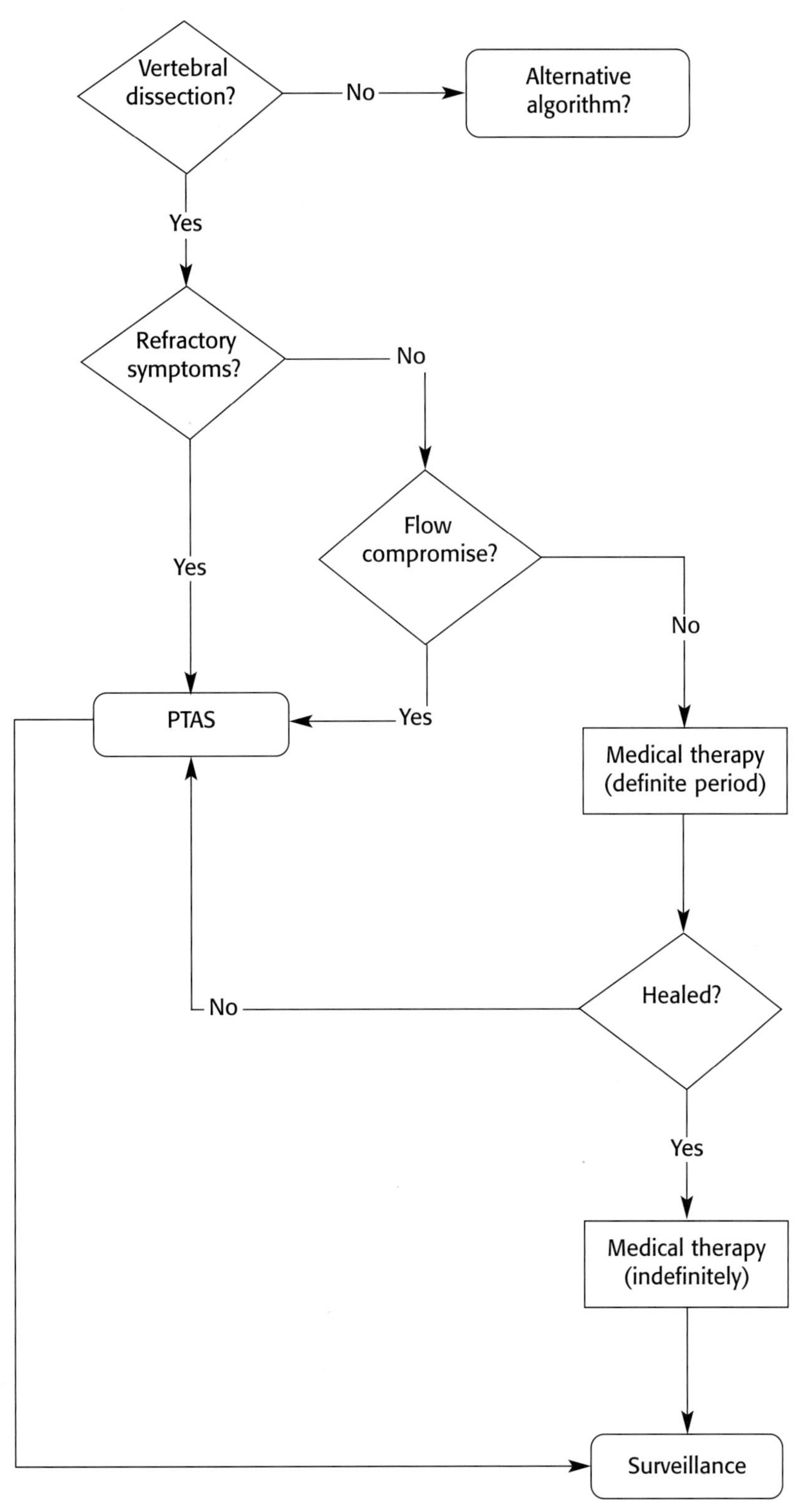

PTAS, percutaneous transluminal angioscopy.

CHAPTER

12 Management of Intracranial Atherosclerosis

CAMILO R. GOMEZ AND JAMES D. GEYER

OBJECTIVES

- What are the goals of therapy in patients with intracranial atherosclerotic pathology?
- What criteria need to be used to decide how to treat patients with intracranial atherosclerotic lesions?
- When is endovascular therapy of the intracranial arterial lesions indicated?
- Which patients should be considered for revascularization?
- What is the best approach to the asymptomatic patient?

Traditionally, the search for vascular lesions capable of causing stroke was limited to the extracranial portions of the carotid artery, since carotid endarterectomy (CEA) was considered the only available method for revascularization. During the last decade, however, technologic advances have resulted in the introduction of endovascular techniques for the management of many different vascular beds, and cerebral circulation is no exception. In other chapters of the book, we have addressed the use of endovascular techniques in the management of extracranial carotid and vertebral pathology. The present chapter is a review of the various options available for the treatment of patients who are found to have atherosclerotic lesions of the intracranial cerebral arteries, with particular attention to the use of endovascular techniques.

The optimal preventive treatment of patients with intracranial lesions is a matter of heated debate, including the choice of antithrombotic agents. This chapter addresses the subject of endovascular therapy for intracranial lesions. However, the authors believe that endovascular therapy must be applied *in addition to* optimal medical therapy, including risk factor modification by all possible means. Keeping this in mind, endovascular therapy (i.e., balloon angioplasty and stenting) must be always considered as an option for the treatment of patients with hemodynamically significant and symptomatic intracranial lesions. The authors position is based on the following assumptions: (a) Intracranial stenosis is hardly a homogeneous process, and the amalgamation of all lesions into one category that equates to one treatment strategy represents an artificial oversimplification of the subject. In fact, lesion location and severity must be taken into consideration when planning therapy for any patient. (b) In general, intracranial stenoses carry a relatively high risk for stroke, regardless of their medical treatment; underscoring the need for a better alternative therapeutic strategy. (c) Finally, technological advances and experience of interventionalists have appreciably reduced the risk of endovascular therapy for intracranial stenotic lesions.

BACKGROUND AND RATIONALE

Heterogeneity of Intracranial Atherosclerotic Lesions

It is estimated that intracranial stenoses are the direct cause of approximately 10% or more of all ischemic strokes, and of approximately 8% of transient ischemic attacks (TIA). In fact, older reports of angiographic assessments of various stroke subpopulations have shown that intracranial stenotic lesions could be found in approximately 5% to 23% of cases. The differences in prevalence between these reports depend on the criteria for patient inclusion.

There is inadequate attention paid to the heterogeneous nature of intracranial stenoses, particularly as it relates to differences in clinical behavior, symptom formation, prognosis, and response to treatment. Intracranial atherosclerotic lesions are most common in the following locations: (a) the petrous portion of the intracranial internal carotid artery (ICA), (b) the cavernous-siphon portions of the intracranial ICA, (c) the clinoid portion of the intracranial ICA, (d) the main trunk of the middle cerebral artery (MCA), (e) the distal (portions V3 and V4) of the vertebral artery (VA), and (f) the basilar artery (BA). Data regarding the frequency with which these are found are scant, are mostly found in older studies, but suggest that the most frequent locations involve the intracranial VA and the BA. In the intracranial ICA, stenoses are most frequently found in the cavernous (98.5%) portion, followed by the petrous (21.2%), and clinoid (9.0%) segments, with multiple tandem lesions being present in a minority of patients.

Current clinical perspective supports the notion that not all of these intracranial lesions have the same importance. Because they are located distal to major points of collateral support, stenoses of the BA or the MCA are theoretically more ominous than those of the terminal VA or the intracranial ICA, which benefit from collateral support. Consistent with this projected risk, occlusion of the MCA is almost unequivocally associated with stroke, while occlusion of the ICA leads to stroke in only approximately 60% of the cases. Despite this difference, it has been reported that, at the end of a 30-month follow-up period, only one third of patients with symptomatic intracranial ICA stenosis remain alive and free of strokes, while approximately 30% suffered a stroke (one third of them being fatal). The prognosis of BA stenosis is less well-known, but as evidenced by the various series reported in the literature, the outcome of acute BA occlusion is almost invariably fatal. Furthermore, patients with lesions of the intracranial VA or BA have been shown to have approximately a 22% risk for stroke during a of period slightly >1 year. Therefore, it seems unreasonable to recommend any one type of treatment for intracranial stenosis, implying that it is equally efficacious for all type of lesions. Their particular location, severity, and cerebrovascular context must be taken into consideration.

Another aspect that differentiates between intracranial stenoses is their hemodynamic severity, also reflected in their pathogenic potential. Although certainly capable of inducing distal embolization, intracranial stenotic lesions most commonly become symptomatic through flow stagnation, perfusion compromise, and ultimately *in situ* thrombotic occlusion. As an illustration, a residual lumen of 0.5 mm diameter, representative of a 90% diameter reduction in a 5 mm wide vessel (i.e., typical extracranial ICA), only amounts to a 75% diameter reduction in a 2 mm wide vessel (i.e., typical MCA). Nevertheless, the flow stagnation and pressure gradient produced by both lesions are comparable. Thus, the hemodynamic significance of lesions of the intracranial arteries is likely to become evident earlier and in more severe manner, explaining the higher risk of stroke and emphasizing the potential benefit of lumen enlargement by endovascular therapy.

The Natural History and Effectiveness of Medical Treatment

The information presented in this section underscores the importance of stratifying all intracranial atherosclerotic lesions into different diagnostic or therapeutic categories, since some of them appear to have a more ominous prognosis. The natural history of patients with these lesions is poorer than that of patients with extracranial lesions, with annual stroke rates that approximate 8% or greater. Unlike extracranial stenoses, intracranial lesions have a greater tendency to produce unheralded strokes, and when these patients present with TIA, there is a high incidence of subsequent stroke in a short period, usually months.

There are no conclusive answers about the best medical management of intracranial stenotic lesions. Retrospective data previously suggested that long-term anticoagulation with warfarin was more effective than antiplatelet therapy, but the results of a randomized prospective study did not support such an approach. The Warfarin-Aspirin Symptomatic Intracranial Disease (WASID) study compared the effectiveness of warfarin (titrated for international normalized ratio [INR] = 2 to 3) versus aspirin (1,300 mg per day) in reducing the risk of stroke, death, and intracerebral hemorrhage in patients with TIA or stroke secondary to an angiographically documented intracranial atherosclerotic lesion. Even though the original design of the study planned for slightly >800 patients among the two groups, enrollment was stopped after 569 patients had been entered. The main concern was about the safety of the patients receiving warfarin, who displayed higher rates of adverse events including death, major hemorrhages, and myocardial infarction compared to the patients treated with aspirin. Interestingly, the absolute difference of secondary end points was approximately 3% across the board in favor of warfarin (Table 12.1). This, of course, was offset by the greater number of adverse events.

Still, if we take into consideration the comments made earlier, it should not be surprising that we have failed to show general superiority of one or another treatment, since, in fact, we may be comparing apples and oranges. To compound the problem, even if we considered that there may be subsets of patients who may benefit from anticoagulation more than they do from antithrombotic therapy (e.g., patient with very severe stenoses and evidence of flow stagnation), chronic anticoagulation is not a panacea, as evidenced by the WASID study results. Nevertheless, other series highlight the ill-fated future of patients with intracranial atherosclerotic lesions who fail medical therapy, estimating stroke rates as high as 40% to 50% within weeks of diagnosis. All of these observations serve as a framework for rationalizing the study and application of elective intracranial angioplasty and stenting as strategies for stroke prevention.

The Evolution of Endovascular Therapy

Balloon angioplasty of the intracranial arteries has been a feasible option for a number of years. Its application has primarily relied on techniques and instrumentation from other vascular beds (e.g., coronary balloons). Over the last decade, technologic advances and operators' experience have resulted in increased success rates and lower complications. Since the flow within a vessel is determined by the square of the lumen radius, small dilatations of intracranial arteries by means of balloon angioplasty have the potential to result in significant improvement of flow and reduction of stroke risk. For intracranial balloon angioplasty, performed by experienced interventionalists, success rates have increased from approximately 60% to >90%, while complication rates remain consistently <10%, making the procedure more attractive for clinical use. In fact, the

TABLE 12.1 Comparison of the Secondary Endpoints of the Warfarin-Aspirin Symptomatic Intracranial Disease (WASID) Study, Suggesting Benefit of Warfarin

Secondary Endpoint	Aspirin (n = 280) Patients (%)	Warfarin (n = 289) Patients (%)
Ischemic stroke	57 (20.4)	49 (17.0)
Ischemic stroke in target territory	42 (15.0)	35 (12.1)
Disabling or fatal stroke	25 (8.9)	18 (6.2)

These results were offset by the higher number of adverse events in the warfarin group.

figures quoted are probably affected by adverse selection, since many of the reported patients already had failed medical therapy. Despite the recent advances in technology and experience, there are potential technical problems with the performance of balloon angioplasty, including the risk of dissection, elastic recoil, and acute closure, all of which fueled the interest in intracranial stenting.

The conceptual advantages of stenting over balloon angioplasty include (a) lesser risk of acute closure from intimal dissection and thrombus formation and (b) improved long-term patency rates from larger postprocedural lumen diameters and avoidance of recoil. The main limiting factor for the utilization of stents to treat intracranial lesions has been the availability of stents that could be tracked and deployed within the intracranial cavity. In spite of such a limitation, the published major intracranial stenting series (excluding small case reports) report better results than balloon angioplasty. The small sample size of all of these series precludes a generalization of the results. However, series reporting the natural history or effect of medical therapy in intracranial stenoses are only slightly larger and are subject to similar criticism.

It is important to consider in our discussion the results of the Stenting of Symptomatic Atherosclerotic Lesions in the Vertebral or Intracranial Arteries (SSYLVIA) study, since they are relevant to the recommendations we are bound to make later in the chapter. The SSYLVIA study was designed to investigate the effectiveness of a stenting system designed for neurologic use (i.e., NEUROLINK). Enrollment of 61 patients (43 with intracranial lesions and 18 with extracranial vertebral lesions) resulted in one of the largest series reported. The rates of complicating strokes were 6.6% at 30 days and 7.3% between 30 days and 1 year. The rates of restenosis at 6 months were 32.4% for intracranial lesions and 42.9% for extracranial vertebral arteries. These results were generally considered lukewarm at best, and no additional investigation of the NEUROLINK system has been conducted since then.

Several important comments must be made about the SSYLVIA results, particularly because there is such a disparity between the results of the study and our experience of >10 years in elective intracranial stenting. The first comments have to do with the NEUROLINK system itself. The original design of the NEUROLINK stent was that of a balloon-expandable 316L stainless steel stent that, by design, had significantly less metal than the existing coronary stents. In retrospect, this was probably a mistake, particularly for treating extracranial VA lesions, which *cannot be compared* with intracranial stenoses. In addition, the shaft of the balloon catheter was excessively long, a problem that became evident in the only patient we treated under this protocol, as we found it impossible to perform an over-the-wire exchange using standard 300 cm microwires. This forced us to have to recross the lesion, a step commonly avoided in endovascular treatment.

The second set of comments is technical, relating to the variability of the procedures performed. Operators were allowed to use either local or general anesthesia, the latter presenting a separate variable in the therapeutic equation. Over the years, the authors have almost invariably performed elective intracranial stenting under local anesthesia, a technique that allows for monitoring the patients during the procedure. Review of the data also shows that, in general, the degree of diameter enlargement achieved in the study was suboptimal. This is a problem, for there is a large body of literature that correlates the postprocedural diameter with the risk of restenosis in other vascular beds, particularly the coronary arteries. Finally, predilation was left up to the discretion of the operator. Therefore, predilation should be performed in all cases, particularly as it allows the operator to test the vessel before deploying a stent and improves the ability to measure the ultimate target vascular segment before choosing the size of the stent to be used.

Finally, the rate of postdischarge strokes is concerning. In the authors' experience, once the patient leaves the catheterization laboratory, it is very unusual to see a complicating stroke. This is even rarer after 30 days following the procedure. This raises the question of whether the treatment of the patient following the procedure should have been handled differently. For example, the patients in the SSYLVIA study were kept on clopidogrel alone for about 4 weeks, but these patients should be maintained on double antiplatelet therapy indefinitely.

Experience with the Wingspan Stent

More recently, additional research has allowed the introduction of a self-expandable stent designed specifically for intracranial deployment (i.e., Wingspan, Boston Scientific, Boston, MA). The attractiveness of this stent, from the beginning, has been its deliverability to distal intracranial locations (i.e., the stent is delivered via a microcatheter). Also, since it does not require a balloon for deployment, the radial force exerted is not as large as that of balloon-expandable stents. The initial experience in the United States has shown a high rate of procedural success (98.8%), with a 6.1% rate of 30-day stroke and death rate. The latter statistics makes this procedure much more competitive than previously recognized.

CLINICAL APPLICATIONS AND METHODOLOGY

General Considerations

The application of endovascular techniques to the treatment of intracranial atherosclerotic pathology involves two different issues: feasibility and reasonableness. The former relates to whether a procedure *can be performed* as the treatment of a specific lesion, while the latter relates to whether such a procedure *should be performed*, even if feasible. The discussion in the previous section should illustrate to the reader that, at present, the quality of technology and operator's expertise makes endovascular treatment of these lesions feasible. However, the ability to revascularize a lesion should not automatically translate into a procedure that may or may not be needed.

Candidacy for Endovascular Intervention

The heterogeneity of intracranial stenoses is also reflected in their potential for endovascular therapy. Thus, treatment of lesions in the petrous and cavernous portions of the ICA, at present, represents little technical challenge (see Fig. 12.1). However, the ability to track the stents beyond the carotid artery siphon into the clinoid portion of the carotid, or even the MCA, has become reliable only following the introduction of self-expandable stents. Stenting of the intracranial portions of the vertebrobasilar system, namely the V3 and V4 portions of the VA, has also been shown to be feasible and relatively safe and has proved to be an easier system in which to work than the carotid territory (see Fig. 12.2).

Then there is the BA. One of the potential risks of deploying stents intracranially is that of jailing perforating branches from the

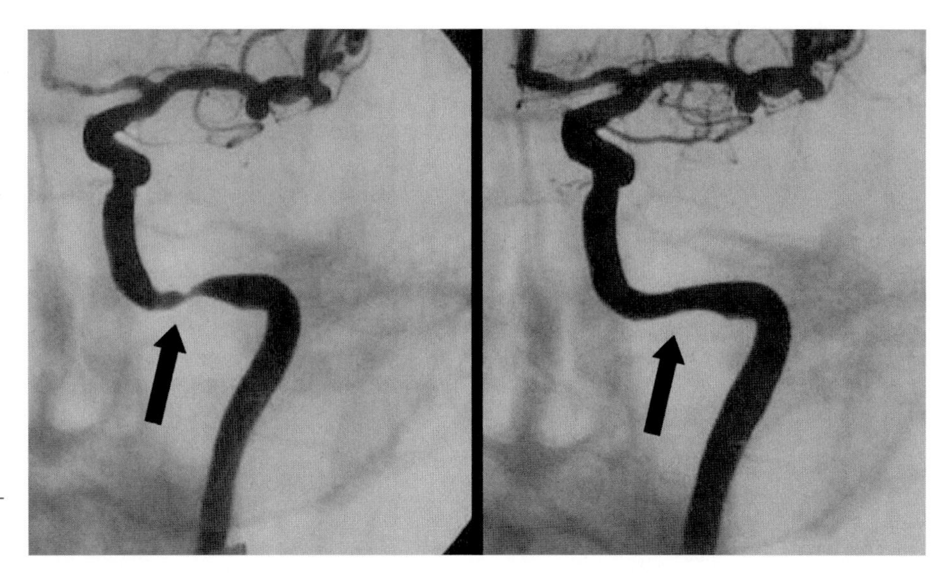

FIGURE 12.1. Successful stenting of a left internal carotid artery stenosis in the petrous segment. The arrows demonstrate the point of stenosis and the final results following stent deployment.

vessel being treated, causing ischemic stroke along the territory of these small vessels. This concept has been traditionally bothersome in patients with BA stenosis, in whom closing of the perforators can lead to devastating consequences. The low incidence of complicating ischemic stroke in patients undergoing intracranial stenting suggests that this risk may be less than originally suspected. Nevertheless, caution is recommended in selecting patients for the treatment of lesions located in vascular segments known for the presence of perforators (see Fig. 12.3).

In general, each patient should be considered from the perspective of the following criteria: (a) location of the lesion (i.e., segment with or without perforators), (b) severity of the lesion (i.e., hemodynamic significance), (c) collateral support (i.e., proximal or distal to major collaterals), (d) symptom formation (i.e., symptomatic or not), and (e) access difficulty (i.e., status of the proximal arterial vessels). Since each of these criteria lends itself suitable for the construction of a dichotomy, and these can be assigned a numeric value, it is possible to construct a scale of interventional complexity (see Table 12.2). This is useful because of the implications for the risk–benefit analysis, but also because of the procedural planning.

Operator's Expertise

Operator's expertise is perhaps the single most important variable that affects the outcome of endovascular treatment of intracranial lesions. The success of prospective trials is directly related to the technical expertise of the operators. Typically they are handpicked, screened for a number of months before the study, and closely monitored. In daily practice, on the other hand, this may or may not be the case. Conversely, it is possible to learn from the experience with carotid stenting trials in which the operators' expertise was not optimal, leading to unusually high procedural complication rates (e.g., Wallstent and SPACE studies).

Three major features characterize expert operators: (a) patient selection skills, (2) phenotypic and genotypic interventional attributes, and (c) high volume of cases (i.e., experience). The best operators spend considerable amount of time making sure that the patient in question is as close an ideal candidate for the procedure as possible. They do not take chances by operating on patients who may not benefit from the procedure, or whose circumstances are such that they pose an unusually high procedural risk. To be able to select patients properly, operators must have fundamental knowledge of neuroanatomy, neurophysiology, clinical neurology, neuroimaging, neuropathology, and neuropharmacology.

The phenotypic characteristics of an operator derive from his or her procedural education, that is, having performed a large number of procedures under the supervision of a qualified mentor, affording him or her the ability to learn all aspects of the procedure. More important, procedural education must be then translated in learning the principles that would allow the operator to troubleshoot when confronted with a situation not previously encountered. The supervised experience must be sufficient to facilitate the learning curve, while conferring the operator fundamental knowledge about cerebral catheterization, neuroangiography, and specific competence with the devices to be used. The other set of characteristics, genotypic, constitute a subject that is not often addressed: Not everyone who wants to operate should! In addition to clinical judgment (i.e., for patient selection) and procedural knowledge (i.e., phenotypic skills), the operator must possess the hand–eye coordination that is inborn and cannot be taught. Just as Michael Jordan was born to play basketball, everyone is born with inherent skills that separate excellence from mediocrity. In our opinion, it is incumbent on postgraduate program directors to see that individuals without natural aptitudes do not advance thinking that they can operate just as their mentors do.

The final aspect of the operator's expertise is related to the volume of procedures performed. There is absolutely no substitute for experience, and the literature shows that consistently for nearly every therapeutic procedure investigated.

Practical Experience

On the basis of the principles outlined, a treatment protocol has been implemented that has allowed for considerable experience in this field. The authors' uncontrolled single-center series accumulated over a period of approximately 8 years includes 95 patients (76 men; 87 white; mean age = 63.7 years) with 102

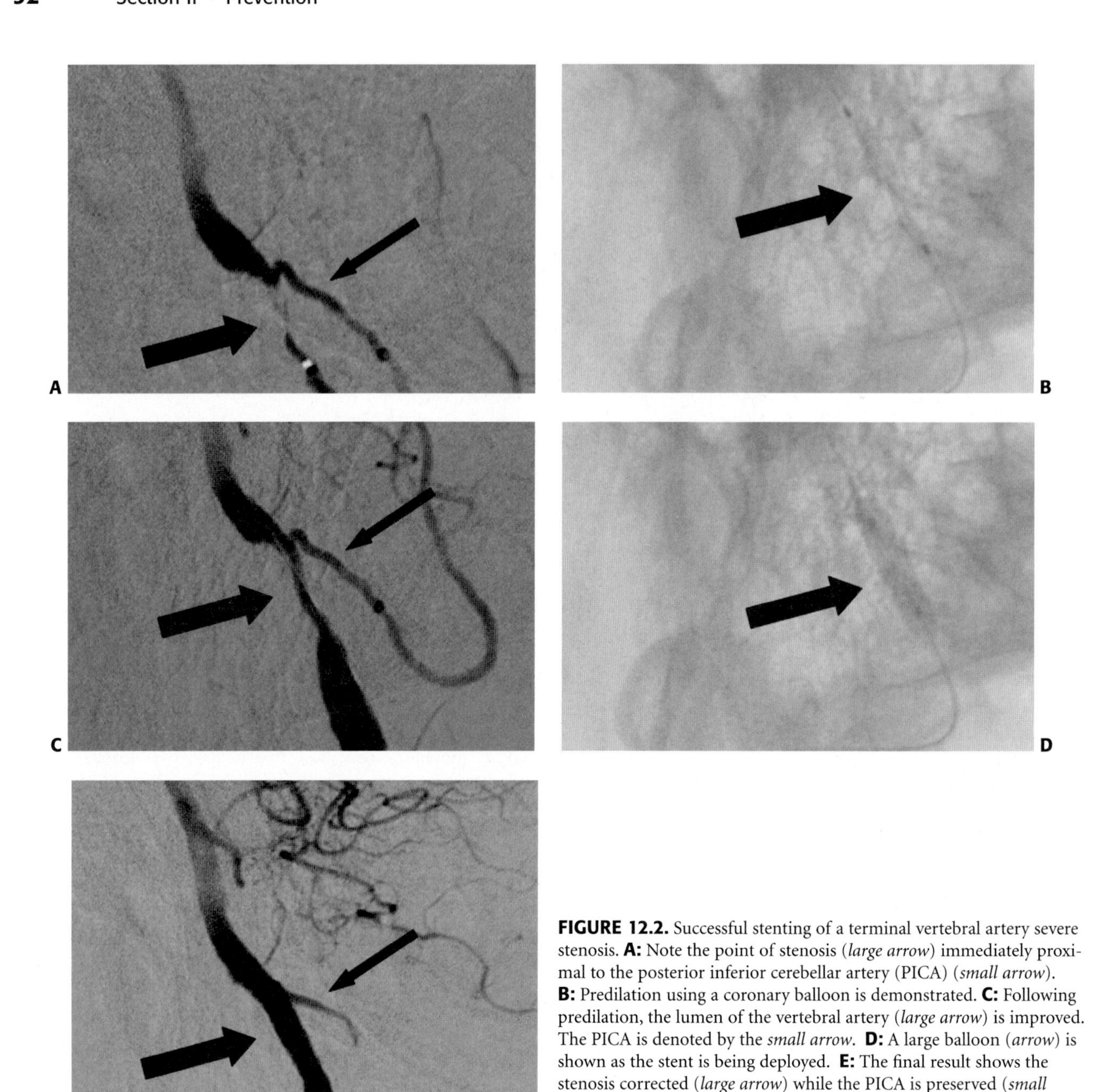

FIGURE 12.2. Successful stenting of a terminal vertebral artery severe stenosis. **A:** Note the point of stenosis (*large arrow*) immediately proximal to the posterior inferior cerebellar artery (PICA) (*small arrow*). **B:** Predilation using a coronary balloon is demonstrated. **C:** Following predilation, the lumen of the vertebral artery (*large arrow*) is improved. The PICA is denoted by the *small arrow*. **D:** A large balloon (*arrow*) is shown as the stent is being deployed. **E:** The final result shows the stenosis corrected (*large arrow*) while the PICA is preserved (*small arrow*).

intracranial arterial lesions. All patients presented with either nondisabling stroke or TIA in the territory of the lesion being treated, and they all demonstrated >50% stenosis in the lesion to be treated. Rather than waiting for medical failure the authors used a complexity scale as a tool to select good candidates for revascularization. All procedures were carried out under local anesthesia, without any sedation. This series includes only the use of coronary stents. The results of the interventions were competitive, with a procedural stroke rate of 3.9%, and a total rate of adverse events of 8.8% (see Table 12.3). The majority of these were of no long-term consequence to the patients. These results are similar to those of published series. It is important to point out that just as it was recently published with the Wingspan stent, the postprocedural lumen diameters in our patients were significantly larger than the preprocedural diameters ($p = 0.0001$) (see Fig. 12.4). Also, after a mean follow-up >36 months, we have only had two cases of restenosis, an experience substantially different from the published data.

PRACTICAL RECOMMENDATIONS

Endovascular techniques must be always considered as a primary form of therapy for patients with identified intracranial stenotic lesions and applied to those who are most likely to benefit from them (see Fig. 12.5). In doing so, issues related to the location and severity of the lesion, its cerebrovascular context (e.g., patterns of collateral flow), the production of symptoms, the response or potential for medical therapy, and the local technical

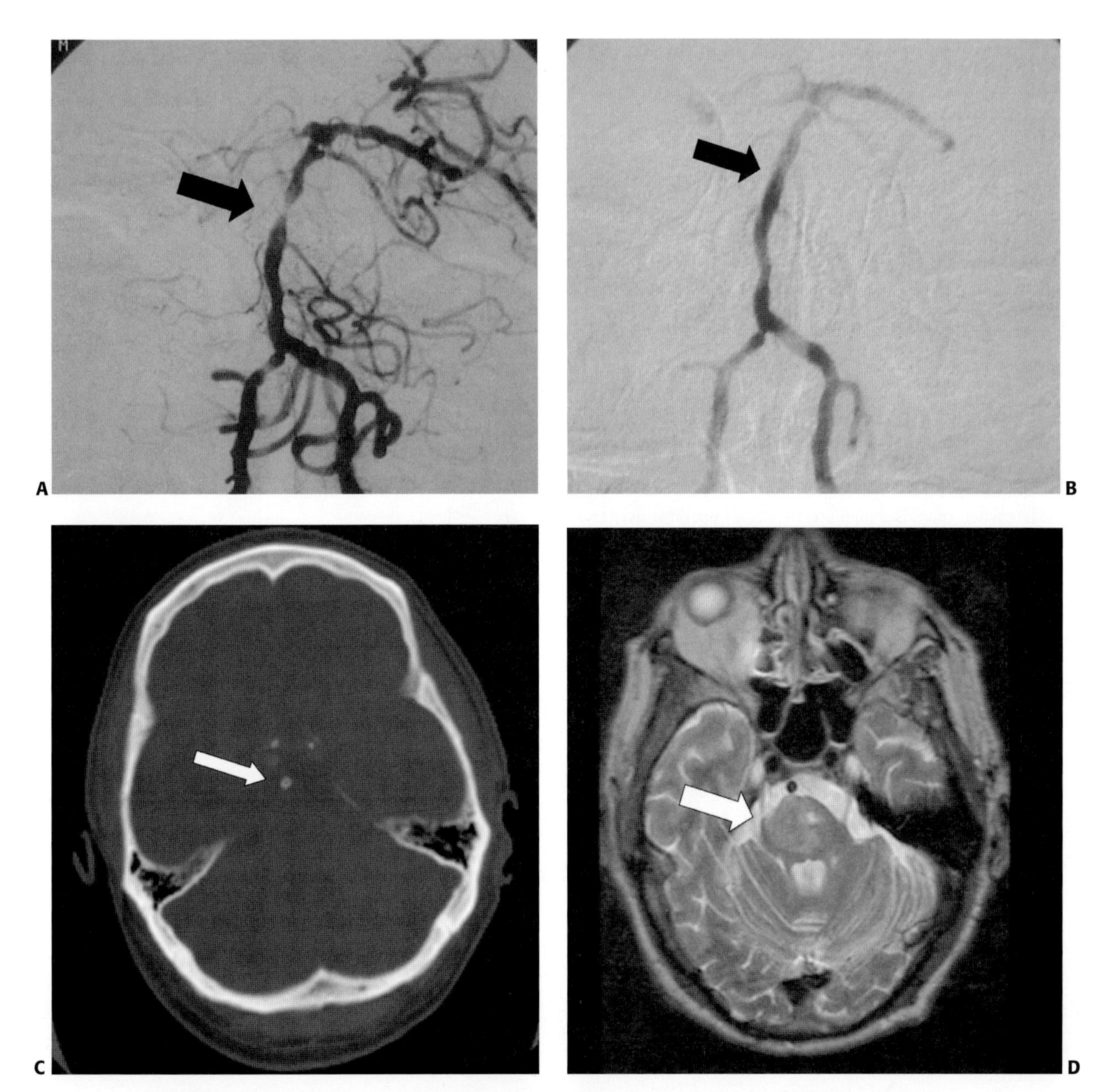

FIGURE 12.3 Basilar artery stenting complicated by closure of perforators. **A:** The original stenosis is demonstrated (*arrow*). This was a symptomatic patient, with recurrent transient ischemic attacks. **B:** The stent has been deployed, and its location noted (*arrow*). Immediately following deployment, the patient became hemiplegic and dysarthric. **C:** Computed tomography was performed on the patient, which demonstrated the stent (*arrow*), best visualized with bone windows. **D:** Later the same day, magnetic resonance imaging (MRI) was done on the patient, which shows a new pontine infarction.

TABLE 12.2 Criteria Used by the Authors' Group to Assess the Interventional Complexity of Intracranial Lesions

Criterion	Favorable Score = 0	Unfavorable Score = 1
Vascular segment location	Minimal perforators	Numerous perforators
Severity of stenosis	<50% diameter reduction	>50% diameter reduction
Collateral support	Proximal to communicating	Distal to communicating
Symptom formation	No	Yes
Access difficulty	No	Yes

Assigning scores to each of the dichotomies is possible to obtain grades between 1 and 5.

TABLE 12.3 Complications in Series of Elective Intracranial Stenting

Deaths: 1 (0.98%)
- Major ischemic stroke: 3 (2.94%)
- Transient ischemic attack: 1 (0.98%)
- Subacute stent thrombosis: 1 (0.98%)
- Other:
  - Wire perforation: 1 (0.98%)
  - Transient double vision: 1 (0.98%)
  - Transient VI to VII nerve pareses: 2 (1.96%)
  - Asymptomatic CCSF: 1 (0.98%)

expertise must factor in the decision process, and the patients must be evaluated accordingly. At present, the ideal situation involves a patient with a severely stenotic (e.g., >75%) symptomatic lesion, in a technically simple location (e.g., V4 segment), particularly when there is a highly experienced operator available (see Fig. 12.6).

In considering endovascular therapy for intracranial lesions, there is no surgical alternative, and thus, the only conceivable comparison of these techniques is with the best medical treatment. Currently there is no consensus about what constitutes optimal medical therapy. Nor is there evidence that medical therapy is better than endovascular therapy. Therefore, physicians accustomed to offering angioplasty and stenting *only* to patients who have failed medical therapy (i.e., have had recurrent symptoms despite optimal levels of anticoagulation), or who have a contraindication for long-term anticoagulation, need to address the question: *What is the price of waiting until best medical therapy fails?* Recent data suggest that this price may be quite high.

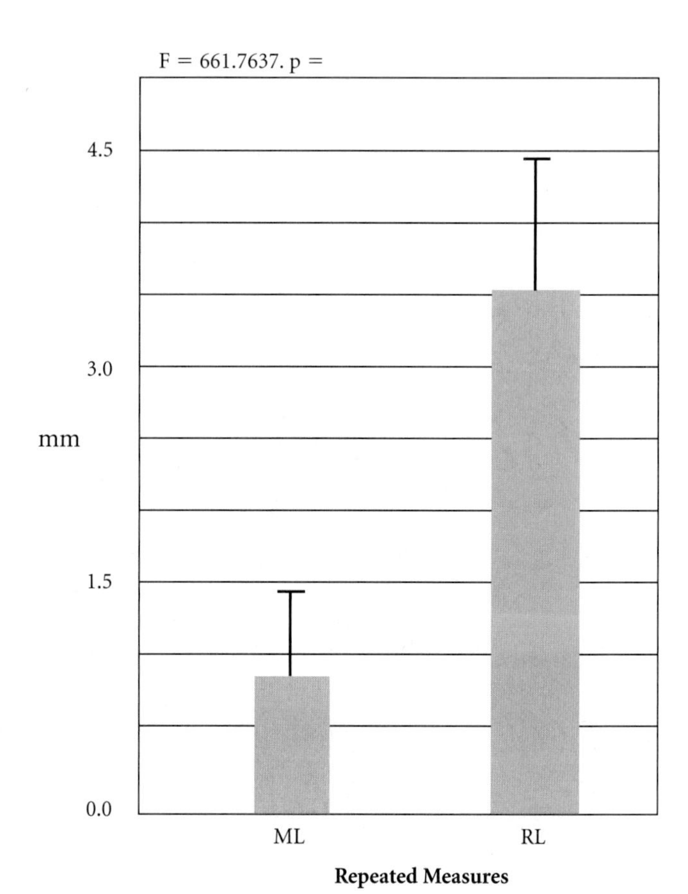

FIGURE 12.4. A comparison between the minimal lumen diameters (MLDs) of the authors' patient series before stenting with the residual lumen diameter (RLD) immediately following stenting. The difference is significant ($p = 0.0001$).

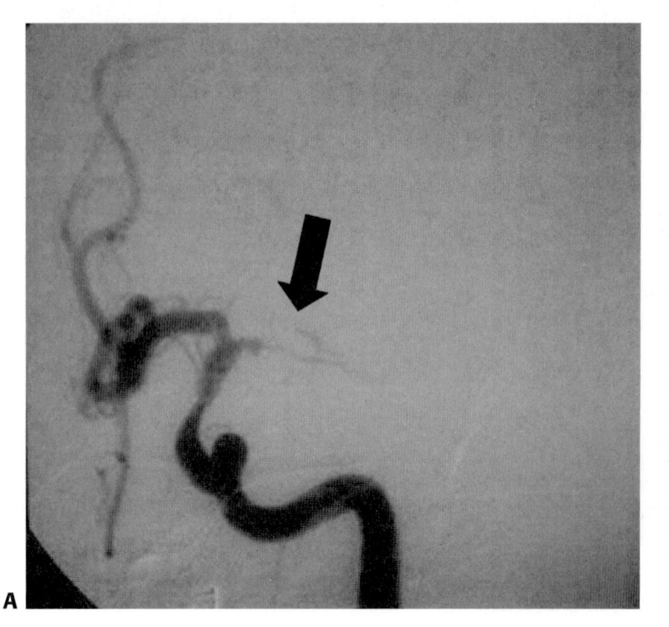

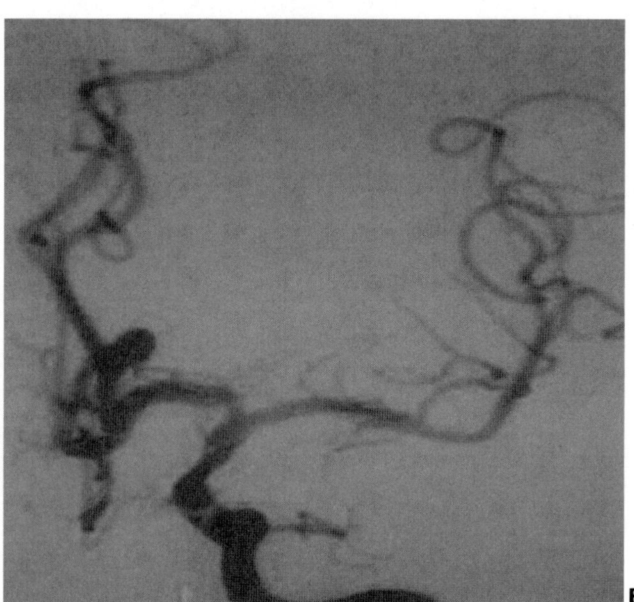

FIGURE 12.5 A–E Successful stenting of a symptomatic middle cerebral artery (MCA). **A:** The procedural angiogram demonstrates severe stenosis (*arrow*). **B:** Poststenting image shows success in restoring flow. *(Continued)*

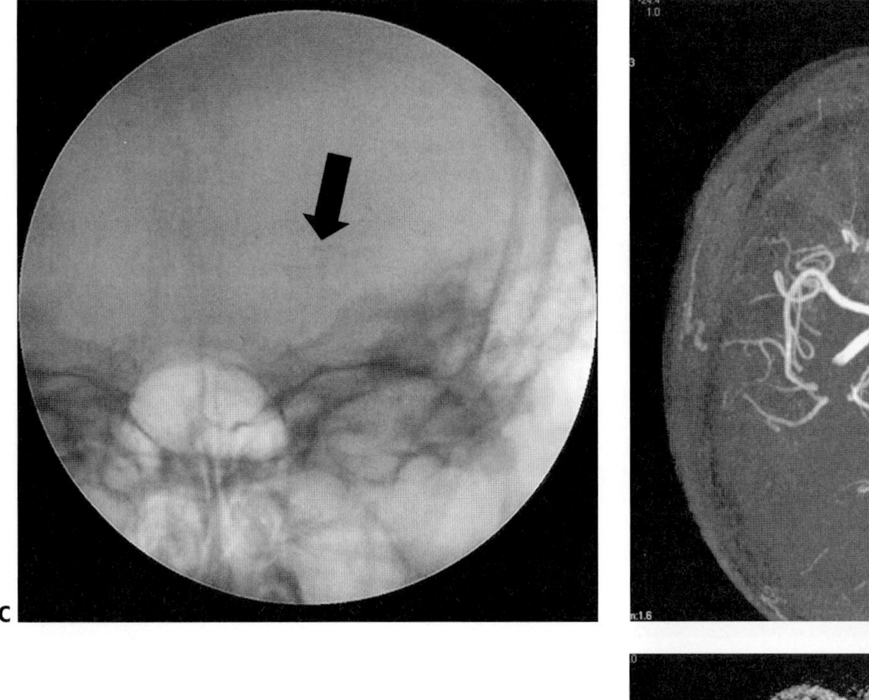
C

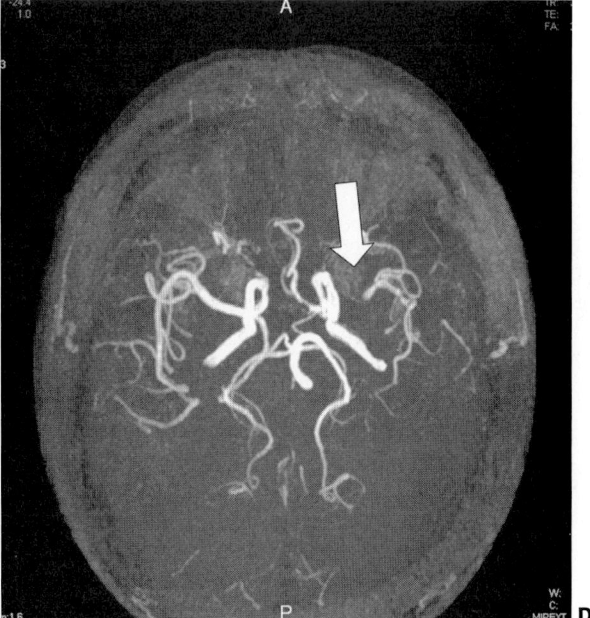

D

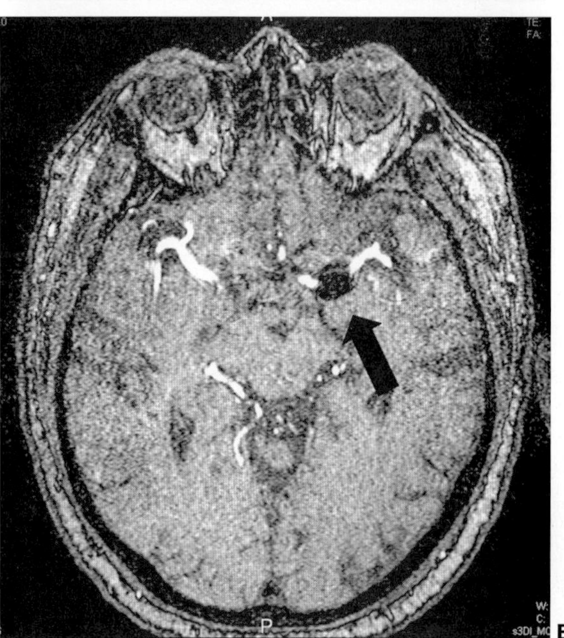

E

FIGURE 12.5 *(continued)* **C:** Fluoroscopy allows visualization of the tent. **D:** Magnetic resonance angiography (MRA) shows a signal gap, suggesting restenosis. **E:** However, source images display the metallic susceptibility artifact.

On the basis of our experience, patients with intracranial atherosclerotic pathology present via one of two routes. The first is the patient who has had a focal nondisabling neurologic deficit presumably resulting from ischemia (transient or not) and the other is the patient referred because of a lesion found in the course of his or her treatment. Although our approach to either of these patients is fundamentally similar, the weight of the choices at each node of the decision tree vary somewhat.

Symptomatic Patient

A patient who has developed a nondisabling deficit from an intracranial arterial lesion must be taken seriously with a sense of urgency that cannot be overemphasized (see Fig. 12.7). The reason is simple, the symptoms constitute the only opportunity to preempt what could be a catastrophic cerebral infarction. The first step is to examine the evidence for the presence of intracranial atherosclerotic pathology. Then a decision must be made about the degree of hemodynamic compromise for, if no significant hemodynamic compromise is evident, medical therapy alone is the recommended strategy. Details about the various components of medical therapy are discussed in other chapters of this book. Nevertheless, the use of double antiplatelet therapy is recommended as the primary pharmacologic intervention. This may be accompanied by the combination of statins (e.g., atorvastatin) and renin–angiotensin system modulators (i.e., angiotensin-converting enzyme inhibitors or angiotensin receptor blockers) for patients with dyslipidemia and hypertension, respectively. In any case,

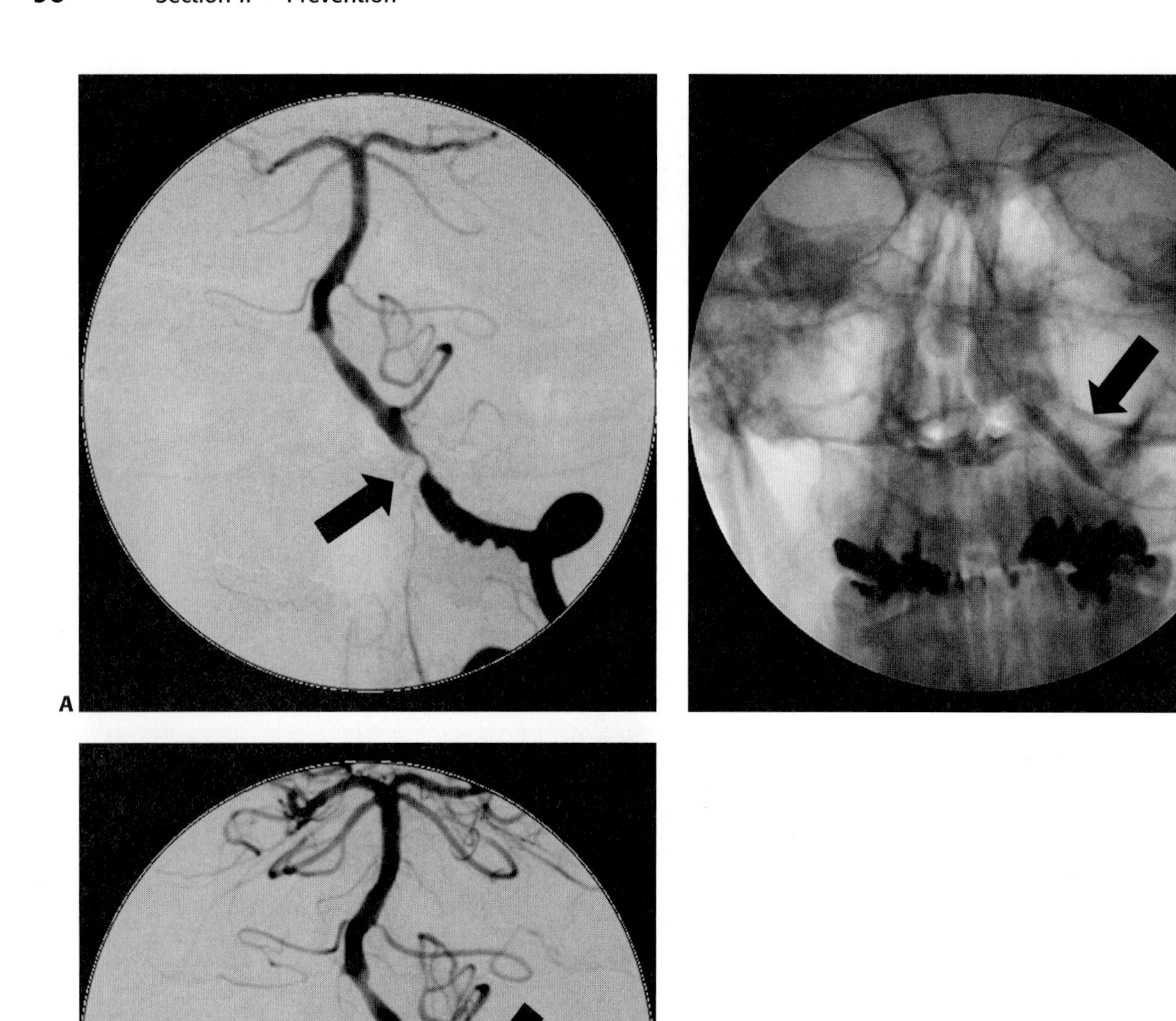

FIGURE 12.6 Successful stenting of an eccentric terminal vertebral stenosis. **A:** Initial images demonstrate a severe lesion in the terminal vertebral artery (*arrow*). **B:** Stent being deployed (*arrow*). **C:** Final image demonstrates correction of the stenosis (*arrow*). No meaningful collaterals from the contralateral vertebral artery are noted.

patients with intracranial arterial lesions and no evidence of significant hemodynamic compromise must be placed in an imaging surveillance program to ensure early detection of progression of the underlying process. An important practical point about the aforementioned recommendation has to do with the definition of significant hemodynamic compromise. This subject is covered extensively in Chapter 22 later in the book but suffice to say, it is imperative that the limitations of every imaging technique are understood, as well as the inherent inadequacy of using diameter stenosis as a surrogate for flow compromise (the actual variable to consider) (see Fig. 12.8).

The management of symptomatic intracranial atherosclerotic lesions that cause significant hemodynamic compromise should always include a consideration for stenting. This should follow the guidelines outlined earlier. A final word about medical therapy for all patients undergoing stenting: It is imperative for these individuals to be treated with aspirin and clopidogrel prior to the procedure to remove the risk of acute stent thrombosis. Once the procedure is completed, both antiplatelet agents must be continued for at least 4 weeks, but preferably indefinitely. Also, with regard to the follow-up of these patients, the myth that following intracranial stent deployment they cannot undergo magnetic resonance imaging (MRI) is simply not true. The authors have performed MRI studies within hours of deployment in up to 3.0 Tesla instruments, without any complications. The only limitation is the metallic susceptibility artifact caused by the stent (Fig. 12.5).

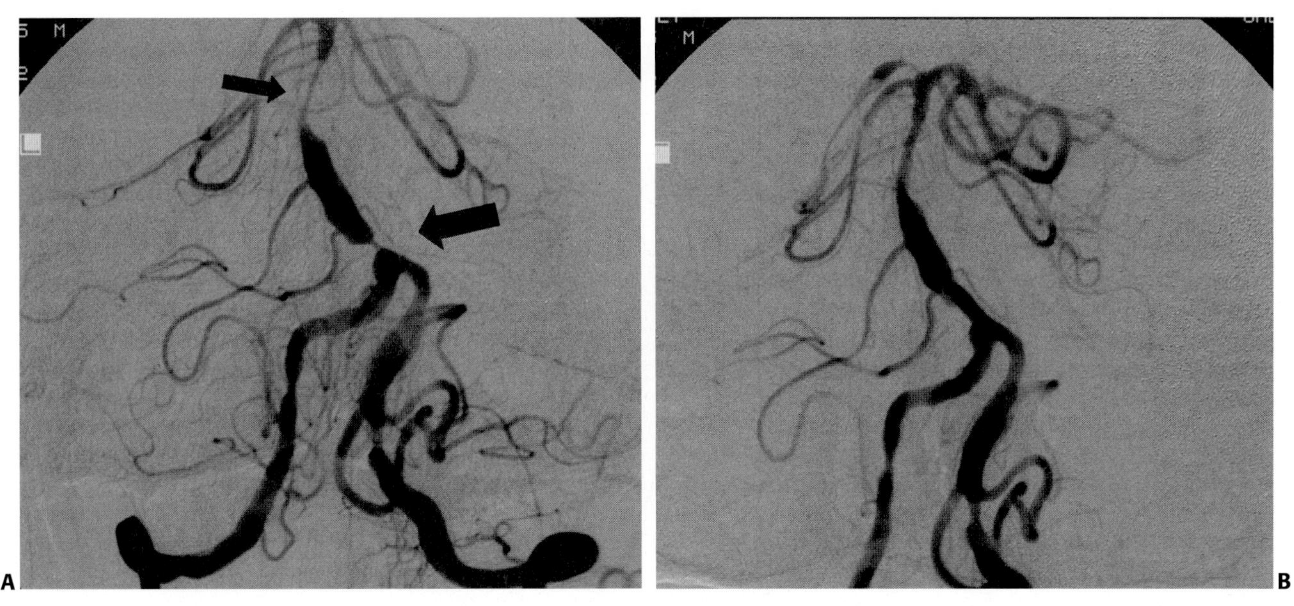

FIGURE 12.7 Tandem basilar artery lesions, both of severe degree. **A:** The proximal (*large arrow*) is at the most proximal portion of the basilar artery. The distal is close to the top of the vessel (*small arrow*). **B:** Final image shows the correction of both lesions, yet the tendency to maintain a smaller size than the native vessel.

Asymptomatic Patient

The approach to the asymptomatic patient with an intracranial arterial lesion, although following a path similar to that described for symptomatic patients, requires considerable more thought and a different threshold within the decision tree. In general, the fact that the lesion has been found without ever having caused any symptoms must be balanced with two other issues: the tendency of intracranial lesions to cause unheralded stroke and the characteristics of the lesion that makes it more or less suitable for treatment. In one extreme, a Grade 0 to 2 is more likely to catch our attention for early treatment than a Grade 3 to 4. Here is another example of a situation where clinical expertise is of extreme importance.

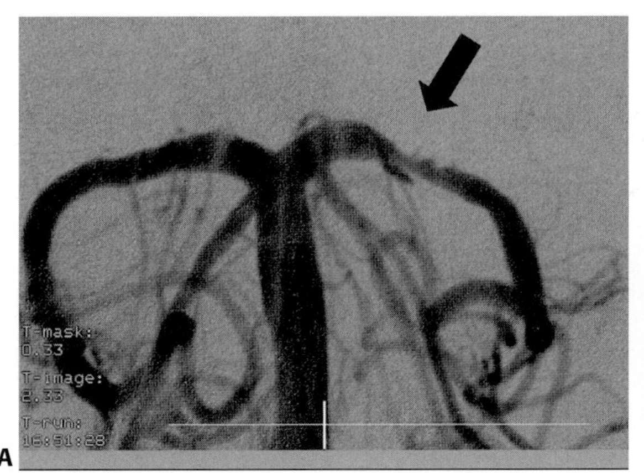

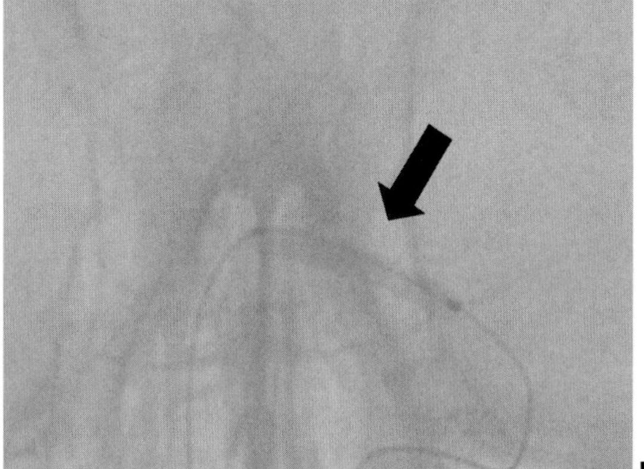

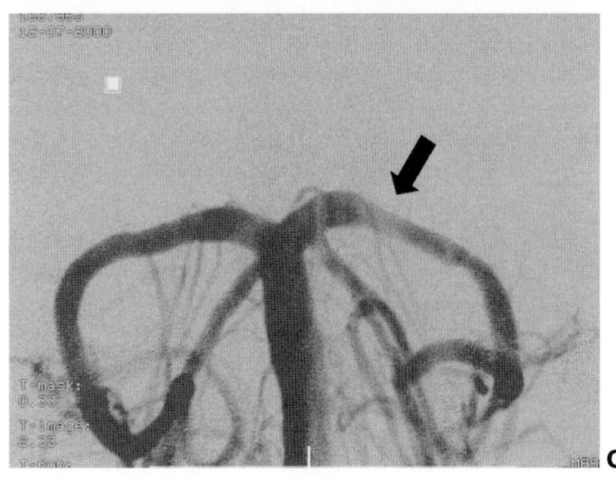

FIGURE 12.8. Successful stenting of a very symptomatic left posterior cerebral artery. **A:** The initial images display the stenosis (*arrow*). Note the difficulty of measuring the degree of stenosis in a vessel this small. **B:** Stent deployment is demonstrated. **C:** The final image displays correction of the stenosis.

SELECTED REFERENCES

Abruzzo TA, Tongc FC, Waldropb ASM, et al. Basilar artery stent angioplasty for symptomatic intracranial athero-occlusive disease: complications and late midterm clinical outcomes. *AJNR Am J Neuroradiol* 2007;28(5):808–815.

Akins PT, Pilgram TK, Cross DT, III, et al. Natural history of stenosis from intracranial atherosclerosis by serial angiography. *Stroke* 1998;29 (2):433–438.

Al-Mubarak N, Gomez CR, Vitek JJ, et al. Stenting of symptomatic stenosis of the intracranial internal carotid artery. *AJNR Am J Neuroradiol* 1998;19(10):1949–1951.

Bose A, Hartmann M, Henkes H, et al. A novel, self-expanding, nitinol stent in medically refractory intracranial atherosclerotic stenoses: the Wingspan study. *Stroke* 2007;38(5):1531–1537.

Callahan AS, III, Berger BL. Balloon angioplasty of intracranial arteries for stroke prevention. *J Neuroimaging* 1997;7(4):232–235.

Clark WM, Barnwell SL, Nesbit G, et al. Safety and efficacy of percutaneous transluminal angioplasty for intracranial atherosclerotic stenosis. *Stroke* 1995;26(7):1200–1204.

Connors JJ, III, Wojak JC. Intracranial angioplasty. *J Invasive Cardiol* 1998;10(5):298–303.

Connors JJ, III, Wojak JC. Percutaneous transluminal angioplasty for intracranial atherosclerotic lesions: evolution of technique and short-term results. *J Neurosurg* 999;91(3):415–423.

Feldman RL, Trigg L, Gaudier J, et al. Use of coronary Palmaz-Schatz stent in the percutaneous treatment of an intracranial carotid artery stenosis. *Cathet Cardiovasc Diagn*1996;38(3):316–319.

Fiorella D, Levy EI, Turk AS, et al. US multicenter experience with the wingspan stent system for the treatment of intracranial atheromatous disease: periprocedural results. *Stroke* 2007;38(3):881–887.

Gomez CR, Orr SC. Angioplasty and stenting for primary treatment of intracranial arterial stenoses. *Arch Neurol* 2001;58(10):1687–1690.

Honda S, Mori T, Fukuoka M, et al. Successful percutaneous transluminal angioplasty of the intracranial vertebral artery 1 month after total occlusion—case report. *Neurol Med Chir (Tokyo)* 1994;34(8):551–554.

Jiang W-J, Srivastava T, Gao F, et al. Perforator stroke after elective stenting of symptomatic intracranial stenosis. *Neurology* 2006;66(12):1868–1872.

Jiang W-J, Xub, X-T, Jinc M, et al. Apollo stent for symptomatic atherosclerotic intracranial stenosis: study results. *AJNR Am J Neuroradiol* 2007;28(5):830–834.

Kang H-S, Han, MH, Kwon O-K, et al, Intracranial hemorrhage after carotid angioplasty: a pooled analysis. *J Endovasc Ther* 2007; 14(1): 77–85.

Leung TW, Mak H, Yu SCH, et al. Perforator stroke after elective stenting of symptomatic intracranial stenosis. *Neurology* 2007;68(15):1237; author reply 1237.

Mori T, Kazita K, Chokyu K, et al. Short-term arteriographic and clinical outcome after cerebral angioplasty and stenting for intracranial vertebrobasilar and carotid atherosclerotic occlusive disease. *AJNR Am J Neuroradiol* 2000;21(2):249–254.

Mori T, Kazita K, Mori K. Cerebral angioplasty and stenting for intracranial vertebral atherosclerotic stenosis. *AJNR Am J Neuroradiol* 1999;20 (5):787–789.

Nomura, M., Hashimoto N, Nishi S, et al. Percutaneous transluminal angioplasty for intracranial vertebral and/or basilar artery stenosis. *Clin Radiol* 1999;54(8):521–527.

Prognosis of patients with symptomatic vertebral or basilar artery stenosis. The Warfarin-Aspirin Symptomatic Intracranial Disease (WASID) Study Group. *Stroke* 1998;29(7):1389–1392.

Qureshi AI, Kirmani JF, Hussein HM, et al. Early and intermediate-term outcomes with drug-eluting stents in high-risk patients with symptomatic intracranial stenosis. *Neurosurgery* 2006;59(5):1044–1051.

Stenting of Symptomatic Atherosclerotic Lesions in the Vertebral or Intracranial Arteries (SSYLVIA): study results. *Stroke* 2004;35(6):1388–1392.

Takis C, Kwan ES, Pessin MS, et al. Intracranial angioplasty: experience and complications. *AJNR Am J Neuroradiol* 1997;18(9):1661–1668.

Wojak JC, Dunlapc DC, Hargravec KR, et al. Intracranial angioplasty and stenting: long-term results from a single center. *AJNR Am J Neuroradiol* 2006;27(9):1882–1892.

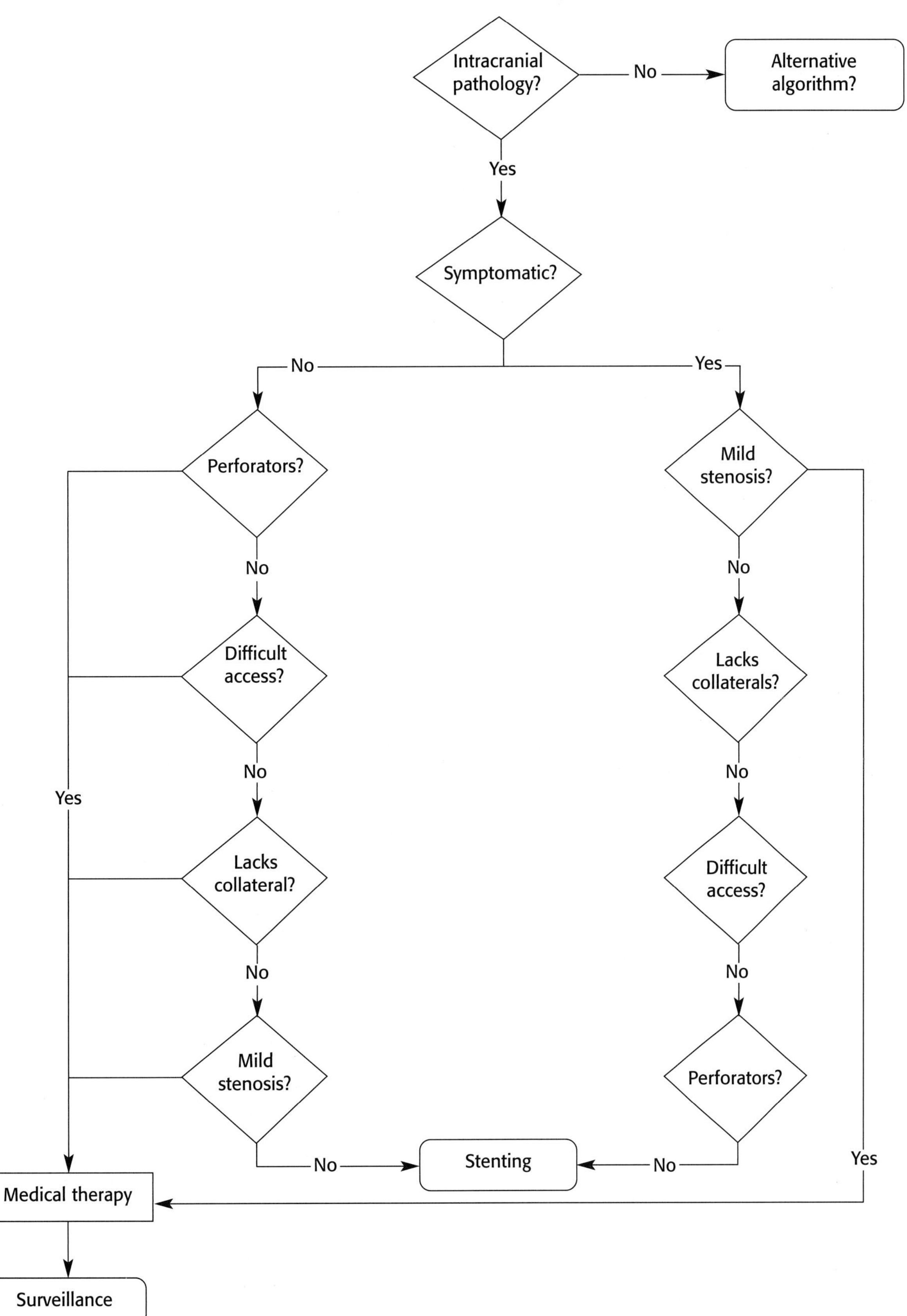
CRITICAL PATHWAY
Intracranial Stenosis Management
Intracranial pathology?
No
Alternative algorithm?
Yes
Symptomatic?
No
Yes
Perforators?
No
Difficult access?
No
Lacks collateral?
No
Mild stenosis?
No
Yes
Mild stenosis?
No
Lacks collaterals?
No
Difficult access?
No
Perforators?
No
Yes
Stenting
Medical therapy
Surveillance

CHAPTER

13 Sleep and Vascular Disorders

JAMES D. GEYER, PAUL R. CARNEY, STEPHENIE C. DILLARD, AND JULIE C. TSIKHLAKIS

OBJECTIVES

- What is obstructive sleep apnea?
- What is the relationship between sleep and hypertension?
- What is the relationship between sleep and stroke?
- What is the relationship between sleep and congestive heart failure?
- What is the effect of treatment of sleep related breathing disorders with positive airway pressure on vascular disease?

Vascular diseases, including myocardial infarction, stroke, cerebrovascular disease, congestive heart failure (CHF), and cardiac arrhythmias, are the most common cause of morbidity and mortality in industrialized countries. Sleep-related breathing disorders are also widespread and increasing in prevalence, in part because of the increasing incidence of obesity. Approximately 20 million Americans suffer from obstructive sleep apnea. Given the frequency of sleep disorders and vascular disorders, it is not surprising that the two conditions often coexist. The interaction between the obstructive sleep apnea/hypopnea syndrome and vascular diseases is much more complex than originally thought, and their comorbidity is more than mere coexistence. Sleep-related breathing disorders, insomnia, and even normal autonomic changes associated with rapid eye movement (REM) sleep can adversely affect vascular diseases. This chapter reviews the normal autonomic processes that occur during sleep and discusses the role that sleep disorders may play in heart disease, hypertension, and stroke.

INTRODUCTION TO SLEEP MEDICINE

Normal Autonomic Physiology of Sleep

The autonomic nervous system regulates the involuntary, automatic functions of the visceral organs. It is composed of the parasympathetic and sympathetic divisions, the two opposing systems, the balance of which determines autonomic function. The sympathetic system has a stimulant effect and is responsible for the so-called fight or flight response. Its primary neurochemical mediator is noradrenaline, an adrenalinelike substance that results in increased heart rate, increased respiratory rate, vasoconstriction of visceral organs with concomitant vasodilatation of skeletal muscles, increased blood pressure, pupillary dilation, and inhibition of digestion, urination, and defecation. In contrast, the parasympathetic system counterbalances these effects. Its primary neurotransmitter is acetylcholine, and its effects include slowing of the heart rate and respirations, vasodilatation of visceral organs with decreased blood pressure, pupillary constriction, increased peristalsis, and emptying of the bladder and the rectum.

Since vasoconstriction and hypertension are major contributors to myocardial infarction and stroke, it is useful to examine the body's normal sympathetic and parasympathetic responses during sleep. In general, at sleep onset there is a decrease in sympathetic tone and an increase in parasympathetic tone, which causes a lowering of the heart rate, blood pressure, respiratory rate, and tidal volume. These changes continue during non-REM (NREM) sleep. With the transition to tonic REM sleep, the portion of REM sleep that occurs without REMs, the parasympathetic activity continues to increase and the sympathetic activity is further suppressed. During phasic REM sleep, the portion of REM sleep that has accompanying REMs, there are bursts of sympathetic activity.

During normal inspiration, the heart rate has a brief acceleration to accommodate venous return and increased cardiac output. During expiration, there is a progressive decrease in heart rate. This normal variability in cardiac rhythm is a marker for cardiac health, and its absence is associated with increasing age and/or cardiac disease. During REM sleep, it is normal for the heart rate to become increasingly variable with episodes of moderate tachycardia and bradycardia. Respiratory patterns are also irregular and may result in mild oxygen desaturations even in healthy subjects. The neurons controlling the principal diaphragmatic respiratory muscles typically are not significantly inhibited during REM sleep, but accessory airway muscles in the ribcage and neck may have partial muscle atonia, causing the diaphragm to bear most of the load of respiration. This may lead to partial diaphragmatic fatigue, hypoventilation, and decreased oxygenation, which can last for several minutes. These episodes are referred to as *REM sleep hypoventilation episodes* and are not necessarily pathologic.

Bursts of sympathetic activity may produce a transient increase in the baseline heart rate up to 35%, especially during phasic REM sleep. β-blockers such as atenolol tend to reduce this phenomenon. Increased parasympathetic activity during NREM sleep contributes to cardiac electrical stability and helps decrease cardiac metabolic activity, decreasing the risk of cardiac arrhythmia; however, the decreased blood pressure produced by the parasympathetic system can contribute to decreased blood flow into the coronary arteries and result in myocardial hypoperfusion, increasing the risk of infarction in patients with significant coronary atherosclerosis. The surges in autonomic activity and increased heart rate during REM sleep increase the risk for ventricular arrhythmias. Sympathetic activity results in increased oxygen consumption by the cardiac muscle and also produces coronary vasoconstriction, decreasing the blood flow to the heart and increasing the risk of cardiac ischemia. It has been documented that a significant number of myocardial infarctions occur in the early morning hours, upon awakening or shortly after awakening; however, the relationship between sleep state, cardiac ischemia, and myocardial infarction is incompletely understood at this time.

Cerebral blood flow is, of course, closely linked to cardiac output, and the factors described in the preceding text also affect blood flow to the brain. In addition, during REM sleep, there is an increase in blood flow to the limbic system and the brain stem, with circulation to these structures decreasing during NREM sleep. As brain activity increases during REM sleep, the cerebral requirements for glucose and oxygen both increase, and there is a compensatory increase in oxygenated hemoglobin delivery, which accompanies the transition from NREM sleep to REM sleep. Mild hypercapnea develops during NREM sleep and appears to counteract the circulatory effect of the decreased cerebral metabolic rate during NREM sleep. $PaCO_2$ is an important determinant of respiration and cerebral blood flow during sleep in patients with obstructive sleep apnea and other related disorders.

Sleep-Disordered Breathing

During wakefulness, upper airway muscle tone maintains upper airway patency. With sleep onset, there is a decrease in voluntary muscle tone with a concomitant increase in upper airway resistance to airflow. Normal REM sleep is associated with relative voluntary muscle atonia, which further worsens the airway constriction. The narrowing of the airway may become pathological in people with anatomically crowded or weakened airways. Causes for this upper airway crowding include enlarged tonsils, macroglossia, low soft palate, micrognathia (typically manifested as an overbite), large neck circumference, and a large uvula.

Upper airway narrowing or collapse during sleep results in obstructive sleep apnea. *Apnea* is defined as complete upper airway obstruction lasting for at least 10 seconds in an adult. A partial airway obstruction with increased work of breathing and sleep disruption or oxygen desaturation is known as a *hypopnea.* Since the physiologic effects are the same, patients with hypopneas may present with the same symptoms as those with complete apneas.

The apnea-hypopnea index (AHI) is defined as the number of apneas and hypopneas per hour of sleep and is one of the measures of the severity of obstructive sleep apnea. An AHI >5 is considered abnormal, and if occurring with complaints of sleepiness or related symptoms, it defines obstructive sleep apnea-hypopnea syndrome. Symptoms of obstructive sleep apnea may include excessive daytime sleepiness, unrefreshing sleep, cognitive dysfunction, morning headaches, nocturnal sweating, nocturia, loud snoring, and insomnia.

Most patients with obstructive sleep apnea do not have oxygen desaturations or hypoventilation during wakefulness. Obesity hypoventilation syndrome, previously known as the *Pickwickian syndrome,* occurs in patients with hypoventilation but no primary lung disease. This is a heterogeneous disorder with components of upper airway obstruction, impaired respiratory compliance secondary to mechanical factors related to the obesity, and abnormalities of ventilatory drive. Most of these patients with obesity hypoventilation have severe obstructive sleep apnea with marked oxygen desaturation, but some patients have prolonged nocturnal oxygen desaturation unrelated to apnea or hypopnea.

Vascular Pathology and Sleep

Hypertension

The Sleep Heart Health Study was designed as a prospective cohort study to investigate obstructive sleep apnea and other sleep-disordered breathing as risk factors for the development of hypertension and cardiovascular disease. The results of the study suggest that the elevated sympathetic activity associated with sleep-related breathing disorders likely represents the primary mechanism in the pathogenesis of developing subsequent hypertension. This would typically begin as a loss of nocturnal dipping, the normal drop in blood pressure that occurs during sleep. Normal nocturnal dipping may result in a 20 mm Hg decrease in systolic blood pressure. Following the loss of nocturnal dipping, some patients develop elevated nocturnal arterial blood pressure that can then progress to an elevated daytime blood pressure. Obstructive sleep apnea is an independent risk factor for the development of both nocturnal and daytime arterial hypertension. There appears to be a linear association between the severity of obstructive sleep apnea and the likelihood of developing subsequent hypertension. According to the Wisconsin Sleep Cohort Study, a patient with an AHI >15 events per hour has a 2.9-fold relative risk of developing hypertension. This implies that many patients thought to have essential hypertension may actually have hypertension secondary, at least in part, to obstructive sleep apnea.

The Joint National Committee on Prevention, Detection, Evaluation, and Treatment of High Blood Pressure has recommended that obstructive sleep apnea should be excluded as a contributing cause of medically refractory hypertension. With the new tighter controls recommended for the treatment of hypertension, screening for these contributing causes becomes increasingly important, especially in patients who have already had a heart attack or stroke.

Nasal continuous positive airway pressure (CPAP) in hypertensive patients with moderate to severe obstructive sleep apnea leads to a significant reduction in the daytime and nocturnal arterial blood pressure, with the effect being more pronounced in patients with severe obstructive sleep apnea. Since patients with only a 50% reduction in apneas on the AHI do not have a significant reduction in blood pressure, the goal of therapy to is decrease the AHI to >5 apneas or hypopneas per hour, underscoring the importance of appropriate titration of the CPAP and excellent patient compliance with treatment.

Congestive Heart Failure

CHF is frequently associated with stroke. Patients with CHF have a significantly increased risk of sleep-disordered breathing, with obstructive sleep apnea occurring in 11% to 37% of patients, and patients with obstructive sleep apnea often have coexisting central sleep apnea, a cessation of airflow with no associated respiratory effort lasting for at least 10 seconds. Central apnea, periodic breathing, and Cheyne-Stokes breathing are also frequently associated with CHF. The Sleep Heart Health Study identified a 2.38-fold increased relative risk for the development of CHF in patients with obstructive sleep apnea, which was independent of all other recognized risk factors for heart failure. Symptoms classically associated with CHF such as paroxysmal nocturnal dyspnea may in fact be related, in part, to obstructive sleep apnea.

Central sleep apnea occurs more frequently in patients with severe CHF and may in some cases contribute to the progression of the heart failure. Patients with CHF and central sleep apnea have higher levels of catecholamines than do patients with CHF without central sleep apnea, and this catecholamine effect can have negative effects on cardiac function.

In patients with CHF, aggressive treatment of obstructive sleep apnea results in a reduction of systolic blood pressure and improvement of left ventricular function with improvement of the left ventricular ejection fraction and left ventricular end systolic diameter, and augmentation of the heart's stroke volume. Furthermore, the risk of ventricular tachycardia decreases as does the frequency of premature ventricular contractions (PVCs).

Cardiac Arrhythmias

Tachyarrhythmias commonly occur with obstructive sleep apnea, usually occurring at the end of an apnea or hypopnea episode during the period of increased respiratory effort and airflow and often in association with an electroencephalographic (EEG) arousal. Several studies have indicated that the frequency of atrial fibrillation is increased in patients with obstructive sleep apnea and other sleep-related breathing disorders. Ventricular tachycardia becomes more likely as the oxygen saturation falls below 60%.

Bradyarrhythmias are also frequently associated with obstructive sleep apnea. Sinus bradycardia, which can be severe, is common during apnea or hypopnea. Rarely, patients may develop sinus arrest or atrioventricular block. Patients with nocturnal bradycardia should be screened for obstructive sleep apnea.

Coagulation and Platelet Activity

Thrombus formation is the most common clinical event that leads to cerebral and myocardial infarction. The process of clot formation is complex, which involves the interaction of platelets, circulating coagulation factors, and the surface of endothelial cells lining the blood vessels. When a blood vessel is injured, circulating platelets adhere to the wall forming a loose aggregate that occludes the lumen of the vessel. The platelet aggregate then activates the coagulation cascade resulting in the production of fibrin, which strengthens the loose aggregate, thereby forming a thrombus. The tendency for platelets to aggregate increases with obstructive sleep apnea, mediated at least in part by the increased levels of catecholamines in these patients. Furthermore, these patients may also have abnormally increased daytime levels of fibrinogen, the precursor to fibrin.

Hematocrit is defined as the volume percent of erythrocytes in whole blood. While plasma, or the liquid component of blood, can flow freely, the cellular components of blood produce increased blood viscosity with a decreased rate of flow, especially in small blood vessels and in arteries narrowed by atherosclerotic plaque. As the rate of flow decreases, the tendency to form circulating platelet aggregates increases, increasing the risk of thrombosis. When patients with moderate to severe obstructive sleep apnea experience chronic nocturnal hypoxia, the body attempts to compensate by producing more erythrocytes, thereby increasing the oxygen-carrying capacity of the blood. This produces a state of hyperviscosity, which when coupled with the increased tendency to produce platelet aggregates places these patients at a greatly increased risk of heart attack and stroke.

There is evidence that treatment of obstructive sleep apnea with CPAP can improve the nocturnal hypoxemia and therefore help decrease hematocrit and blood viscosity. Furthermore, lessening the episodes of catecholamine release would reduce the relative increase in platelet aggregation. CPAP may also reduce the activity of some circulating clotting factors.

Metabolic Syndrome X

Metabolic syndrome X is a recently recognized constellation of metabolic abnormalities that are associated with an increased risk of vascular diseases. The symptoms include central obesity with fat deposits centered on the abdomen, glucose intolerance/insulin resistance, hypertension, hypercholesterolemia, and clotting abnormalities. Although syndrome X is not a vascular disease, it greatly increases a patient's risk of heart attack and stroke and is therefore included for discussion in this chapter. The previous section discussed the possible role sleep-related breathing disorders may have on two of the components of syndrome X, hypertension and clotting abnormalities. We now examine the possible role of sleep disorders and two of the other abnormalities: glucose intolerance and obesity.

Obstructive sleep apnea has been shown to produce glucose intolerance, with the severity of the apnea correlating with the degree of insulin resistance. Obstructive sleep apnea is associated with higher blood glucose levels, higher insulin levels, and higher glycosylated hemoglobin levels. Unfortunately, treatment of obstructive sleep apnea with CPAP has not been associated with consistent improvement of glucose tolerance. Further study of the exact metabolic effects of CPAP is needed.

There may also be an association between obstructive sleep apnea and obesity. Leptin, a hormone produced by fat cells, is seen in increased levels in obese patients. Males with obstructive sleep apnea have relatively higher levels of leptin than do males of similar weight but without obstructive sleep apnea. Leptin may increase the production of platelet aggregates (see Section on Coagulation and Platelet Activity) and may serve as an independent marker for the risk of vascular disease. Studies have shown that leptin levels fall following treatment with CPAP, and therapy for obstructive sleep apnea may not only improve the patient's difficulty with weight gain but also decrease the risk of heart attack and stroke by decreasing the tendency toward platelet aggregation.

Ischemic Heart Disease

Obstructive sleep apnea and coronary artery disease frequently coexist, with at least 50% of patients with heart disease having significant obstructive sleep apnea. Obstructive sleep apnea is an independent risk factor for myocardial infarction with the relative risk similar to hypertension and smoking. The sympathetic activity during normal REM sleep increases blood pressure and heart rate with an increase in cardiac oxygen consumption. Significant oxygen desaturations in a patient with obstructive sleep apnea further contribute to nocturnal angina and nocturnal ischemic changes in the electrocardiogram (ECG).

Treatment of obstructive sleep apnea with CPAP in patients with coronary artery disease has been shown to improve ECG changes. There is also evidence of fewer incidences or lesser degree of nocturnal angina, but large clinical trials are lacking. Obstructive sleep apnea syndrome also appears to affect outcome following myocardial infarction. Patients with untreated obstructive sleep apnea have a higher mortality following myocardial infarction than patients with cardiac disease but without obstructive sleep apnea (38% versus 9%).

Cerebrovascular Disease

More than 750,000 strokes occur in the United States each year with approximately 150,000 fatalities. Tremendous resources are required to care for the >3 million stroke survivors in the United States alone. Numerous studies have demonstrated that 31% to 54% of strokes occur during sleep, and the most common time of onset during wakefulness is in the first several hours following awakening. The Sleep Heart Health Study identified an increase in the prevalence of stroke in patients with obstructive sleep apnea, and other studies have shown the frequency of coexisting sleep apnea and stroke in 62.5% to 80% of stroke patients.

Cerebral autoregulation is the process by which the brain attempts to control intracranial blood pressure to maintain adequate cerebral blood flow. Obstructive sleep apnea interferes with this process. While the change has not been shown to cause stroke, the inability of the brain to alter pressures to ensure adequate circulation may result in decreased cerebral perfusion and produce enlargement of an acute stroke that originated from other causes. Treatment of obstructive sleep apnea with CPAP results in improvement of the cerebral autoregulation and overall cerebral blood flow measured by transcranial Doppler ultrasound.

Obstructive sleep apnea inter-reacts with multiple stroke risk factors and appears to significantly increase the risk of cerebral infarction. Aggressive management of obstructive sleep apnea is an important component in stroke prevention.

CLINICAL APPLICATIONS AND METHODOLOGY

Evaluation

All patients with vascular disease including stroke, cerebrovascular disease, hypertension, CHF, and myocardial ischemia should be screened for sleep disorders. A number of complaints may accompany obstructive sleep apnea syndrome including sleepiness, fatigue, tiredness, and perceived laziness. A history of loud snoring, snorts, nocturnal coughing and gasping, and witnessed apneas can commonly be obtained from bed partners. Although uncommon, some patients may not have snoring or may be unaware of the nocturnal symptoms. Table 13.1 contains a more detailed list of symptoms associated with obstructive sleep apnea syndrome.

TABLE 13.1 Symptoms of Sleep Apnea

Excessive daytime somnolence
Unrefreshing sleep
Loud snoring
Witnessed apneas
Choking or coughing during sleep
Nocturnal reflux
Nocturnal perspiration
Nocturia
Morning headaches
Irritability
Cognitive impairment
Difficulty falling asleep
Difficulty staying asleep

The physical examination may also be helpful in the identification of sleep-related breathing disorders. A neck circumference >16.5 inches is associated with an increased risk of obstructive sleep apnea. A low soft palate, large tonsils, long or thick uvula, large tongue, or an overbite may constrict the airway and contribute to an increased risk of upper airway collapse. Table 13.2 contains a list of physical findings associated with obstructive sleep apnea syndrome. Some patients, especially those with pharyngeal/bulbar weakness, may have an otherwise unremarkable airway anatomy. Patients with bulbar and hemifacial weakness are at even higher risk of a sleep-related breathing disorder.

An overnight screening study with oximetry, capnography, and nasal pressure monitoring can be helpful in borderline or questionable cases. Unfortunately, these monitoring devices are not in widespread use. Overnight pulse oximetry provides information about the degree of oxygen desaturation but can miss significant obstructive sleep apnea and evidence of upper airway resistance syndrome. A negative oximetry study does not eliminate obstructive sleep apnea syndrome from the differential diagnosis.

Overnight laboratory-based polysomnography is the gold standard for evaluation of a possible sleep-related breathing disorder. A standard polysomnogram should include limited EEG, electro-oculography (EOG), ECG, limb movement, snore monitoring, respiratory effort, and measurement of airflow. Additional monitoring with capnography and nasal pressure monitoring provides further information about hypoventilation and respiratory event–related arousals (RERAs). Table 13.3 outlines some of the typical polysomnographic findings associated with obstructive sleep apnea syndrome. Overnight polysomnography should be obtained for any patient with a suspected sleep-related breathing disorder. Given the extremely high rate of obstructive sleep apnea in the stroke population, strong consideration should be given to formal polysomnography for these patients.

TABLE 13.2 Factors Influencing Upper Airway Compromise

Impaired upper airway motor function
Supine posture
Variable ventilatory drive
Increased extraluminal pressure
Decreased lung volume
Decreased pressure reflexes
Anatomically small airway

TABLE 13.3 Polysomnographic Findings in Obstructive Sleep Apnea Syndrome

AHI >5
AHI REM >AHI NREM
Apnea duration longer in REM
AHI supine >AHI lateral
Snoring
Reduced deep sleep (stages 3, 4)
Reduced REM sleep
Oxygen desaturations
Tachycardia with arousal
Bradycardia with apnea onset

AHI, apnea-hypopnea index; REM, rapid eye movement; NREM, non–rapid eye movement.

TREATMENT

Identifying the subpopulation of patients requiring treatment for a sleep-related breathing disorder can be challenging. The threshold for initiating therapy in patients with stroke or other vascular disorders should be lower than that in the general population. In this group, even relatively mild sleep apnea may warrant treatment, even if there is little or no associated daytime sleepiness. Special attention should be given to the severity of the obstructive sleep apnea during REM sleep and in each sleep position. The detrimental aspects of obstructive sleep apnea are frequently worse during REM sleep. In most patients, the severity of the sleep-related breathing disorder is worst in the supine position. Following strokes with hemiparesis, one lateral position may be associated with severe apnea while the other may be associated with relatively normal sleep.

Nasal CPAP is the treatment of choice for most patients with obstructive sleep apnea (see Table 13.4). Positive airway pressure (PAP) treatment maintains upper airway patency via a pneumatic splint, with the air pressure preventing airway collapse. CPAP maintains a constant pressure throughout the respiratory cycle. Bilevel PAP provides a higher pressure on inhalation than on exhalation, which may be more comfortable, especially in patients with weakness from stroke or neuromuscular disease.

Empiric selection of a pressure setting for these devices is fraught with danger (see Table 13.5 for a review of problems associated with PAP theory). An inadequate setting will leave the patient undertreated and an excessive pressure may result in patient noncompliance (see Table 13.6 for methods of improving compliance) or central apnea. The patient should be evaluated with formal polysomnography and then with a CPAP titration. In select patients this can be accomplished during a combined or split-night study.

There is a limited role for surgical treatment of obstructive sleep apnea in the stroke patient. Tracheostomy bypasses the upper airway and therefore the region of obstruction. This procedure should be reserved for patients with severe obstructive sleep apnea who are unable to tolerate or use CPAP or similar devices. The more commonly used surgical procedures such as uvulopalatopharyngoplasty (UPPP), mandibular advancement, and maxillomandibular advancement may be associated with significant morbidity and prolonged recovery times, and should be used judiciously in the stroke population.

Obesity is commonly associated with obstructive sleep apnea. Weight loss can significantly decrease the severity of obstructive sleep apnea in terms of AHI and oxygen desaturation. Maintaining weight loss can often be difficult for the patient. Weight loss in the nonobese patient is of little clinical utility.

Positional therapy is an option for patients with abnormal breathing isolated to a single position. Avoiding that position will then allow normal nocturnal respiration. This positional response should be documented by formal polysomnography. A wedge pillow can also be added to CPAP therapy to decrease the pressure requirement.

Supplemental oxygen alone is typically ineffective in treating the respiratory events and may actually prolong the duration of

TABLE 13.4 Benefits of Positive Airway Pressure Treatment

Decreased sleepiness and fatigue
Improved sleep quality
Improved quality of life
Decreased sympathetic tone
Decreased systemic blood pressure
Decreased pulmonary blood pressure
Decreased platelet activation
Decreased C-reactive protein
Decreased fibrinogen level
Decreased overall vascular risk
Improved cognitive function
Reduced insulin resistance

TABLE 13.5 Continuous Positive Airway Pressure Problems and Their Treatments

Claustrophobia	Pressure intolerance
Desensitization	Ramp setting
Nasal prong interface	C-flex
Anxiolytics	Bilevel pressure
Mask leaks	Wedge pillow
Careful mask fit	Skin breakdown
Education	Adjust straps
Nasal congestion	Change mask styles
Heated humidity	Tape barrier for skin protection
Nasal steroid spray	Mouth dryness
Nasal saline spray	Humidifier
Decongestants	Chinstrap
Full face mask	Full face mask
Oral mask	Lower pressure setting
	Treat nasal congestion

TABLE 13.6 Methods to Improve Positive Airway Pressure Compliance

Patient education
Family education
Telephone follow-up
Objective compliance monitoring
Regular clinic visits
Early treatment of problems with CPAP

individual events. The use of stimulant medications to treat the degree of daytime sleepiness has little effect on the degree of obstructive sleep apnea. Treating the symptoms without addressing the primary problem does not significantly improve the quality of life or lower the associated vascular morbidity.

PRACTICAL RECOMMENDATIONS

The sleepiness and snoring associated with obstructive sleep apnea are frequently the presenting symptoms and those about which the patients are most concerned. The effect of sleep apnea on a variety of vascular disorders is largely unappreciated by the patient and the treating physician. Identification and aggressive treatment of sleep-related breathing disorders not only decrease vascular risk but also improve functional status. This medical information can also be used to encourage the patient toward better CPAP compliance. Given the importance of effective treatment, patient compliance with CPAP therapy should be monitored closely.

Sleep disorders are frequently overlooked in the general patient population and may be recognized even less often in patients with vascular disease. The coexisting medical disorders, limitation of movement, and medication side effects can all obscure the presence of a sleep disorder. Identification and appropriate management of obstructive sleep apnea is critical for improved quality of life, decreased risk of recurrent stroke, and improved functional outcome. The patient and the family should be asked about the presence of fatigue, tiredness, laziness, sleepiness, snoring, and apnea.

Sleep-disordered breathing, including obstructive sleep apnea, occur so frequently in patients with stroke and transient ischemic attack that strong consideration should be given to formal sleep evaluation with polysomnography in all cerebrovascular patients.

Screening questions take only seconds to ask and can dramatically improve the patients' outcome. Patients may have had a sleep-related breathing disorder before the stroke or may develop it as a consequence of the associated weakness, so screening should occur both during the acute phase of stroke treatment and during follow-up examinations.

In our experience, even patients with severe hemiparesis and aphasia can tolerate PAP treatment well. The importance of patient and family education cannot be overemphasized, since compliance with treatment is closely related to the degree of improvement in symptoms and stroke risk reduction.

SELECTED REFERENCES

Ancoli-Israel S, Stepnowsky C, Dimsdale J, et al. The effect of race and sleep-disordered breathing on nocturnal BP "dipping": analysis in an older population. *Chest* 2002;122(4):1148–1155.

Babu AR, Herdegen J, Fogelfeld L, et al. Type 2 diabetes, glycemic control, and continuous positive airway pressure in obstructive sleep apnea. *Arch Intern Med* 2005;165(4):447–452.

Bassetti C, Aldrich MS. Sleep apnea in acute cerebrovascular diseases: final report on 128 patients. *Sleep* 1999;22(2):217–223.

Becker HF, Jerrentrup A, Ploch T, et al. Effect of nasal continuous positive airway pressure treatment on blood pressure in patients with obstructive sleep apnea. *Circulation* 2003;107(1):68–73.

Berry R, Carney P, Geyer J, eds. *Clinical Sleep Disorders.* Philadelphia, PA: Lippincott, Williams & Wilkins; 2005.

Borgel J, Sanner BM, Keskin F, et al. Obstructive sleep apnea and blood pressure: interaction between the blood pressure-lowering effects of positive airway pressure therapy and antihypertensive drugs. *Am J Hypertens* 2004;17(12 Pt 1):1081–1087.

Culebras A. Cerebrovascular disease and sleep. *Curr Neurol Neurosci Rep* 2004;4(2):164–169.

Dhillon S, Chung SA, Fargher T, et al. Sleep apnea, hypertension, and the effects of continuous positive airway pressure. *Am J Hypertens* 2005;18 (5 Pt 1):594–600.

Diaz J, Sempere AP. Cerebral ischemia: new risk factors. *Cerebrovasc Dis* 2004;17(Suppl 1):43–50.

Doherty LS, Kiely JL, Swan V, et al. Long-term effects of nasal continuous positive airway pressure therapy on cardiovascular outcomes in sleep apnea syndrome. *Chest* 2005;127(6):2076–2084.

Dursunoglu N, Dursunoglu D, Cuhadaroglu C, et al. Acute effects of automated continuous positive airway pressure on blood pressure in patients with sleep apnea and hypertension. *Respiration* 2005;72(2): 150–155.

Geiser T, Buck F, Meyer BJ, et al. In vivo platelet activation is increased during sleep in patients with obstructive sleep apnea syndrome. *Respiration* 2002;69(3):229–234.

Guardiola JJ, Matheson PJ, Clavijo LC, et al. Hypercoagulability in patients with obstructive sleep apnea. *Sleep Med* 2001;2(6):517–523.

Harsch IA, Hahn EG, Konturek PC. Insulin resistance and other metabolic aspects of the obstructive sleep apnea syndrome. *Med Sci Monit* 2005;11(3):RA70–RA75.

Kanagala R, Murali NS, Friedman PA, et al. Obstructive sleep apnea and the recurrence of atrial fibrillation. *Circulation* 2003;107(20):2589–2594; epub May 12, 2003.

Kenchaiah S, Narula J, Vasan RS. Risk factors for heart failure. *Med Clin N Am* 2004;88(5):1145–1172.

Larkin EK, Elston RC, Patel SR, et al. Linkage of serum leptin levels in families with sleep apnea. *Int J Obes (Lond)* 2005;29(3):260–267.

Nachtmann A, Stang A, Wang YM, et al. Association of obstructive sleep apnea and stenotic artery disease in ischemic stroke patients. *Atherosclerosis* 2003;169(2):301–307.

Naughton MT. The link between obstructive sleep apnea and heart failure: underappreciated opportunity for treatment. *Curr Cardiol Rep* 2005; 7(3):211–215.

Nelson CA, Wolk R, Somers VK. Sleep-disordered breathing: implications for the pathophysiology and management of cardiovascular disease. *Compr Ther* 2005;31(1):21–27.

Parish JM, Somers VK. Obstructive sleep apnea and cardiovascular disease. *Mayo Clin Proc* 2004;79(8):1036–1046.

Phillips B. Sleep-disordered breathing and cardiovascular disease. *Sleep Med Rev* 2005;9(2):131–140.

Phillips C, Hedner J, Berend N, et al. Diurnal and obstructive sleep apnea influences on arterial stiffness and central blood pressure in men. *Sleep* 2005;28(5):604–609.

Punjabi NM, Shahar E, Redline S, et al. Sleep-disordered breathing, glucose intolerance, and insulin resistance: the Sleep Heart Health Study. *Am J Epidemiol* 2004;160(6):521–530.

Svatikova A, Wolk R, Gami AS, et al. Interactions between obstructive sleep apnea and the metabolic syndrome. *Curr Diab Rep* 2005;5(1): 53–58.

Weinstein MD. Continuous positive airway pressure in patients with heart failure. *N Engl J Med* 2003;349(1):93–95; author reply 93–95.

Yaggi H, Mohsenin V. Sleep-disordered breathing and stroke. *Clin Chest Med* 2003;24(2):223–237.

CRITICAL PATHWAY
Evaluation and Mangement of Sleep Disorders in the Stroke Patient

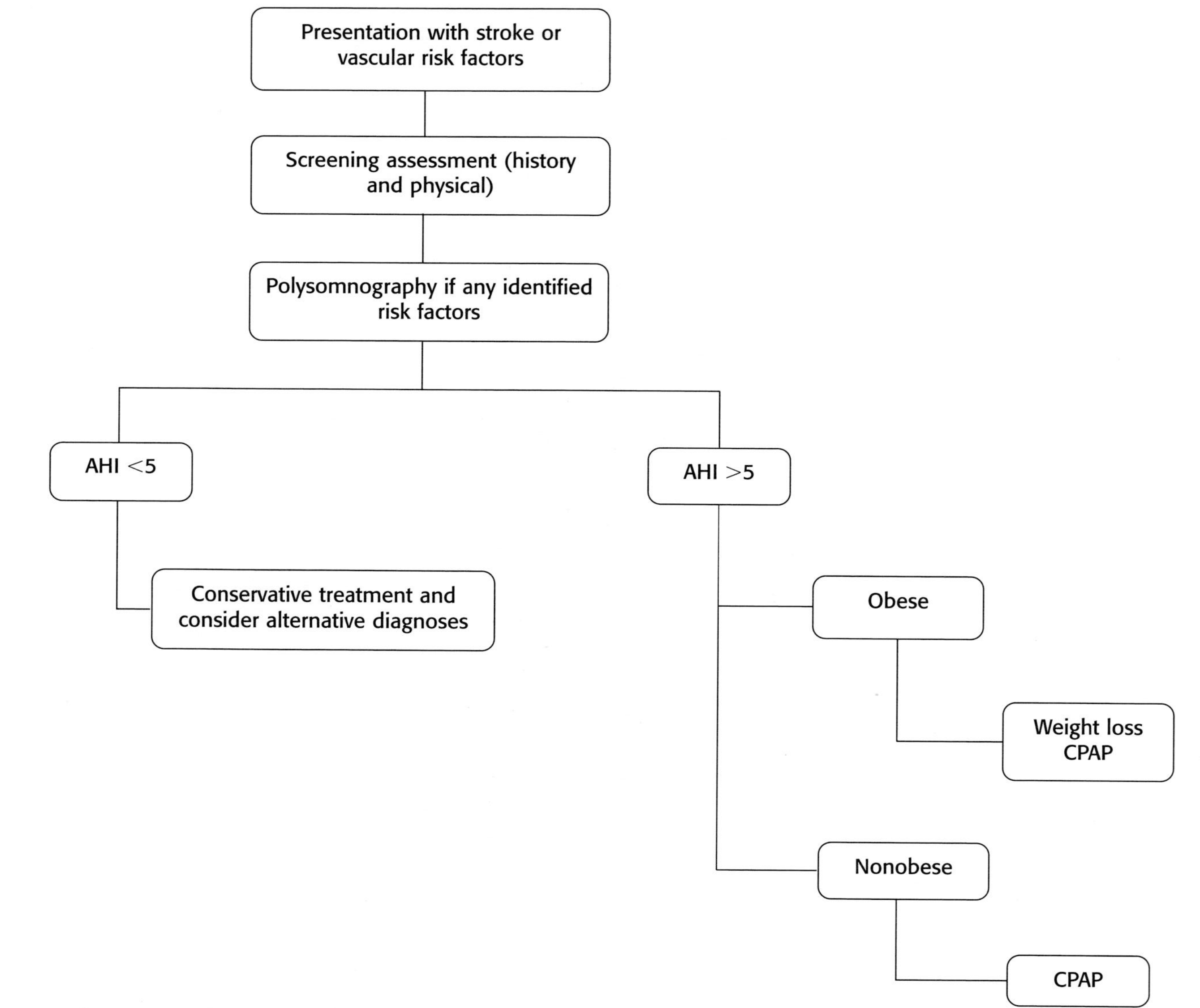

AHI, apnea-hypopnea index; CPAP, continuous positive airway pressure.

Prothrombotic States and Stroke

SHANTHI SIVENDRAN AND JOSEPH DRABICK

OBJECTIVES

- What does the literature currently recommend for hypercoagulable testing and stroke?
- What criteria should be used when selecting the appropriate patient population for testing?
- What is the current diagnostic testing available and when should they be employed?
- What are the current guidelines for antiplatelet and anticoagulation therapy?

Each year in the United States about 700,000 people are affected by stroke. The common risk factors include hypertension, diabetes, elevated lipid levels, excessive alcohol consumption, cigarette smoking, sedentary lifestyle, and obesity. The pathologic subcategories of stroke are divided into atherosclerotic infarction in larger arteries, small vessel disease, cardiac embolism, determined causes (dissection, hypercoagulable states, sickle cell disease), and undetermined causes. This chapter focuses on stroke secondary to hypercoagulable states. Patients who are hypercoagulable or prothrombotic are more likely to develop arterial or venous thromboembolism. Deep venous thrombosis secondary to hypercoagulable states is well documented. Arterial thrombosis, although a recognized complication, is quite uncommon particularly in the setting of stroke. In the nearly 40% of stroke cases in which there is an unclear etiology, investigation of hypercoagulable states is a common next step for clinicians. Unfortunately, the current literature demonstrating associations between prothrombotic states and stroke is both limited and conflicting. This makes it difficult for clinicians to know when it is appropriate to screen for hypercoagulable states in the setting of stroke, which diseases to screen for, and what the appropriate treatment entails. In this chapter, we review the current literature for the most common hypercoagulable states—the factor V Leiden (FVL) mutation, the prothrombin gene G20210A mutation, the methylenetetrahydrofolate reductase (MTHFR T) mutation, and antiphospholipid (aPL) antibody syndrome and their association with stroke. Given these studies, a framework is provided for selecting appropriate patients to screen and for potential treatments for these patients.

BACKGROUND AND RATIONALE

The Factor V Leiden Mutation

The FVL gene mutation is a well-recognized risk factor for venous thromboembolism. This specific gene mutation in the gene coding for FVL makes it more resistant to breakdown by activated protein C. The evidence for whether this mutation increases arterial thrombosis is less clear. An early study by Ridker et al. described a large-scale prospective study in which healthy men were screened for the factor V mutation and followed up over an 8.6-year period. This study showed no association between the factor V mutation and stroke from all causes or myocardial infarction (MI). The advantage of this study is that it is a large-scale study allowing for prospective evaluation of arterial thrombosis and factor V mutation.

A British study in 1998 investigated the association between FVL (as well as other inherited deficiencies) and children presenting with arterial stroke between 1990 and 1996. This study showed no significant difference between the prevalence of FVL mutation in the control population 5.2% (4/77) and the study population 12% (6/50). The pitfalls of this study are the low numbers of patients evaluated and the use of children evaluated at the hospital who did not have any thrombotic problems as the "normal" control group. This study did raise the question that FVL in conjunction with other abnormalities (such as hyperhomocysteinemia) may confer more of a risk than the isolated mutation on its own.

Another study by Longstreth et al. in 1998 investigated the association between FVL mutation and thrombotic risk in women younger than 45. This was a case-controlled study with case patients being women aged 18 to 44 with first stroke (n = 106) and control subjects being recruited randomly from the same geographic region. The study showed FVL in 0.9% of case patients and 4.1% of control subjects. Thus, this study did not show a strong association between stroke and FVL mutation. The blood samples used in this study were collected at some point after the acute event, leading to the question of whether FVL levels at the time of presentation would be significantly different. This study cites a previous study in which samples were collected at the time of presentation in which there was no association between FVL mutation and increased risk of arterial thrombosis.

Hankey et al. investigated the relationship of inherited thrombophilias, including FVL, and the different pathogenic subtypes of stroke (large artery, small artery, cardiac embolism, etc.). Case studies were patients presenting with first ever ischemic stroke (IS) from March 1996 to June 1998 at a western Australian teaching hospital. Control subjects were randomly selected in the same region and stratified by age, group, sex, and postal code; 219 case patients were identified and 205 controls. The result was no significant difference between the control and case groups for the risk of arterial thrombosis. This study suggested that one in seven patients with first presentation of stroke will have prothrombotic factors but that this would be unlikely to be relevant to the pathogenesis of stroke.

Another small study investigating the association between inherited thrombophilias, including FVL, and IS in young adults showed no increased risk. This study performed by Voetsch et al. compared patients of both white and African descent in Brazil. Case patients were survivors of a first cerebral ischemic event occurring when they were aged between 15 and 45 years of age and who did not have cancer or systemic disease. Control groups were 225 healthy adults matched to age and sex. The prevalence of FVL in the white control group was 5.8% and in the case group 4.4% ($p = 0.83$). Among those of African origin, 0.9% of control patients and 0% of the case patients carried FVL.

The Copenhagen City Heart Study looked at the relationship between arterial thrombosis [MI, IS, non-MI ischemic heart disease (IHD)] and FVL in three case-controlled studies and three prospective studies with a 21-year follow-up. This study suggested no association.

The last study discussed here that shows no association between FVL and cryptogenic IS is by Aznar et al. in 2004. Forty-nine patients younger than 50 with no evidence of atherosclerosis, heart disease, foramen ovale, or vessel occlusive disease were age, gender, and ethnically matched to healthy controls. The odds ratio (OR) for cryptogenic stroke compared with the control group for FVL was 2.62 (95% CI, 0.49 to 13.95), which was not considered significant.

There are a few studies that show a positive correlation between FVL and IS. A 2003 study by Pezzini et al. investigated the association between inherited thrombophilic disorders and patent foramen ovale (PFO)-related strokes. The study found that in the 36 patients in whom the PFO was thought to be related to the stroke (PFO+), 19.4% had FVL mutation. This is compared to the 3.3% of the 89 patients in whom the PFO was not considered to be related to the stroke (PFO−).

A 1999 study from Italy investigated sex difference in association with FVL and premature IS. The study showed that compared with noncarriers, carriers were independently more likely to have an IS (OR 2.56). This higher risk is more pronounced in women with an OR of 3.95. The study population in this group was patients younger than 50 years with first occurrence of IS.

Two meta-analyses have been done on current published studies. The first by Kim et al. (2003) analyzed studies from 1990 to 2002 that investigated the relationship between FVL and arterial thrombosis. Only studies in which the initial ischemic event occurred were included and patients younger than 55 years were grouped and analyzed separately. A total of 56 studies (54,547 patients) were analyzed. Of these, 25,053 were investigated for the relationship between FVL and arterial thrombosis. There was a modest increased risk for arterial thrombosis—OR of 1.21 (95% CI, 0.99 to 1.49). For patients younger than 55 the risk was greater with an OR of 1.37 (95% CI, 0.96 to 1.97). Three studies also provided data on sex differentiation in relation to FVL and arterial thrombosis. The OR was higher in women than in men.

The second meta-analysis looked at 32 genes, including FVL Arg506Gln, in >18,000 cases and 58,000 controls. The electronic database was searched for all case-controlled and nested case-controlled strokes up to January 2003. Only studies of white adults from 120 studies were included. Statistically significant associations were identified for patients with IS and FVL Arg506Gln (OR 1.33; 95% CI, 1.12 to 1.58).

The Prothrombin (G20210A) Gene Mutation

The G20210A mutation in the prothrombin gene is the second most common inherited risk factor for venous thrombosis. The defect is a single point mutation in the 3' untranslated region of the prothrombin gene. At nucleotide position 20210 there is a G-to-A transition. This is associated with increased prothrombin levels leading to a prothrombotic state particularly in venous thrombosis. As with FVL, its role in arterial thrombosis is less well understood and conflicting data appears in the literature.

Ridker et al., in a study published in 1999, followed up 22,071 healthy male US physicians aged between 40 and 84 over a prospective 10-year period for the occurrence of both arterial and venous thrombotic events. Of the study participants, 833 had some thrombotic event and were analyzed for the mutation; 1,774 control subjects were matched to these patients. This study showed no evidence of an association between the prothrombin mutation and the risk for stroke.

Another study investigated the same association with a different cohort of subjects. In 1998, in a study by Longstreth et al. a population of women aged 18 to 44 years was used in a population-based, case-controlled study of 149 patients with identified stroke (first case) and 526 control subjects matched by age. Blood specimens were typed for the prothrombin variant. No strong association was found between G20210A and stroke with an OR of 1.2 (95% CI, 0.1 to 6.9).

In 2001 Hankey et al. investigated the relationship between inherited thrombophilias in the different pathogenic subtypes of IS. The details of the design set up are discussed in The Factor V Leiden Mutation section. The study showed no association between G20210 and any pathological subtype of stroke (larger artery, small artery, cardiac embolism, etc.).

One study attempted to tease out a relationship between ethnicity, the G20210 mutation, and IS. As with previously discussed studies, the authors in this study also examined FVL, and the details of study design can be found in the previous section. Among 119 white controls 2.5% had the mutation and 5.3% of the white stroke patients had the mutation, although this higher frequency was not statistically significant ($p = 0.33$). Among patients of African origin 1.9% of controls and 2.6% of patients with stroke had the mutation, which again was not statistically significant ($p = 1.0$).

For each study showing no relationship between G20210 and IS there is one that does show an association. Aznar et al. investigated the relationship between multiple inherited thrombophilias and stroke including G20210 as outlined in The Factor V Leiden Mutation section. Although there was no association between FVL and IS in this study, there was a positive correlation between G20210 and IS in Mediterranean patients younger than 50 (OR 3.75; 95% CI, 1.05 to 13.34). The drawback to this study was the small population size of 49 patients.

The previously discussed meta-analysis by Kim et al. also included G20210A. A pooled analysis of studies included 16,945 patients and only showed a modest association between G20210A and IS (OR, 1.32; 95% CI, 1.03 to 1.69). A subset of patients older than 55 years was examined and the association was slightly stronger (OR, 1.66; 95% CI, 1.13 to 2.46).

Another meta-analysis previously discussed by Casas et al. investigated the genetic basis of IS. They found a statistically significant association between IS and G20210A (OR, 1.44; 95% CI, 1.11 to 1.86). Finally, the Pezzini et al. study discussing the pathogenic link between PFO, inherited thrombophilic disorders, and stroke showed a higher frequency of G20210A in stroke patients with PFO in comparison to controls with no strokes (11% versus 2%; 95% CI, 0.04 to 0.94). It also showed a higher frequency of G20210A among stroke patients with PFOs than that in stroke patients without PFOs (19.4% versus 3.3%; 95% CI, 1.45 to 26.1; $p = 0.021$).

The Methylenetetrahydrofolate Reductase Mutation

Another more controversial inherited thrombophilia is homozygosity for a thermolabile variant of MTHFR-T that results in a C-to-T substitution at nucleotide 677. This then leads to a substitution of alanine by valine. When this mutation occurs there is a defect in a folic acid–binding site of MTHFR. This binding defect causes mild hyperhomocysteinemia, which is more pronounced when the circulating levels of plasma folate are already low. Mild hyperhomocysteinemia has already been described as an independent risk factor for peripheral, coronary, and cerebral vascular disease. The role of the MTHFR-T defect in IS is controversial. A study by Voetsch et al. (2000) demonstrated that Brazilian patients of African descent with IS were more likely to be homozygote for the thermolabile variant of MTHFR than controls (OR 5.9). However, the sample population was small. No association was shown in the white population. A meta-analysis of genetic studies by Casas et al. in 2004 demonstrated a statistically significant association between MTHFR and IS (OR 1.24; 95% CI, 1.08 to 1.42). In a study by Margaglione et al. (1999) there was a borderline significant association between the MTHFR gene and IS.

Antiphospholipid Syndrome

Primary aPL antibody syndrome describes patients with elevated anticardiolipin (aCL) antibody (ACA) levels or other antibodies directed toward anionic phospholipids or their associated plasma proteins and venous or arterial thrombosis. The presence of these autoantibodies is associated with the development of arterial and venous thrombosis. The prevalence of aPL antibody, specifically the aCL subtype (ACA), was studied by Vila et al. (1994) among 552 normal blood donors randomly selected from a blood bank. The prevalence of IgG ACA was 6.5 % and that of IgM ACA was 9.4% in the donor population.

The association between aPL antibodies and cerebral vascular events is strong. One of the early large studies published by the Antiphospholipid antibodies in Stroke Study (APASS) group in 1993 studied 255 first IS patients and 255 age-/sex-matched hospitalized nonstroke patients. aCL antibodies were found in 9.7% of stroke patients and 4.3% of control patients. The OR for this was adjusted for cigarette smoking, coronary artery disease, age, gender, ethnicity, diabetes mellitus, and hypertension and was statistically significant at 2.31 (95% CI, 1.09 to 4.90; $p = 0.029$). Among the patients who had a stroke, the presence of antibodies did not predict stroke etiology. An even higher rate of aPL positivity was found in the Antiphospholipid Antibodies in Stroke Substudy, with 41% of 1,770 IS patients testing positive for aPL antibodies.

aPL antibodies also appear to result in a higher recurrence rate of stroke in young patients. A 1997 study by Levine et al. showed that patients with higher levels of IgG aCL at the time of first stroke (GPL >40) may have more frequent recurrent thrombo-occlusive events and death, and these events may also happen sooner. This is compared to patients with first time stroke who have lower levels of IgG aCL (10 to 40 GPL). The study population was 132 patients with focal cerebral ischemia who had at least 10 GPL units of aCL at time of first stroke. They were then followed up prospectively.

In 1992, Levine et al. also studied 75 patients with aPL antibody syndrome who were followed up prospectively and they showed a stroke recurrent rate of 18.7% per year and 15.2% per year for transient ischemic attack (TIA). Nencini et al. showed similar results in their study of 44 young patients (aged 15 to 44) followed up prospectively over 3 years. Of these, 18% had aPL antibodies and these patients had significantly more prior cerebral events and were more likely to have recurrent thrombotic events than the patients without aPL antibodies.

CLINICAL APPLICATIONS AND METHODOLOGY

Patient Selection

As described in the previous section, the literature on the relationship between inherited thrombophilias is varied. This paucity of knowledge makes it difficult for the physician to identify which patients should undergo testing for coagulopathic states. Although thrombophilia is a recognized cause of IS, the incidence is rare. In addition, physicians often find these tests difficult to interpret as there is no gold standard and in the setting of acute thrombosis the results can be equivocal. Finally, the cost of testing can be exorbitant, with a 2001 study from Duke hospital quoting the cost of ordering activated protein C, aCL antibodies, and lupus anticoagulant (LA) to be $1,014. Still, given all of these negatives, detecting coagulation disorders can guide the physician with the choice of treatment and help predict recurrent events. This information can be a valuable patient education counseling tool.

A 2002 study by Bushnell et al. investigated physician's knowledge and practices in evaluating coagulation disorders and stroke. The investigators surveyed 59 neurologists (academic faculty, residents/fellows, and community-based practitioners) with interesting results. First, neurologists recognized that the diagnostic yield of these coagulation tests is low in patients with stroke, and most test subjects indicated that in <25% of their patients, these tests would influence management. However, less than half of the neurologists followed the recommended guidelines of repeating certain coagulopathy tests after 2 to 3 months because of false positives associated with an acute thrombotic event. The study also found that although physicians recognized potential risk factors that improve the yield of these tests (miscarriage, recurrent thrombosis), these factors were poorly documented in the medical record. The study also found that one third of patients who underwent testing had other clearly defined reasons for undergoing anticoagulation therapy and that the results of the coagulation tests would not have affected management.

As can be expected, there is no consensus in the literature about which patients should be screened for thrombophilias. Commonly, one finds that patients with stroke from unexplained causes, stroke in the young, and recurrent stroke patients end up undergoing coagulation testing. With any patient who undergoes testing, the physician must recognize the potential benefits of the test. In essence, will the result of the test change the management plan to improve patient morbidity and mortality? Another point to consider is whether there are acceptable treatments for a positive result. Several groups have reviewed the role of diagnostic testing for coagulopathies in IS.

In 2000 Bushnell et al. attempted to find a quantitative method to assess the diagnostic yield of various coagulation tests in reference to IS. In this study, they calculated the pre- and post-test probabilities of common coagulation deficiencies [prothrombin gene mutation, activated protein C resistance (APCR)/FVL mutation, aCL antibodies, LA] in IS. The pretest probabilities calculated ranged from 3% to 21%, but these percentages were increased in patients younger than 50 years. Still, from previous studies, these numbers fall below the range of 40% to 60%, which is considered the range of pretest probability where a diagnostic test would provide information leading to diagnosis and management. Using historical features of these diseases, Bushnell et al. provide a scheme of factors that increase pretest probability and thus increase post-test probability (ratio of patients who have coagulopathy testing positive). For patients in whom aCL and LA are considerations, factors increasing pretest probability included idiopathic thrombocytopenia, multiple miscarriages, venous or arterial thrombosis, livedo reticularis, early age of symptom onset (<45), sterile endocarditis with embolism, and diagnosis of or suspicion of systemic lupus erythematosus (SLE). For patients in whom FVL and the prothrombin gene mutation are being considered, factors increasing pretest probability included cerebral or venous thrombosis without precipitating factors, thrombosis during pregnancy, and family history of thrombosis. In patients with a family history of hereditary coagulation defects of protein C, protein S, and antithrombin III the pretest probability was difficult to calculate because of a paucity of data. Again, common history and physical findings were included to increase the probability of a patient having the disease including venous or arterial thrombosis by age 45, recurrent thrombosis without precipitating factors, thrombosis in unusual locations, warfarin-induced skin necrosis, family history of thrombosis, thrombosis during pregnancy, and resistance to heparin. The authors of this study attempt to provide a systematic approach to choosing the patients who are appropriate for diagnostic testing. They acknowledge that systematic testing of the general stroke population is unwarranted. However, using their provided schematic, we can identify a small subset of stroke patients for evaluation. They also carefully go through the limitations of the study including combining heterogeneous studies and difficulty in obtaining sensitivity and specificity measurements in some studies. They also recommend prospective studies using the scheme they have identified.

In 2003, Hankey et al. proposed that there is no justification for routinely testing stroke patients for thrombophilias. As previous authors have, they argue that the incidence of thrombophilia-related IS is low and that there is no reliable data linking pathological subtypes of stroke with specific thrombophilias. In addition, with the lack of randomized-controlled trials on antiplatelet versus anticoagulation therapy in these patients, screening for thrombophilias would be unlikely to change management.

A recent 2007 article by Rahemtullah et al. reviewed the published literature and made recommendations on which IS patients should undergo testing for hypercoagulability. The authors did not recommend generalized testing for all IS patients because of the low incidence of IS and inherited thrombophilias in patients. For stroke patients with cerebral vein thrombosis, testing could be considered for aPL antibodies, prothrombin G20210A, FVL, protein C, protein S, and antithrombin deficiencies. For recurrent stroke they recommend testing for aPL antibodies. For young patients with stroke or patients with a personal or family history of paradoxical emboli or venous thrombosis they recommend testing for protein C, protein S, or antithrombin deficiencies. They also make some recommendations for pediatric patients presenting with stroke and recommend testing for the prothrombin G20210A and FVL in these populations.

Diagnostic Testing

Once the patient population appropriate for testing is determined, the adequate lab tests must be ordered. When testing for the FVL mutation, a screening assay for APCR is done first. When screening for APCR, a dilution of the patient's plasma with factor V–depleted plasma or the original can be used. Several outside factors can influence the results including but not limited to acute thrombosis, deep vein thrombosis and pulmonary embolism (DVT/PE), aging, female sex, pregnancy, oral contraceptives, and heparin. Once this assay is complete, the FVL mutation can be amplified by using polymerase chain reaction (PCR).

The prothrombin gene mutation is also done by using PCR to amplify the guanine-to-arginine mutation found on the 3′ untranslated region of the gene at position 20210.

Testing for the aPL antibody syndrome is more complex. The testing should include the LA, the IgG, and IgM immunoglobulin subclasses of aCL antibodies, and the anti-B2-glycoprotein I. The LA requires at least two different screening assays such as the direct Russell viper venom time and the activated partial thromboplastin time. The aCL antibodies are measured via an enzyme-linked immunosorbent assay (ELISA). As with the FVL mutation, both of these can be influenced by extrinsic factors. The LA can be affected by diabetes or the use of warfarin or heparin. The aCL screen can be affected by diabetes, aging, multiparity, rheumatoid factor, and hypergammaglobulinemia.

Protein C, protein S, and antithrombin III are tested using specific screening functional assays, the results of which are then confirmed with a quantitative assay. These assays are sensitive to acute phase reactants and acute thrombosis and should be used at least 3 months after the initiating event when the patient is healthier.

The MTHFR mutation is detected using PCR, which amplifies the MTHFR C-to-T677 substitution.

Treatment Modalities

There is very little information available in the published literature on how to treat patients with IS secondary to inherited thrombophilia. The primary issue is whether antiplatelet therapy is satisfactory or whether long-term anticoagulant therapy is warranted. A lot of data are available for patients with aPL antibodies. The Warfarin-Aspirin Recurrent Stroke Study WARSS/APASS study looked at secondary stroke prevention in patients with aPL antibody syndrome. Patients were randomly assigned to either 325 mg of aspirin or to warfarin with a target INR of 1.4 to 2.8. The study reviewed 720 patients and showed no difference in thrombotic events between those treated with warfarin and those with aspirin. According to the American Heart Association/American Stroke Association (AHA/ASA) Council on Stroke, antiplatelet therapy is recommended for treating cases of IS or TIA in patients with positive aPL antibodies (Class IIa, Level of Evidence B). In contrast, they recommend oral anticoagulation therapy (INR 2 to 3) for patients with aPL antibody syndrome.

Treatment of the other hypercoagulable states associated with stroke (FVL, prothrombin G20210A, MTHFR) is more ambiguous. The AHA/ASA recommends that these patients should be evaluated for DVT, an indication for anticoagulation therapy in the correct clinical context (class I, level of evidence A). They also recommend that patients be fully evaluated for other mechanisms of stroke. For patients with uncomplicated stroke with underlying inherited thrombophilia, the guidelines suggest antiplatelet therapy or long-term anticoagulants (class IIa, level of evidence C).

PRACTICAL RECOMMENDATIONS

From our experience the most common reasons for further evaluating a stroke patient are unexplained stroke and stroke at a young age. Although thrombophilias are a rare cause of IS, in the appropriate clinical setting, detection of these disorders guides the physician in prevention of recurrent stroke, prevention therapies, screening, and counseling. The challenge, as discussed earlier, is a combination of low frequency of cases, difficulty of patient selection, lack of gold standards in testing, cost of testing, and ambiguity of some test results. Despite the paucity of information on the subject, we have provided some practical recommendations here for approaching the evaluation of a stroke patient with a suspected coagulation disorder.

There is no evidence to suggest that routine testing of all patients for hypercoagulable states is warranted. In unexplained stroke cases, stroke in the young, and recurrent stroke patients testing may be beneficial depending on the clinical context. As outlined in the Bushnell study, factors that increase the pretest probability of a coagulapathy include idiopathic thrombocytopenia, multiple miscarriages, venous or arterial thrombosis, livedo reticularis, early age of symptom onset, sterile endocarditis with embolism, diagnosis or suspicion of SLE, cerebral or venous thrombosis without precipitating factors, thrombosis during pregnancy, and a family history of thrombosis.

A diagnostic workup can include a screening assay for activated protein C resistance (if positive this is followed up with PCR to amplify the FVL mutation); PCR for the prothrombin gene mutation; LA, IgG, and IgM immunoglobulin subclasses of aCL; anti-B2-glycoprotein I; protein C functional assay; protein S functional assay; antithrombin III functional assay; and PCR to amplify the MTHFR mutation. In acute thrombosis protein C, protein S, and antithrombin III should be repeated three months after the initiating event.

Treatment options depend on the individual diagnosis. In general, antiplatelet therapy is adequate for those with positive aPL antibodies or uncomplicated stroke. In patients with aPL antibody syndrome, recurrent strokes, or concurrent deep venous thrombosis, anticoagulation therapy should be considered.

SELECTED REFERENCES

The Antiphospholipid Antibodies in Stroke Study (APASS) Group. Anticardiolipin antibodies are an independent risk factor for first ischemic stroke. *Neurology* 1993;43:2069–2073.

Aznar J, Mira Y, Vaya A, et al. Factor V Leiden and prothrombin G20210A mutation sin young adults with cryptogenic ischemic stroke. *Thromb Haemost* 2004;91:1031–1034.

Bushnell CD, Goldstein LB. Diagnostic testing for coagulopathies in patients with ischemic stroke. *Stroke* 2000;31:3067–3078.

Bushnell CD, Goldstein LB. Physician knowledge and practices in the evaluation of coagulopathies in stroke patients. *Stroke* 2002;33:948–953.

Bushnell CD, Siddiqi Z, Goldstein LB. Improving patient selection for coagulopathy testing in the setting of acute ischemic stroke. *Neurology* 2001; 57:1333–1335.

Bushnell CD, Siddiqi Z, Morgenlander JC, et al. Use of specialized-coagulation testing in the evaluation of patients with ischemic stroke. *Neurology* 2001;56:624–627.

De Stefano V, Chiusolo P, Paciaroni K, et al. Prothrombin G20210A mutant genotype is a risk factor for cerebrovascular ischemic disease in young patients. *Blood* 1998;91:3562–3565.

Hankey GJ, Eikelboom JW. Routine thrombophilia testing in stroke patients is unjustified. *Stroke* 2003;34:1826–1827.

Hankey GJ, Eikelboom JW, van Bockxmeer FM, et al. Inherited thrombophilia in ischemic stroke and its pathogenic subtypes. *Stroke* 2001; 32:1793–1799.

Juul K, Tybjaeg-Hansen A, Steffensen R, et al. Factor V Leiden: the Copenhagen City Heart Study and 2 meta-analyses. *Blood* 2002;100:3–10.

Kim RJ, Becker RC. Association between factor V leiden, prothrombin G20210A, and methlenetetrahydrofolate reductase C677T mutation and events of the arterial circulatory system: a meta-analysis of published studies. *Am Heart J* 2003;146:948–957.

Levine SR, Brey RL, Sawaya KL, et al. Recurrent stroke and thrombo-occlusive events in the antiphospholipid syndrome. *Ann Neurol* 1995; 38:119–124.

Levine SR, Brey RL, Tilley BC, et al. Antiphospholipid antibodies and subsequent thrombo-occlusive events in patients with ischemic stroke. *JAMA* 2004;291:576–584.

Longstreth WT, Jr, Koepsell TD, Reitsma PH. Risk of stroke in young women and two prothrombotic mutations: factor V leiden and prothrombin gene variant (G20210A). *Stroke* 1998;29:577–580.

Margaglione M, D'Andrea G, Giuliani N, et al. Inherited prothrombotic conditions and premature ischemic stroke: sex difference in the association with factor V leiden. *Arterioscler Thromb Vasc Biol* 1999; 19:1751–1756.

Martinelli I, Franchi F, Akwan S, et al. The transition G to A at position 20210 in the 3'-untranslated region of the prothrombin gene is not associated with cerebral ischemia. *Blood* 1997;90:3806.

Pezzini A, Del Zotto E, Magoni M, et al. Inherited thrombophilic disorders in young adults with ischemic stroke and patent foramen ovale. *Stroke* 2003;34:28–33.

Rahemtullah A, Van Cott, EM. Hypercoagulation testing in ischemic stroke. *Arch Pathol Lab Med* 2007;131:890–901.

Ridker PM, Hennekens CH, Lindpainter K, et al. Muation in the gene coding for coagulation factor V and the risk of myocardial infarction, stroke, and venous thrombosis in apparently healthy men. *N Engl J Med* 1995; 332:912–917.

Ridker PM, Hennekens CH, Miletich JP. G20210A mutation in prothrombin gene and risk of myocardial infarction, stroke, and venous thrombosis in a large cohort of US men. *Circulation* 1999;99:999–1004.

Sacco RL, Adams R, Albers G, et al. Guidelines for prevention of stroke in patients with ischemic stroke or transient ischemic attack. *Circulation* 2006;113:e409–e449.

Voetsch B, Damasceno BP, Camargo EC, et al. Inherited thrombophilia as a risk factor for the development of ischemic stroke in young adults. *Thromb Haemost* 2000;83:229–233.

CHAPTER

15 Unruptured Intracranial Aneurysms

AARON S. DUMONT, R. WEBSTER CROWLEY, AND NEAL F. KASSELL

OBJECTIVE

- What is the prevalence and incidence of intracranial aneurysms and what conditions are associated with a higher prevalence of aneurysms?
- What are the most common presentations for patients with unruptured intracranial aneurysms?
- What is the annual risk of rupture for unruptured intracranial aneurysms and what factors increase the risk of rupture?
- What are the treatment options for patients with unruptured intracranial aneurysms and how are patients selected for treatment with these methods?
- What are the risks of treatment associated with unruptured intracranial aneurysms?

Unruptured intracranial aneurysms (UIAs) are being detected with increased frequency because of the widespread availability of high-quality, noninvasive brain imaging techniques. Fortunately, the increased detection of unruptured aneurysms has been accompanied by an increased (although incomplete) understanding of the natural history of UIAs and improvement in therapeutic options, particularly with the development and implementation of endovascular techniques.

UIAs may pose a significant threat to patients harboring these lesions. However, clearly not all UIAs need to be treated. In formulating a management plan for an individual patient, the risks posed by the natural history of the aneurysm (the incidence of rupture and its consequences) must be balanced by the risks posed by the intervention (morbidity and mortality associated with the putative treatment option). Ideally, those treating patients with UIAs should consider all clinical, pathophysiological, and radiological data to select those patients who will most highly benefit from treatment—those who are at highest risk of rupture who can be treated with acceptably low risk. This remains a significant challenge, even when equipped with increased knowledge provided by contemporary, high-quality studies and modern advances in treatment. This chapter reviews UIAs focusing on issues important for the management of patients harboring these lesions.

CLINICAL APPLICATIONS AND METHODOLOGY

Epidemiology

Intracranial aneurysms are common in the general population. The prevalence of UIAs has been largely determined through autopsy studies and through angiographic series. Taken collectively, the prevalence ranges from 0.2% to 9%, with a mean of approximately 2%.

The incidence of aneurysm rupture or subarachnoid hemorrhage (SAH) (number of aneurysm ruptures per 100,000 population per year) varies depending on factors such as the population being studied (Finnish and Japanese persons have a greater disposition) or the age distribution of the population (a younger population has a lower incidence) among others. The incidence of aneurysmal SAH ranges from approximately 7 to 21 per 100,000 persons per year, with an average of 10 per 100,000 persons per year. In the United States alone, there are approximately 28,000 new patients with SAH each year. The incidence of SAH has remained stable over the last three decades.

Aneurysms are more common with increasing age, with a peak incidence occurring between the ages of 50 and 60. There is a clear female gender predilection (approximately 1.6 times higher incidence in females). Smoking and hypertension may predispose to aneurysm formation and/or rupture.

Although most cases of SAH are sporadic, in families with a history of SAH in more than one family member, the prevalence of unruptured aneurysms in other family members is markedly increased (a 4- to 10-fold increased prevalence). Autosomal polycystic kidney disease is unequivocally associated with a higher prevalence of intracranial aneurysms. Other conditions that may predispose to intracranial aneurysm formation include Ehlers-Danlos syndrome Type IV, α_1-antitrypsin deficiency, Marfan syndrome, neurofibromatosis type I, and pseudoxanthoma elasticum, although the association is less well determined in some of these conditions.

Presentation

UIAs may be found incidentally (during the evaluation of unrelated symptoms or conditions) or may be detected during the evaluation of symptoms directly attributable to the aneurysm itself.

UIAs are most frequently discovered during the evaluation of unrelated symptoms or conditions, particularly with the widespread availability of noninvasive imaging techniques such as computed tomographic (CT) scanning, CT angiography, magnetic resonance imaging (MRI) and MR angiography (see Fig. 15.1). Alternatively, they may be discovered during the treatment of a patient with SAH from a different aneurysm. These would be classified as asymptomatic UIAs.

UIAs may also produce symptoms due to mass effect or as the source of thromboembolism. When aneurysms enlarge they can produce a local mass effect. For example, aneurysms arising at the origin of the posterior communicating artery on the internal carotid artery can compress the third cranial nerve, causing an oculomotor palsy. In general, the acute onset of third cranial nerve palsy must be urgently evaluated to rule out aneurysm as the cause. When aneurysms of the cavernous sinus enlarge or acutely develop thrombus within them (increasing their local mass effect), they may also produce cranial neuropathies, leading to isolated palsies or a complete cavernous sinus syndrome. When aneurysms reach a giant size (>25 mm in diameter) they can compress the adjacent brain or brainstem, producing correlative neurological symptoms. When lesions of the posterior circulation enlarge, they can compress and distort the brainstem, producing ataxia, gait difficulty, weakness, numbness, and/or cranial neuropathies (see Fig. 15.2).

Diagnosis

UIA may be diagnosed clinically (e.g., a posterior communicating artery aneurysm producing an acute third nerve palsy), although they are confirmed with imaging techniques. Noninvasive techniques such as CT angiography and MR angiography are being increasingly used. The sensitivity and specificity of these techniques are generally excellent, and source data can be used to create two- and three-dimensional reconstructions (see Fig. 15.3). Catheter-based angiography has long been considered the gold standard. Catheter-based angiography can generally detect the smallest aneurysms, can provide superb resolution, and can provide three-dimensional reconstructed images. Angiography is the basis for endovascular treatment of intracranial aneurysms. However, diagnosis and most treatment decisions can be initially formulated based on noninvasive techniques. Angiography can be reserved for select cases where the noninvasive studies leave doubt or in any case where endovascular therapy will be attempted.

Natural History

Aneurysm rupture is associated with a high fatality rate. In a recent, large series of UIA, aneurysm rupture during the study period

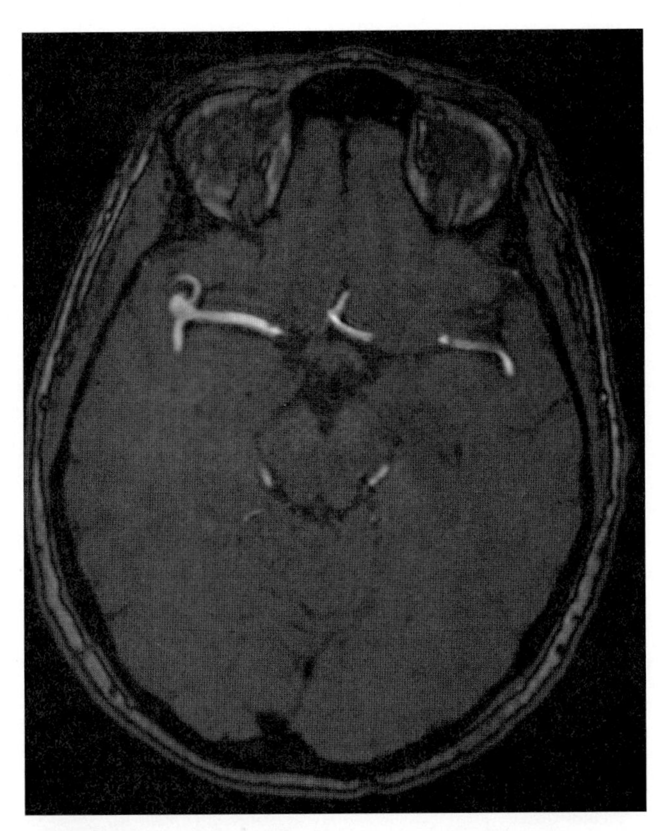

FIGURE 15.1. Unruptured, right middle cerebral artery bifurcation aneurysm found in a 56-year-old female who tripped and sustained a ground level fall.

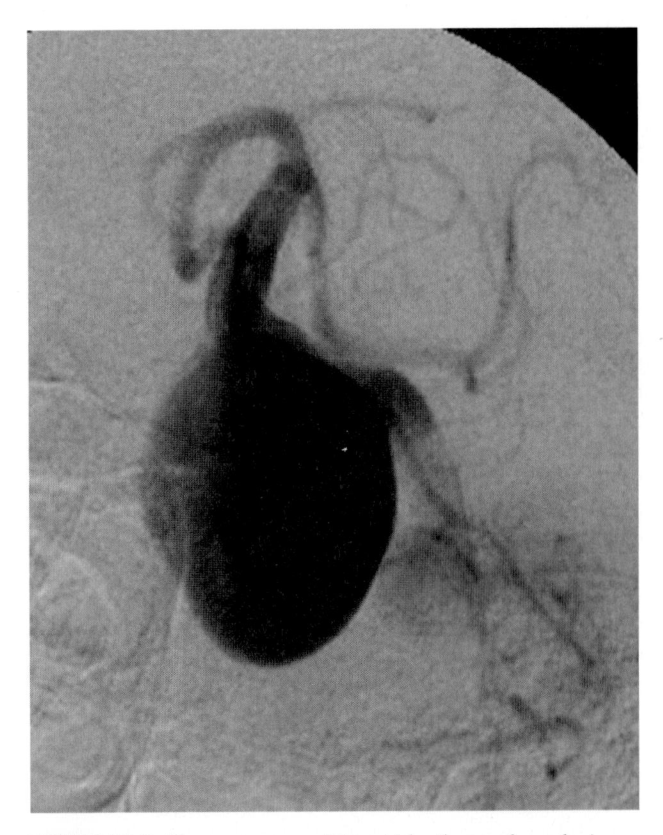

FIGURE 15.2. Giant aneurysm of the mid-basilar trunk producing brainstem compression resulting in ataxia, dizziness, and gait disturbance.

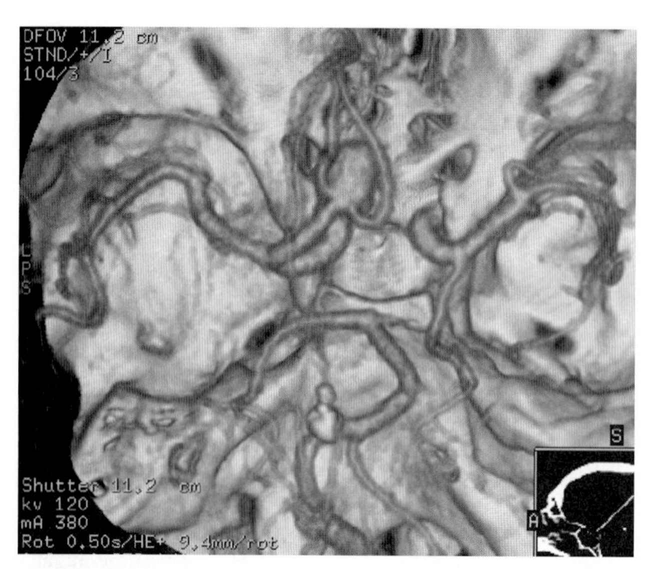

FIGURE 15.3. Three-dimensional reconstruction of a CT-angiogram (superior view). This broad-necked, anterior communicating artery aneurysm was found during the workup for headaches. It is fed by a dominant left A1 segment and there is a hypoplastic right A1 segment.

carried a 52% to 86% mortality rate. A major challenge in evaluating patients with UIA is to determine the risk of rupture and its consequences on the patient's lifetime and to balance this with the risks associated with various treatment options. Understanding the natural history of UIA is therefore critical in this decision-making process.

The International Study of Unruptured Intracranial Aneurysms (ISUIA) is a landmark study that has had an enormous impact on contemporary thoughts about the natural history of UIA and the risks associated with prophylactic intervention. In the first report, the study included both a retrospective and prospective component based on 2,621 enrolled patients from 53 participating centers from across the world. In the retrospective component, the natural history of UIA was evaluated and 1,449 patients (with 1,937 aneurysms) were enrolled and divided into two groups. Group 1 was composed of 727 patients with no history of prior SAH and Group 2 consisted of 722 patients with a history of SAH from a different aneurysm that had been repaired successfully. The data obtained from this component are summarized in Table 15.1. A main point emanating from the data is that small aneurysms in the anterior circulation in patients with no prior history of SAH appear to have an extremely low rate of annual rupture.

In the prospective component of this study, treatment-related morbidity and mortality were evaluated in 1,172 patients in whom UIAs had been newly diagnosed. These patients were divided into two groups as before (those with and without a prior history of SAH). Results from the prospective component are summarized in Table 15.2. The overall morbidity and mortality at 1 year was 15.7% in Group 1 patients and 13.1% in Group 2 patients (including neurocognitive outcomes). The only significant predictor of poor surgical outcome was increasing age, as there was insufficient power to examine other potential predictors such as aneurysm location and size. In addition, insufficient numbers of patients were treated with endovascular techniques to allow meaningful analyses.

TABLE 15.1 ISUIA (1998) Retrospective Component

Group I (No prior history of SAH) (n = 727)	**Group II** (History of SAH) (n = 722)
Rates of Rupture <10 mm: 0.05%/y >10 mm: ~1%/y >25 mm: 6% in first year	**Rates of Rupture** <10 mm: 0.5%/y >10 mm: ~1%/y >25 mm: insufficient data (n = 3)
Predictors of Rupture Increasing size Location (basilar tip, posterior cerebral artery, posterior communicating artery)	**Predictors of Rupture** Location (basilar tip) Older age

ISUIA, International Study of Unruptured Intracranial Aneurysms; SAH, subarachnoid hemorrhage.

The low rates of rupture for certain aneurysms (small, anterior circulation aneurysms in patients with no prior history of SAH) found in the retrospective component were met with some skepticism. Many ruptured aneurysms treated were <10 mm and the patients included in the retrospective study were those who were seen between 1970 and 1991 and they had not received treatment for their aneurysm. The possibility of surgical selection bias arose (as the study population enrolled represented only 40% of the patients with UIAs evaluated at participating centers during that same period). Some patients obviously were treated during that period, creating the possibility that the nontreated study group was composed of those patients left after surgical selection. Nevertheless, this study represented a seminal contribution and the best study to date.

The second phase of ISUIA was reported 5 years later. Four thousand and sixty patients were enrolled prospectively from those who were evaluated at participating centers between 1991 and 1998. One thousand six hundred and ninety-two patients did not have aneurysmal repair, 1,917 patients had open surgery, and 451 patients underwent endovascular procedures. A summary of the rupture rates for aneurysms that were not treated can be found in Table 15.3. The combined morbidity and mortality associated with

TABLE 15.2 ISUIA (1998) Prospective Component

Group I (No prior history of SAH) (n = 961)	Group II (History of SAH) (n = 211)
Treatment modality Surgery: 798 (83%) Endovascular: 163 (17%)	Treatment modality Surgery: 198 (94%) Endovascular: 13 (6%)
Overall morbidity and mortality At 1 mo – 17.5% At 1 y: 15.7%	Overall morbidity and mortality At 1 mo: 13.6% At 1 y: 13.1%
Predictor of poor surgical outcome: age	Predictor of poor surgical outcome: age

ISUIA, International Study of Unruptured Intracranial Aneurysms; SAH, subarachnoid hemorrhage.

TABLE 15.3 ISUIA (Wiebers 2003): 5-Year Cumulative Rupture Rates of Untreated Aneurysms

Location	<7 mm Group 1	<7 mm Group 2	7–12 mm	13–24 mm	≥25 mm
Cavernous carotid (*n* = 210)	0%	0%	0%	3.0%	6.4%
Post-Pcomm (*n* = 445)	0%	1.5%	2.6%	14.5%	40%
AComm/MCA/ICA (*n* = 1,037)	2.5%	3.4%	14.5%	18.4%	50%

Post-PComm, vertebrobasilar, posterior cerebral artery, posterior communicating artery; AComm, anterior communicating artery; MCA, middle cerebral artery; ICA, internal carotid artery.
Cumulative rupture rates were not shown for Group 2 aneurysms separately for aneurysms ≥7 mm due to low numbers.

treatment is summarized in Table 15.4. Increasing age was found to be a predictor for poor outcome. Size >12 mm and location in the posterior circulation were predictors of poor outcome for both the surgical and endovascular cohorts. In summary, this study provided very important data on the natural history of UIAs and the risks associated with treatment.

Other population-based studies have provided additional information on the natural history of UIA. Juvela et al provided a retrospective report based on 142 patients (with 181 aneurysms) with long-term follow-up (average of 18.1 years per patient). They found an annual incidence of bleeding of 1.3%, with increasing aneurysm size, age at diagnosis (inversely), and cigarette smoking emerging as predictors of rupture. Interestingly, 29 of 33 aneurysms that ruptured were <10 mm at the time of the original diagnosis. Although in the retrospective most patients had a prior history of SAH from another aneurysm, this study circumvented the problem of surgical selection bias, as surgery was never offered for patients with unruptured aneurysms during the study period (1956 to 1978). A further study by Tsutsumi et al enrolled 62 patients with an average follow-up of 4.3 years. They found an approximately 2% per year risk of rupture (22.1% 10-year cumulative risk). This study was small and retrospective, and consisted of primarily elderly patients with a relatively high incidence of concomitant ischemic and hemorrhagic disease. Nevertheless, numerous studies such as those described in the preceding text generally find the rate of rupture to be 1% to 2% per year for unruptured aneurysms.

A meta-analysis was recently performed by Wermer et al to delineate the risk of rupture of UIA in relation to patient and aneurysm characteristics. They included 19 studies with 4,705 patients and 6,556 unruptured aneurysms. They found that the overall annual rupture risks were 1.2% (follow-up <5 years), 0.6% (follow-up 5 to 10 years), and 1.3% (follow-up >10 years). Risk factors for rupture included age >60 years, female gender, Japanese or Finnish descent, size >5 mm, posterior circulation aneurysm, and symptomatic aneurysm.

In summary, the landmark ISUIA and additional studies have provided important information on the natural history of UIA, predictors of rupture, and the risks associated with prophylactic treatment.

PRACTICAL RECOMMENDATIONS

Treatment Options and Outcomes

Treatment options include observation (with or without serial imaging), microsurgery with craniotomy and clipping, or endovascular therapy.

Observation is employed in instances where the risks of treatment appear to be higher than the risks of rupture and its consequences. Most aneurysms of the cavernous carotid artery are observed (as they pose little risk of SAH owing to their being confined in the dural envelope of the cavernous sinus) unless they are acutely symptomatic causing disabling cranial nerve symptoms from compression. For small aneurysms of the anterior circulation in the elderly or for those with short life expectancies, observation may also be indicated. Periodic surveillance imaging can be performed to evaluate for changes in aneurysm size or configuration.

Urgent treatment is generally indicated for patients with acutely symptomatic UIA. In the case of an acute third nerve palsy caused by compression from a posterior communicating artery aneurysm, the aneurysm should be treated with the same urgency as for a ruptured aneurysm. The earlier the aneurysm is treated, the greater the chance of recovery of cranial nerve function. The fact that a neurological deficit has arisen acutely implies that the aneurysm has changed in some way and may herald an impending rupture.

Microsurgery with clipping of the aneurysm has traditionally been accepted as the treatment of choice for unruptured aneurysms that are thought to require treatment. This conceptualization is changing, however, with the development and validation of endovascular therapy as a treatment alternative for intracranial aneurysms. Aneurysms of the middle cerebral artery bifurcation are frequently difficult to treat endovascularly and are often better suited for craniotomy and clipping. Many aneurysms of the posterior circulation are associated with significant morbidity when treated with microsurgery and frequently are treated effectively with endovascular techniques. Aneurysms of the ophthalmic segment (ophthalmic artery and superior hypophyseal artery) may also be effectively treated with endovascular therapy, while microsurgical clipping frequently requires removal of the anterior clinoid

TABLE 15.4 ISUIA (Wiebers 2003): Outcome Following Treatment for UIA—Overall Morbidity and Mortality

Time Point	Open Surgical		Endovascular	
	Group 1 (*n* = 1,591)	Group 2 (*n* = 326)	Group 1 (*n* = 409)	Group 2 (*n* = 42)
At 30 d	13.7%	11.0%	9.3%	7.1%
At 1 y	12.6%	10.1%	9.8%	7.1%

ISUIA, International Study of Unruptured Intracranial Aneurysms.

process, opening of the distal dural ring, and performance of a neck incision to obtain proximal control, which collectively make this treatment option more complex compared to coiling, which does not normally require unique techniques. For aneurysms of other locations, such as the anterior communicating artery and posterior communicating artery, recommending microsurgical clipping or endovascular therapy depends on different factors including the age of the patient, medical comorbidities, configuration of the aneurysm (size, neck size, dome-to-neck ratio, presence of calcification), and the patient and their families' wishes.

Endovascular therapy has emerged as an accepted alternative to craniotomy and clipping for the treatment of intracranial aneurysms. Coil embolization is a minimally invasive option and has enjoyed dramatic improvements in technology and technique. New microcatheters, microguidewires, complex coil shapes, and coated coils (to improve aneurysm healing) have been developed and are widely used. For the treatment of complex, wide-necked aneurysms, balloon or stent assistance has been employed to treat aneurysms that were not previously treatable with endovascular techniques.

Long-term follow-up with endovascular techniques is beginning to emerge but is presently incomplete. Concerns on the durability have long been raised as coil compaction and recanalization are known to occur following coil embolization. Patients undergoing these procedures must be made aware of the need for post-treatment follow-up and the potential for retreatment for significant recurrences.

The risks associated with treatment have been outlined in the preceding section from the ISUIA studies. Endovascular therapy for UIA is associated with a 5% to 10% risk of morbidity and an exceptionally low mortality rate. The risks associated with microsurgery reported by the ISUIA may be representative, although reports from specialized centers have revealed lower rates of morbidity and mortality (2% or less in some series). A recent study examining detailed cognitive outcomes following microsurgery for UIA did not reveal any significant detrimental long-term cognitive effects of repair.

It should be emphasized that both microsurgery and endovascular therapy are complementary and not competitive tools that are used to treat the same condition. Once a decision is made that a patient should undergo treatment for aneurysm, the safest and most effective treatment should be applied. Sometimes, challenging aneurysms may require a multimodal approach involving surgery (e.g., construction of a bypass) followed by endovascular therapy (occlusion of the aneurysm and parent vessel) (Fig. 15.4).

CONCLUSION

UIAs are common in the general population and are being detected with increasing frequency because of widespread implementation of noninvasive imaging studies. The rupture of an intracranial aneurysm is associated with high rates of death and disability, although most intracranial aneurysms do not rupture. The challenge of those evaluating patients harboring UIA is to select patients who will benefit significantly from treatment after carefully analyzing all clinical, physiological, and radiological data and balancing the risks of treatment with the risks posed by the natural history of that particular aneurysm.

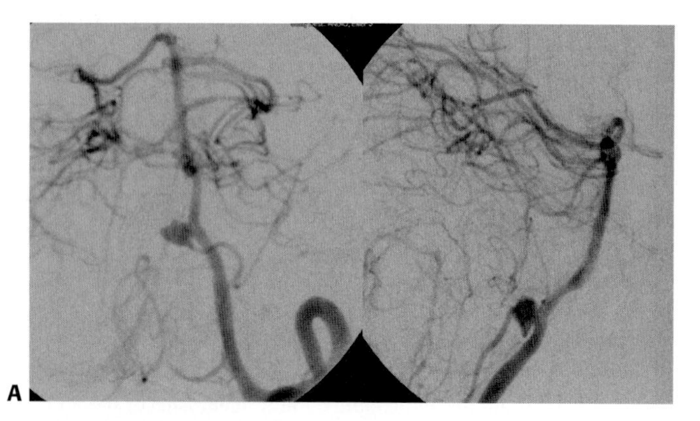

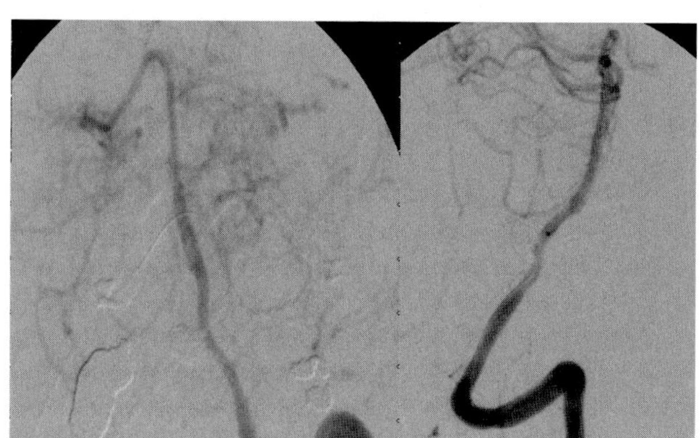

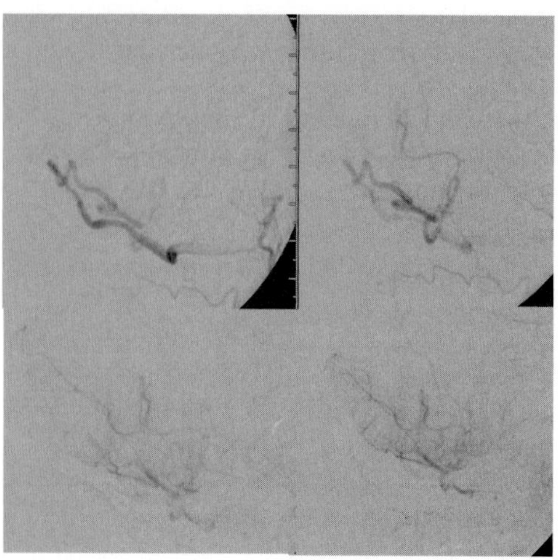

FIGURE 15.4. A: A 46-year-old female was found to have a fusiform aneurysm of the proximal left posterior inferior cerebellar artery (PICA) that was not amenable to either direct neck clipping or coil embolization. **B:** The patient underwent a left occipital to PICA bypass followed by endovascular occlusion of the aneurysm and parent vessel. The *arrow* denotes complete occlusion of the aneurysm and the parent left PICA. **C:** The patent bypass can be seen providing blood flow to the left cerebellar hemisphere. The *arrow* indicates the site of anastomosis.

Considerable progress has been made over the last decade in noninvasive imaging techniques, in the understanding of the natural history of UIA, in treatment options for UIA (particularly with endovascular therapy), and in delineation of the actual risks (including cognitive morbidity) associated with treatment. However, additional work is still needed in the area of UIA that will hopefully translate into improved outcomes for patients harboring UIA.

SELECTED REFERENCES

Chen PR, Amin-Hanjani S, Albuquerque FC, et al. Outcome of oculomotor nerve palsy from posterior communicating artery aneurysms: comparison of clipping and coiling. *Neurosurgery* 2006;58(6): 1040–1046.

Gerlach R, Beck J, Setzer M, et al. Treatment related morbidity of unruptured intracranial aneurysms—results of a prospective single centre series with an interdisciplinary approach during a 6 year period (1999–2005). *J Neurol Neurosurg Psychiatr* 2007;78(8):864–871.

International Study of Unruptured Intracranial Aneurysms Investigators. Unruptured intracranial aneurysms—risk of rupture and risks of surgical intervention. *N Engl J Med* 1998;339(24):1725–1733.

Jane JA, Kassell NF, Torner JC, et al. The natural history of aneurysms and arteriovenous malformations. *J Neurosurg* 1985;62(3):321–323.

Juvela S, Porras M, Poussa K. Natural history of unruptured intracranial aneurysms: probability of and risk factors for aneurysm rupture. *J Neurosurg* 2000;93(3):379–387.

Kang HS, Han MH, Kwon BJ, et al. Repeat endovascular treatment in post-embolization recurrent intracranial aneurysms. *Neurosurgery* 2006; 58(1):60–70.

Leivo S, Hernesniemi J, Luukkonen M, et al. Early surgery improves the cure of aneurysm-induced oculomotor palsy. *Surg Neurol* 1996; 45(5):430–434.

Murayama Y, Nien YL, Duckwiler G, et al. Guglielmi detachable coil embolization of cerebral aneurysms: 11 years' experience. *J Neurosurg* 2003;98(5):959–966.

Nussbaum ES, Madison MT, Myers ME, et al. Microsurgical treatment of unruptured intracranial aneurysms. A consecutive surgical experience consisting of 450 aneurysms treated in the endovascular era. *Surg Neurol* 2007;67(5):457–464.

Pouratian N, Oskouian RJ, Jr, Jensen ME, et al. Endovascular management of unruptured intracranial aneurysms. *J Neurol Neurosurg Psychiatr* 2006;77(5):572–578.

Ronkainen A, Hernesniemi J, Puranen M, et al. Familial intracranial aneurysms. *Lancet* 1997;349(9049):380–384.

Ronkainen A, Hernesniemi J, Ryynanen M. Familial subarachnoid hemorrhage in east Finland, 1977–1990. *Neurosurgery* 1993;33(5):787–796.

Ronkainen A, Hernesniemi J, Ryynanen M, et al. A ten percent prevalence of asymptomatic familial intracranial aneurysms: preliminary report on 110 magnetic resonance angiography studies in members of 21 Finnish familial intracranial aneurysm families. *Neurosurgery* 1994;35(2): 208–212; discussion 212–213.

Tsutsumi K, Ueki K, Morita A, et al. Risk of rupture from incidental cerebral aneurysms. *J Neurosurg* 2000;93(4):550–553.

Tuffiash E, Tamargo RJ, Hillis AE. Craniotomy for treatment of unruptured aneurysms is not associated with long-term cognitive dysfunction. *Stroke* 2003;34(9):2195–2199.

Weir B. Unruptured intracranial aneurysms: a review. *J Neurosurg* 2002;96(1):3–42.

Wermer MJ, van der Schaaf IC, Algra A, et al. Risk of rupture of unruptured intracranial aneurysms in relation to patient and aneurysm characteristics: an updated meta-analysis. *Stroke* 2007;38(4):1404–1410.

Wiebers DO, Whisnant JP, Huston J, III, et al. Unruptured intracranial aneurysms: natural history, clinical outcome, and risks of surgical and endovascular treatment. *Lancet* 2003;362(9378):103–110.

Winn HR, Jane JA, Sr, Taylor J, et al. Prevalence of asymptomatic incidental aneurysms: review of 4568 arteriograms. *J Neurosurg* 2002;96 (1): 43–49.

CHAPTER 16

Cavernous Malformations and Developmental Venous Anomalies

STYLIANOS RAMMOS AND GIUSEPPE LANZINO

OBJECTIVES

- What are the most common presenting symptoms in patients with cavernous malformations and developmental venous anomalies?
- What is the natural history of cavernous malformations and developmental venous anomalies?
- What are the indications for the treatment of cavernous malformations?
- Should surgery be recommended to a patient with a cavernous malformation and seizures?
- What should the patient with an incidental cavernous malformation or developmental venous anomaly be told?

Cavernous malformations (CMs) and developmental venous anomalies (DVAs) are two of the four classic categories of intracranial vascular malformations described by McCormick. This classification includes arteriovenous malformations, venous malformations (now more correctly defined as DVAs), CMs, and capillary telangiectasiae.

BACKGROUND AND RATIONALE

Cavernous Malformations

CMs are one of the four classic categories of intracranial vascular malformations described by McCormick. CMs have been variously described in the literature as cavernous angiomas, cavernous hemangiomas, cavernomas, and classically included in the group of occult or cryptic vascular malformations. This latter definition was used before the introduction of magnetic resonance imaging (MRI) and refers to the characteristic lack of visualization of CMs on conventional catheter angiography.

Intracranial CMs have been reported in all age-groups. Nevertheless, they are more commonly diagnosed in the fourth and fifth decades of life. Autopsy studies and review of a large number of consecutive MRIs have established the incidence of CMs to be somewhere between 0.37% and 0.5% of the general population. Once considered congenital, serial MRIs have demonstrated a dynamic behavior with de novo CM formation, growth, and regression. Growth is usually ascribed to intracapsular or extracapsular hemorrhage. De novo CMs have also been observed after radiation therapy, especially in the pediatric population. CMs occur in sporadic and familial forms. Familial CMs have been associated with different gene mutations and are characterized by multiple lesions in the same patient. The frequent association between CMs and other intracranial vascular malformations, such as DVAs and capillary telangiectasiae, raises interesting questions about a possible mutual, causal relationship between these vascular anomalies.

CMs of the brain occur in different areas of the neuraxis. In the supratentorial compartment, CMs are typically located in a cortical/subcortical distribution. However, they can also be located in deep structures such as the basal ganglia. In the infratentorial compartment, they frequently involve the brainstem (the pons in particular), the cerebellum, and the spinal cord. CMs in less typical areas, such as the ventricles and the cranial nerves, are also encountered. Lesions involving the cavernous sinus, despite sharing some pathological features with other brain CMs, have distinct clinical behavior and therapeutic implications and are considered a different form of the disease.

On gross inspection, CMs have the typical appearance of mulberrylike lesions. Their size ranges from a few millimeters to giant lesions measuring several centimeters in diameter. Section of the lesion reveals a honeycomb of dilated vascular spaces filled with blood of different ages (caverns). There is no intervening brain parenchyma intermingled with the dilated vascular channels. The surrounding brain is often gliotic and hemosiderin stained; hence it is yellow or brown tinged.

The most common mode of presentation of supratentorial CMs is seizures, reported in 40% to 80% of patients. Approximately 30% of patients present with overt hemorrhage. Given the low pressure of blood flowing through the endothelial channels forming the

CM, hemorrhage from these lesions is unlikely to cause catastrophic neurological deficits. Not unusually, patients complain of subacute onset of tedious, persistent, lateralizing headache. A significant number of lesions are discovered incidentally in the course of investigations done for a variety of reasons. In the brainstem and spinal cord, the acute/subacute onset of a neurological deficit with or without headache is the most common presentation. This is usually related to intra- or extracapsular hemorrhage.

The natural history of CMs is related to the mode of presentation and lesion location. The risk of hemorrhage is significantly higher after a first hemorrhagic episode. In a series of 122 patients with CMs followed up for a mean of 34 months, the hemorrhage rate was 0.6% per year in patients with incidental lesions. It was much higher (4.5% per year) in those with a prior history of hemorrhage. The risk of recurrent hemorrhage is higher in patients with blood dissecting and violating the capsule of the CM and extending in the surrounding brain parenchyma. In such patients, there seems to be a temporal clustering of rebleedings in the first 2 years following the first hemorrhagic episode. Symptomatic hemorrhages are not uncommon in the brainstem, basal ganglia, and spinal cord. Given the eloquence of such areas, even very small volumetric increases in size may become symptomatic.

The diagnosis of CMs is based on their typical MRI appearance (see Fig. 16.1). On T2-weighted sequences, CMs display a hypointense rim consisting of a hemosiderin ring and a heterogeneous hyperintense internal core representing the endothelial caverns filled with blood of different ages. Zabramski et al. have divided CMs in four different types based on their MRI characteristics, which relate to different pathological states. On CT, CMs appear as hyperdense lesions because of hemorrhage or calcifications. Cerebral angiography is not necessary for diagnosis. These lesions are not usually visualized on conventional catheter angiography, hence the past definition of occult or cryptic vascular malformations.

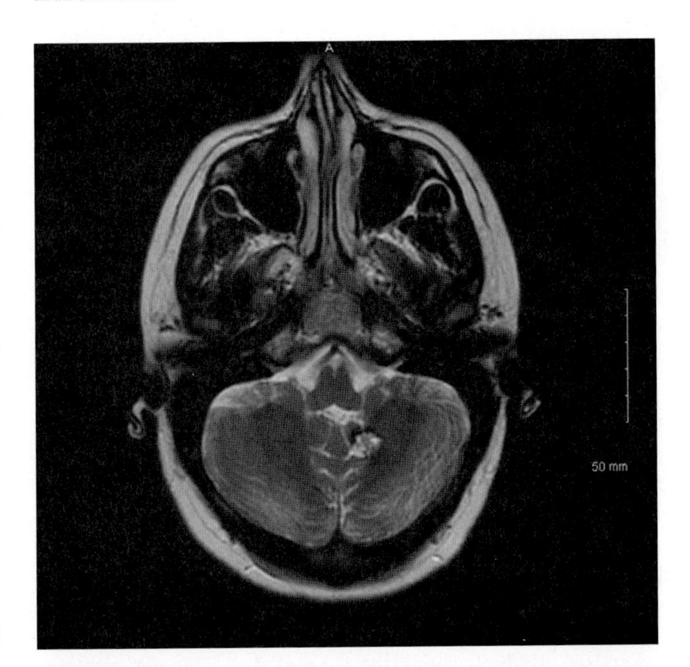

FIGURE 16.1. Characteristic T2-weighted magnetic resonance image (MRI) depicting incidentally discovered vermian cavernous malformation (CM) with hypointense hemosiderin rim and hyperintense core.

Developmental Venous Anomalies

Similar to CMs, a multiplicity of terms has been employed in the literature to define DVAs. These various names have stressed particular aspects of the same clinical entity: their angiographic appearance (*caput medusae*, *star cluster*), the anatomic/pathological features (*medullary venous malformation*), and their non-neoplastic nature (*venous angioma* and *venous malformation*). *DVA* is a term introduced by Lasjaunias in 1986 in an attempt to indicate their congenital origin and the lack of malformed venous elements. This is the currently recommended term and the one adopted in this chapter.

DVAs represent congenital cerebrovascular anomalies with mature venous vessel walls that lack arterial or capillary elements. They are composed of radially arranged, dilated medullary veins, which converge into an enlarged, transcortical or subependymal, draining vein. These collateral venous channels coalesce to form a physiologically normal venous outflow tract and are separated by intervening normal neuropil. In this context, DVAs may be viewed as extreme anatomic variants of medullary venous drainage. DVAs are most commonly solitary, but may be multiple. They are located at the junction of superficial and deep venous systems, adjacent to the cortical surface or near the ependymal surface of the ventricles. Two thirds are supratentorial and one third infratentorial.

DVAs were once thought to be rare lesions. Current literature though supports that DVAs are the most commonly identified intracranial vascular malformation (63% and 50% of all malformations in autopsy and MRI series, respectively). Their cited prevalence in retrospective imaging and autopsy studies is 0.5% to 0.7% and 2.6%, respectively. There is no gender preference. Initial diagnosis is usually established in the fourth and fifth decades. There is no familial aggregation and a recent report identifies a distinct (from CMs) genetic origin.

Historically, DVAs were diagnosed by their characteristic appearance on cerebral angiography. The pathognomonic angiographic appearance is visualized entirely during the late venous phase and consists of wedge- or umbrella-shaped collections of dilated medullary veins (caput medusae) converging into an enlarged transcortical/subependymal collector vein. DVAs are rarely identified on noncontrast enhanced CT, unless they are associated with a CM. Contrast-enhanced MRI is currently the imaging modality of choice. DVAs exhibit strong enhancement, with stellate, tubular vessels converging into a collector vein, which drains into a dural sinus or ependymal vein (see Fig. 16.2).

In the pre-MRI era, DVAs were considered an underestimated cause of intracerebral hemorrhage (ICH). Up to 43% of DVAs were thought to eventually lead to ICH, especially when infratentorial and encountered in young patients. For this reason, aggressive surgical management was pursued. Unfortunately, surgical excision led to disastrous postoperative complications due to venous infarction and cerebral edema after excision of the DVA. With the introduction of MRI, it has become evident that most, if not all, of the ICHs that were once attributed to DVAs are indeed related to an associated CM. Resection of the CM alone, with sparing of the associated DVA, is sufficient to prevent further hemorrhage. Thus, the previously reported high morbidity of DVAs is now accounted for by the coexistence of the angiographically occult CM that might have been unidentified before the advent of MRI. It is strongly suggested that if a patient with a known DVA presents with ICH, a second lesion should be sought.

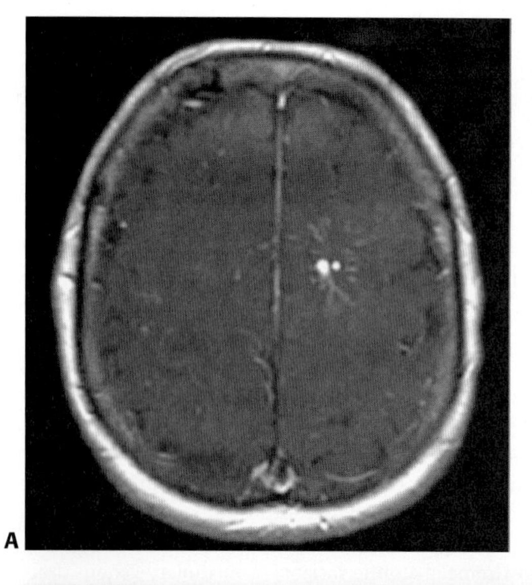

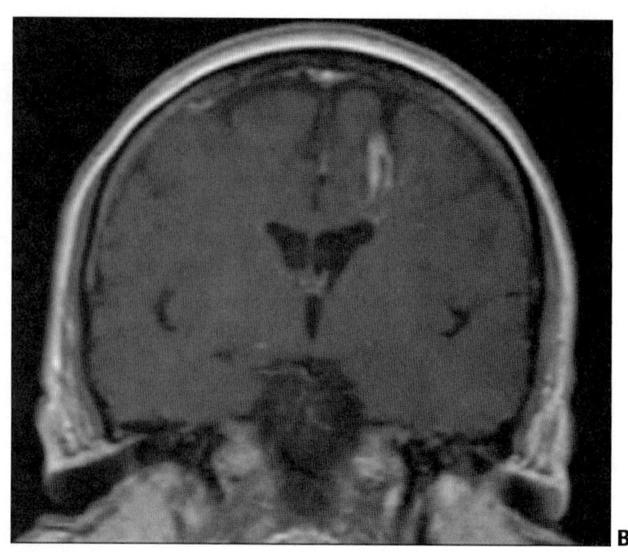

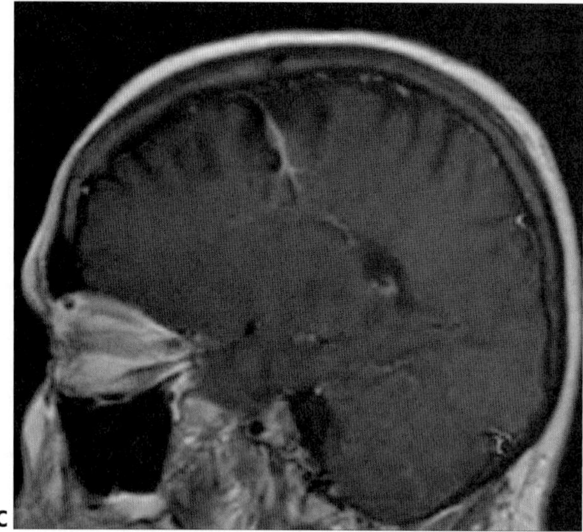

FIGURE 16.2. Contrast-enhanced magnetic resonance imaging (MRI) depicting right frontal developmental venous anomaly (DVA) with caput medusae draining through collector vein to the superior sagittal sinus in a patient presenting with headache. **A:** axial view, **B:** coronal view, and **C:** sagittal view.

Currently, DVAs are most commonly diagnosed in young adults presenting with a variety of symptoms, which are frequently not related to the DVA per se. Most patients are asymptomatic, with the DVA being an incidental finding. Symptoms and signs that lead to acquisition of a diagnostic MRI include headache, dizziness, and seizures. Headache is the most common presenting symptom but most likely appears to be an incidental finding, since it is likely to resolve over time with no intervention in the patient harboring a DVA. It is speculated that new-onset and transient headache that localizes to the general area of a DVA might be related to focal thrombosis of the collector venous channels forming the DVA. However, no convincing proof of this latter statement exists.

The second most common symptom associated with a DVA is seizure. Usually, no correlation between the location of the DVA and the epileptogenic focus can be identified. When a positive association is found, there usually is a coexisting CM or hippocampal sclerosis in the same patient. Notably, there is a rare prevalence of DVAs in large epileptic populations. A negative correlation of DVAs and seizure activity is also indirectly supported by the fact that seizure control can usually be achieved after surgical excision of the coexisting lesion with preservation of the DVA or with the use of antiepileptics only. Multiple other symptoms have been reported in association with DVAs, but a causal relationship has been usually refuted or very difficult to be ascertained.

CLINICAL APPLICATIONS AND METHODOLOGY

The goals of treatment of CMs are prevention of future hemorrhage and seizure control in symptomatic patients. Neurosurgical treatment is usually indicated in the presence of overt, symptomatic hemorrhage; in patients with seizures; and exceptionally, in select asymptomatic patients with enlarging lesions as evidenced by serial MRI imaging. Many CMs are discovered incidentally and treatment is not recommended in the absence of symptoms directly related to the CM. Asymptomatic patients can be followed up conservatively. It should be stressed that CMs are very low flow lesions, and especially in the supratentorial, nonbasal ganglia location, large hemorrhages causing permanent, disabling symptoms are uncommon.

In patients with supratentorial CMs, treatment is indicated in the presence of a prior, recent hemorrhage. This recommendation must be weighed against the risks of surgery. With advances in image guidance, intraoperative monitoring, and functional MRI, surgical resection can be achieved with a very low morbidity even in such difficult and eloquent areas as the motor strip, the speech areas, and the insula. Surgery should be considered early, especially in patients with hemorrhage, which violates the boundaries of the CM capsule. In these patients, as indicated before, temporal clustering of hemorrhages can occur within the first 2 years of the first episode. In patients with recent hemorrhage, we prefer to operate after 10 to 14 days to allow for the clot to liquefy, thus providing a cushion protecting the surrounding brain during manipulation. The parenchyma surrounding CMs is quite often gliotic and hemosiderin stained. It is usually not necessary to resect the hemosiderin-stained brain, provided the entire CM is excised.

The treatment of patients presenting with seizures from supratentorial CMs is controversial. If the seizure is related to frank hemorrhage, surgical resection should be considered. Patients with refractory seizures should be considered for surgical resection even in the absence of demonstrated hemorrhage. Most of the controversy is related to surgical resection of CMs in the patients with medically controlled seizures without frank hemorrhage. In such cases, we consult with the patients and their family extensively on the risks of surgery as well as the possible long-term side effects of chronic anticonvulsants. We tend to recommend surgery for young patients with one seizure or seizures of recent onset and a CM present in a location easy to access surgically. The type and extent of surgical resection in these patients is also debatable. Some authors, including us, recommend simple lesionectomy (i.e., resection of only the CM) in patients with recent-onset seizures as opposed to the more extensive epilepsy surgery with resection of the surrounding gliotic, hemosiderin-laden brain. Most retrospective studies have reported good outcomes after lesionectomy alone, with improvement of seizure control in up to 92% of patients and complete seizure control in >80% of patients. Success of seizure control after surgery is related to the interval between seizure onset and surgical excision. Longer duration of seizures before surgery is associated with a lower success rate. This observation underscores the importance of early CM resection. Patients with chronic epilepsy and CMs do not respond well to lesionectomy alone. In these patients extensive neurophysiological studies are necessary to define the source of seizures and the extent of the focus, which quite often is not limited to the CM per se. The results of surgery in patients with chronic epilepsy and CMs are not quite as satisfactory as in patients with CMs and seizures of recent onset.

Patients with symptomatic CMs of the brainstem and spinal cord can undergo surgical resection with good results in most cases. Surgical treatment should be considered in symptomatic CM abutting the brainstem or spinal cord surface so that no noble parenchyma is traversed to approach the lesion. After surgical resection of CMs in these locations, patients often experience transient neurological deterioration with aggravation of their presenting symptoms. Most commonly, these postoperative deficits regress within a few weeks.

PRACTICAL RECOMMENDATIONS

CMs and DVAs have become a common reason for office consultation in neurological and neurosurgical practices. They are usually an incidental finding encountered during diagnostic evaluation for a wide range of symptoms, which are rarely attributable to the DVA or CM itself. As a general rule, patients with an incidentally found lesion do not need invasive treatment. Patients with incidental DVAs can be reassured about the benign nature of this finding, and no imaging or clinical follow-up is usually indicated. Patients with incidental CMs can also be reassured about the relatively benign natural history of these lesions. They also need to be informed that in the unlikely event of a hemorrhage, this is not as devastating as other high-flow vascular lesions such as aneurysms and intraparenchymal arteriovenous malformations.

Patients with symptomatic hemorrhage from a CM should be considered for surgical excision. Exceptions include patients with deep-seated lesions not abutting the brain or ependymal surface, whose resection would expose the patient to unacceptable surgical risks. Patients with significant medical risk factors should also be considered for conservative treatment, even after frank hemorrhage. In considering surgical indications, it is important to realize the temporal clustering of hemorrhages and the interval from the last hemorrhagic episode. Patients with a history of hemorrhage >2 years before evaluation should be considered asymptomatic from a practical point of view. CMs with recent hemorrhage are relatively easier to resect as opposed to chronic lesions, which are quite often calcified and require more manipulation of the surrounding parenchyma.

Patients who present with seizure have to be counseled about the potential benefit of surgery. Most supratentorial CMs can be resected with very low morbidity. A growing body of literature suggests that surgery is more effective if performed earlier, and the likelihood of seizure control with anticonvulsants is highest among patients with only one or a few seizures and a short interval between onset and surgery. In these patients, resection of the CM alone (lesionectomy) without resection of the surrounding hemosiderin-stained parenchyma is usually sufficient to achieve effective seizure control. Patients with chronic epilepsy should undergo a full preoperative investigation with consideration of invasive monitoring to better localize the focus of the seizure. In these patients a true seizure operation with resection of the lesion along with the epileptogenic brain might be necessary to achieve seizure control. In patients with established, chronic epilepsy and CMs, the results of surgery are not necessarily as good as in patients with one or a few recent seizures undergoing simple lesionectomy.

Frequently asked questions involve the issue of pregnancy and anticoagulation. There a few reported cases of CMs increasing in size during pregnancy. These cases are rare and constitute the exception rather than the rule. In general, we counsel patients with asymptomatic CMs to proceed with normal pregnancy. Patients with symptomatic CMs should be treated as indicated irrespective of their pregnancy status. There is no contraindication in patients with CMs to undergo vaginal delivery and a C-section is usually not warranted. Patients with asymptomatic and incidental CMs can be placed on anticoagulation if clinically necessary. While anticoagulation does not trigger bleeding in patients with CMs, there is the theoretical concern of a larger hemorrhage should the CM bleed while the patients are on anticoagulation. Once again, patients with CMs without prior history of bleeding have a benign natural history, and this very low risk of bleeding must be weighed against the potential benefits of anticoagulation.

SELECTED REFERENCES

Aiba T, Tanaka R, Koike T, et al. Natural history of intracranial cavernous malformations. *J Neurosurg* 1995;83:56–59.

Barker FG, Amin-Hanjani S, Butler WE, et al. Temporal clustering of hemorrhages from untreated cavernous malformations of the central nervous system. *Neurosurgery* 2001;49:15–24.

Broggi G, Ferroli P, Franzini A. Cavernous malformations and seizures: lesionectomy or epilepsy surgery? In: Lanzino G, Spetzler RF, eds. *Cavernous Malformations of the Brain and Spinal Cord*. New York: Thieme; 2007.

Deshmukh VR, Spetzler RF. Management of atypical cavernous malformations. In: Lanzino G, Spetzler RF, eds. *Cavernous Malformations of the Brain and Spinal Cord*. New York: Thieme; 2007:102–107.

Feiz-Erfan I, Zabramski JM, Kim LJ, et al. Natural history of cavernous malformations of the central nervous system. In: Lanzino G, Spetzler RF, eds. *Cavernous Malformations of the Brain and Spinal Cord*. New York: Thieme; 2007.

Gonzalez LF, Lekovic GP, Eschbacher J, et al. Are cavernous sinus hemangiomas and cavernous malformations different entities? *Neurosurg Focus* 2006;15;21(1):e6.

Guclu B, Ozturk AK, Pricola KL, et al. Cerebral venous malformations have distinct genetic origin from cerebral cavernous malformations. *Stroke* 2005;36(11):2479–2480.

Klopfenstein JD, Feiz-Erfan I, Spetzler RF. Brainstem cavernous malformations. In: Lanzino G, Spetzler RF, eds. *Cavernous Malformations of the Brain and Spinal Cord*. New York: Thieme;2007:78–87.

Lasjaunias P, Burrows P, Planet C. Developmental venous anomalies (DVA): the so-called venous angioma. *Neurosurg Rev* 1986;9: 233–242.

Lee C, Pennington MA, Kenney CM, III. MR evaluation of developmental venous anomalies: medullary venous anatomy of venous angiomas. *AJNR Am J Neuroradiol* 1996;17:61–70.

Malik GM, Morgan JK, Boulos RS, et al. Venous angiomas: an underestimated cause of intracranial haemorrhage. *Surg Neurol* 1988;30:350–358.

McCormick WF. The pathology of vascular ("arteriovenous") malformations. *J Neurosurg* 1966;24:807–816.

McLaughlin MR, Kondziolka D, Flickinger JC, et al. The prospective natural history of cerebral venous malformations. *Neurosurgery* 1998;43: 195–200.

Morioka T, Hashiguchi K, Nagata S, et al. Epileptogenicity of supratentorial medullary venous malformation. *Epilepsia* 2006;47(2):365–370.

Nimjee SM, Powers CJ, Bulsara KR. Review of the literature on de novo formation of cavernous malformations of the central nervous system after radiation therapy. *Neurosurg Focus* 2006;15;21(1):e4.

Perrini P, Lanzino G. The association of venous developmental anomalies and cavernous malformations: pathophysiological, diagnostic, and surgical considerations. *Neurosurg Focus* 2006;15;21(1):e5.

Pozzati E, Marliani AF, Zucchelli M, et al. "The neurovascular triad: mixed cavernous, capillary and venous malformations of the brainstem. *J Neurosurg* 2007;107(6):1113–1119.

Thai QA, Pradilla G, Rigam onti D. Capillary telangiectasis, cavernous malformations, and developmental venous anomalies: different expressions of the same disease process? In: Lanzino G, Spetzler RF, eds. *Cavernous Malformations of the Brain and Spinal Cord*. New York: Thieme; 2007: 48–53.

Zabramski JM, Wascher TM, Spetzler RF, et al. The natural history of familial cavernous malformations: results of an ongoing study. *J Neurosurg* 1994;80:422–432.

CRITICAL PATHWAY
Diagnosis of Cavernous Malformations

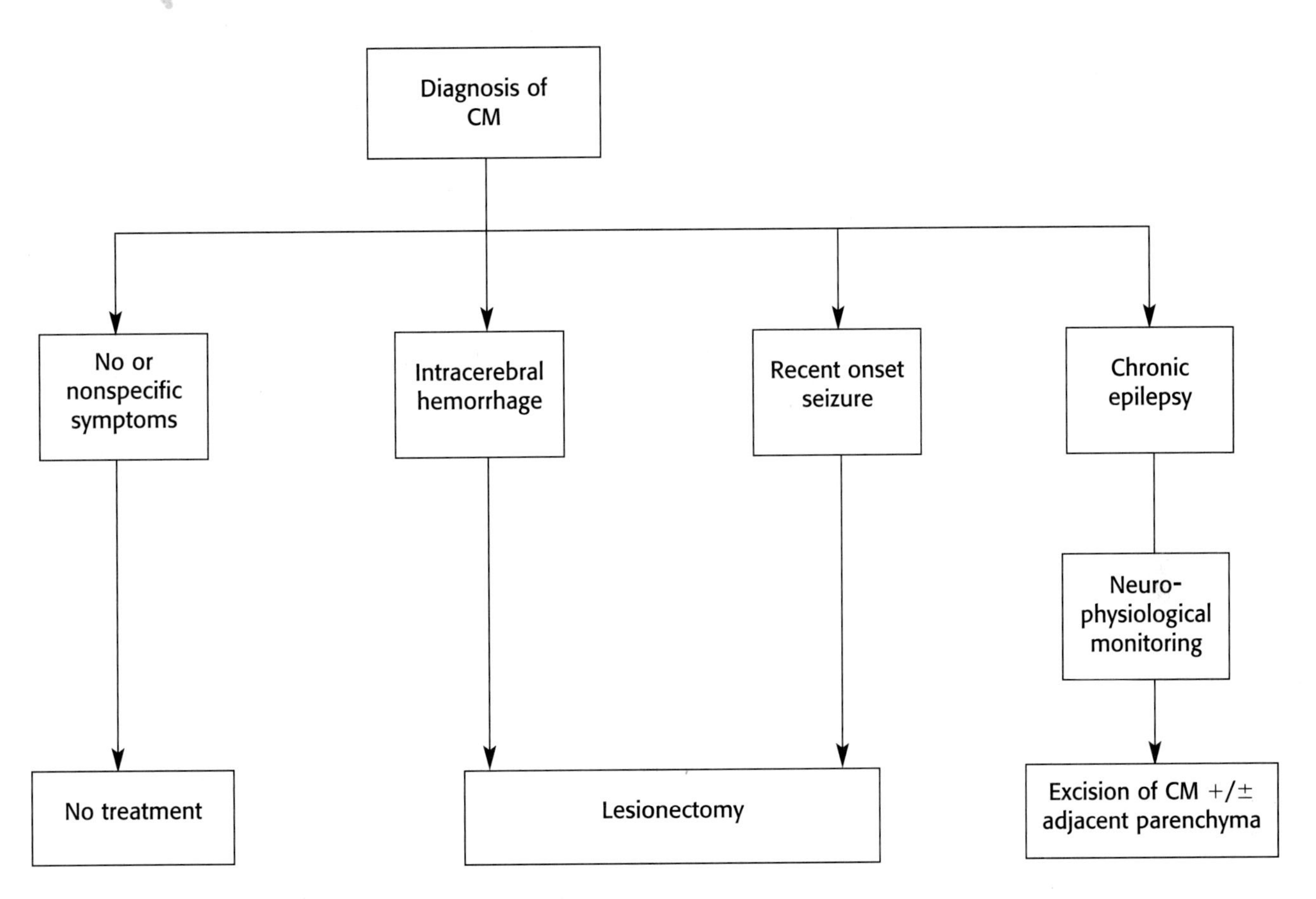

CM, cavernous malformations.

CHAPTER

17 Stroke in Pregnancy

DARA G. JAMIESON

OBJECTIVES

- How can stroke be prevented in women?
- What is the risk of stroke in pregnancy?
- How can cerebrovascular disease be prevented and treated in women?

Stroke is a major cause of death and disability in women, with greatest risk in the later decades of life. According to the 2006 report of the American Heart Association, each year about 46,000 more women than men have a stroke. The differential stroke risk between men and women changes with age. More boys than girls have strokes, and incidence of stroke is greater in men in their 60s and 70s, but stroke is more common in women after age 80 years. Because women live longer than men, more women than men die of stroke each year. Women accounted for 61% of all stroke deaths in 2003.

While women share many of the same stroke risk factors as men, hormonal changes such as pregnancy increase a woman's risk of stroke. Stroke in pregnancy may be specifically related to the pregnancy or it can be due to an unrelated superimposed condition. Causes of stroke are generally the same in men and women but some types of strokes found in both, such as cerebral venous thrombosis (CVT) and subarachnoid hemorrhage (SAH), are more commonly seen in women. Prevention of stroke in pregnancy begins with recognition and treatment of modifiable stroke risk factors prior to pregnancy. The most obvious, but rather impractical, way to prevent stroke associated with pregnancy is to avoid pregnancy. Barrier methods of contraception are essentially risk-free, but hormonal manipulation to prevent pregnancy may pose its own cerebrovascular risk. Prevention of stroke in women in general is outlined in this chapter with the realization that although some features of antiplatelet therapy are unique to women the majority of stroke risk reduction strategies are not gender-specific. The increased risk of stroke associated with pregnancy is reviewed in relation to ways of preventing and treating in women during and after their pregnancies.

STROKE IN WOMEN

In 2006, a National Institute of Neurological Disorders and Stroke (NINDS) sponsored multidisciplinary working group published an overview of our current understanding of the role of estrogen, both endogenous and exogenous, in stroke risk, as well as recommendations for future investigation. Exogenous hormones, oral contraceptives, or hormone replacement therapy increases the risk of venous thrombosis, especially in women with underlying coagulation abnormalities. The factor V Leiden and the prothrombin 20210A gene mutations are especially common and are associated with thrombosis, including CVT. In the setting of a right-to-left cardiac shunt, these thrombophilias, which are generally not associated with intra-arterial thrombosis, can lead to ischemic stroke. The risk appears greatest during the first year of treatment with exogenous hormones.

Diseases more prevalent in women may be associated with stroke risk. Approximately 21 million American women have migraine headaches. The Women's Health Study (WHS) analyzed the correlation between migraine of different types and vascular events. Migraine with aura was found to increase the risk of ischemic stroke, as well as myocardial infarction (MI), coronary revascularization, and angina. Migraine without aura and nonmigraine headaches were not associated with increased vascular risk.

Oral Contraception

While the correlation between oral contraceptives and stroke risk has been debated for decades, the evidence for an association, independent of traditional vascular risk factors, is not clear. The oral contraceptives in current use have lower doses of estrogen than in the earlier studies that showed increased risk. Meta-analyses of studies published up to 2000 (with patient data collection up to 1995) reported variable risk depending on study design, with risk found with case–control, but not cohort, studies. Doses of estrogen >50 μg were associated with greater risk than lower dosages. The absolute risk was noted to be low, with only an additional 4.1 ischemic strokes per 100,000 nonsmoking, normotensive women using low-dose estrogen oral contraceptives.

A population-based cohort study in the Netherlands, the Risk of Arterial Thrombosis in Relation to Oral Contraceptives (RATIO) study, reported that current oral contraceptive use was associated with a risk of stroke twice that of nonusers (OR 2.1; 95% CI, 1.5 to 3.1), even with risk factor adjustment. Smoking, hypertension, hypercholesterolemia, diabetes, and obesity conferred significantly increased risk in combination with oral contraception.

Thrombophilias, specifically factor V Leiden and the G20210A mutation for the prothrombin gene, increase the risk of CVT with oral contraceptives. Ischemic stroke risk, in association with oral contraceptives, has also been shown to be increased with factor V Leiden and methylenetetrahydrofolate reductase (MTHFR) 677TT polymorphism.

Pregnancy

The risk of stroke, both ischemic and hemorrhagic, in pregnancy is unclear with estimates in the range of 4 to 11 cerebral infarctions and 5 to 9 hemorrhagic strokes per 100,000 births. Greater risk of cerebral infarction and hemorrhagic stroke is found in the postpartum period as compared to the prepartum trimesters. Stroke risk associated with pregnancy is discussed in more detail below.

Menopause

The increase stroke risk in postmenopausal woman appears to be due to a combination of age and hormonal changes with decreasing estrogen levels. Primary prevention studies have not shown benefit with hormone replacement therapy (HRT). Some primary and secondary prevention trials have suggested that HRT may increase the risk of cerebrovascular events. The Women's Health Initiative (WHI) found a 44% increased incidence in ischemic, but not hemorrhagic, stroke with estrogen plus progestin treatment of healthy women who were on average a decade into menopause. In women in WHI who were treated with estrogen alone, because of prior hysterectomy, ischemic stroke risk was increased by 39%. In women with increased vascular risk due to coronary heart disease, HRT offered no protection against ischemic stroke, as found in the Heart and Estrogen/Progestin Replacement study. A nested case–control study of >158,000 women, aged 50 to 69 years, in the United Kingdom General Practice Research Database, found that a combined odds ratio for transient ischemic attack (TIA), ischemic stroke, and hemorrhagic stroke associated with the use of HRT was 1.34 (95% CI, 1.11 to 1.61) with individual statistical significance for TIA only. The increased TIA risk was dependent on an increased dose of estrogen and oral delivery. The data suggested increased risk during the first year of treatment. Estrogen supplementation has not been shown of benefit in secondary stroke prevention. The Women's Estrogen for Stroke Trial (WEST) was a randomized placebo-controlled trial of women with prior TIA or ischemic stroke to study if 17β-estradiol reduced the rate of recurrent stroke. The results showed that estrogen alone had no overall benefit in preventing recurrent stroke of fatality, but there was an increase in the overall stroke rate in the first 6 months of treatment. The estrogen-treated women with nonfatal strokes had worse neurological deficits compared to women with strokes in the placebo group.

STROKE PREVENTION IN WOMEN

Almost all recommendations for primary and secondary stroke prevention apply equally to both men and women. Lifestyle issues, long recognized for their role in cardiovascular disease, have recently been evaluated in women as risk factors for hemorrhagic and ischemic stroke. In general, the same lifestyle advocated for decrease in cardiovascular risk benefits cerebrovascular risk. Kurth et al. (2006) used data from the WHS of almost 38,000 healthy female health professionals aged 45 years and older to look at lifestyle and weight as risk factors for stroke. A composite healthy lifestyle was associated with a significantly reduced total and ischemic stroke risk, but not hemorrhagic stroke risk (see Table 17.1). The association was apparent even after controlling for hypertension, diabetes, and elevated cholesterol. Analysis of the individual components of the healthy lifestyle showed substantial reduction of stroke risk in nonsmokers and women with lower body mass indices. The associations with alcohol consumption and physical activity were weaker. The healthier diet paradoxically increased risk of ischemic and hemorrhagic stroke, but the overall risk outcomes were unchanged with removal of diet data. Obesity is a strong risk factor for ischemic stroke, with a less clear relationship with hemorrhagic stroke. The Northern Manhattan Stroke Study found that waist-to-hip ratio measurement of abdominal fat predicted ischemic stroke risk, especially in young people. In the WHS there was a statistically significant trend for increased risk of total and ischemic stroke with increasing body mass index.

TABLE 17.1 Healthy Lifestyle for Women

- Abstinence from smoking
- Body mass index <22 kg per m^2
- Exercise ≥4 times per wk
- Alcohol consumption of 4 to 10.5 drinks/wk
- Diet high in cereal fiber, folate, omega-3 fatty acids; high polyunsaturated to saturated fat ratio; low in *trans* fat; low in glycemic load

As defined in the Women's Health Study.

Women have different degrees of risk reduction with medical and surgical therapy for stroke prevention. Women may respond differently to aspirin therapy than men, at least in primary prevention. Women appear to benefit from aspirin for prevention of a first stroke, an effect not as striking in men. The WHS, the first primary prevention trial of aspirin therapy specific to women, found that low dose aspirin (100 mg every other day) protected women against a first stroke, but generally offered no protection against MI and vascular death. Women aged 65 years and older accounted for only 10% of the WHS population but experienced 31% of the major cardiovascular events in the trial. An older subgroup did show a significant benefit from aspirin in the prevention of primary cardiovascular events, including ischemic stroke, and MI. A sex-specific meta-analysis of aspirin therapy for the primary prevention of cardiovascular events evaluated studies of aspirin in over 95,000 individuals, including 51,342 women. The analysis noted that the women had relatively few MIs but increased strokes, as compared to men. Aspirin therapy was associated with a 24% reduced rate of ischemic stroke (OR 0.76; 95% CI, 0.63 to 0.93; $p = 0.02$), with no apparent effect on hemorrhagic stroke in women.

PREGNANCY AND STROKE

Ischemic Stroke and Intracerebral Hemorrhage in Pregnancy

Kittner et al. (1996) reviewed data from the Baltimore–Washington Cooperative Young Stroke Study, a hospital-based registry initiated to study the incidence and causes of stroke in young adults. All female patients aged 15 through 44 years who were discharged from 46 hospitals in the central Maryland and the Washington, D.C.,

TABLE 17.2 Cerebrovascular Disease in Pregnancy

Ischemic stroke
Artery-to-artery embolization
Cardioembolic embolization
Fluid/air/venous thrombus embolization
Cerebral vasoconstriction
Pre-eclampsia/eclampsia/HELLP
Hemorrhagic stroke
Subarachnoid hemorrhage
Intracerebral hemorrhage
Spinal epidural hemorrhage
Subdural hematoma
Venous thrombosis
Cerebral venous thrombosis

HELLP, hemolysis, elevated liver enzymes, low platelet count.

metropolitan area were identified in 1988 or 1991. For cerebral infarction, the adjusted relative risk during pregnancy was 0.7 (95% CI, 0.3 to 1.6), but increased to 8.7 (95% CI, 4.6 to 16.7) for the postpartum period (after a live birth or stillbirth). For intracerebral hemorrhage (ICH), the adjusted relative risk was 2.5 (95% CI, 1.0 to 6.4) during pregnancy but 28.3 (95% CI, 13.0 to 61.4) for the postpartum period. The excess risk for either type of stroke during or within 6 weeks after pregnancy was 8.1 strokes per 100,000 pregnancies (95% CI, 6.4to 9.7). The risks of cerebral infarction and ICH were increased in the 6 weeks after delivery but not during pregnancy itself.

There is an increased hemorrhagic, as compared to ischemic, stroke risk with pregnancy. The results of a study of women in French public hospitals, the French Stroke in Pregnancy Study Group, also found that the risk of cerebral infarction or ICH was higher during the postpartum period than during any trimester of pregnancy. In contrast to the overall incidence of cerebrovascular disease in young women in France with increased risk of ischemic stroke as compared to ICH, rates of cerebral infarction and ICH during pregnancy and the postpartum period were similar. A study of peripartum stroke in Taiwanese women found that ICH was twice as common as ischemic stroke, a relative incidence that was higher than that in Western countries. The most common causes of ICH were vascular anomaly, pre-eclampsia/eclampsia, coagulopathy, and undetermined.

TABLE 17.3 Risk Factors for Stroke in Pregnancy and the Puerperium

Advanced maternal age (>35 y old)
African-American ethnicity
Pre-eclampsia/eclampsia (current or historical)
Traditional vascular risk factors (hypertension, diabetes, heart disease, smoking)
Lupus
Anemia/blood transfusion
Migraine headaches
Thrombophilias
Sickle cell disease

Bateman et al. used an administrative data set of hospital discharges from 1993 to 2002 to identify women, 15 to 44 years of age, who had pregnancy-related ICH. They found a rate of 7.1 pregnancy-related ICH per 100,000 at-risk person-years compared to 5.0 per 100,000 person-years for nonpregnant women in the same age range. The increased risk was largely associated with ICH in the postpartum period. ICH accounted for 7.1% of all pregnancy-related mortality in the database. Significant independent risk factors included advanced maternal age, African-American ethnicity, preexisting or gestational hypertension, pre-eclampsia/eclampsia, coagulopathy, and tobacco use.

Therapy for Acute Ischemic Stroke in Pregnancy

Pregnant woman with cerebrovascular disease should undergo an investigation that focuses on diagnosing and treating their medical condition. While the fetus should be protected when possible, the need to preserve neurological functioning of the woman is the primary consideration. While magnetic resonance imaging (MRI) and magnetic resonance angiography (MRA) studies without contrast are preferable, a computed tomography (CT) scan with pelvic shielding may be used when diagnosis must be made rapidly before initiation of treatment.

Thrombolytic therapy can be considered in pregnant women with acute ischemic stroke, assuming that the usual inclusion and exclusion criteria have been considered. The hemorrhagic risk of treatment should be considered if delivery appears imminent during the time of thrombolysis. Thrombolytic therapy should not be used for ischemic strokes occurring in the period immediately after delivery, because of the risk of uterine bleeding. Intra-arterial treatment of documented arterial thrombosis may confer decreased systemic risk. Thrombolytic therapy has also been delivered locally to pregnant women with CVT.

Since it is a large molecule (7,200 kDA) recombinant tissue plasminogen activator (rt-PA) does not cross the placenta and has no known tetratogenicity. Anecdotal reports of success with rt-PA given either IV or IA in all trimesters indicate that thrombolysis may be an option when the neurological deficit warrants the risk to the mother and the fetus.

Spinal Cord Cerebrovascular Disease in Pregnancy

While most CNS vascular complications of pregnancy are cerebral, hemorrhage and infarction of the spinal cord can occur. Spinal epidural hemorrhage may occur spontaneously or as a result of vascular malformation leakage with the increased vascular volume of pregnancy. Elevated venous pressure in the epidural space, in association with the hemodynamic changes of pregnancy, may result in spontaneous hemorrhage from the engorged extradural venous plexus. Prompt surgical decompression and evacuation predicts a generally good functional recovery. Infarction of the spinal cord is more likely to be related to embolic material unique to pregnancy than to be due to atherosclerotic material.

Subarachnoid Hemorrhage and Pregnancy

SAH is the third leading cause of maternal mortality during pregnancy, with high fetal mortality as well. SAH is more common in women of childbearing age or older. A wide range of frequencies have been reported for SAH during pregnancy. Increased risk of SAH with pregnancy is controversial, with speculation that hormonal and hemodynamic changes predispose to aneurysm formation and rupture. While the risk of SAH has been theorized to increase with the hemodynamic changes of stages of pregnancy, scientific correlation is lacking. The notion that rupture is more likely to occur during vaginal delivery has been questioned.

Roman et al. reviewed eight women who presented with aneurysmal SAH (six women) or aneurysmal compression (two women). As expected, maternal and perinatal mortality rates were correlated with the maternal Hunt and Hess score. When gestational age allows, delivery by sectioning is suggested before aneurysmal treatment. This recommendation may change with the increased use of endovascular management for symptomatic, and incidental, aneurysms.

Neurosurgical intervention takes precedence over obstetric considerations. Endovascular aneurysmal coiling has changed the management of SAH in the past decade. The risk of poor obstetrical outcome may be decreased with nonsurgical obliteration, with little risk of fetal radiation exposure.

The primary goal of medical management is decreasing vasospasm and delayed cerebral ischemia. Placental blood flow fluctuates with mean arterial pressure, without autoregulation. Nimodipine does not have any clear deleterious effect on the fetus but may cause maternal hypotension and fetal hypoxia. Aminocaproic acid, mannitol, and high dose steroids, which may have deleterious effects on the fetus, are rarely used in SAH patients. Angiotensin receptor blockers should be avoided for blood pressure management because of teratogenic effects.

Once the aneurysm has been successfully obliterated, then vaginal delivery may be considered in neurologically stable women. However, labor trauma should be lessened by epidural anesthesia, shortening the second stage, and by delivery with instruments. A recently or partially obliterated aneurysm may dictate elective sectioning.

Other Cerebrovascular Disorders in Pregnancy and Puerperium

Pregnancy and the puerperium convey unique features to syndromes that may also occur at other times of a woman's life. Reversible cerebral vasoconstriction syndromes are a diverse set of syndromes that characteristically produce headache and focal neurological deficits due to angiographically evident vasoconstriction. These syndromes, more common in women, are distinct from primary angiitis of the central nervous system, which is more common in men. These vasoconstriction syndromes occur in nonpregnant women but can present as overlapping syndromes during pregnancy. Eclampsia, posterior reversible encephalopathy syndrome (PRES), and primary postpartum angiopathy are probably all variations of these reversible cerebral vasoconstriction syndromes. Venous thrombosis syndromes may be diagnosed with hypercoagulopathy during pregnancy, posing challenges for treatment. Ischemic stroke may be due to emboli unique to pregnancy.

Pre-eclampsia and Eclampsia

Pre-eclampsia and eclampsia are leading causes of maternal and perinatal mortality and are important risk factors for both hemorrhagic and ischemic stroke. They complicate about 5% to 8% of pregnancies with about 5 in 1,000 pregnancies associated with severe consequences. About half of eclampsia cases occur antenatally; up to 20% occur during labor and delivery, and approximately 30% are postpartum. In the Baltimore–Washington, D.C., study pre-eclampsia or eclampsia was found in 24% of women with cerebral infarction and 14% of women with ICH. Forty-seven percent of the French women with cerebral infarction and 44% of the women with cerebral hemorrhage had pre-eclampsia or eclampsia.

Treatment with intravenous magnesium sulfate, while scientifically ambiguous, decreases risk of seizures in women with pre-eclampsia and eclampsia. The increased risk of eclampsia and pre-eclampsia with antiphospholipid antibodies is unclear. The deleterious effect of eclampsia and pre-eclampsia extends beyond the pregnancy period. Risk of ischemic stroke not associated with pregnancy and the puerperium is increased in women with a history of pre-eclampsia, as compared to women without a history of pre-eclampsia.

Posterior Reversible Encephalopathy Syndrome

PRES) describes a syndrome of headaches, seizures, visual changes, and accelerated hypertension. Imaging shows increased signal intensity on FLAIR and T2-weighted imaging in the posterior cortical-subcortical regions bilaterally. Lesions, which reflect vasogenic edema, can also be seen in the frontal and cerebellar regions and are not always reversible. While PRES may be associated with pregnancy or the postpartum period, many other conditions are also linked with the syndrome. Early recognition of the condition and prompt lowering of elevated blood pressure can prevent cerebral hemorrhage. Magnesium sulfate can be administered intravenously, in addition to delivery if possible, to treat the vasogenic edema and seizure risk.

Primary Postpartum Angiopathy

Primary postpartum angiopathy (Fleming's syndrome) is a rare, generally reversible, cerebral vasoconstriction syndrome that presents with headaches and focal neurological deficits. Seizures, and rarely cerebral hemorrhages, may occur. Imaging shows reversible multifocal brain ischemia due to segmental narrowing of large and medium-sized cerebral arteries. Spinal fluid is normal, distinct from cerebral angiitis. These patients generally recover without immunosuppressive treatment, although an ICH may cause a permanent deficit. The lack of peripheral edema, proteinuria, and hypertension distinguish Call Fleming syndrome from eclampsia. The MRI scan may be normal or may show cortical lesions. Angiography shows vasoconstriction that reverses parallel to clinical improvement.

Cerebral Venous Thrombosis

CVT has been associated with pregnancy and the postpartum period, especially in association with congenital or acquired coagulation disorders. Anticoagulation acutely with intravenous unfractionated heparin, while problematic with venous infarction and ICH, appears to improve outcome. Because of the teratogenic effects of warfarin, body weight–adjusted subcutaneous low molecular weight heparin should be used for chronic anticoagulation in pregnancy. Local thrombolyis for CVT has been attempted in pregnant women; however, there is not enough experience to make recommendations about intravascular therapy. In general, postpartum CVT has a good prognosis for survival. Risk of recurrence of CVT with subsequent pregnancies is unclear with the suggestion that risk is greatest when the next pregnancy occurs within the next 2 years.

Thrombophilias

A hypercoagulable state causing thrombosis, more commonly venous than arterial, may be diagnosed in pregnancy. Antiphospholipid antibodies, lupus anticoagulants (LA) and anticardiolipin antibodies (aCL), are associated with premature birth and fetal loss occurring after 10 weeks. Increased aCL is independently associated with an increased risk of ischemic stroke or TIA in women but not men. Women with antiphospholipid antibodies and a history of pregnancy losses without prior thrombosis can be treated with combination of aspirin and heparin during pregnancy. Aspirin (81 mg daily) is started before conception and subcutaneous heparin (5,000–10,000 units every 12 hours) or LMWH (enoxaparin 1 mg/kg or 40 to 80 mg daily; dalteparin 5,000 units daily; or nadroparin 3,800 units daily) can be started with documentation of a viable pregnancy.

Thrombophilias, specifically factor V Leiden, the G20210A mutation for the prothrombin gene, and MTHFR 677TT polymorphism increase the risk of CVT. They may be initially diagnosed with a pregnancy-related CVT and indicate risk with subsequent pregnancies. Patients with thrombophilia and CVT should be treated with subcutaneous heparin or LMWH for the duration of the pregnancy.

Embolic Stroke

Embolic ischemic stroke associated with pregnancy may be related to increased risk of paradoxical embolization in the setting of deep vein thrombosis. Cardiomyopathy associated with pregnancy can result in embolic stroke. Engorgement of pelvic veins, with increased vascular volume that may increase intracardiac shunting, make the pregnant woman vulnerable to multiple types of emboli including fat, amniotic fluid, air from orogenital sex, and choriocarcinoma. Percutaneous device closure of a patent foramen ovale, an option that avoids chronic anticoagulation, has been described during pregnancy.

Cerebrovascular Complications of Labor and Delivery

The physical exertion of vaginal delivery, either spontaneous or pharmacologically induced, can lead to cerebral complications including headaches due to intracranial hypotension and subdural hematomas. New, daily persistent postural headache due to intracranial hypotension may be caused by spontaneous, or anesthesia related, dural rupture during the effort of labor and delivery. These headaches are characterized by pain while upright and that are relieved while recumbent. Intracranial subdural hematomas may complicate epidural catheter placement with or without obvious dural puncture.

SELECTED REFERENCES

Arana A, Varas C, Gonzalez-Perez A, et al. Hormone therapy and cerebrovascular events: a population-based nested case-control study. *Menopause* 2006;15:730–736.

Baillargeon J-P, McClish DK, Essah PA, et al. Association between the current use of low-dose oral contraceptives and cardiovascular arterial disease: a meta-analysis. *J Clin Endo Metab* 2005;90:3863–3870.

Bateman BT, Schumacher HC, Bushnell CD, et al. Intracerebral hemorrhage in pregnancy; frequency, risk factors, and outcome. *Neurology* 2006; 67:424–429.

Berger JS, Roncaglioni MC, Avanzini F, et al. Aspirin for the primary prevention of cardiovascular events in women and men. *JAMA* 2006;295:306–313.

Bernstein RA. Reversible cerebral vasoconstriction syndromes. *Curr Treat Opt Cardio Med* 2006;8:229–234.

Bleeker CP, Hendriks IM, Booij LHDJ. Postpartum post-dural puncture headache: Is your differential diagnosis complete? *Br J Anesth* 2004;93: 461–464.

Brown DW, Dueker N, Jamieson DJ, et al. Preeclampsia and the risk of ischemic stroke among young women: results from the Stroke Prevention in Young Women Study. *Stroke* 2006;37:1055–1059.

Burling JE. Aspirin prevents stroke but not MI in women; vitamin E has no effect on CV disease or cancer. *Clev Clin J Med* 2006;73:863–870.

Bushnell CD. Hormone replacement therapy and stroke: the current state of knowledge and directions for future research. *Semin Neurol* 2006; 26:123–130.

Bushnell CD. Oestrogen and stroke in women: assessment of risk. *Lancet Neurol* 2005;4:743–751.

Bushnell CD, Hurn P, Colton C, et al. Advancing the study of stroke in women: summary and recommendations for future research from an NINDS-sponsored multidisciplinary working group. *Stroke* 2006;37: 2387–2399.

Call GK, Fleming MC, Sealfon S, et al. Reversible cerebral segmental vasoconstriction. *Stroke* 1988;19:1159–1170.

Chan W-S, Ray J, Wai EK, et al. Risk of stroke in women exposed to low-dose oral contraceptives. *Arch Int Med* 2004;164:741–747.

Cywinski JB, Parker BM, Lozada LJ. Spontaneous spinal epidural hematoma in a pregnant patient. *J Clin Anesth* 2004;16:371–375.

Ehtisham A, Stern BJ. Cerebral venous thrombosis. *The Neurologist* 2006;12:32–38.

ESHIRE Capri Workshop Group. Hormones and cardiovascular health in women. *Human Reprod Update* 2006;12:483–497.

Henderson VW. The neurology of menopause. *The Neurologist* 2006;12: 149–159.

James AH, Bushnell CD, Jamison MG, et al. Incidence and risk factors for stroke in pregnancy and the puerperium. *Obstet Gynecol* 2005;106: 509–516.

Johnson DM, Kramer DC, Cohen E, et al. Thrombolytic therapy for acute stroke in late pregnancy with intra-arterial recombinant tissue plasminogen activator. *Stroke* 2005;36:e53–e55.

Kemmeren JM, Tanis BC, van den Bosch, MAAJ, et al. Risk of arterial thrombosis in relation to oral contraceptives (RATIO) study: oral contraceptives and the risk of ischemic stroke. *Stroke* 2002;33:1202–1208.

Kittner S, Stern BJ, Feeser BR, et al. Pregnancy and the risk of stroke. *New Engl J Med* 1996;335(11):768–774.

Kurth T, Gaziano, JM, Cook NR, et al. Migraine and risk of cardiovascular disease in women. *JAMA* 2006;296:283–291.

Kurth T, Gaziano JM, Rexrode KM, et al. Prospective study of body mass index and risk of stroke in apparently healthy women. *Circulation* 2005;111:1992–1998.

Kurth T, Moore SC, Gaziano JM, et al. Healthy lifestyle and risk of stroke in women. *Arch Int Med* 2006;166:1403–1409.

Lam PM, Chung TK, Haines C. Where are we with postmenopausal hormonal therapy in 2005? *Gyn Endo* 2005;21(5):248–256.

Leonhardt G, Gaul C, Nietsch HH, et al. Thrombolytic therapy in pregnancy. *J Thromb Thrombolysis* 2006;21(3):271–276.

Liang CC, Chang SD, Lai SL, et al. Stroke complicating pregnancy and the puerperium. *Eur J Neurol* 2006;13:1256–1260.

Lim W, Crowther MA, Eikelboom JW. Management of antiphospholipid antibody syndrome. *JAMA* 2006;295:1050–1057.

Murugappan A, Coplin WM, Al-Sadat AN, et al. Thrombolytic therapy of acute ischemic stroke during pregnancy. *Neurology* 2006;66:768–770.

Pathan M, Kittner SJ. Pregnancy and stroke. *Curr Neurol Neurosci Reports* 2003;3:27–31.

Ridker PM, Cook NR, Lee IM, et al. A randomized trial of low-dose aspirin in the primary prevention of cardiovascular disease in women. *N Eng J Med* 2005;352:1293–1304.

Roman H, Descargues, G, Lopes M, et al. Subarachnoid hemorrhage due to cerebral aneurysmal rupture during pregnancy. *Acta Obstet Gynecol Scand*, 2004;83:330–334.

Rosendaal FR, Helmerhorst FM, Vandenbroucke JP. Female hormones and thrombosis. *Arterioscler Thromb Vasc Biol* 2002;22:201–210.

Schrale RG, Omerod J, Ormerod OJM. Percutaneous device closure of the patent foramen ovale during pregnancy. *Cath Cardiovasc Intervent* 2007;69:579–583.

Selo-Ojeme DO, Marshman LAG, Ikomi A, et al. Aneurysmal subarachnoid hemorrhage in pregnancy. *Eur J Ob Gyn Repro Bio* 2004;116:131–143.

Sharshar T, Lamy C, Mas JL. Incidence and causes of strokes associated with pregnancy and puerperium: a study in public hospitals of Ile de France. *Stroke* 1995;26:930–936.

Suarez JI, Tarr RW, Selman WR. Aneurysmal subarachnoid hemorrhage. *N Engl J Med* 2006;354:387–396.

Suk SH, Sacco RL, Boden-Albala B, et al. Abdominal obesity and risk of ischemic stroke: the Northern Manhattan Stroke Study. *Stroke* 2003;34: 1586–1592.

Szkup P, Stoneham G. Spontaneous spinal and epidural haematoma during pregnancy: case report and review of the literature. *Br J Rad* 2004:77; 881–884.

Thom T, Haase N, Rosamond W. Heart disease and stroke statistics—2006 update: a report from the American Heart Association statistics committee and stroke statistics subcommittee. *Circulation* 2006;113:85–151.

Tincani A, Branch W, Levy RA, et al. Treatment of pregnant patients with antiphospholipid syndrome. *Lupus* 2003;12;499–503.

Wiese KM, Talkad A, Mathews M, et al. Intravenous recombinant tissue plasminogen activator in a pregnant woman with cardioembolic stroke. *Stroke* 2006;37:2168–2169.

Pediatric Stroke

PAUL R. CARNEY, JAMES D. GEYER, MATTHEW A. SAXONHOUSE, CAMILO R. GOMEZ AND IRENE MALATY

OBJECTIVES

- Why are things done as they are?
- What are the issues to be considered?
- What has been the prior experience?

Stroke in the pediatric population is increasingly being recognized. Estimates of incidence range between 2 and 8 per 100,000, with neonates being disproportionately affected. A recent population-based study found that perinatal arterial ischemic stroke (PAS) was recognized in 1 in 2,300 term infants. The rise in the diagnosis of stroke is in part attributable to improved diagnostic techniques and to greater survival of susceptible children.

BACKGROUND AND RATIONALE

In the past it was felt that children generally recover from stroke with minimal long-term deficit (due to plasticity of the young brain). More recently, however, it was demonstrated that only 31% of children with ischemic stroke regained a normal neurological examination. Approximately 17% had persistent cognitive deficits. Long-term disability can derive from physical, cognitive, behavioral, and psychiatric sequelae. Despite significant advances in management, stroke continues to be one of the leading causes of death among children.

Current treatment guidelines are hampered by the lack of controlled clinical trials. Unfortunately the evidence-based interventions established for adults cannot be directly extrapolated to pediatric patients. Differences in the hemodynamic and coagulation pathways as well as in the significant risk factors that contribute to cerebrovascular accidents distinguish the two types of patients. For instance, atherosclerosis, one of the most common sources of adult stroke, rarely contributes to stroke risk in the pediatric population.

Two sets of guidelines have recently been proposed that may help guide neurologists and generalists treating pediatric stroke. In the United States, the American College of Clinical Pharmacy guidelines (ACCP) published in *Chest* addressed both neonatal and childhood arterial ischemic stroke and cerebral sinus venous thrombosis. The Scottish Intercollegiate Guidelines from the United Kingdom (UK Royal College of Physicians pediatric working group) addressed pediatric patients aged 1 month to 18 years. Both sets of guidelines contain a review of the literature and inputs from pediatric hematologists. The UK guidelines add the involvement of pediatric neurologists. The two sets of guidelines have several areas of agreement, and also variation on several points.

To know when to evoke these guidelines, the acutely presenting pediatric stroke patient must be recognized in a timely fashion. Unfortunately, the average delay between symptom onset and first diagnostic study is 28.5 hours, largely prohibiting the consideration of hyperacute interventions. This delay stems from the often nonspecific symptoms with which pediatric stroke patients present. Neonates with underlying stroke frequently present with seizures as well as lethargy and apnea, whereas older children may present with more focal neurological deficits such as speech abnormalities, visual or sensory changes, or hemiparesis. The differential diagnosis can be vast, including infections and metabolic imbalances. A few key stroke masqueraders should also be considered. Familial hemiplegic migraine is an autosomal dominant migraine variant characterized by hemiplegia during the aura phase. There is often a positive family history, and electroencephalogram (EEG) pattern of unilateral slow background rhythm. Postictal or Todd paralysis is a consideration when focal weakness occurs after a seizure and can closely mimic stroke. Patients should be treated with the urgency of an acute cerebral infarction until proven otherwise.

Physicians must be aware of predisposing conditions and risk factors to have the index of suspicion required to diagnose stroke. This involves awareness of three main categories of cerebrovascular events: arterial ischemic, hemorrhagic, and sinovenous thrombosis. Risk factors overlap for stroke subtypes, but treatment may differ.

Perinatal Stroke

A number of ischemic and hemorrhagic insults may affect the developing fetal or neonatal brain. It is therefore important for the clinician to be aware of the different types of events that can cause perinatal stroke, as the evaluation, management, and expected outcome depend on the type of lesion. PAS refers to a cerebrovascular event occurring during fetal or neonatal life, within 28 days of birth, with pathological or radiological evidence of focal arterial infarction of brain. Sinovenous thrombosis describes thrombosis in one or more of the cerebral venous sinuses and may be associated with secondary hemorrhage. Primary hemorrhagic stroke and other types of intracranial hemorrhages (ICHs) that tend to affect near-term and term infants tend to be associated with specific risk factors. Periventricular hemorrhagic infarction (PVHI), a lesion that mainly affects preterm infants, is a serious complication of germinal matrix–intraventricular hemorrhage. Although these lesions tend to have significant overlap in terms of being hemorrhagic or ischemic, the results may very widely from immediate or eventual death to other long-term consequences, including the effects of these types of events on the neonate may result in immediate or eventual death with other long-term complications including cerebral palsy, epilepsy, blindness, behavioral disturbances, and cognitive dysfunction. Despite the type of lesion, symptoms may be subtle and are often nonspecific. The acute and chronic manifestations of perinatal stroke are reviewed in Table 18.1.

Hemorrhage

Primary hemorrhagic stroke and other types of ICH include subdural, primary subarachnoid, intracerebellar, and intraventricular hemorrhage (IVH), and other miscellaneous types such as focal hemorrhages into the thalamus, basal ganglia, brainstem, or spinal cord. Figure 18.1 shows a hemorrhage in the thalamic region on computed tomography (CT). In general, primary subarachnoid hemorrhages are more frequently seen in the premature infant but tend to be clinically benign, in contrast to intracerebellar hemorrhages that, although also more frequently observed in premature infants, tend to be serious. Subdural and other miscellaneous types of hemorrhages tend to affect full-term infants, and their outcome is variable. Although IVHs tend to predominately occur in premature infants (discussed later), they have been reported to occur in term infants as well. Most of these types of hemorrhages tends

TABLE 18.1 The Acute and Chronic Manifestations of Perinatal Stroke

Signs of Acute Stroke
Seizures
Apnea
Encephalopathy
Poor feeding
Thrombocytopenia
Anemia
Focal neurological symptoms—typically difficult to identify
Murmurs, bruits, tachypnea—absent distal pulses may suggest cardiac anomalies
Skin lesions—may suggest infections or embolic disease
Placental thrombosis—may suggest infectious or embolic disease
Signs of Chronic Infarction
Cerebral palsy
Epilepsy
Cognitive dysfunction
Early hand preference may be indicative of hemiparesis
Abnormal head circumference
Delayed milestones
Hemiparesis
Language dysfunction
Cognitive impairments
Behavioral problems

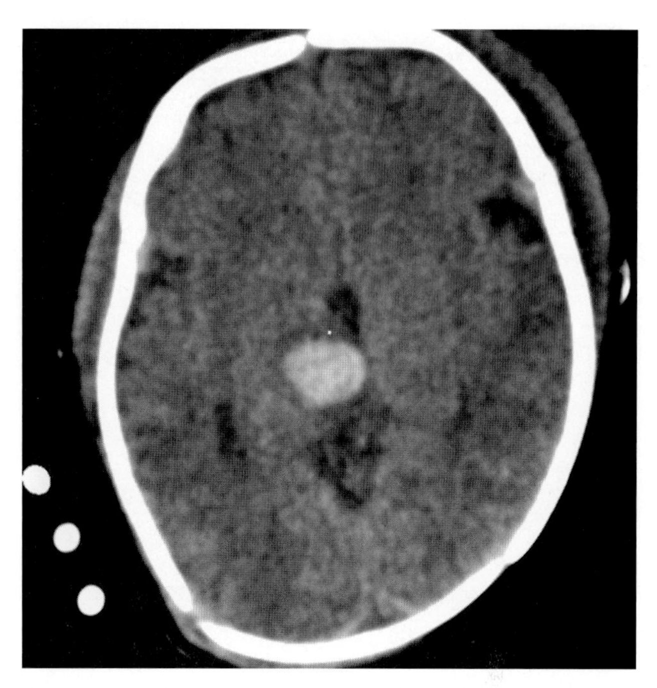

FIGURE 18.1. Computed tomography of the head with a right thalamic hemorrhage. There is also some apparent hypodensity in the right hemisphere.

to be antepartum or occur during the stresses of delivery and are associated with specific risk factors as outlined in Table 18.2.

PVHI usually accompanies a large germinal matrix-IVH. Figure 18.2 illustrates examples of PVHI. The current understanding is that this type of lesion is a venous hemorrhagic infarct in the drainage area of the periventricular terminal vein—a complication mainly associated with prematurity. A recent study found that 1% of infants weighing <2,500 g met the diagnostic criteria for PVHI, with the highest percentage (9.9%) being those weighing

TABLE 18.2 Causes of Perinatal Intracranial Hemorrhage

Coagulation factor deficiencies
Factor V deficiency
Factor X deficiency
Congenital fibrinogen deficiency
Hemophilia (factors VIII and IX)
Hyperhomocystinemia
Hypoprothrombinemia
Alloimmune thrombocytopenia
Vitamin K deficiency
Birth asphyxia
Congenital arterial aneurysm
Arteriovenous malformation
Coarctation of the aorta
Cerebral tumor
Extracorporeal membrane oxygenation
Maternal factors
Idiopathic thrombocytopenic purpura
Warfarin use
Substance abuse
von Willebrand's disease

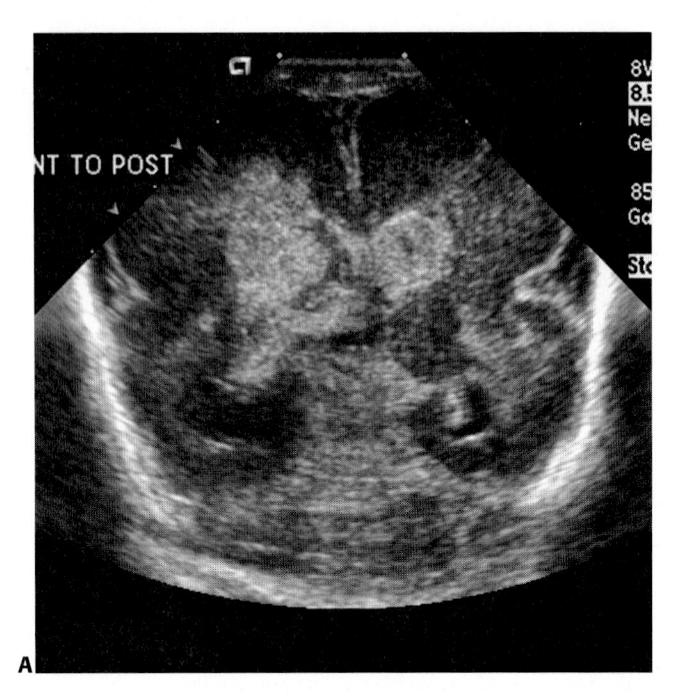

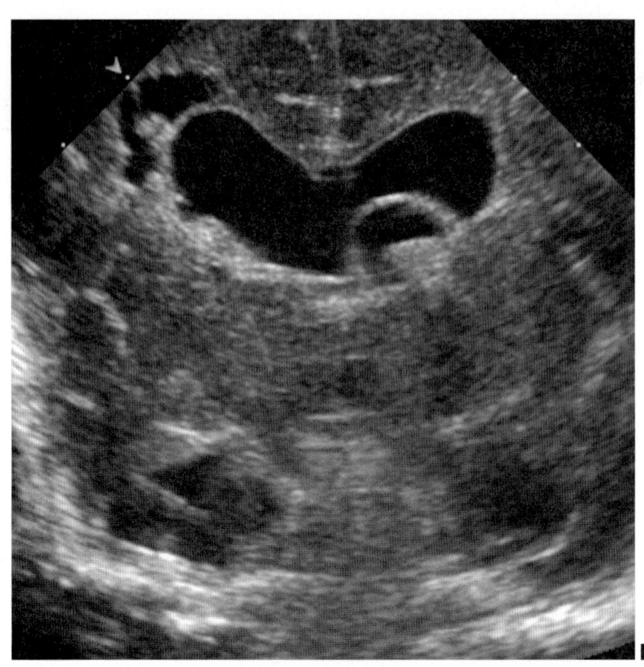

FIGURES 18.2 A AND B. Ultrasonography with periventricular hemorrhagic infarction.

<750 g. Intrapartum risk factors associated with the development of PVHI include emergent cesarean section, low Apgar scores, and need for respiratory resuscitation, while postnatal factors include pneumothorax, pulmonary hemorrhage, patent ductus arteriosus, acidosis, hypotension requiring pressure support, and significant hypercarbia. Although an exact cause–effect relationship of these risk factors and correct knowledge of when these events occur have been difficult to prove, it is felt that disturbances in systemic and cerebral hemodynamics occurring around the intrapartum and early neonatal period are important in the development of PVHI.

Perinatal Arterial Ischemic Stroke

PAS, occurring more frequently in the near-term and term infant, has a prevalence ranging from 17 to 93 per 100,000 live births. Most lesions occur in the left hemisphere within the distribution of the middle cerebral artery. Rarely, multifocal lesions occur but tend to be embolic in origin. The difficulty with identifying PAS in the neonate is that symptoms tend to be nonspecific and are often difficult to identify. In many cases, the symptoms may not become evident until quite some time after the stroke. The acute and chronic manifestations of PAS are reviewed in Table 18.1. Figure 18.3 reveals a multifocal infarction on diffusion-weighted magnetic resonance imaging (MRI) involving the pons and temporal lobe.

There has been a wide range of risk factors that have been implicated in the etiology of PAS. These are listed in Table 18.3. However, some studies report no finding of an obvious precipitating event in as many as 25% to 77% of cases. The difficulty with identifying a specific risk factor for the development of the lesion is that neonates often have multiple risk factors, making it likely that a combination of environmental risk factors interacting with genetic vulnerabilities is often responsible for the ischemic event.

The exact role of genetic thrombophilias in the pathogenesis of PAS is yet to be defined, but disorders such as factor V Leiden mutation, the prothrombin 20210 promoter mutation, hyperhomocystinemia, elevated lipoprotein (a) levels, antiphospholipid antibodies, and relative protein C deficiency have been described with increased frequency in infants who have PAS when compared with healthy control subjects. Other genetic thrombophilias have also been implicated and are provided in Table 18.3. Further studies are required to better define the potential role of infantile thrombophilia in the pathogenesis and outcome of PAS but experts in the field do recommend a comprehensive thrombophilia

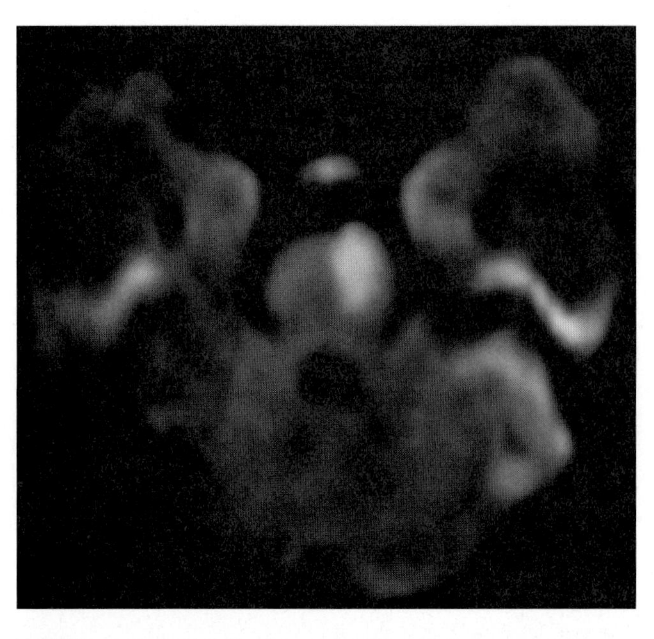

FIGURE 18.3. Axial diffusion-weighted images, $b = 1{,}000$, demonstrate multiple areas of high signal in the left temporo-occipital lobe, left thalamus, and left pons.

TABLE 18.3 Risk Factors Associated with Perinatal Arterial Ischemic Stroke

Risk Factors
Male sex
African-American race
Oligohydramnios
Chorioamnionitis
Prolonged rupture of membranes
Birth trauma
Birth asphyxia
Cesarean delivery
Congenital heart disease
Bacterial meningitis
Anemia
Polycythemia (hyperviscosity)
Hereditary endotheliopathy with retinopathy, nephropathy, and stroke
Inherited or acquired prothrombotic disorders
Factor V Leiden mutation
Prothrombin 20210 promoter mutation
Hyperhomocysteinemia
Elevated lipoprotein (a)
Antiphospholipid antibody syndrome
Protein C deficiency
Protein S deficiency
Antithrombin III deficiency
Methylenetetrahydrofolate reductase deficiency
Maternal factors
Primiparity
History of infertility
Maternal diabetes
Pre-eclampsia

assessment for all infants presenting with PAS, regardless of other risk factors present.

Management of PAS is mainly supportive. Current guidelines from the American College of Chest Physicians suggest that neonates with proven cardioembolic stroke should receive treatment with unfractionated heparin (UFH) or low-molecular-weight heparin (LMWH). The guidelines do not recommend anticoagulant therapy for neonates with noncardioembolic stroke. However, the guidelines do not mention whether the number of blood vessels affected should be taken into consideration or whether noncardiac-related embolism warrants anticoagulation. In addition, there is a lack of information on how to properly anticoagulate neonates who are found to have a genetic thrombophilia.

Sinovenous Thrombosis

Most cases of sinovenous thrombosis occur in term infants and present with nonspecific clinical features as listed in Table 18.1. The superficial and lateral sinuses are most frequently involved and venous infarction has been reported in up to 30% of cases. Figure 18.4 reveals a normal magnetic resonance venogram (MRV). Risk factors for the development of sinovenous thrombosis are similar to those for PAS and are listed in Table 18.3, although a significant number of cases are reported as idiopathic. Management of neonates with sinovenous thrombosis is controversial and is limited by the fact that there are no current clinical trials evaluating the use of anticoagulation. Current guidelines from the American College of Chest Physicians recommend the use of either LMWH or UFH only for neonates with sinovenous thrombosis but without large ischemic infarctions or evidence of intracerebral hemorrhage due to the theoretical risk of bleeding. Radiological monitoring and initiation of anticoagulation only if extension occurs is recommended for the remainder of cases.

Pediatric and Young Adult

Arterial Ischemic Stroke

Arterial ischemic stroke can be related to a number of vascular, hematologic, cardiac, and metabolic risk factors. Potential causes of ischemic stroke in children are presented in Table 18.4.

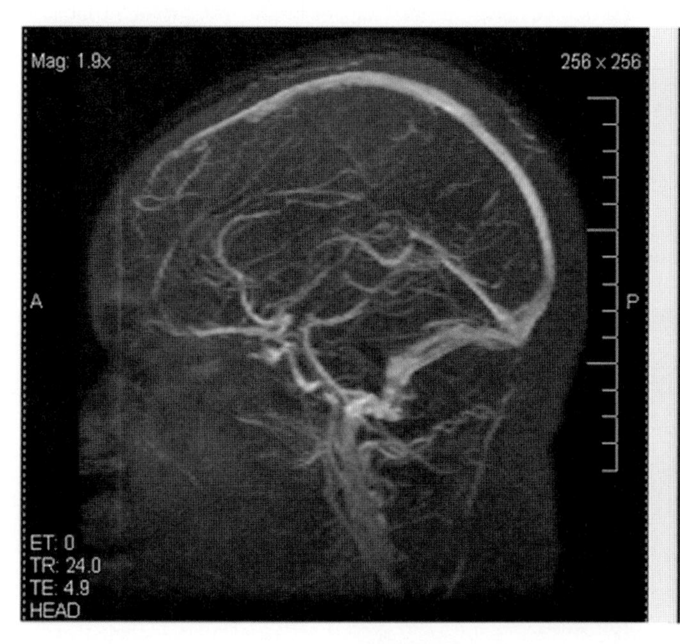

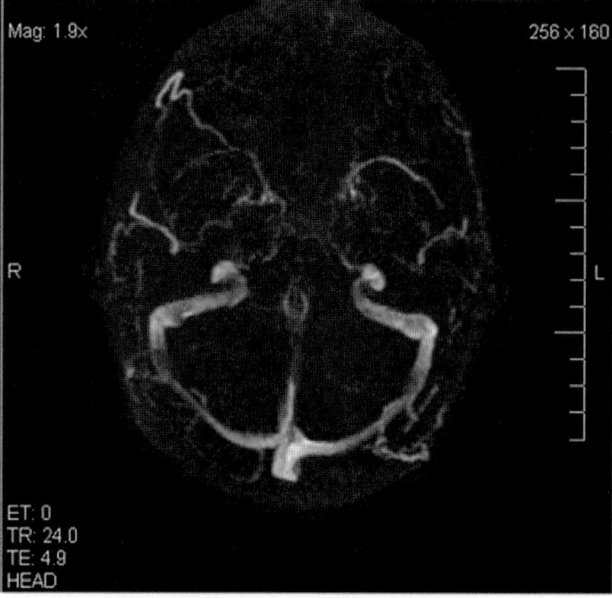

FIGURE 18.4. Magnetic resonance venogram in a healthy individual.

TABLE 18.4 Causes of Ischemic Stroke in Children and Young Adults

1. Vascular dissection (trauma, strangulation, arthritis)
2. Moya-moya disease (large vessel occlusions)
3. Fibromuscular dysplasia
4. Vasculitis
   a. Infectious
   b. Necrotizing
      (1) PAN, Wegener syndrome, Churg-Strauss syndrome, lymphomatosis
   c. Collagen vascular disease
      (1) SLE, RA, Sjögren's disease, scleroderma
   d. Systemic disease
      (1) Behçet's disease, sarcoid, ulcerative colitis
   e. Giant-cell arteritis
      (1) Takayasu syndrome, temporal
   f. Hypersensitivity (drug, chemical)
   g. Neoplastic
   h. Primary CNS vasculitis
5. Migraine (diagnosis of exclusion)
6. Cardiac embolism, patent foramen ovale
7. Hypercoaguable state (primary)
   a. Antithrombin III deficiency
   b. Protein C deficiency
   c. Protein S deficiency
   e. Dysfibrinogenemia
   f. Factor XII deficiency
   g. Antiphospholipid antibodies
   h. Fibrinolytic abnormalities
   i. Activated protein C resistance, factor V Leiden mutation (gene on 1q23)
   j. Hyperhomocysteinemia (gene on 1q36)
   k. CADASIL (gene on 19p13)—Recurrent subcortical infarcts with spared U fibers
   l. MTHFR polymorphism
8. Hypercoaguable state (secondary)
   a. Malignancy
   b. Pregnancy
   c. Oral contraceptives
   d. Disseminated intravascular coagulation
   e. Nephrotic syndrome
   f. Dehydration
9. Platelet abnormalities
   a. Myeloproliferative disease
   b. Diabetes mellitus
   c. Heparin-induced thrombocytopenia
10. Rheology
   a. Homocystinuria (cystathione synthase deficiency)
   b. Polycythemia vera
   c. Sickle cell disease
   d. Thrombotic thrombocytopenia purpura
11. Hyperlipidemia
12. Connective tissue disease (Ehlers-Danlos syndrome, Menkes syndrome, homocystinuria)
13. Organic academia
14. Mitochondrial myopathy (MELAS)
15. Fabry's disease (a-galactosidase A deficiency)
16. Vasospasm (cocaine)

PAN, polyarteritis nodosa; SLE, systemic lupus erythematosus; RA, rheumatoid arthritis; CNS, central nervous system; CNS, central nervous system; CADASIL, Cerebral autosomal dominant arteriopathy with subcortical infarcts and leukoencephalopathy; MTHFR, Methylenetetrahydrofolate reductase; MELAS, mitochondrial encephalopathy with lactic acidosis and strokelike.

Arterial dissection most commonly occurs after trauma. These injuries occur more frequently in boys than in girls. Traumatic dissection can result from head or cervical trauma, including whiplash, shaken baby, or intraoral trauma such as falling with a pencil in the mouth. Rarely, dissection occurs atraumatically from a connective tissue disease such as fibromuscular dysplasia (see Table 18.5). Diagnosis is made via characteristic findings on MRI and magnetic resonance angiography (MRA) of the head and neck, extracranial vascular ultrasound, or cerebral angiography. Findings of a double lumen, intimal flap, or bright crescent on T1 fat suppression images confirm the diagnosis. Also, the finding of occlusion or segmental narrowing of an artery within 6 weeks of a known trauma, or of vertebral artery occlusion at the C2 vertebral level even without trauma should raise the possibility of dissection. This is because the C1-2 vertebral level is the most common location for a vertebral artery dissection. Artery-to-artery embolism from the site of endothelial injury is the usual pathogenic mechanism for infarction. In one meta-analysis, 15% of posterior circulation and 5% of anterior circulation dissections were followed by recurrent ischemic events.

TABLE 18.5 Causes of Arterial Dissection

Traumatic
Head trauma
Cervical trauma, including whiplash, shaken baby
Intraoral trauma such as falling with a pencil (or popsicle) in the mouth
Trauma related to tonsillectomy
Nontraumatic
Fibromuscular dysplasia
Marfan Syndrome
Ehlers-Danlos syndrome
Klippel-Feil syndrome

Moya-Moya

Moya-moya is a vascular condition with risk of recurrent stroke. Primary moya-moya disease is an autosomal dominant disease most common in Japanese patients, hence the Japanese name meaning *puff of smoke*. This describes the angiographic blush that occurs because of extensive collateralization in response to occlusion of large intracranial arteries, often with bilateral carotid artery occlusion. Moya-moya syndrome can also occur secondary to sickle cell disease (SCD), Down syndrome, cranial radiation, or neurofibromatosis.

Vasculitis

Vasculitis is another source of stroke risk in the pediatric population. Primary vasculitides include those affecting large and medium vessels, such as Takayasu arteritis, and those affecting small vessels, such as primary central nervous system (CNS) angiitis and Wegener granulomatosis. Unique to children is the importance of secondary, postinfectious vasculitis. In one study of acute ischemic stroke, varicella zoster infection was detected in the preceding 12 months in 31% of children as opposed to 9% of healthy controls. Strokes typically involved the basal ganglia with typical vascular abnormalities of focal stenosis of the distal internal carotid and proximal segments of anterior cerebral (A1), middle cerebral (M1), and posterior cerebral (P1) arteries. Other pathogens including human immunodeficiency virus (HIV) and cytomegalovirus (CMV) may produce similar vasculitis and stroke risk. Radiation to the brain can also be a risk factor for secondary vasculitis.

Sickle Cell Disease

SCD is one of the most prevalent hematologic risk factors for pediatric stroke. An astounding 9% of patients with SCD will have an acute ischemic stroke by the age of 14, and approximately 20% will have MRI evidence of silent ischemic insults. Risk is greatest during the younger years (from 2 to 8), and two thirds of the patients will have a recurrent event if untreated. The sickled erythrocytes can cause thrombosis in large blood vessels or occlusion of small blood vessels leading to hypoperfusion in watershed areas. SCD is the only area of pediatric stroke for which clear evidence-based guidelines exist. The Stroke Prevention Trial in Sickle Cell Anemia (STOP) trial in 1998 was aborted early due to a clear demonstration of 92% relative risk reduction in stroke with exchange transfusion for cerebral blood flow velocities >200 cm per second on transcranial Doppler. This has led to clear recommendations by the American Academy of Neurology for screening SCD patients with transcranial Doppler ultrasound. The frequency of screening has not been established. Sicklers with frequent transfusions are at risk for iron overload, and alternative therapies including hydroxyurea can also be considered in the long-term maintenance of patients with SCD.

Other Hematologic Conditions

Further hematologic variables relevant to ischemic stroke include high concentrations of lipoprotein A, protein C deficiency, and factor V Leiden mutation. These hypercoaguable states are most highly associated with risk of recurrent stroke. Other prothrombotic states include positivity for antiphospholipid antibodies including anticardiolipin antibodies and lupus anticoagulant, protein S deficiency, factor V Leiden mutation, prothrombin gene mutation (G20210A), and antithrombin III deficiency. Extensive discussion of each of these is beyond the scope of this chapter. Hyperviscosity or sludging effect can also be caused by dehydration, thrombocytosis, and polycythemia. Malignancies including leukemia and lymphoma can also create hypercoaguable states with increased risk of stroke. Several chemotherapeutic agents have also been implicated in cerebral infarction, including adriamycin, asparaginase, and methotrexate. Severe anemia, often seen in developing countries, can result in cerebral infarction secondary to the poor oxygen-carrying capacity.

Cardiac Risk Factors

Cardiac risk factors rise in importance in pediatric stroke relative to the adult population. Congenital heart disease is one of the major risk factors for stroke in pediatric patients. The Canadian Pediatric Ischemic Stroke Registry reported that 19% of children with arterial ischemic stroke had heart disease. The risk is particularly high during surgical procedures. Right-to-left shunting can lead to hypoxia and polycythemia, creating a hyperviscous state. Infective endocarditis additionally poses risk for embolic stroke, and patent foramen ovale (PFO) is a risk for thromboembolic strokes due to venous–arterial communication. PFO is three times more prevalent in pediatric stroke patients than in the general population.

Other etiologies to consider are toxic or iatrogenic sources such as cocaine or oral contraceptive pills. Metabolic sources of stroke risk include homocysteinuria, ornithine transcarbamylase deficiency, and mitochondrial encephalopathy with lactic acidosis and strokelike (MELAS) episodes. MELAS is a heritable mitochondrial disease that presents in childhood with proximal muscle weakness, episodic vomiting and lactic acidosis, migraine headaches, and strokelike episodes. The areas of infarction can be inconsistent with any single vascular distribution. Diagnosis is made by muscle biopsy finding ragged red fibers, and the disease is usually progressive. Hearing and visual loss may occur as well. Cerebral autosomal dominant arteriopathy with subcortical infarcts and leukoencephalopathy (CADASIL) and hyperhomocyteinemia can lead to endothelial damage and platelet aggregation, which are treated with folate and vitamin B. Neurocutaneous diseases of childhood such as Sturge Weber and neurofibromatosis I can be associated with increased risk of stroke.

Hemorrhagic Stroke

Hemorrhagic stroke in children, in contrast to adults, occurs with a frequency equal to that of ischemic stroke. Trauma and bleeding diathesis are important risk factors for hemorrhagic stroke. Risk factors for hemorrhagic stroke are outlined in Table 18.6.

Aneurym in Subarachnoid Hemorrhage

Intracranial aneurysms are common in the general population. The prevalence of unruptured intracranial aneurysms has been largely determined through autopsy studies and through angiographic series. In adults, the prevalence ranges from 0.2% to 9%, with a

TABLE 18.6 Risk Factors for Hemorrhagic Stroke

Hypertension
Aneurysm
Infection
Autoimmune disorders
Vasculitis
Trauma
Surgery
Vascular malformations (see Fig. 18.5)
Telangiectasias
Sickle cell disease
Leukemia
Thrombocytopenia
Cocaine or amphetamine use
Ephedra
Warfarin
Antiplatelet agents
Alagille syndrome

mean of approximately 2%. The prevalence is thought to be lower in children.

The incidence of aneurysm rupture or subarachnoid hemorrhage (number of aneurysm ruptures per 100,000 population per year) varies depending on factors such as the population being studied (Finnish and Japanese persons have a greater disposition) or the age distribution of the population (a younger population will have a lower incidence) among others. The incidence of aneurysmal subarachnoid hemorrhage ranges from approximately 7 to 21 per 100,000 persons per year with an average of 10 per 100,000 persons per year. In the United States alone, there are approximately 28,000 new patients with subarachnoid hemorrhage each year. The incidence of subarachnoid hemorrhage has remained stable over the last three decades.

Aneurysms are relatively uncommon in children and become more common with increasing age, with a peak incidence occurring in between the ages of 50 and 60. There is a clear female gender predilection (approximately 1.6 times higher incidence in females). Smoking and hypertension may predispose to aneurysm formation and/or rupture.

Although most cases of subarachnoid hemorrhage are sporadic, in those families with a history of subarachnoid hemorrhage in more than one family member, the prevalence of unruptured aneurysms in other family members is markedly increased (a 4- to 10-fold increased prevalence). Autosomal polycystic kidney disease is unequivocally associated with a higher prevalence of intracranial aneurysms. Other conditions that may predispose to intracranial aneurysm formation include Ehlers-Danlos syndrome Type IV, α_1-antitrypsin deficiency, Marfan syndrome, neurofibromatosis I, and pseudoxanthoma elasticum, although the association is less well determined in some of these conditions.

The diagnosis of ICH is suggested by the rapid onset of neurological dysfunction and signs of increased intracranial pressure (ICP), such as headache, vomiting, and decreased level of consciousness. The symptoms of ICH are related primarily to the etiology, anatomical location, and extension of the expanding hematoma. Abnormalities in the vital signs such as hypertension, tachycardia or bradycardia (Cushing response), and abnormal respiratory patterns are common effects of elevated ICP and brainstem compression. Approximately 90% of adult patients have systolic blood pressure $\geq$160 mm Hg and/or diastolic blood pressure $\geq$100 mm Hg at the onset. Confirmation of ICH cannot rely solely on the clinical examination and requires the use of emergent CT scan or MRI.

Widespread use of nonenhancing CT scan of the brain has dramatically changed the diagnostic approach of this disease, becoming the method of choice to evaluate the presence of ICH. CT scan evaluates the size and location of the hematoma, extension into the ventricular system, degree of surrounding edema, and anatomical disruption. Hematoma volume may be easily calculated from CT scan images by using the ABC÷2 method. This method multiplies the greatest hemorrhage diameter (A) by the diameter 90 degrees to it (B), multiplied by (C), which is the number of CT slices on which the hemorrhage appears multiplied by slice thickness (cm). Contrast-enhanced CT scan is not done routinely in most centers, but may prove helpful in predicting hematoma expansion and outcome. MRI techniques such as gradient-echo (GRE, T2*) are highly sensitive for the diagnosis of ICH but may be more difficult to obtain in the pediatric patient (often requiring sedation). Sensitivity of MRI for ICH is 100%. In the Hemorrhage and Early MRI Evaluation (HEME) study, MRI and CT were equivalent for the detection of acute ICH but MRI was significantly more accurate than CT for the detection of chronic ICH.

Further discussion of unruptured aneurysms and subarachnoid hemorrhage is undertaken in the chapters on these disorders.

CLINICAL APPLICATIONS AND METHODOLOGY

The child presenting with acute stroke will require careful history and physical examination including perinatal history and developmental milestones. As discussed earlier, the diagnosis of acute stroke in childhood can be challenging. The physician must have a high index of suspicion. Stroke should not be considered an adult disease, but a neurological disorder with different manifestations in different age-groups. Table 18.7 highlights many of the physical findings associated with stroke in the pediatric age-group.

Clearly the most crucial initial interventions are those of stabilizing airway, breathing, and circulation. Adequate oxygenation and ventilation are crucial to reducing the metabolic demand of the ischemic brain. Oxygen should be applied via 100% mask and intubation performed for hypoxia, failure to protect airway, decompensated shock, status epilepticus, or Glasgow Coma Scale (GCS) <8. Core temperature should be kept between approximately 36°C and 37°C. Normoglycemia should be maintained, and seizures should be treated aggressively. Cardiac monitoring with telemetry or Holter monitor should be applied, and initial laboratory reports should be sent to evaluate the glucose levels, electrolyte levels, liver function test results, complete blood count [white blood cell (WBC), hematocrit, platelets], coagulation profile [prothrombin time (PT)/partial thromboplastin time (PTT)/international normalized ratio (INR)], erythrocyte sedimentation rate, antinuclear antibodies, and toxicology screen. This can help identify a metabolic acidosis, which can be seen in MELAS, a concurrent infection, or gross hematologic abnormalities. In general, a chest radiograph and electrocardiogram (ECG) are obtained because of the significance of cardiac disease to risk of pediatric stroke.

TABLE 18.7 Signs of Acute Stroke and Chronic Infarction

Signs of Acute Stroke
Respiratory failure
Seizures
Focal neurological symptoms are typically difficult to identify
Murmurs may suggest cardiac anomalies
Skin lesions may suggest infections or embolic disease
Signs of Chronic Infarction
Cerebral palsy
Epilepsy
Cognitive dysfunction
Early hand preference may be indicative of hemiparesis
Head circumference
Delayed milestones
Hemiparesis
Language dysfunction
Cognitive impairments
Behavioral problems

Because a key initial branch point in the approach to stroke is the distinction between a hemorrhagic and an ischemic event, CT of the head should be performed immediately. Although MRI with diffusion-weighted imaging is better equipped to detect the acute ischemic event, the study takes longer and often requires sedation of the child. CT, although insensitive to infarction in the first 2 days and inferior for evaluating the posterior fossa, is more readily available and quickly obtained. A negative CT scan acutely does not, however, rule out ischemia and requires follow-up imaging in 24 to 48 hours.

When MRI is performed after the CT, diffusion imaging helps age the stroke. Perfusion and proton magnetic resonance spectroscopy images are variations that can help determine the territory of ischemia in addition to infarction. MRA is a noninvasive way to detect vascular occlusions or abnormalities but may overestimate degree of stenosis. MRI and MRA should be sought in arterial ischemic or hemorrhagic strokes. In the latter, arterial venous malformations or aneurysms may be detected and may possibly be amenable to treatment. When dissection is suspected, fat suppression MRI of the neck or MRA of the cervical arteries can make the diagnosis. Figure 18.5 shows an MRA with occlusion of the right internal carotid artery (RICA) and a poorly visualized basilar system. MRV is useful for detecting cerebral sinus thromboses. Conventional angiography is the gold standard as therapeutic interventions may be possible with the procedure, but because it is more time consuming and invasive, it is usually reserved for those cases in which MRA is nondiagnostic.

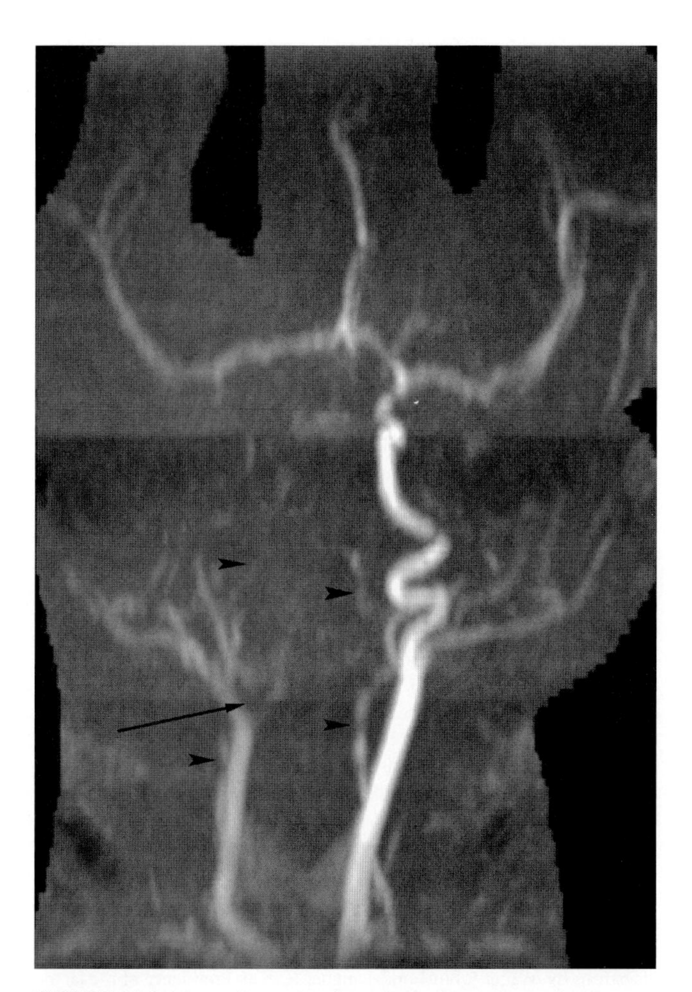

FIGURE 18.5. Three-dimensional maximum intensity projection (MIP) image from a 3-D time-of-flight magnetic resonance angiogram demonstrates occlusion of the right internal carotid artery at its origin (*arrow*). The vertebral arteries are diminutive (*arrowheads*) and the basilar artery is not visualized.

ECG should be obtained to evaluate for congenital heart disease or for thrombotic source. A bubble contrast study with agitated saline should be part of the evaluation to detect intracardiac shunting due to a PFO. Transthoracic ECG is less invasive, but transesophageal ECG allows visualization of the aortic arch and ascending aorta.

If the initial tier of investigations fails to identify a cause for stroke, further evaluation is indicated for known hypercoaguable states (Table 18.4). These investigations should be made 3 to 6 months after the acute stroke. Hemoglobin electrophoresis is used to detect sickle cell, and arterial pyruvate, cerebrospinal fluid (CSF), and arterial lactate are used to evaluate for mitochondrial disease. Lipid profile and serum and urine homocysteine can help detect predisposition to thrombosis. HIV testing should also be considered.

Hemorrhagic Stroke

Hemorrhagic stroke or intracerebral hemorrhage requires close observation, likely in the intensive care unit. Tight control of blood pressure is vital. The target blood pressure should be identified after consultation between the neurologist and the neurosurgeon. If significant mass effect is present, surgical evacuation or craniotomy for decompression may be indicated. Children should be emergently transported to a tertiary care center if necessary.

Anticonvulsant Therapy

The 30-day risk of clinically evident seizures after ICH is approximately 8%. Convulsive status epilepticus may be seen in 1% to 2% of patients, and the risk of long-term epilepsy ranges from 5% to 20%. Lobar location is an independent predictor of early seizures. Acute seizures should be treated with intravenous lorazepam (0.05 to 0.1 mg per kg) followed by an intravenous loading dose of phenytoin or fosphenytoin (20 mg per kg). Critically ill patients with ICH may benefit from prophylactic antiepileptic therapy, but no randomized trial has addressed the efficacy of this approach. Some centers prophylactically treat ICH patients with large supratentorial hemorrhages and depressed level of consciousness during the first week, based on evidence that this practice reduces the frequency of seizures from 14% to 4% during the first 7 days after severe traumatic brain injury. The American Heart Association (AHA) guidelines recommend antiepileptic medication for up to 1 month, after which therapy should be discontinued in the absence of seizures. This recommendation is supported by the results of a recent study that showed that the risk of early seizures was reduced by prophylactic antiepileptic drug (AED) therapy.

Electroencephalogram Monitoring

Continuous electroencephalographic (cEEG) monitoring has been shown to detect nonconvulsive seizures or status epilepticus in 28% of stuporous or comatose ICH patients, a finding consistent with studies of patients with other types of severe acute brain injury. Moreover, ictal activity detected by cEEG after ICH is associated with neurological deterioration and increased midline shift. It is our practice to perform surveillance cEEG monitoring for at least 48 hours in all comatose ICH patients and to treat nonconvulsive seizures and status with midazolam starting at 0.2 mg/kg/hour. However, the management of nonconvulsive status epilepticus is controversial.

Fever Control

Fever after ICH is common, particularly after IVH, and should be treated aggressively. Sustained fever after ICH has been shown to be independently associated with poor outcome, and even small temperature elevations have been shown to exacerbate neuronal injury and death in experimental models of ischemia. As a general standard, acetaminophen and cooling blankets should be given to all patients with sustained fever in excess of 38.3°C (101.0°F), but evidence for the efficacy of these interventions in neurological patients is meager. Newer adhesive surface cooling systems (Arctic Sun, Medivance, Inc.) and endovascular heat exchange catheters (Cool Line System, Alsius, Inc.) have been shown to be much more effective for maintaining normothermia. However, clinical trials are needed to determine whether these measures improve clinical outcome.

Nutrition

As is the case with all critically ill neurological patients, enteral feeding should be started within 48 hours to avoid protein catabolism and malnutrition. A small-bore nasoduodenal feeding tube may reduce the risk of aspiration events.

Ischemic Stroke

In ischemic stroke, maintaining normothermia, a temperature of 36°C to37°C, and normogylcemia is advisable (Hutchison). In general, the treatment guidelines suggested in *Chest* recommend UFH or LMWH for 5 to 7 days regardless of etiology, and the U.K. guidelines suggest aspirin 5 mg per kg immediately. Neither guideline recommends the use of alteplase. Specific situations merit further interventions (deVeber-c).

In patients with SCD, both guidelines suggest exchange transfusion to sickle hemoglobin (HbS) <30%, and intravenous hydration is indicated. Transcranial Doppler ultrasonography is used to screen periodically for increased cerebral flow suggesting need for exchange. Long-term therapy does carry a risk for iron overload, which may require chelation. Possible alternative therapies are hydroxyurea and bone marrow transplantation.

In patients without SCD, noninvasive arterial imaging of extracranial and intracranial arteries should be obtained. Carotid Doppler ultrasonography can quickly evaluate for dissection in suspected cases. Both guidelines recommend anticoagulation for 3 to 6 months after dissection. The *Chest* guidelines specify 5 to 7days of UFH or LMWH followed by LMWH or warfarin for 3 to 6 months, whereas the UK guidelines generally suggest anticoagulation for up to 6 months or until vessel healing.

CT angiography or MRA of the head and neck provide additional information about the patency of vessels and evidence of vasculitis. Vasculitis is usually acutely treated with steroids, with consideration for long-term immunosuppression. The *Chest* guidelines suggest aspirin 2 to 5 mg/kg/day after initial UFH or LMWH for 5 to 7 days in patients with other vasculopathies. The UK guidelines recommend continued aspirin 1 to 3 mg/kg/day after 5 mg per kg on the first day.

ECG should be obtained as soon as possible to evaluate for congenital heart disease and for evidence of a cardioembolic source. Both the guidelines support anticoagulation for cardiogenic embolism, and the *Chest* guidelines specify recommendations for UFH or LMWH for 5 to 7 days followed by LMWH or warfarin for 3 to 6 months.

For suspected cerebral sinus thrombosis— such as in patients with unexplained lethargy, seizure, or headache— MRI/MRV, CV, or cerebral angiography should be obtained. Both the guidelines suggest anticoagulation as therapy. The *Chest* guidelines specify UFH or LMWH for 5 to 7 days, then LMWH or warfarin with target INR 2 to 3 for 3 to 6 months.

PRACTICAL RECOMMENDATIONS

There is a paucity of evidence-based medicine to clearly direct our intervention. The general guidelines for evaluation and management are outlined in this chapter. The diagnosis requires a high level of clinical suspicion, and it is important for the clinician to be mindful of these possibilities.

SELECTED REFERENCES

Adams FJ, McKie VC, Hsu L, et al. Prevention of first stroke by transfusion in children with sickle cell anemia and abnormal results on transcranial Doppler ultrasonography. *N Engl J Med* 1998;339:5–11.

Askalan R, Laughlin S, Mayank S, et al. Chickenpox and stroke in childhood: a study of frequency and causation. *Stroke* 2001;32:1257–1262.

Bassan H, Feldman HA, Limperopoulos C, et al. Periventricular hemorrhagic infarction: risk factors and neonatal outcome. *Pediatr Neurol* 2006;35(2):85–92.

Carlin TM, Chanmugam A. Stroke in children. *Emerg Med Clin N Am* 2002;20:671–685.

Chalmers EA. Perinatal stroke—risk factors and management. *Br J Haematol* 2005;130(3):333–343.

de Veber G. Arterial ischemic strokes in infants and children: an overview of current approaches. *Semin Thromb Hemos* 2003;29(6):567–573.

de Veber G. Canadian Pediatric Ischaemic Stroke Registry. *Pediatr Child Health* 2000b;*A17*.

de Veber G. In pursuit of evidence-based treatments for paediatric stroke: the UK and Chest guidelines. *Lancet Neurol* 2005;4:432–436.

de Veber G, Adams M, Andrew M. Cerebral thromboembolism in neonates: clinical and radiographic features. *Blood* 1998;92:2959.

de Veber G, Adams C, Andrew M, et al. Canadian Pediatric Ischemic Stroke Registry. *Canad J Neurol Sci* 1995;22(Suppl 1):S24.

Fullerton HJ, Claiborne Johnston S, Smith WS. Arterial dissection and stroke in children. *Neurology* 2001;57:1155–1160.

Fullerton HJ, Wu YW, Sidney S, et al. Risk of recurrent childhood arterial ischemic stroke in a population-based cohort: the importance of cerebrovascular imaging. *Pediatrics* 2007;119(3):495–501.

Gabis LV, Yangala R, Lenn NJ. Time lag to diagnosis of stroke syndromes. *Pediatr Infect Dis J* 2000;19:624–628.

Golomb MR, MacGregor DL, Domi T, et al. Presumed pre- or perinatal arterial ischemic stroke: risk factors and outcomes. *Ann Neurol* 2001;50(2):163–168.

Govaert P, Matthys E, Zecic A, et al. Perinatal cortical infarction within middle cerebral artery trunks. *Arch Dis Child Fetal Neonatal Ed* 2000; 82:F59–F63.

Gunther G, Junker R, Strater R, et al. Symptomatic ischemic stroke in full-term neonates: role of acquired and genetic prothrombotic risk factors. *Stroke* 2000;31(10):2437–2441.

Hagstrom JN, Walter J, Bluebond-Langner R, et al. Prevalence of the factor V leiden mutation in children and neonates with thromboembolic disease. *J Pediatr* 1998;133(6):777–781.

Hartel C, Schilling S, Sperner J, et al. The clinical outcomes of neonatal and childhood stroke: review of the literature and implications for future research. *Eur Neurol* 2004;11:431–438.

Harum KH, Hoon AH, Jr, Kato GJ, et al. Homozygous factor-V mutation as a genetic cause of perinatal thrombosis and cerebral palsy. *Dev Med Child Neurol* 1999;41(11):777–780.

Hogeveen M, Blom HJ, Van Amerongen M, et al. Hyperhomocysteinemia as risk factor for ischemic and hemorrhagic stroke in newborn infants. *J Pediatr* 2002;141(3):429–431.

Hunt RW, Inder TE. Perinatal and neonatal ischaemic stroke: a review. *Thromb Res* 2006;118(1):39–48.

Hutchison JS, Ichord R, Guerguerian A, et al. Cerebrovascular disorders. *Semin Pediatr Neurol* 2004;11(2):139–146.

Jordan LC. Stroke in childhood. *The Neurologist* 2006;12(2):94–102.

Kenet G, Nowak-Gottl U. Fetal and neonatal thrombophilia. *Obstet Gynecol Clin N Am* 2006;33(3):457–466.

Kirkham FJ. Stroke in childhood. *Arch Dis Child* 1999;81:85–89.

Kirkham FJ, Sebire G, Steinlin M, et al. Arterial ischemic stroke in children. *Thromb Haemos* 2004;92:697–706.

Lee J, Croen LA, Backstrand KH, et al. Maternal and infant characteristics associated with perinatal arterial stroke in the infant. *JAMA* 2005; 293(6):723–729.

Lynch JK. Cerebrovascular disorders in children. *Curr Neurol Neurosci Reports* 2004;4:129–138.

Lynch JK, Hirtz DG, DeVeber G, et al. Report of the National Institute of Neurological Disorders and Stroke workshop on perinatal and childhood stroke. *Pediatrics* 2002;109(1):116–123.

Lynch JK, Pavlakis S, deVever (check Vever or Veber) G. Treatment and prevention of cerebrovascular disorders in children. *Curr Treatment Opt Neurol* 2005;7:469–480.

Miller V. Neonatal cerebral infarction. *Semin Pediatr Neurol* 2000;7(4): 278–288.

Monagle P, Chan A, Massicotte P, et al. Antithrombotic therapy in children: the Seventh ACCP Conference on Antithrombotic and Thrombolytic Therapy in Children. *Chest* 2004;126;645S–687S.

Nelson KB. Perinatal ischemic stroke. *Stroke* 2007;38(2 Suppl):742–745.

Nowak-Gottl U, Duering C, Kempf-Bielack B, et al. Thromboembolic diseases in neonates and children. *Pathophysiol Haemost Thromb* 2003; 33(5–6):269–274.

Nowak-Gottl U, Gunther G, Kurnik K, et al. Arterial ischemic stroke in neonates, infants, and children: an overview of underlying conditions, imaging methods, and treatment modalities. *Semin Thromb Hemost* 2003;29(4):405–414.

Paediatric Stroke Working Group. Stroke in childhood: clinical guidelines for diagnosis, management and rehabilitation, 2004. http://www.rcplondon.ac.uk/pubs/books/childstroke

Sebire G, Fullerton H, Riou E, et al. Toward the definition of cerebral arteriopathies of childhood. *Curr Opin Pediatr* 2004;16:617–622.

Schulzke S, Weber P, Luetschg J, et al. Incidence and diagnosis of unilateral arterial cerebral infarction in newborn infants. *J Perinat Med* 2005; 33(2):170–175.

Sloan MA, Alexandrov AV, Tegeler CH, et al. Assessment: transcranial Doppler ultrasonography: report of the Therapeutics and Technology Assessment Subcommittee of the American Academy of Neurology. *Neurology* 2004;62:1468.

Thorarensen O, Ryan S, Hunter J, et al. Factor V Leiden mutation: an unrecognized cause of hemiplegic cerebral palsy, neonatal stroke, and placental thrombosis. *Ann Neurol* 1997;42(3):372–375.

Varelas PN, Sleight BJ, Rinder HM, et al. Stroke in a neonate heterozygous for factor V Leiden. *Pediatr Neurol* 1998;18(3):262–264.

Volpe JJ. *Neurology of the Newborn*. 4th ed. Philadelphia, PA: W.B. Saunders; 2001.

Wu YW, Hamrick SE, Miller SP, et al. Intraventricular hemorrhage in term neonates caused by sinovenous thrombosis. *Ann Neurol* 2003;54(1): 123–126.

Wu YW, Lynch JK, Nelson KB. Perinatal arterial stroke: understanding mechanisms and outcomes. *Semin Neurol* 2005;25(4):424–434.

SECTION III

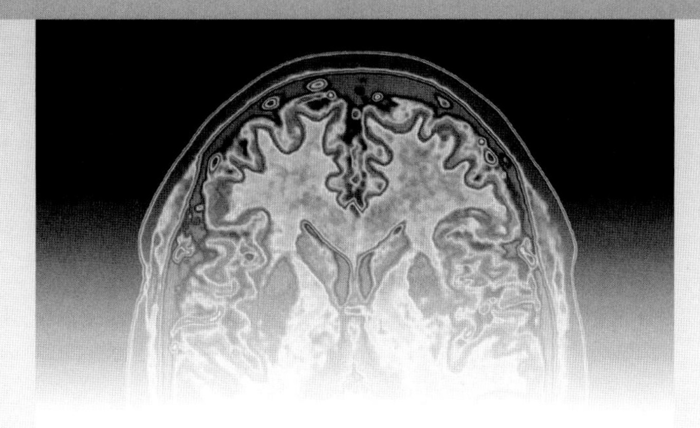

Urgent Stroke Management

CHAPTER

19 Urgent Clinical Assessment of Acute Stroke

KERRI S. REMMEL

OBJECTIVES

- What do EMS personnel need to do for the urgent assessment of a stroke patient?
- What are the essential elements in the initial assessment and management of acute stroke patients?
  - What is initial urgent assessment in the rapid response room?
  - What comprises urgent clinical assessment and management of acute hemorrhagic stroke?
  - How is patient eligibility for thrombolytic therapy or other immediate interventions for acute ischemic stroke rapidly assessed?
  - What are the essential elements in the assessment and management of acute stroke patients *not* eligible for thrombolytic therapy?
- What is the role of a written protocol for assessment and initial care of a stroke patient?

Acute stroke, including ischemic or hemorrhagic subtypes, is a medical emergency. Rapid identification and transportation of the acute stroke patient to the nearest primary stroke center (PSC) or comprehensive stroke center (CSC) has been shown to increase the chances of an acute stroke patient receiving appropriate therapy. Determining whether an acute stroke case is ischemic or hemorrhagic needs to be done shortly after the patient's arrival in the emergency department (ED) to decide the appropriate medical management.

The nonemergent approach to treating acute ischemic stroke, which was commonly used in the past, should be replaced by a rapid and systematic approach. Intravenous tissue plasminogen activator (tPA) has been approved by the Food and Drug Administration (FDA) for thrombolysis in acute ischemic stroke within 3 hours of the onset of symptoms. However, the limitation of a 3-hour window for administration of intravenous (IV)-tPA along with the reluctance of ED physicians to administer the medication without neurology consultation has resulted in only 3% to 5% of ischemic stroke patients receiving this medication nationally. Many advancements in endovascular reperfusion techniques such as clot retrieval devices, intra-arterial thrombolysis, angioplasty, and stenting have provided more treatment options for acute stroke patients. Therefore, a multidisciplinary approach and the establishment of stroke systems of care are essential elements to overcoming obstacles in the delivery of care for acute stroke patients. In April 2003 (with an update in 2005), the American Stroke Association (ASA) published a scientific statement guideline for the early management of patients with ischemic stroke. The purpose of the statement is to provide updated recommendations that can be used by neurologists or other physicians who provide acute stroke care.

Currently, there is no FDA-approved pharmacological treatment for hemorrhagic stroke. Hemorrhagic stroke patients are managed medically or surgically. The need for surgical intervention needs to be discussed among the patient or his/her legal guardian, the stroke neurologist, and the neurosurgeon.

CLINICAL APPLICATIONS

Early Identification and Urgent Assessments of a Stroke Patient

Nationwide efforts have been made to develop systems of care to improve the efficacy and effectiveness of stroke treatment. The Stroke Chain of Survival described by ASA includes

- rapid recognition and reaction to stroke warning signs (and use of 9-1-1 for notification),
- rapid emergency management of stroke (EMS) dispatch,
- rapid EMS system transport and prearrival notification to the nearest PSC or CSC,
- rapid diagnosis and treatment in the hospital.

One of the main goals of the stroke awareness program is to educate the community on the signs and symptoms of stroke and on seeking treatment immediately. Studies have shown that educating the community and EMS personnel on the need to seek medical attention immediately will increase the number of acute stroke patients receiving thrombolytic therapy. A 9-1-1 system should be used to activate EMS. The advantages of using EMS for transporting acute stroke patients include prearrival assessment and notification, which allow the stroke team to prepare for the upcoming acute stroke case. The initial assessments that should be done by trained EMS personnel are shown in Tables 19.1 and 19.2 and Figure 19.1.

Several studies show improvements in stroke patient identification by EMS after training (with sensitivity range from 86% to 97%). Therefore, routine and updated training of EMS personnel should play an important part in the care of stroke patients.

Urgent Assessment of the Acute Stroke Patient in the Emergency Department Setting

Failure to identify stroke patients immediately on their arrival to the ED may result in expiration of the time window for IV-tPA administration. In the overcrowded ED setting, the patient may not be evaluated by an ED physician until hours after his/her arrival. One multicenter study in the United Kingdom showed that 86% of ED patients' vital signs will be measured in 15 minutes, but only 22% will be evaluated by an ED physician in 15 minutes and 38% in 30 minutes. In a stroke center, one member of the stroke team should be at patients' bedside within 15 minutes of arrival. Coordinated care in the ED is a critical step in the management of acute stroke patients.

Utilization of a rapid assessment room, usually designated for trauma victims, shortens the time of initial stabilization and assessment. The acute stroke team should be activated before the patients' arrival if possible or on their arrival at triage without waiting for full assessment and stabilization of the patient by ED physicians. A system should be in place, sometimes referred to as a stroke code, to rapidly notify the acute stroke team. A parallel stroke pager system can be used to notify several stroke team members at one time. Table 19.3 outlines the activities that should take place in the rapid response room.

The algorithm for urgent assessment and timeline of acute stroke patients is summarized in Figure 19.2.

Computed tomography (CT) scan of the brain without contrast should be completed within 25 minutes of patient arrival in the ED and be read within 45 minutes of arrival in the ED. CT scan of the brain without contrast will identify most cases of hemorrhage, and it helps discriminate nonvascular causes of strokelike symptoms such as a brain tumor (Grade B). In most cases of acute ischemic stroke, a CT scan of the brain will not show any abnormalities. Signs of early ischemia on a CT scan are as follows:

- Hyperdense middle cerebral artery (MCA) sign, which is indicative of a thrombus or a clot in the first portion of the MCS. Although this sign is highly specific, false positives of hyperdense MCA signs have been reported in patients with a high hematocrit or severe calcification. It also has a low sensitivity (27% to 34% in large case series) and should not be used for prognostic value or as a prediction of responsiveness to IV-tPA.
- Loss of the gray–white differentiation in the cortical ribbon at the lateral margin of the insula (loss of the insular ribbon signs) or the lentiform nucleus, and sulcal effacement of cerebral cortex from cytotoxic edema (class C).
- The sylvian dot signs, which may indicate distal occlusion of the MCA. It has a specificity of 38% to 46%.

The Alberta Stroke Program Early CT Score (ASPECTS) was used to identify patients who are unlikely to recover fully despite thrombolytic therapy. However, this scoring system has not been assessed in clinical practice and has limited use for evaluating the ischemic area in the MCS distributions.

Magnetic resonance imaging (MRI) of the brain is superior to CT scan of the brain for detection of hemorrhagic and ischemic stroke. However, the use of MRI should not delay treatment of patients who are eligible for IV-tPA (Grade B).

On the basis of the interpretation of a noncontrast CT scan of the brain, further assessment and management of the acute stroke patient can be differentiated as shown in Fig. 19.3.

TABLE 19.1 EMS Initial Assessment of the Acute Stroke Patient

1. Perform ABCs per basic life support or advanced cardiac life support protocol
2. Recognize stroke signs and symptoms
3. Perform a rapid stroke assessment [The Cincinnati Prehospital Stroke Scale (Table 19.2) or LAPSS (Fig. 19.1)]
4. Determine time of onset or last known to be normal time
5. Transport the patient rapidly to the nearest stroke center. If possible, bring a witness or family member to confirm time of onset and provide more information on past medical history, surgical history, and medications list
6. Provide prearrival notification to the receiving ED of possible acute stroke patient
7. Assess and monitor neurological status during transport
8. Check blood glucose if possible

ABC, airway/breathing/circulation; LAPSS, Los Angeles Prehospital Stroke Screen; ED, emergency department.

Management of the Acute Ischemic Stroke Patient

The Acute Stroke Patient Who Qualifies for IV-tPA

The assessment and management of acute stroke patient who qualifies for IV-tPA involves the following steps:

1. Confirmation of time of onset: It is critical to determine the time of onset or time last known at baseline. Unfortunately, time of onset is not always easy to obtain because of decreased level of consciousness, confusion, difficulty with speech (severe slurring or aphasia), and no family or witnesses available.

   Common mistakes in identifying the time of onset are as follows:
   - The time when the patient wakes up with symptoms is recorded instead of the time when the patient was last known to be at baseline.
   - For patients who wake up with symptoms, it is common to document the time of onset as the time when they went to sleep the previous night. It is critical to not assume this time of onset to be accurate and to question the patient, family, or witnesses as to whether the patient was seen normal at any other time, for example, when getting up to go to the bathroom, or getting up for a drink of water. It may change the time of onset significantly.
   - When the patient is unable to give history, phone calls should immediately be made to any potential witness who will be able to help determine the time of onset.
   - It is not necessary to obtain consent before administering IV-tPA. However, the physician should always inform the patient and/or family of the potential risks and benefits of this medication.

TABLE 19.2 The Cincinnati Prehospital Stroke Scale

	Test	Normal	Abnormal
Facial Droop			
Left: normal *Right:* stroke patient with facial droop (right side of face)	Have patient show teeth or smile	Both sides of face move equally	One side of face does not move as well as the other side
Arm Drift			
	Patient closes eyes and holds both arms straight out for 10 seconds	Both arms move to the same extent or both arms do not move at all (other findings, such as pronator drift, may be helpful)	One arm does not move or one arm drifts down compared with the other
Abnormal Speech			
	Have the patient say "you can't teach an old dog new tricks"	Patient uses correct words with no slurring	Patient slurs words, uses the wrong words, or is unable to speak

From Kothari R, Hall K, Brott T, et al. Early stroke recognition: developing an out-of-hospital NIH Stroke Scale. *Acad Emerg Med* 1997;4(10):986–990 and American Heart Association Guidelines for Cardiopulmonary Resuscitation and Emergency Cardiovascular Care. *Circulation* 2005;112(24)(suppl):IV1–IV203.

2. Evaluation of inclusion and exclusion criteria: Rapid evaluation of the inclusion and exclusion criteria is important to ensure that patients meet all inclusion criteria and have no past or present conditions that would exclude them from receiving IV-tPA (see Table 19.4).
   Several disorders have symptoms that can mimic those of an acute ischemic stroke and are important to consider when evaluating a patient with sudden onset of focal neurological deficits. Some of the conditions that can mimic symptoms of ischemic stroke are metabolic conditions such as hyperglycemia or hypoglycemia, hypothyroidism, complex partial seizure with Todd paralysis, and complex migraine.
3. See Table 19.5 for management of blood pressure in the ischemic stroke patient who is eligible for thrombolytic therapy.
4. In addition to the stroke neurologist or his/her designee, the role of the nurse in the urgent care of an acute stroke patient is critical. The nurse will need to make sure that the patient has two large-bore IVs and Foley catheter before administration of IV-tPA. The nurse is also often responsible for calculating the dose based on the patient's weight. They may also be responsible for mixing the drug. The nurse will also need to record frequent vital signs and neurological assessment during and after administering thrombolytic therapy. Patients will require monitoring in the intensive care unit for at least the first 24 hours. No needlesticks or invasive procedures are allowed for 24 hours after administration of the drug. Separate preprinted orders for patients who receive thrombolytic therapy should be available in the ED.

The Acute Stroke Patient Who Does Not Qualify for IV-tPA but May Benefit from Endovascular Procedures

Intra-arterial thrombolysis or other endovascular procedures should be done within 6 hours of the onset of stroke symptoms. A longer period has been recommended for the posterior circulation because of its devastating morbidity and mortality and its reversibility. Although it did not meet the FDA approval, urokinase, alteplase (tPA), or prourokinase is currently offered by many stroke centers for intra-arterial thrombolysis in acute stroke patients who do not meet the criteria for IV-tPA or in whom the time from onset of symptoms is >3 hours. Studies to evaluate the feasibility of combined intravenous and local intra-arterial recombinant tPA (rt-PA) have shown promising results. The Merci clot retrieval device was approved by the FDA in 2004. Mechanical disruption of the clot with angioplasty or stent was also done to achieve vascular reperfusion.

The Acute Stroke Patient Who Does Not Qualify for Acute Thrombolysis or Endovascular Procedure

Ineligibility for acute thrombolysis could be due to conditions such as:

Criteria	Yes	Unknown	No
1. Age >45 years	☐	☐	☐
2. History of seizures or epilepsy absent	☐	☐	☐
3. Symptom duration <24 hours	☐	☐	☐
4. At baseline, patient is not wheelchair bound or bedridden	☐	☐	☐
5. Blood glucose between 60 and 400	☐	☐	☐
6. Obvious asymmetry (right vs left) in any of the following 3 exam categories (must be unilateral):	☐	☐	☐
	Equal	**R Weak**	**L Weak**
Facial smile/grimace	☐	☐ Droop	☐ Droop
Grip	☐	☐ Weak grip ☐ No grip	☐ Weak grip ☐ No grip
Arm strength	☐	☐ Drifts down ☐ Falls rapidly	☐ Drifts down ☐ Falls rapidly

One-sided motor weakness (right arm)

If items 1 through 6 are all checked "Yes" (or "Unknown"), provide prearrival notification to hospital of potential stroke patient.

If any item is checked "No," return to appropriate treatment protocol.

Interpretation: 93% of patients with stroke will have a positive LAPSS score (sensitivity=93%), and 97% of those with a positive LAPSS score will have a stroke (specificity=97%).

Note that the patient may still be experiencing a stroke if LAPSS criteria are not met.

FIGURE 19.1. Los Angeles Prehospital Stroke Screen (LAPSS): for the evaluation of an acute, noncomatose, nontraumatic neurologic complaint. Note that the patient may still be experiencing a stroke if LAPSS criteria are not met. (Kidwell CS, Saver JL, Schubert GB, et al. Design and retrospective analysis of the Los Angeles Prehospital Stroke Screen (LAPSS). *Prehosp Emerg Care* 1998;2(4):267–273; Kidwell CS, Starkman S, Eckstein M, et al. Identifying stroke in the field. Prospective validation of the Los Angeles prehospital stroke screen (LAPSS). *Stroke* 2000;31(1):71–76.)

- ischemic stroke symptoms rapidly improving and resolving,
- prior or present conditions in which IV or intra-arterial thrombolysis may do more harm than benefit (see Table 19.2),
- hemorrhagic conversions of a large ischemic stroke,
- patient refusing thrombolytic therapy,
- no vascular stenosis was found during evaluation for endovascular procedures.

Additional assessment and management of an acute stroke patient who is not a candidate for thrombolytic therapy include the following techniques:

- Table 19.6 lists methods of management of blood pressure in ischemic stroke patients who are not eligible for thrombolytic therapy.
- After acute ischemic stroke, blood flow loses its normal autoregulation. Underlying large vessels stenosis could result in cerebral blood flow becoming pressure dependent.

TABLE 19.3 Assessment of Acute Stroke Patient in the Rapid Response Room

1. Assess ABCs and evaluate baseline vital signs.
2. Provide oxygen. Oxygen supplementation via nasal canula or non-rebreather mask should be used on patients with low oxygen saturation (<92%) (grade I) or nonhypoxemia (grade IIB) (2005 AHA Guidelines).
3. Establish IV access and obtain blood samples including platelet count and coagulation studies. It is important to notify the laboratory staff about the acute stroke case so that the results can be obtained and provided directly to the physician. Label the thrombolysis case with the pager or cell phone number of the physician attached to the case or direct communications with the laboratory personnel will also emphasize the importance of rapid processing.
4. Check blood glucose levels and promptly treat hypoglycemia. Hyper- or hypoglycemia affects the morbidity and mortality of stroke patients. Therefore, it should be treated promptly, although it should not delay the administration of IV-tPA.
5. Perform a neurological screening assessment. Use the NIHSS Stroke Scale or similar tool.
6. Obtain a stat CT scan of the brain without contrast.
7. Obtain a 12-lead ECG and portable chest x-ray. Do not delay CT scan to obtain these procedures and do not delay CT scan to treat hemodynamically stable patient with arrhythmia (2005 AHA guidelines).

ABCs, airway/breathing/circulation; IV, intravenous; NIHSS, National Institute of Health Stroke Scale; ECG, electrocardiogram; CT, computed tomography.

- Reducing blood pressure in either situation may precipitate a larger ischemic area. If patients seem pressure dependent with recurrent symptoms after blood pressure is reduced, IV vasopressors such as norepinephrine, phenylephrine, dopamine, or dobutamine can be used with close monitoring.
- Blood glucose
- As mentioned earlier, hypoglycemia or hyperglycemia can mimic stroke symptoms. An accucheck should be performed immediately by EMS or in the ED.
- A patient with atrial fibrillation should receive anticoagulants unless he or she is a candidate for thrombolytic therapy or has a contraindication to anticoagulation.
- Temperature reduction in case of fever in a stroke patient has been shown to improve the outcome. Acetaminophen (up to 4 g per day in divided doses) or cooling blankets should be used as necessary.
- Acute ischemic stroke patients who showed signs or symptoms of cerebral herniation or hemorrhagic transformation also need to have immediate consideration for surgical intervention.

Obtaining Cerebral Vascularization Imaging

It is essential that vascular studies are done on acute stroke patients as soon as possible. For acute stroke patients who receive IV-tPA, imaging can be done during or shortly after thrombolytic therapy is completed. For a stroke patient who may be candidate for endovascular procedures, the availability of immediate noninvasive imaging may help identify appropriate candidates for intra-arterial

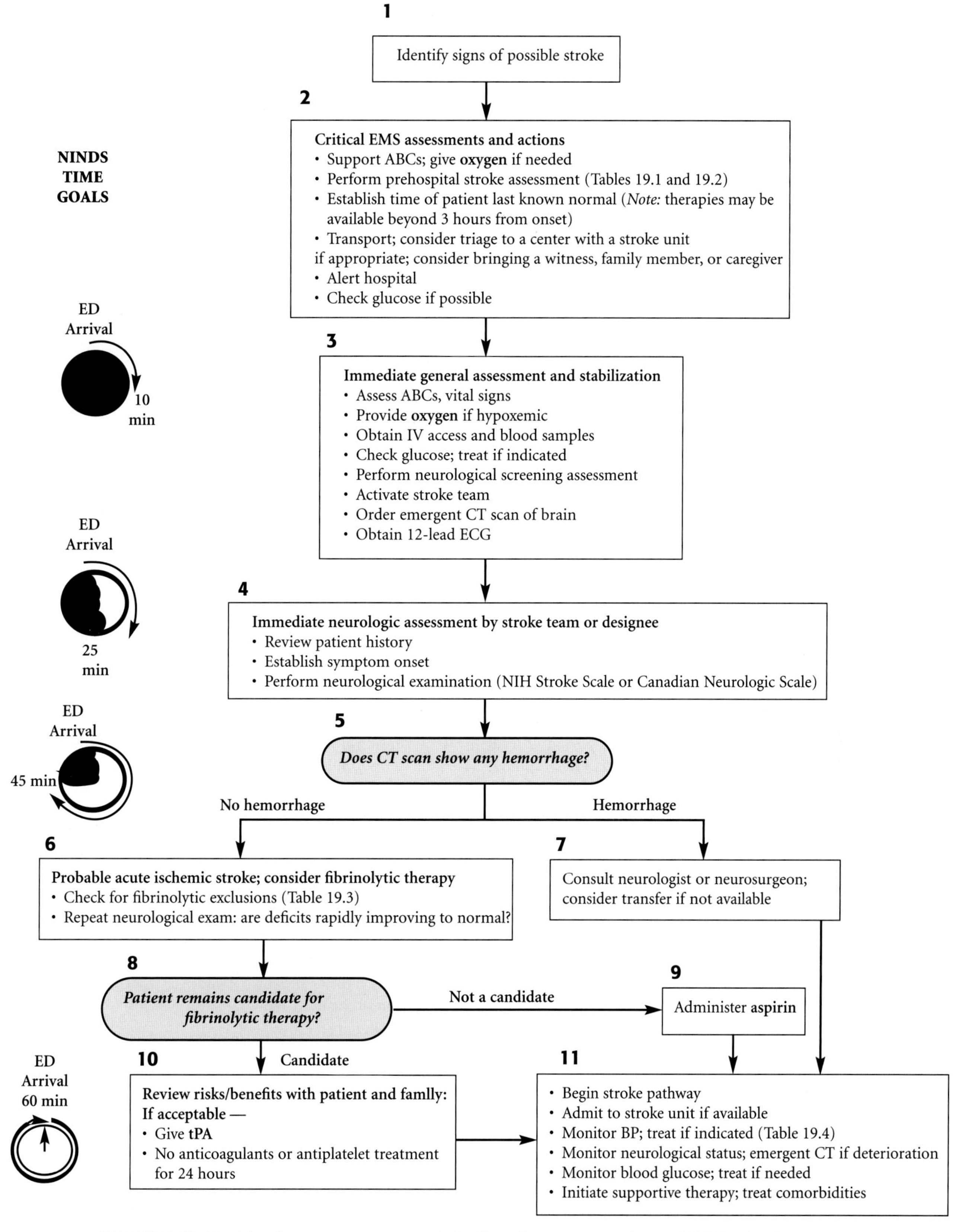

FIGURE 19.2. Algorithm for urgent assessment and timeline of acute stroke patients. NINDS, National Institute of Neurological Disorders and Stroke IV, intravenous access; CT, computed tomography; ECG, electrocardiogram; NIH, National Institutes of Health; tPA, tissue plasminogen activator; BP, blood pressure.

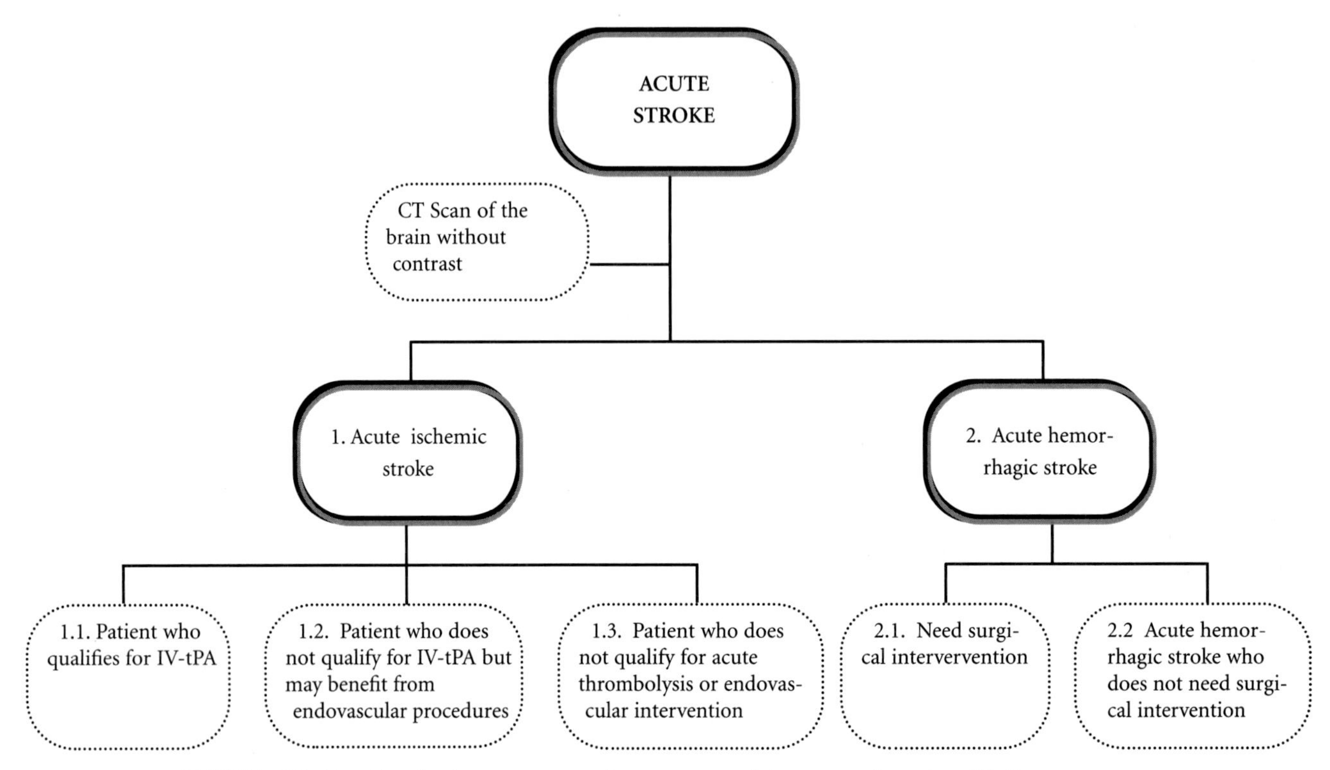

FIGURE 19.3. Algorithm for the assessment and management of the aute stroke patient. IV-tPA, intravenous tissue plasminogen activator.

thrombolysis and eliminate the need to activate the endovascular intervention team if no stenosis is found.

Not every facility has MRI or magnetic resonance angiography (MRA) in their facility. However, MRI is still the most preferred non-invasive imaging for the assessment of stroke patients. Use of MRI is limited by the table weight limit, severe claustrophobia, and field incompatibility with patient devices (e.g., metal-tip catheters, pace-makers, or other implanted metal that is not compatible with MRI)

CT angiography (CTA) requires less acquisition time than MRI and can be used if patients are unable to get an MRI/MRA for any of the aforementioned reasons. CTA assesses for stenotic or occluded vessels. CT perfusion can be utilized to assess for hypop-erfusion of brain tissue.

Management of Acute Hemorrhagic Stroke

Hemorrhagic stroke is associated with 30% to 50% of mortality(see Table 19.7). Only 20% of patients with intracranial hemorrhage (ICH) was able to regain functional independence at 6-month fol-low-up.

Identification of Type, Location, and Severity of Intracranial Hemorrhage on the CT Scan of the Head

CT scan of the head will classify the type and severity of hemor-rhage, which include intraparenchymal hemorrhage, intraventricu-lar hemorrhage, and subarachnoid hemorrhage. We also need to identify the presence of subdural or epidural hematoma, which may be present because of head trauma. The type and location of hemorrhage on CT scan of the brain may helps in determining the etiology of ICH.

Determination of the Etiology of Intracranial Hemorrhage

Common causes of hemorrhagic stroke are as follows:

1. Hypertension: Hypertension is the most common etiology of hemorrhagic stroke. It is attributed to up to 75% of the etiology of ICH. Elevated blood pressure is found in the 46% to 68% of patients with ICH. History of hypertension is reported up to 93% of patients with ICH. Possible mech-anisms of hypertension-causing ICH are lipohyalinosis and lipofibrinoid necrosis of the small or medium arterioles in the brain due to chronic hypertension, as well as the pres-ence of arteriolar microaneurysms (Charcot-Bouchard aneurysm), which may result in spontaneous rupture. A recent study in initially healthy men with hemorrhagic stroke showed that systolic blood pressure was a consistent and significant predictor of hemorrhagic stroke. Adequate control of blood pressure decreases the risk of ICH and the risk of recurrence. Hypertension is also associated with a higher body mass index (BMI), cigarette smoking, and dia-betes. Typical sites of ICH due to hypertension on the CT scan of the head are:
   - Putamen (50%)
   - Thalamus (15%)
   - Lobar (15%)
   - Cerebellum (10%)
   - Pons (10%)
2. Cerebral amyloid angiopathy: Cerebral amyloid angiopathy is caused by disposition and infiltration of amyloid β-pep-tide protein into the media and adventitia of the cortical arterioles of the brain. The prevalence of cerebral amyloid angiopathy increases with age. Recurrent hemorrhage is reported in 5% to 15% of cases.
3. Aneurysm
4. Vascular malformations such as arteriovenous malformation

TABLE 19.4 Inclusions and Exclusions Criteria for IV-tPA

Inclusion Criteria

- ☐ Age 18 or older
- ☐ Stroke symptom onset <3 h
- ☐ Clinical diagnosis of ischemic stroke causing a measurable neurological deficit

Exclusion Criteria

- ☐ Evidence of ICH on CT
- ☐ Symptoms minor or isolated
- ☐ Symptoms clearing spontaneously
- ☐ Symptoms causing severe deficits
- ☐ Symptoms of SAH
- ☐ Onset to treatment >3 h or time of onset unknown
- ☐ Previous head trauma or stroke in last 3 mo
- ☐ MI within the last 3 mo
- ☐ GI or urinary tract hemorrhage previous 21 d
- ☐ Major surgery in last 14 d
- ☐ Arterial puncture at a noncompressible site in the previous 7 d
- ☐ History of intracranial hemorrhage
- ☐ Blood pressure >185/110 mm Hg requiring aggressive treatment
- ☐ Evidence of active bleeding or acute trauma
- ☐ INR >1.7
- ☐ Platelet count <100,000 mm^3
- ☐ Blood glucose <50 mg/dL
- ☐ Heparin within previous 24 h, PTT must be within normal range
- ☐ Seizure at onset with postictal neurologic impairments
- ☐ > one third hypodensity on CT

ICH, intracranial hemorrhage; CT, computed tomography; SAH, subarachnoid hemorrhage; MI, myocardial infarction; GI, gastrointestinal; INR, international normalized rate; PTT, partial thromboplastin time.

5. Brain tumor
6. Anticoagulant-associated intracerebral hemorrhage.
   When taking a history from patients with hemorrhagic stroke, it is important to obtain the history of other medical problems and a list of current medications. Warfarin is the predominant cause of anticoagulant-associated ICH, and the most common clinical indication for warfarin use is atrial fibrillation. Other common indications for use of warfarin are deep venous thrombosis or pulmonary embolism.
7. Ischemic stroke with hemorrhagic conversion or hemorrhagic venous thrombosis.

Management of the Blood Pressure in the Acute Hemorrhagic Stroke

It is important to control blood pressure immediately after the diagnosis of ICH is established to prevent increase of hematoma expansion, which will correlate with a poor outcome. The last American Heart Association (AHA) guidelines for treatment of blood pressure in hemorrhagic stroke were published in 1999 and are thought to be outdated. Most common practice at present is to keep systolic blood pressure <160 mm Hg.

TABLE 19.5 Management of Blood Pressure in the Ischemic Stroke Patient Who Is Eligible for Thrombolytic Therapy

BP Level (mm Hg)	Treatment
Pretreatment	
SBP >**185** or DBP >**110**	**Labetalol** (may repeat once) or **nitropaste** If BP is not reduced and maintained, do **not** administer rt-PA
During and After rt-PA	
SBP **180–230** or DBP **105–120**	**Labetalol**
SBP >**230** or DBP **121–140**	**Nicardipine** or **labetalol** If BP not controlled consider nitroprusside
DBP >**140**	**Nitroprusside**

BP, blood pressure; SBP, systolic blood pressure; DBP, diastolic blood pressure; rt-PA, recombinant tissue plasminogen activator.
From Adams HP, Jr, Adams RJ, Brott, T, et al. Guidelines for the early management of patients with ischemic stroke: a scientific statement from the Stroke Council of the American Stroke Association. *Stroke* 2003;34(4):1056–1083, with permission.

The perihematoma zone, previously thought to be an ischemic area, experiences metabolic and perfusion changes in the acute and subacute hemorrhagic periods. The stages of changes in metabolism and perfusion in the perihematoma area are as follows:

- *Within the first 48 hours (hibernation phase)*: An acute period of decreased metabolism with coupled reduction in blood flow;
- *Between 48 hours to 14 days (reperfusion phase)*: A heterogeneous pattern due to mixed features of persistent hypoperfusion, normoperfusion, and hyperperfusion;
- *After 14 days (normalization phase)*: with normal perfusion except in the area of nonviable tissue

Even with hypoperfusion, the low metabolism in the acute hibernation phase probably prevents development of ischemia and may allow safe reduction of systolic blood pressure in the acute setting.

TABLE 19.6 Management of Blood Pressure in Ischemic Stroke Patient Who Is Not Eligible for Thrombolytic Therapy

BP Level (mm Hg)	**Treatment**
SBP <**220** or DBP <**120**	No treatment unless end organ involvement
SBP >**220** or DBP >**121–140**	**Nicardipine** or **labetalol** to 10%–15% in BP
DBP >**140**	**Nitroprusside** to 10%–15% in BP

BP, blood pressure; SBP, systolic blood pressure; DBP, diastolic blood pressure.

TABLE 19.7 Initial Assessment of Acute Hemorrhagic Stroke Patient in the Rapid Response Room

1. Assess ABCs and evaluate baseline vital signs, establish unresponsiveness.
2. Provide oxygen. Oxygen supplementation via nasal canula or non-rebreather mask should be used on patients with low oxygen saturation (<92%) (grade I) or nonhypoxemia (grade IIB) (2005 AHA guidelines).
3. Establish IV access and obtain blood samples including platelet count and coagulation studies, and blood type and screen. Start intravenous fluid (preferably normal saline).
4. Perform a neurologic screening assessment. Use the NIHSS or similar tool.
5. Obtain a stat CT scan of the brain without contrast.
6. Control systolic blood pressure.
7. Obtain a 12-lead ECG and portable chest x-ray. Do not delay CT scan to obtain these procedure and do not delay CT scan to treat hemodynamically stable patient with arrhythmia (2005 AHA guidelines).
8. Obtain neurosurgical and/or neurology consult to determine whether patient would benefit from surgical procedure. Include patient and/or his or her legal guardian on the decision-making process. Surgical procedure that need to be considered include craniotomy for removal of clot, prevention of herniation, or ventriculostomy.
9. Start seizure prophylaxis and mannitol (if there is mass effect on the CT scan of the brain). Reverse anticoagulation if needed.
10. Identify the etiology of the acute hemorrhage.
11. Admit to neurointensive care unit. Obtain stat repeat CT head with worsening of neurological status.

ABCs, airway/breathing/circulation; NIHSS, National Institute of Health Stroke Scale; electrocardiogram; IV, intravenous; CT, computed tomography.

Choice of Antihypertensive Agents in the Acute Hemorrhagic Stroke Setting Several studies showed safety and efficacy of the use of intravenous nicardipine in the acute setting of ICH.

Prognosis of the ICH

Poor predictors of the outcome include the following:

1. The Glasgow Coma Scale (GCS)
2. Volume of the hematoma: ICH volume can be estimated by selecting the largest area of hematoma on the CT scan of the brain and then multiplying the diameter of the hematoma in three dimensions and dividing by two. Patients with hematoma volume 0 to 29 had a mortality of 19%, 30 to 60 cm^3 had mortality of 46% to 74%, and >60 cm^3 had up to 91% mortality.
3. Intraventricular extension
4. Age (worse in patients older than 80 years)
5. Early hematoma growth
6. International normalized ratio (INR) level: INR level of 2.5 to 4.5 will increase risk of ICH by 10-fold.

Measurement and Management of Intracranial Pressure

Measurement of ICP is appropriate on ICH patients with rapid declining in mental status, stuporous or comatose. Other common management procedures in the acute ICH setting is elevation of the head of bed to 30 degrees and triple H therapy, which include hypervolemia (preferably normal saline), hyperventilation to pCO_2 of 28 to 32 mm Hg and hyperosmolarity by rapid IV mannitol 20% infusion.

Hemostatic Therapy

The eptacog alfa, which is a recombinant activated factor VII (rFVIIa) (Novoseven, NovoNordisk A/S), is currently used for patients with hemophilias. Study of use of this drug for hemostatic therapy in ICH patients with a normal coagulation system initially showed promising results, but the results of the next phase of the study were still not sufficient for FDA approval. A recent study showed the efficacy of this drug for the rapid reversal of INR in ICH patients who are taking coumadin.

Acute Hemorrhagic Stroke Patients Who Require Neurosurgical Intervention

In some cases, an acute stroke patient may need a hemicraniectomy or surgical decompression as a life-saving procedure. Acute hemorrhagic stroke patients need to have an immediate evaluation by the neurologist and neurosurgeon to determine the need for surgical intervention. This procedure is usually done after medical management procedures such as hyperosmolar therapy with IV mannitol or hyperventilation have failed. A meta-analysis of 12 prospective randomized controlled trials of neurosurgical intervention in spontaneous intracerebral hemorrhage shows a strong trend toward reduced mortality (0.85; 95% CI, 0.71 to 1.02). However, in the setting of dominant hemisphere infarction, a significant morbidity effect on language and dominant extremities should be considered. The patients' wishes should be considered and discussed thoroughly with their next of kin or legal guardian.

Acute Hemorrhagic Stroke Patients Who Do Not Require Neurosurgical Intervention

See Figure 19.4 for an algorithm for stabilization and monitoring of acute hemorrhagic stroke patients who do not need surgical intervention on the initial evaluation.

Anticonvulsants

Seizure prophylaxis is recommended for up to 1 month after ICH and should be discontinued in the absence of seizures. The 30-day risk of clinically evident seizures after ICH is about 8%. Convulsive status epilepticus may be seen in 1% to 2% of patients, and the risk or epilepsy is 5% to 20%.

Written Protocol and Telemedicine for Assessment and Initial Care of Stroke Patients

The narrow time window, as well as the relationship between time to treatment and outcome, has led to the development of a number of strategies (e.g., clinical pathways, standing orders) to be able to administer treatment drug as soon as possible.

In the ED without a stroke center facility, ED physicians can evaluate patients for eligibility to receive IV-tPA. Consultation

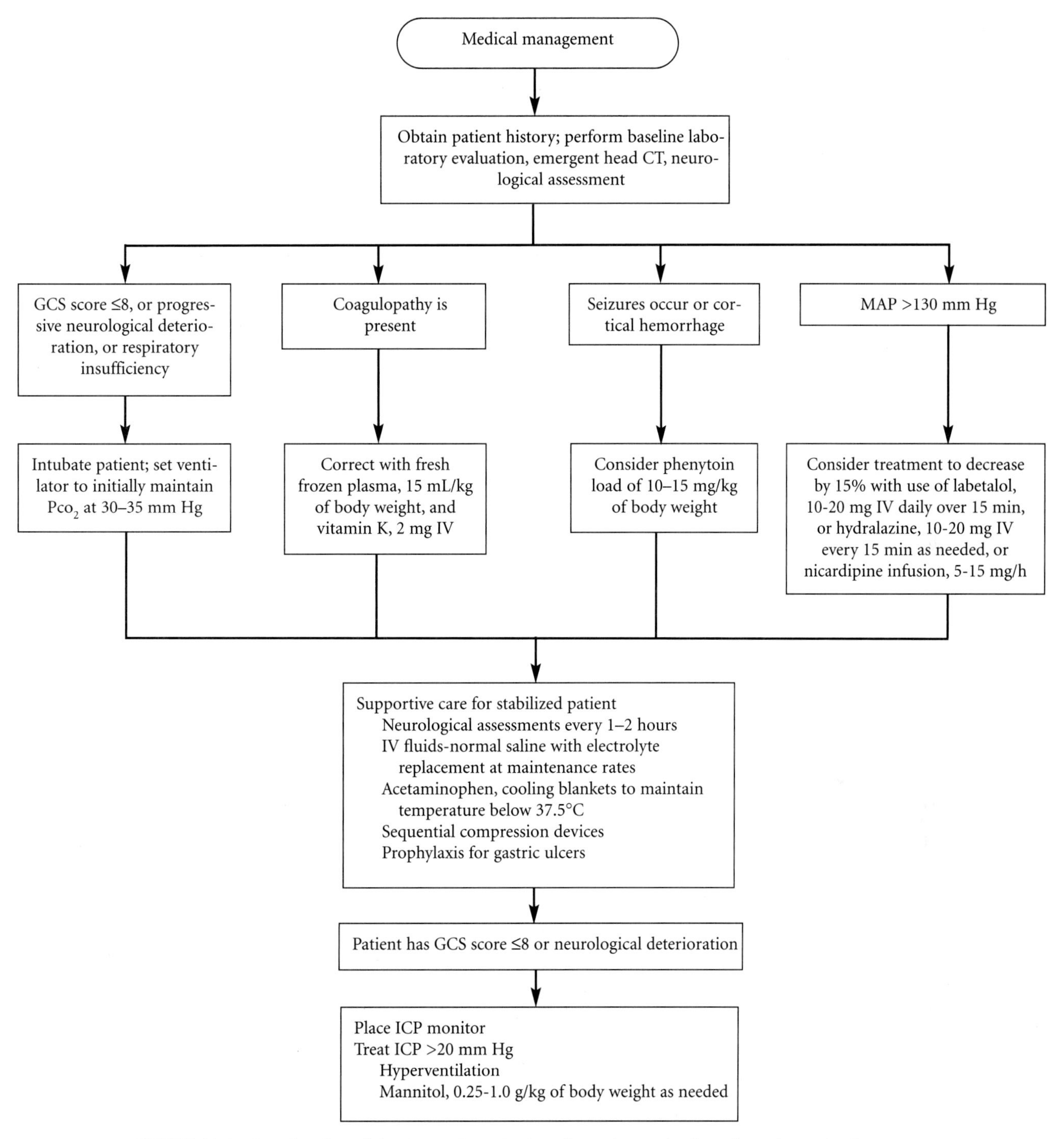

FIGURE 19.4. Algorithm for stabilization and monitoring of acute hemorrhagic stroke patients who do not need surgical intervention on the initial evaluation. CT, computed tomography; GCS, Glasgow Coma Scale; MAP, mean arterial pressure; IV, intravenous.

through telemedicine or teleradiology may be obtained for complex cases. Although protocol deviations for IV-tPA have been shown to be higher when given by ED physicians compared to when given by neurologists (30% versus 5%), these protocol deviations were reduced with staff education. Several studies have already shown that IV-tPA can be safely and effectively administered by ED physicians.

Every ED, especially EDs with the capability of giving IV thrombolysis, should have a written clinical pathway on the management of acute stroke patients. This written pathway should include the roles of health care personnel, criteria and pathway for acute thrombolytic therapy, and if applicable the process of transferring the patient to comprehensive stroke center (see Fig. 19.5).

PHYSICIAN'S ORDERS
UNIVERSITY OF LOUISVILLE STROKE TEAM

HEIGHT CM	WEIGHT KG
ALLERGIES	☐ NKA

DATE & TIME	ORDERS FOR TEST REQUIRE AN ACCOMPANYING INDICATION, SIGN OR SYMPTOM SMALL OR LARGE VESSEL ISCHEMIC STROKE ADMISSION	√ & INITIAL THAT ORDER WAS "WRITTEN, READ BACK AND VERIFIED"
	DATE: PHYSICIANS ORDERS:	☐
	Instructions: Place check in box if you desire to order and signature at bottom. Fill in blanks to specify doses.	
	ADMISSION DIAGNOSIS:	☐
	Admit to: ☐ Intermediate bed on PCU Date:_____Time of Symptom onset:_____	
	☐ Neuro ICU to Dr.__________, Stroke Service ■ Notify Primary Care Physician of patient admission	☐
	TREATMENTS:	
	☐ O_2 by nasal cannula to maintain saturations >95% ☐ Blood glucose twice a day for 2 days. Call Stroke Team for blood sugar >150.	☐
	☐ Blood glucose before meals and at bedtime ☐ Foley to straight bag drainage	
	☐ Intake and Output per routine ☐ Tum every 2 hours	☐
	■ Continuous cardiac monitoring ■ Vital signs with neurologic checks every 30 minutes x 2 hours, then every hour x 24 hours, then routine.	
	■ TED/SCD ■ Oral (Yankeur) suction at bedside	☐
	■ Notify Stroke Team if: Temp. 101° F, Pulse <80 or >110, Respirations <12 or >30. Call Stroke Team if SBP_____<____. DPB >100. ■ No peripheral IV sticks to affected stroke side	
	DIET:	☐
	☐ Nothing by mouth ☐ Healthy heart diet	
	☐ Regular ☐ No concentrated sweets	☐
	☐ DHT placement with K.U.B. for confirmation ☐ Tube feeds__________	
	ACTIVITIES/PRECAUTIONS:	☐
	☐ Bed rest ☐ Aspiration precaution	
	☐ Fall precaution ☐ Seizure precaution	☐
	MEDICATIONS: (Specify dosages and route)	
	■ Call Stroke Team prior to starting any oral antihypertensives ■ Avoid sedatives, narcotics, and neuroleptics	☐
	■ Call Stroke Team before giving IV glucose solutions or Lactated Ringers ■ Do not use sublingual Nifedipine	
	☐ IV fluid. 0.9% NS @_____mL/hour ☐ Give labetalol 10 mg IV x 1 for SBP >220 or DBP >120 and call Stroke Team	☐
	☐ Start nicardipidine drip 5 mg/hour, titrate max 15 mg/hour to keep BP_____	
	Physician's Signature: Date	
	Physicians ID # Pager#	

FIGURE 19.5. Stroke admission orders. *(continued)*

PHYSICIAN'S ORDERS
UNIVERSITY OF LOUISVILLE STROKE TEAM

HEIGHT CM	WEIGHT KG
ALLERGIES	□ NKA

DATE & TIME	ORDERS FOR TEST REQUIRE AN ACCOMPANYING INDICATION, SIGN, OR SYMPTOM ALTEPLACE (TPA) PROTOCOL/ORDERS	☑ INITIAL THAT ORDER WAS "WRITTEN, READ BACK AND VERIFIED"
	Admit Stroke Team	□
	□ Administer IV TPA 0.9 mg/kg (maximum dose of 90 mg). Give 10% as a bolus over one minute, followed by remaining 90% as a continuous infusion over 60 minutes.	□
	Patient weight_____ Time of initial bolus_____ GTT infusion started_____	
	□ No arterial punctures, IM injections, or invasive procedures for 24 hours following infusion. □ No anticoagulants or antiplatelet agents for 24 hours following TPA infusion.	□
	□ If considering antiplatelet agents or anticoagulants in first 24 hours, verify fibrinogen >100, and PTT <80.	
	□ No F/C, NG tube, arterial catheter or central venous catheter for 24 hours. □ Admit to ICU by:______________________________	□
	□ Vital signs with neuro checks every 15 minutes for 2 hours, then every 30 minutes for 6 hours, then every 1 hour for 16 hours.	
	□ O2 by nasal cannula to maintain saturations >95% □ STAT head CT for any change in mental status or neurologic condition and notify Stroke Team	□
	MEDICATIONS:	□
	□ 0.9% NS @_____mL/hour	
	□ Acetaminophen 650 mg by mouth every 4 hours as needed for temperature >99.4°F; cooling blanket as needed for temperature >102°F to avoid shivering.	□
	□ Acetaminophen 650 mg per rectum every 4 hours as needed for temperature > 99.4°F;	
	□ If SBP is 180-230 mmHg or DBP is 105-120 mmHg for two or more readings 5-10 minutes apart: notify Stroke Team.	□
	Give IV labetalol 10 mg over 1-2 minutes. The dose may be repeated or doubled every 10 minutes up to a total dose of 150 mg.	
	Monitor blood pressure every 15 minutes during labetalol treatment and observe for development of hypotension.	□
	□ If SBP > 230 mmHg or if DBP is 121-140 mmHg for two or more readings 5-10 minutes apart: notify Stroke Team	
	Give IV labetalol 20 mg over 1-2 minutes. The dose may be repeated or doubled every 10 minutes up to a total dose of 150 mg.	
	Monitor blood pressure every 15 minutes during labetalol treatment and observe for development of hypotension.	
		□
		□
		□
	Physician's signature: Date	
	Physicians ID # Pager #	

FIGURE 19.5. *(continued)*

SELECTED REFERENCES

2005 American Heart Association Guidelines for Cardiopulmonary Resuscitation and Emergency Cardiovascular Care. *Circulation* 2005;112 (24 Suppl):IV1–IV203.

Adams H, Adams RJ, Brott, T, et al. Guidelines for the early management of patients with ischemic stroke: 2005 guidelines update a scientific statement from the Stroke Council of the American Heart Association/American Stroke Association. *Stroke* 2005;36(4):916–923.

Adams HP, Jr, Adams RJ, Brott, T, et al. Guidelines for the early management of patients with ischemic stroke: a scientific statement from the Stroke Council of the American Stroke Association. *Stroke* 2003;34(4): 1056–1083.

Akins PT, Delemos C, Wentworth D, et al. Can emergency department physicians safely and effectively initiate thrombolysis for acute ischemic stroke? *Neurology* 2000;55(12):1801–1805.

Alberts MJ, Latchaw RE, Selman WR, et al. Recommendations for comprehensive stroke centers: a consensus statement from the Brain Attack Coalition. *Stroke* 2005;36(7):1597–1616.

Alberts, M.J., Hademenos G, Latchaw RE, et al. Recommendations for the establishment of primary stroke centers. Brain Attack Coalition. *JAMA* 2000;283(23):3102–3109.

Alberts MJ. tPA in acute ischemic stroke: United States experience and issues for the future. *Neurology* 1998;51(3 Suppl 3):S53–S55.

Arakawa S, Saku Y, Ibayashi S, et al. Blood pressure control and recurrence of hypertensive brain hemorrhage. *Stroke* 1998;29(9):1806–1809.

Bowman TS, Gaziano JM, Kase CS, et al. Blood pressure measures and risk of total, ischemic, and hemorrhagic stroke in men. *Neurology* 2006;67 (5):820–823.

Broderick JP, Adams HP Jr, Barsan W, et al. Guidelines for the management of spontaneous intracerebral hemorrhage: a statement for healthcare professionals from a special writing group of the Stroke Council, American Heart Association. *Stroke* 1999;30(4):905–915.

Broderick JP, Brott TG, Duldner JE, et al. Volume of intracerebral hemorrhage. A powerful and easy-to-use predictor of 30-day mortality. *Stroke* 1993;24(7):987–993.

Brott T, Broderick J, Kothari R, et al. Early hemorrhage growth in patients with intracerebral hemorrhage. *Stroke* 1997;28(1):1–5.

Choi JH, Bateman BT, Mangla S, et al. Endovascular recanalization therapy in acute ischemic stroke. *Stroke* 2006;37(2):419–424.

Combined intravenous and intra-arterial recanalization for acute ischemic stroke: the Interventional Management of Stroke Study. *Stroke* 2004;35(4):904–911.

del Zoppo GJ, Higashida RT, Furlan AJ, et al. PROACT: a phase II randomized trial of recombinant pro-urokinase by direct arterial delivery in acute middle cerebral artery stroke. PROACT Investigators. Prolyse in Acute Cerebral Thromboembolism. *Stroke* 1998;29(1):4–11.

Dion JE. Management of ischemic stroke in the next decade: stroke centers of excellence. *J Vasc Interv Radiol* 2004;15(1 Pt 2):S133–S141.

Fisher CM. Pathological observations in hypertensive cerebral hemorrhage. *J Neuropathol Exp Neurol* 1971;30(3):536–550.

Flaherty ML, Kissela B, Woo D, et al. The increasing incidence of anticoagulant-associated intracerebral hemorrhage. *Neurology* 2007;68(2):116–121.

Freeman WD, Brott TG, Barrett KM, et al. Recombinant factor VIIa for rapid reversal of warfarin anticoagulation in acute intracranial hemorrhage. *Mayo Clin Proc* 2004;79(12):1495–1500.

Fulgham JR, Ingall TJ, Stead LG, et al. Management of acute ischemic stroke. *Mayo Clin Proc* 2004;79(11):1459–1469.

Furlan A, Higashida R, Wechsler L, et al. Intra-arterial prourokinase for acute ischemic stroke. The PROACT II study: a randomized controlled trial. Prolyse in Acute Cerebral Thromboembolism. *JAMA* 1999;282(21): 2003–2011.

Furlan AJ, Whisnant JP, Elveback LR. The decreasing incidence of primary intracerebral hemorrhage: a population study. *Ann Neurol* 1979;5(4): 367–373.

Gobin YP, Starkman S, Duckwiler GR, et al. MERCI 1: a phase 1 study of Mechanical Embolus Removal in Cerebral Ischemia. *Stroke* 2004;35(12): 2848–2854.

Harraf F, Sharma AK, Brown MM, et al. A multicentre observational study of presentation and early assessment of acute stroke. *BMJ* 2002;325 (7354):17.

Kidwell CS, Saver JL, Schubert GB, et al. Design and retrospective analysis of the Los Angeles Prehospital Stroke Screen (LAPSS). *Prehosp Emerg Care* 1998;2(4):267–273.

Kidwell CS, Starkman S, Eckstein M, et al. Identifying stroke in the field. Prospective validation of the Los Angeles prehospital stroke screen (LAPSS). *Stroke* 2000;31(1):71–76.

Kothari R, Hall K, Brott T, et al. Early stroke recognition: developing an out-of-hospital NIH Stroke Scale. *Acad Emerg Med* 1997;4(10):986–990.

Kothari RU, Brott T, Broderick JP, et al. The ABCs of measuring intracerebral hemorrhage volumes. *Stroke* 1996;27(8):1304–1305.

Lewandowski CA, Frankel M, Tomsick TA, et al. Combined intravenous and intra-arterial r-TPA versus intra-arterial therapy of acute ischemic stroke: Emergency Management of Stroke (EMS) Bridging Trial. *Stroke* 1999;30(12):2598–2605.

Manno EM, Atkinson JL, Fulgham JR, et al. Emerging medical and surgical management strategies in the evaluation and treatment of intracerebral hemorrhage. *Mayo Clin Proc* 2005;80(3):420–433.

Mayer SA, Rincon F. Treatment of intracerebral haemorrhage. *Lancet Neurol* 20054(10):662–672.

Morgenstern LB, Staub L, Chan W, et al. Improving delivery of acute stroke therapy: The TLL Temple Foundation Stroke Project. *Stroke* 2002;33(1):160–166.

Morgenstern LB, Bartholomew LK, Grotta JC, et al. Sustained benefit of a community and professional intervention to increase acute stroke therapy. *Arch Intern Med* 2003;163(18):2198–2202.

Muir KW, Buchan A, von Kummer R, et al. Imaging of acute stroke. *Lancet Neurol* 2006;5(9):755–768.

Passero S, Rocchi R, Rossi S, et al. Seizures after spontaneous supratentorial intracerebral hemorrhage. *Epilepsia* 2002;43(10):1175–1180.

Qureshi AI, Hanel RA, Kirmani JF, et al. Cerebral blood flow changes associated with intracerebral hemorrhage. *Neurosurg Clin N Am* 2002;13 (3):355–370.

Qureshi AI, Harris-Lane P, Kirmani JF, et al. Treatment of acute hypertension in patients with intracerebral hemorrhage using American Heart Association guidelines. *Crit Care Med* 2006;34(7):1975–1980.

Ronning OM, Guldvog B. Should stroke victims routinely receive supplemental oxygen? A quasi-randomized controlled trial. *Stroke* 1999;30(10): 2033–2037.

Schonewille WJ, Algra A, Serena J, et al. Outcome in patients with basilar artery occlusion treated conventionally. *J Neurol Neurosurg Psychiatr* 2005;76(9):1238–1241.

Schwamm LH, Pancioli A, Acker JE, III, et al. Recommendations for the establishment of stroke systems of care: recommendations from the American Stroke Association's Task Force on the Development of Stroke Systems. *Stroke* 2005;36(3):690–703.

Shaltoni HM, Albright KC, Gonzales NR, et al. Is intra-arterial thrombolysis safe after full-dose intravenous recombinant tissue plasminogen activator for acute ischemic stroke? *Stroke* 2007;38(1):80–84.

Smith WS, Corry MD, Fazackerley J, et al. Improved paramedic sensitivity in identifying stroke victims in the prehospital setting. *Prehosp Emerg Care* 1999;3(3):207–210.

Smith WS. Intra-arterial thrombolytic therapy for acute basilar occlusion: pro. *Stroke* 2007;38(2):701–703.

Sorensen B, Johansen P, Nielsen GL, et al. Reversal of the International Normalized Ratio with recombinant activated factor VII in central nervous system bleeding during warfarin thromboprophylaxis: clinical and biochemical aspects. *Blood Coagul Fibrinolysis* 2003;14(5):469–477.

Wallace JD, Levy LL. Blood pressure after stroke. *JAMA* 1981;246(19): 2177–2180.

Wijdicks EF, Nichols DA, Thielen KR, et al. Intra-arterial thrombolysis in acute basilar artery thromboembolism: the initial Mayo Clinic experience. *Mayo Clin Proc* 1997;72(11):1005–1013.

Woo D, Broderick JP. Spontaneous intracerebral hemorrhage: epidemiology and clinical presentation. *Neurosurg Clin N Am* 2002;13(3): 265–279, v.

CHAPTER

20 Code Stroke

JAMES D. GEYER AND CAMILO R. GOMEZ

OBJECTIVES

- What is a code stroke?
- What are the important components of a code stroke system?
- What are the goals and parameters that guide the code stroke system?

Significant delays often occur in the evaluation of the stroke patient. Most of these delays are entirely avoidable, and they exist because of system failures or needless bureaucracy. Any delay obviously slows the initiation of treatment. With the philosophy of "time is brain," these delays are unacceptable and should not be tolerated.

BACKGROUND AND RATIONALE

The advent of recombinant tissue plasminogen activator (rt-PA) for the treatment of acute cerebral infarction placed the emphasis on speed in the evaluation and management of the acute stroke patient. Rapid evaluation and initial management is very important regardless of the use of thrombolytic therapies, and so the concept of the code stroke was developed to decrease inhospital therapeutic delays.

The code stroke, sometimes referred to as the stroke code, provides a framework for the expedited evaluation and aggressive management of the acute stroke patient. The stroke team should use the code stroke protocols to initiate therapy and begin treatment of the acute stroke patient immediately on presentation.

The Fundamentals of Acute Stroke Treatment (FAST) program is designed to emulate systems available for other disorders, including acute cardiac care [i.e., Advanced Cardiac Life Support (ACLS)], acute trauma [i.e., Advanced Trauma Life Support (ATLS)], and critical care [i.e., Fundamentals of Critical Care Support (FCCS)].

Stroke continues to be a major health problem in our country, and although significant progress has been made in its treatment, treatment protocols are unevenly implemented across health care facilities and communities. The implementation of stroke center guidelines and the creation of regional acute stroke transportation systems demand some standardization of the care that stroke victims receive. Capitalizing on the success other programs such as ACLS, ATLS, and FCCS have had, it seems reasonable to take a similar approach to the educational process and dissemination of information on acute stroke care. The objectives of the FAST program are as follows:

1. To provide some degree of standardization of the basic fundamental care received by stroke victims
2. To disseminate the concept that stroke is not only treatable but its fundamental management is also within the reach of any health care facility
3. To maximize the opportunity for stroke victims to have access to optimal medical care

CLINICAL APPLICATIONS AND METHODOLOGY

The code stroke is initiated after a potential stroke has been identified. The stroke should *not* be verified to initiate the system, it needs to only be suspected. Whether initiated by the emergency medical technician, emergency department triage nurse, hospital-based nurse, or emergency department physician, the code stroke should be called immediately on identifying a potential acute stroke.

The initiation of a code stroke should create a series of standard orders and protocols. These protocols may differ slightly from institution to institution but should all use a similar model. Since the time frame for the use of rt-PA is so short (3 hours from the time of symptom onset), the need for an expedited evaluation and management protocol is manifest. Unfortunately, many patients arrive with very little time remaining in this treatment window.

Presentation/Recognition

The first impediment to expedited care is recognition of the presenting signs and symptoms as being a possible stroke. Complex and arcane neurological syndromes (e.g., ataxia in an alcoholic patient or the preolivary syndrome with ipsilateral tongue weakness) may be difficult to identify as a stroke. These cases, however, represent a tiny minority of the patients presenting with acute stroke. Unfortunately, common presentations such as hemiparesis or monocular blindness are also frequently missed.

The triage nurse and the emergency department physicians and nurses should have a good understanding of the common stroke presentations. Unilateral arm or leg weakness, unilateral arm or leg numbness, unilateral vision loss, ataxia, aphasia, and dysarthria should all be easily recognized as syndromes suggesting a possible stroke. Table 20.1 contains a listing of the common syndromes. Staff should have an in-service on their recognition and these findings should be re-emphasized on a regular basis.

Initiation

Once recognized as a potential stroke the code stroke system should be initiated. This must be a prearranged system that initiates multiple pathways of notification, evaluation, and management seamlessly and with the least amount of oversight and effort. If possible the operator should have the stroke team connected via a group-paging link. By calling the code team, all concerned parties would be simultaneously notified of the stroke. This type of system obviates the possibility of a key member of the team being accidentally missed in the notification process. Important members of the team to be notified include (but not limited to) the on-call neurologist, neurology nurse or nurse practitioner, neuroimager/neuroradiologist, imaging technologist, pharmacist, and chaplain. These individuals should be notified of the stroke, estimated time of arrival (if still in transport), and location.

Initial Evaluation

The emergency department staff should obtain the basic information about the event and the basic background medical history (see Table 20.2) immediately on arrival. The basic background stroke history includes time of symptom onset (the time the patient was last known to be at neurological baseline), symptom description, and symptom course (specifically whether the symptoms are progressing, stable, or improving).

The background medical history is also of vital importance. The list of comorbid medical disorders (including recent head injury, gastrointestinal bleeding, etc.), surgical history, and recent procedures (such as lumbar puncture, endoscopic procedures, etc.), and a full list of medications (specifically asking about the use of antiplatelet agents and anticoagulant therapy) should be obtained and placed on the chart.

Screening Medical Assessment

On arrival, the staff should immediately place the patient on cardiac monitoring and initial vital signs including heart rate, respiratory rate, temperature, and blood pressure should be obtained. The blood pressure should be rechecked intermittently. The patient's weight is an important vital sign, since it may be used in the calculation of rt-PA dose and it will be needed to monitor fluid status.

TABLE 20.1 Common General Stroke Presentations

Unilateral weakness (face, arm, leg, or a combination)
Unilateral numbness (face, arm, leg, or a combination)
Unilateral vision loss (one eye or visual fields from both eyes)
Ataxia or clumsiness
Slurred speech
Aphasia (often mistaken for confusion)

TABLE 20.2 Initial Medical History

Past Medical History

Factors that might be contraindications to rt-PA administration
- Gastrointestinal hemorrhage within the preceding 21 d
- Urinary tract hemorrhage within the preceding 21 d
- Arterial puncture in a noncompressible site within the preceding 7 d
- Serious head trauma within the last 3 mo
- Known history of intracranial hemorrhage
- Received heparin with an elevated PTT within the preceding 48 h

Past Surgical History

Major surgery within the last 14 d

Medication List

Antiplatelet therapy
Warfarin
Heparin
Low-molecular-weight heparinoids

rt-PA, recombinant tissue plasminogen activator; PTT, partial thromboplastin time.

In addition to the cardiac monitoring, a formal 12-lead electrocardiogram (ECG) should be obtained and placed with the chart.

When possible during the evaluation, a portable chest x-ray should be obtained. This may be most conveniently obtained in the emergency department examination room or when the patient is being transported for initial cerebral imaging.

Intravenous access is extremely important and should be obtained immediately after arrival. At this time, initial laboratory studies should be drawn and sent as stat studies. These initial laboratory studies include a comprehensive metabolic profile (basic chemistry studies and hepatic profile), complete blood count, coagulation panel [prothrombin time (PT), partial thromboplastin time (PTT), international normalized ratio (INR)], and pregnancy test if applicable (see Table 20.3). Additional studies such as C-reactive protein and alcohol levels may be of some benefit. In a young adult, additional studies for hypercoagulable states (see Table 20.4)

TABLE 20.3 Initial Imaging and Laboratory Evaluation

ECG 12 lead
Chest x-ray (portable)
Laboratory studies
- Complete blood count with platelets
- Chemistry profile (Na, K, Cl, CO_2, BUN, Cr, glucose)
- Hepatic panel (AST, ALT, total bilirubin, albumin)
- Coagulation panel (PT, PTT, INR)
- Cardiac enzymes (CK, CK-MB, index, troponin)
- Pregnancy test (if applicable)

ECG, electrocardiogram; BUN, blood urea nitrogen; AST, aspartate aminotransferase; ALT, alanine aminotransferase; PT, prothrombin time; PTT, partial thromboplastin time; INR, international normalized ratio; CK, creatine kinase; CK-MB, MB isoenzyme of creatine kinase.

TABLE 20.4 Hypercoagulation Studies (in the Young Adult)

Serum viscosity
Fibrinogen
Antiphospholipid antibodies
Antithrombin III
Protein C (total, free)
Protein S (total, free)
Activated protein C resistance
Factor V Leiden
Lupus anticoagulant
Homocystine
Serum IFE
Anticardiolipin antibody
RPR

IFE, immunofixation electrophoresis; RPR, rapid plasma reagin.

should be drawn, since the administration of rt-PA or heparin can alter the results of the laboratory tests.

Screening Medical and Neurological Examination

The initial medical and neurological examinations are typically quite brief but nevertheless fairly comprehensive. The general medical screening includes cardiac, respiratory, gastrointestinal, and cutaneous assessments. In the time-sensitive environment of the code stroke, these examinations cannot be comprehensive but should still serve to identify factors that might affect initial patient management. The examination should be completed in several minutes.

One of the best known methods for stroke assessment is the National Institutes of Health Stroke Scale (NIHSS). The NIHSS has certain definite advantages: (a) it has become the standard of care for acute stroke assessment, (b) it consists of a 15-item scale with high sensitivity, (c) it has been validated in numerous settings, and (d) it is widely used by practitioners. Unfortunately, it does have some disadvantages in that it is a rather complex and somewhat slow.

Another method of acute stroke assessment, the Cincinnati Scale, again has some advantages, being much simpler to administer than the NIHSS and having been validated against the NIHSS. It is a brief three-item scale that focuses on arm weakness, speech abnormalities, and facial weakness, and therefore, it is relatively easy to administer. Its disadvantage, though, is that it is structured only to identify the stroke, without gauging its severity. The Los Angeles Scale is similar to the Cincinnati Scale, and also includes three items: arm weakness, grip, and facial weakness. Just like the Cincinnati Scale, its disadvantage is that it only provides identification of the stroke, without addressing its severity.

The Stroke Observation Scale (SOS) was derived from the five critical neurological domains covered by the NIHSS:

1. Level of consciousness (LOC)
2. Visual function
3. Facial movements
4. Arm and/or leg strength
5. Language function

Each domain can be scored as either a 0 or a 2 based on whether it is normal or not, leading to a minimum score of 0 (i.e., normal) and a maximum of 10 (i.e., most severe). Its importance is twofold: (a) the more the domains are affected, the greater the chances that the patient has a stroke and (b) the more the domains are affected, the greater the severity of the stroke (i.e., worse deficit). The SOS is outlined in Table 20.5.

Rapid examination is described in the following sections. A more detailed discussion of the medical and neurological examinations is found in the appendices.

Initial Management

The patient should be kept in a supine position with a slight elevation of the head of the bed, typically at an angle of 30 degrees or less. Obviously, exceptions to this rule are not uncommon and must be anticipated for optimal patient care. For example, a patient with severe congestive heart failure may be unable to maintain a supine position with the head of the bed that low. A compromise between the demands of the heart failure and the need to optimize cerebral hemodynamics must be met. The opposite problem may arise in the severely hypotensive patient. In this case, use of the Trendelenburg position (head of bed below the foot of the bed) may be necessary.

As described above, intravenous (IV) access should be obtained on arrival to the emergency department. The patient should be started on IV fluids immediately. The fluid type and drip rate are dependent on individual patient characteristics and are discussed in depth in Chapter 34. The initial IV fluid for most patients is normal saline. Many acute stroke patients are relatively dehydrated on presentation and should be treated accordingly.

Before we discuss how to accomplish this, it is important to point out that the penumbra exists because vessels from adjacent vascular territories, called collaterals, supply some degree of blood flow to the penumbra. In this sense, at the tissue level, the ischemic penumbra behaves as any other tissue in shock [i.e., with abnormally low perfusion pressure and oxygen delivery (Do_2)]. In turn, Do_2 to any tissue is dependent on two factors: (a) blood flow and (b) arterial oxygen content. Therefore, following the shock analogy, the ischemic penumbra is likely to benefit from optimization of flow and oxygen content. These two strategies can be implemented by means of improving cardiovascular performance and promoting full arterial oxygen saturation. It is easy to realize then how managing the stroke patients in the supine position, while administering supplemental oxygen, makes considerable amount of sense. Supplemental oxygen to the point of achieving Sao_2 = 100% is likely to be beneficial and poses no significant risk for the patients. In addition, just like the management of any other patient

TABLE 20.5 Stroke Observation Scale

Domain	Score = 0	Score=2
LOC	Spontaneous	Stimulation required
Visual	No deficit	Any deficit
Facial	Symmetrical	Lateralization
Arm/leg	Normal	Asymmetry
Language	Normal	Aphasia/dysarthria

LOC, level of consciousness.

with shock, placing the patient in a supine position improves cardiovascular performance while minimizing the postural effects of relative hypovolemia. The next step in the code stroke protocol is the administration of isotonic crystalloid fluids as a form of resuscitation. The basis for this is the responsiveness of the collateral arterioles that maintain the penumbra viable to enhanced intravascular volume, as well as the direct relationship between blood flow and pressure in the ischemic tissue. In fact, it is possible to demonstrate mathematically that increasing preload has a beneficial effect on cerebral perfusion pressure. Finally, it must be pointed out that a large percentage of all stroke patients (somewhere between 25% and 30%) have prerenal azotemia on presentation, a fact that further underscores the importance of fluid resuscitation.

Blood Pressure Management

We have discussed earlier about fluid management and oxygen administration for collateral optimization. In addition, it is important to point out that blood pressure is another variable that can be manipulated to improve flow in the ischemic penumbra. Unlike healthy brain tissue, which has autoregulation, flow is directly proportional to blood pressure in the ischemic tissue. Thus, actively lowering blood pressure in patients with acute ischemic stroke is contraindicated because of the negative effects that this is likely to have on collateral flow. There are a few exceptions to this guideline, particularly for patients being treated with IV thrombolysis, whose blood pressure must be controlled on the basis of existing national guidelines. Another exception is that for patients with acute compromise of another end organ (e.g., concurrent myocardial ischemia). For those patients whose blood pressure must be carefully reduced, the ideal blood pressure–reducing agent should allow treatment of the underlying pathophysiology, with a rapid onset of action, a predictable dose response, no effect on other organs, minimal adverse effects, and the capacity to be transitioned to an oral formulation. In general, blood pressure depends on systemic vascular resistance and cardiac output. The only medication class available to directly affect cardiac output is the β-blockers, while the rest of them act on systemic vascular resistance. Excessive hypertension, systolic blood pressure (SBP) >210 mm Hg or diastolic blood pressure (DBP) >120 mm Hg should be treated in most cases. Special care should be taken to avoid overly aggressive blood pressure control, since this has an adverse effect on perfusion of the ischemic penumbra.

Transport

Patient transport within the emergency department and to various other departments is an easily overlooked and underappreciated component of the care of an acute stroke patient. A specific patient transport plan should be developed for the code stroke team. Waiting on transport is not an acceptable situation in the code stroke setting. Patients must be transported by gurney or bed to maintain the supine position. Wheelchair transport, even for relatively intact patients, should not be attempted. The transport team should include a nurse with experience with the acute stroke patient. If necessary, the neurologist may accompany the patient for imaging studies. This affords immediate analysis of the imaging data and institution of the treatment plan.

Initial Imaging

The next step in the urgent evaluation of stroke patients is imaging of the brain. Imaging is a key for the differential diagnosis of stroke, because it often allows the identification of alternative diagnoses. It is also the key to definitive therapy since, for example, it is impossible to administer intravenous thrombolysis without prior imaging of the brain. Imaging also has an effect on prognosis because we know that certain imaging findings are associated with worse outcomes (e.g., dense MCA sign). Finally, imaging is important for monitoring the effects of treatment, through sequential, repeated, and comparative imaging assessment of the brain status. Early in the management of stroke, imaging is most useful to address three specific questions:

1. Is the stroke ischemic or hemorrhagic?
2. Has the brain already undergone damage?
3. Is there an alternative diagnosis?

Imaging is therefore complementary to the clinical assessment, and such a relationship involves a concept that is of of paramount importance in the urgent care of stroke: *clinical imaging mismatch.* This highly important concept requires knowledge of what to expect for each patient when studied using imaging studies. A mismatch between the clinical and the imaging findings must trigger an immediate reconsideration of all possible explanations for the mismatch, including unrealistic expectations from the imaging study, the impact of time and type of stroke on the imaging demonstration of the lesion, and the technical limitations of the imaging modalities. In this context, patients with deficits and normal imaging must be carefully considered, since they may respond readily to treatment or they may be candidates for specific forms of therapy (e.g., intravenous thrombolysis)

Urgent imaging for acute stroke largely depends on the utilization of computed tomography (CT). The reasons for using CT as the main imaging modality are that CT is fast, widely available, sensitive for the information being sought (i.e., hemorrhagic changes, alternative diagnoses), (d) not invasive, and (e) can be easily repeated and compared. The utilization of CT over the years has allowed us to categorize the different results that can be obtained in the context of acute stroke care as follows:

1. *Normal:* This is probably the ideal finding, since a normal-appearing CT indicates an opportunity for the preservation of brain tissue through the implementation of therapy.
2. *Diagnostic for acute ischemic or hemorrhagic strok:.* This is of extreme importance since it defines the presence of hemorrhagic stroke or that of early ischemic damage, having an impact on the benefit–risk ratio assessment of definitive therapy.
3. *Diagnostic for previous strokes:* The importance of this finding is that it may provide insight into cause and mechanism of stroke (e.g., multiple vascular territories affected in patients with atrial fibrillation).
4. *Diagnostic for related processes:* Along the same lines as the previous finding, this sometimes helps identify potential causes for the stroke (e.g., calcifications indicating the presence of atherosclerotic plaques in the brain arteries).
5. *Diagnostic for an alternative or concurrent process:* Part of the concept of triage described earlier involves the recognition that the symptoms of stroke are not exclusive for this condition and that alternative diagnoses will indicate the need for other forms of therapy.

In addition, several of these findings may coexist and present themselves in combination, adding to the amount of information we obtain from urgent imaging and improving our ability to apply immediate therapy to the patients most likely to benefit from it. Finally, it is important to also take into consideration that the disease process is not static, that the appearance of stroke changes over time, and that CT is often the optimal tool to assess and follow these changes.

In a few facilities, by no means most, urgent magnetic resonance imaging (MRI) is available. When this is available, a specific protocol must be in place to obtain the images in a timely fashion without altering time- sensitive treatment options.

In summary, the impact of early imaging on the treatment of acute stroke is that it assists with early recognition, in turn leading to early treatment. This results in better treatment options and better outcomes.

PRACTICAL RECOMMENDATIONS

Every hospital, regardless of size, should have a code stroke system in place. Small hospitals would have a rapid referral system in place for acute stroke patients. Larger hospitals should create comprehensive initial evaluations systems. The initial laboratory and imaging evaluation should follow a carefully choreographed pattern for most patients. The system should, nevertheless, accommodate adjustments for critically ill patients.

SELECTED REFERENCES

2005 American Heart Association Guidelines for Cardiopulmonary Resuscitation and Emergency Cardiovascular Care. Circulation 2005;112(24)(suppl);IV1–IV203.

Adams HP, Jr, Adams RJ, Brott T, et al. Guidelines for the early management of patients with ischemic stroke: a scientific statement from the Stroke Council of the American Stroke Association. *Stroke* 2003;34(4): 1056–1083.

Adams H, Adams R, Del Zoppo G, et al. Guidelines for the early management of patients with ischemic stroke: 2005 guidelines update a scientific statement from the Stroke Council of the American Heart Association/ American Stroke Association. *Stroke* 2005;36(4):916–923.

Akins PT, Delemos, C, Wentworth D, et al. Can emergency department physicians safely and effectively initiate thrombolysis for acute ischemic stroke? *Neurology* 2000;55(12):1801–1805.

Alberts MJ. tPA in acute ischemic stroke: United States experience and issues for the future. *Neurology* 1998;51(3 Suppl 3):S53–S55.

Alberts MJ, Hademenos G, Latchaw RE, et al. Recommendations for the establishment of primary stroke centers. Brain Attack Coalition. *JAMA* 2000;283(23):3102–3109.

Alberts MJ, Latchaw RE, Selman WR, et al. Recommendations for comprehensive stroke centers: a consensus statement from the Brain Attack Coalition. *Stroke* 2005;36(7):1597–1616.

Arakawa S, Saku Y, Ibayashi S, et al. Blood pressure control and recurrence of hypertensive brain hemorrhage. *Stroke* 1998;29(9):1806–1809.

Bowman TS, Gaziano JM, Kase CS, et al. Blood pressure measures and risk of total, ischemic, and hemorrhagic stroke in men. *Neurology* 2006;67(5):820–823.

Broderick JP, Brott TG, Duldner JE, et al. Volume of intracerebral hemorrhage. A powerful and easy-to-use predictor of 30-day mortality. *Stroke* 1993;24(7):987–993.

Broderick JP, Brott TG, Tomsick T, et al. Guidelines for the management of spontaneous intracerebral hemorrhage: a statement for healthcare professionals from a special writing group of the Stroke Council, American Heart Association. *Stroke* 1999;30(4):905–915.

Brott T, Broderick J, Kothari R, et al. Early hemorrhage growth in patients with intracerebral hemorrhage. *Stroke* 1997;28(1):1–5.

Choi JH, Bateman BT, Mangla S, et al. Endovascular recanalization therapy in acute ischemic stroke. *Stroke* 2006;37(2):419–424.

del Zoppo GJ, Higashida RT, Furlan AJ, et al. PROACT: a phase II randomized trial of recombinant pro-urokinase by direct arterial delivery in acute middle cerebral artery stroke. PROACT Investigators. Prolyse in Acute Cerebral Thromboembolism. *Stroke* 1998;29(1): 4–11.

Dion JE. Management of ischemic stroke in the next decade: stroke centers of excellence. *J Vasc Interv Radiol* 2004;15(1 Pt 2):S133–S141.

Fisher CM. Pathological observations in hypertensive cerebral hemorrhage. *J Neuropathol Exp Neurol* 1971;30(3):536–550.

Flaherty ML, Kissela B, Woo D, et al. The increasing incidence of anticoagulant-associated intracerebral hemorrhage. *Neurology* 2007;68(2):116–121.

Freeman WD, Brott TG, Barrett KM, et al. Recombinant factor VIIa for rapid reversal of warfarin anticoagulation in acute intracranial hemorrhage. *Mayo Clin Proc* 2004;79(12):1495–1500.

Fulgham JR, Ingall TJ, Stead LG, et al. Management of acute ischemic stroke. *Mayo Clin Proc* 2004;79(11):1459–1469.

Furlan A, Higashida R, Wechsler L, et al. Intra-arterial prourokinase for acute ischemic stroke. The PROACT II study: a randomized controlled trial. Prolyse in Acute Cerebral Thromboembolism. *JAMA* 1999;282(21): 2003–2011.

Furlan AJ, Whisnant JP, Elveback LR. The decreasing incidence of primary intracerebral hemorrhage: a population study. *Ann Neurol* 1979;5(4): 367–373.

Gobin YP, Starkman S, Duckwiler GR, et al. MERCI 1: a phase 1 study of Mechanical Embolus Removal in Cerebral Ischemia. *Stroke* 2004;35(12): 2848–2854.

Harraf F, Sharma AK, Brown MM, et al. A multicentre observational study of presentation and early assessment of acute stroke. *BMJ* 2002;325(7354):17.

Kidwell CS, Saver JL, Schubert GB, et al. Design and retrospective analysis of the Los Angeles Prehospital Stroke Screen (LAPSS). *Prehosp Emerg Care* 1998;2(4):267–273.

Kidwell CS, Starkman S, Eckstein M, et al. Identifying stroke in the field. Prospective validation of the Los Angeles prehospital stroke screen (LAPSS). *Stroke* 2000;31(1):71–76.

Kothari RU, Brott TG, Broderick JP, et al. The ABCs of measuring intracerebral hemorrhage volumes. *Stroke* 1996;27(8):1304–1305.

Kothari RU, Hall K, Brott T, et al. Early stroke recognition: developing an out-of-hospital NIH Stroke Scale. *Acad Emerg Med* 1997;4(10): 986–990.

Lewandowski CA, Frankel M, Tomsick TA, et al. Combined intravenous and intra-arterial r-tPA versus intra-arterial therapy of acute ischemic stroke: Emergency Management of Stroke (EMS) Bridging Trial. *Stroke* 1999;30(12):2598–2605.

Manno EM, Atkinson JL, Fulgham JR, et al. Emerging medical and surgical management strategies in the evaluation and treatment of intracerebral hemorrhage. *Mayo Clin Proc* 2005;80(3):420–433.

Mayer SA, Rincon F. Treatment of intracerebral haemorrhage. *Lancet Neurol* 2005;4(10):662–672.

Morgenstern LB, Bartholomew LK, Grotta JC, et al. Sustained benefit of a community and professional intervention to increase acute stroke therapy. *Arch Intern Med* 2003;163(18):2198–2202.

Morgenstern LB, Staub L, Chan W, et al. Improving delivery of acute stroke therapy: the TLL Temple Foundation Stroke Project. *Stroke* 2002;33 (1):160–166.

Muir KW, Buchan A, von Kummer R, et al. Imaging of acute stroke. *Lancet Neurol* 2006;5(9):755–768.

Passero S, Rocchi R, Rossi S, et al. Seizures after spontaneous supratentorial intracerebral hemorrhage. *Epilepsia* 2002;43(10):1175–1180.

Qureshi AI, Hanel RA, Kirmani JF, et al. Cerebral blood flow changes associated with intracerebral hemorrhage. *Neurosurg Clin N Am* 2002;13 (3):355–370.

Qureshi AI, Harris-Lane P, Kirmani JF, et al. Treatment of acute hypertension in patients with intracerebral hemorrhage using American Heart Association guidelines. *Crit Care Med* 2006;34(7):1975–1980.

Ronning OM, Guldvog B. Should stroke victims routinely receive supplemental oxygen? A quasi-randomized controlled trial. *Stroke* 1999;30(10): 2033–2037.

Schonewille WJ, Algra A, Serena J, et al. Outcome in patients with basilar artery occlusion treated conventionally. *J Neurol Neurosurg Psychiatr* 2005;76(9):1238–1241.

Schwamm LH, Pancioli A, Acker JE, III, et al. Recommendations for the establishment of stroke systems of care: recommendations from the American Stroke Association's Task Force on the Development of Stroke Systems. *Stroke* 2005;36(3):690–703.

Shaltoni HM, Albright KC, Gonzales NR, et al. Is intra-arterial thrombolysis safe after full-dose intravenous recombinant tissue plasminogen activator for acute ischemic stroke? *Stroke* 2007;38(1):80–84.

Smith WS. Intra-arterial thrombolytic therapy for acute basilar occlusion: pro. *Stroke* 2007;38(2):701–703.

Smith WS, Corry MD, Fazackerley J, et al. Improved paramedic sensitivity in identifying stroke victims in the prehospital setting. *Prehosp Emerg Care* 1999;3(3):207–210.

Sørensen B, Johansen P, Nielsen GL, et al. Reversal of the international normalized ratio with recombinant activated factor VII in central nervous system bleeding during warfarin thromboprophylaxis: clinical and biochemical aspects. *Blood Coagul Fibrinolysis* 2003;14(5): 469–477.

The IMS Study Investigators. Combined intravenous and intra-arterial recanalization for acute ischemic stroke: the Interventional Management of Stroke Study. *Stroke* 2004;35(4):904–911.

Wallace JD, Levy LL. Blood pressure after stroke. *JAMA* 1981;246(19): 2177–2180.

Wijdicks EF, Nichols DA, Thielen KR, et al. Intra-arterial thrombolysis in acute basilar artery thromboembolism: the initial Mayo Clinic experience. *Mayo Clin Proc* 1997;72(11):1005–1013.

Woo D, Broderick JP. Spontaneous intracerebral hemorrhage: epidemiology and clinical presentation. *Neurosurg Clin N Am* 2002;13(3):265–279.

CHAPTER 21

How to Build a Stroke Team

KERRI S. REMMEL AND ANNA WANAHITA

OBJECTIVES

- What is a stroke team?
- Who are the members of a stroke team?
- Why is a stroke team needed?
- What is needed to build a stroke team?

A stroke team is a group of multidisciplinary health care providers with training and experience in stroke care. Each member of the stroke team should share a strong common interest in caring for stroke patients.

BACKGROUND AND RATIONALE

The concept of a stroke team was introduced in California in 1970. It consisted of a physician, a nurse-coordinator, and a physical therapist. Each member of this team received special training at Memorial Hospital of Long Beach (3 days of intensive training for the physician, 3 weeks for the nurse, and 2 weeks for the physical therapist). After completing the training, the team members returned to their institutions to use their expertise and to train fellow workers on the management of stroke patients. The goals were to encourage and aid local communities to assess the specific needs of stroke patients and to build cost-effective mechanisms for the improvement of the quality of stroke care in the area. In 1974, the results of a stroke project in the Sacramento Medical Center were published. It was intended to create an awareness of stroke for physicians and to introduce the concept of a stroke team in the daily care of stroke patients during the inpatient hospitalization and outpatient follow-up. The stroke team was responsible for locating the stroke patient after admission. They began to collect and analyze stroke data, such as types of stroke, signs and symptoms, and demographic distribution of stroke cases by age and gender.

Before the approval of intravenous tissue plasminogen activator (IV-tPA) by the Food and Drug Administration (FDA) in 1996, the management of stroke patients was fragmented. After IV-tPA was approved, the stroke team's role expanded to improving the quality of care for stroke patients during their hospitalization and in the rehabilitation phase of care. IV-tPA treatment has been shown to improve the outcome of acute stroke patients but it is indicated only within 3 hours of the onset of symptoms in ischemic stroke. As a result of this narrow time window, only 3% to 5% of ischemic stroke patients receive this medication. Numerous studies to expand the time window for treatment have been done but have not been approved by the FDA. In 2004, the FDA approved the Mechanical Embolus Removal in Cerebral Ischemia (MERCI) retrieval system, known as the *corkscrew*, to remove blood clots from the brain in patients experiencing an ischemic stroke. Alteplase (tPA) may also be given through an intra-arterial route and has been widely used in stroke centers. Many studies are currently in progress in various clinical phases for intravenous or intra-arterial use of thrombolytics, which will provide more options, with longer time windows and less adverse events, for immediate treatment of stroke patients.

A strong multidisciplinary collaboration makes it possible for stroke patients to receive such immediate treatments. The process will involve emergency medical service (EMS) personnel, nurses and physicians in the emergency department (ED), neurologists, radiologists, neurosurgeons, and neuroendovascular interventionalists. The hospital management of stroke patients will involve a larger variety of multidisciplinary physicians in disciplines such as cardiology, neurocritical care, internal medicine, or its subspecialties. Physical therapists, occupational therapists, speech-language pathologists (SLPs), social workers, dieticians, nurse practitioners, and nurses also play a very important role in caring for stroke patients. Phlebotomists, laboratory technicians, magnetic resonance imaging (MRI) or other radiology technicians, and pharmacists are also needed to provide services in a timely manner (see Fig. 21.1).

CLINICAL APPLICATION

At present, there is no specific guideline for stroke team membership. In *JAMA*, June 2000 issue, the Brain Attack Coalition (BAC) made recommendations for team members and on their functions in primary stroke centers (PSCs) and comprehensive stroke centers (CSCs). PSCs would function to stabilize patients and to provide emergency care for patients with acute stroke. At the minimum, the team in the PSC should include a physician and another health care professional (i.e., nurse, physician's assistant, or nurse practitioner) and they should be available 24/7 for rapid evaluation of stroke patients. On the basis of the clinical condition and the availability

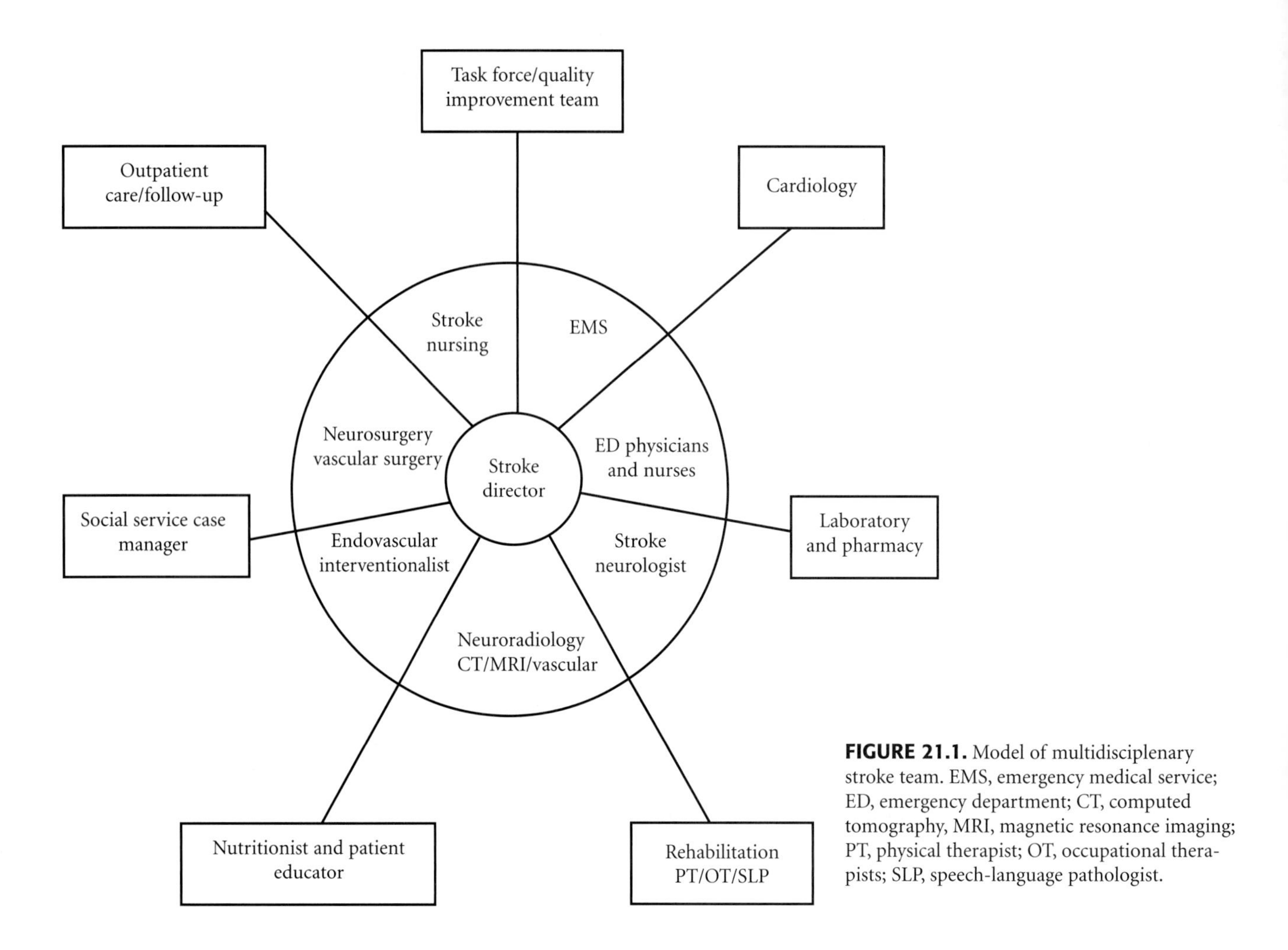

FIGURE 21.1. Model of multidisciplenary stroke team. EMS, emergency medical service; ED, emergency department; CT, computed tomography, MRI, magnetic resonance imaging; PT, physical therapist; OT, occupational therapists; SLP, speech-language pathologist.

of PSC resources, this center would either admit stroke patients or facilitate the patients' transfer to a CSC. A CSC is defined as a facility or system with the necessary personnel, infrastructure, expertise, and programs to diagnose and treat stroke patients who require more complex medical and surgical care, specialized tests, or interventional therapies. A CSC also acts as a resource center for PSCs in their region.

Ideally, a stroke team is led by a stroke neurologist. The 90-day mortality rate is significantly lower when stroke patients are cared for by neurologists when compared to other specialties (grade IIIC). In additon, the disposition of patients treated by neurologists is more likely to be to home or an acute rehabilitation facility rather than to a nursing home, suggesting better functional outcome. In the case of no stroke neurologist, an emergency physician, neurosurgeon, or nurse practitioner can be appointed as a stroke director.

The three basic components of a stroke team are as follows:

1. The acute response stroke team
   - 1.1 EMS personnel
   - 1.2 Emergency department physicians and nurses
   - 1.3 Stroke neurologist and his/her designee
   - 1.4 Neurosurgeons and neuroendovascular interventionalists
2. In-hospital management stroke team
3. Task force stroke team

The Acute Response Stroke Team

The acute response team can be implemented in the setting of PCSs and CSCs. It consists of EMS personnel, ED nurses and physicians, stroke neurologists, and other physicians or advanced practice nurses (APNs). The members of the team may vary depending on the resources of each facility. The acute stroke team will be responsible for rapid identification and a rapid focused history and neurological assessment. The goal of this team is to reduce in-hospital delays in obtaining medical care for stroke patients. The acute stroke team includes the following members.

Emergency Medical Service Personnel

An educational program for paramedics has been shown to improve the accuracy of identification of stroke cases, reduce the transport duration to stroke centers, increase the admission of acute stroke patients, and increase the use of thrombolysis. Patients with stroke symptoms who used EMS had significantly shorter time periods between the time of onset of symptoms and arrival. Integration of EMS with the stroke team reduces prehospital and in-hospital delays [i.e., time to be evaluated by ED physician and neurologist and time to the computed tomography (CT) scanner]. A stroke system should include processes that provide rapid access to EMS (such as 9-1-1) and rapid dispatch of EMS. Rapid identification of stroke cases by EMS and transportation to the nearest PSC or CSC increases the probability of stroke patients receiving

IV-tPA. Diagnostic algorithms and written protocols for EMS ensure the most current management of stroke patients. The protocols should be reviewed by the stroke team at least annually. The ideal protocol will include rapid assessment to minimize the time spent in the field. Medical protocols while en route should include determination of the time of onset, past medical and surgical history, and list of medications taken and medication allergies. To reduce in-hospital delay, EMS can also perform Accu-Chek to determine blood glucose level, initiate IV access, and start an IV infusion with normal saline. EMS personnel should notify ED personnel about a potential stroke patient and their estimated time of arrival while en route, so that the stroke team may be alerted. A single contact number, usually known as a stroke pager, facilitates rapid access to members of the acute stroke team.

Emergency Department Nurses and Physicians

Once stroke patients arrive in the ED, the stroke team is alerted. Rapid assessment and stabilization of the patient is performed by ED physicians and nurses. A stroke neurologist or other member of the acute stroke team should be at the patient's bedside within 15 minutes of being called. According to the BAC and American Stroke Association (ASA) guidelines, patients should have a CT of the head within 25 minutes of arrival and the CT should be interpreted within 45 minutes of placement of the order. The stroke team can facilitate the logistics of these time requirements by calling radiology and by helping transport patients to the scanner. An operation agreement between the stroke team and ED should be made about the existence and operations of the acute response stroke team. For quality improvement monitoring, a log book should be kept to record call times, response times, patient diagnoses, treatments, and outcomes.

Stroke Neurologists or Designee

It is recommended that the CSC should have more than one neurologist or physician with expertise in cerebrovascular disease to ensure 24/7 coverage. They should be available by phone within 20 minutes of being called and be available in-house within 45 minutes if needed. A stroke neurologist usually serves as the stroke service medical director, but also performs direct clinical care of stroke patients. The neurologist mobilizes and coordinates resources, such as laboratory and imaging facilities, for rapid determination of eligibility for IV-tPA or alternative acute stroke treatments.

Neurosurgeons and Neuroendovascular Interventionalists

In some cases, neurosurgeons or neuroendovascular interventionalists may be needed in the acute care of stroke patients. Neurosurgical consult must be available within 2 hours locally or by transfer for stroke patients who receive thrombolytics. A PSC that does not have this infrastructure should have formal procedures in place to transfer patients to a CSC when medically necessary. Neurosurgery and neuroendovascular interventionalist coverage is recommended 24/7 for CSCs.

In-Hospital Management Stroke Team

While the acute response team plays an important role in the acute phase, the inpatient hospital management stroke team will also have a significant effect on the care of stroke patients. In addition to a stroke neurologist, a number of specialty physicians and multidisciplinary health care providers will be involved in the in-hospital management of stroke patients. Substantial evidence shows that during postacute care, stroke patients have a better outcome with a well-organized, multidisciplinary approach (grade A).

Stabilization and Medical Management of Stroke Patient

Medical management including blood pressure management, blood glucose control, and fluid status is also required in the management of acute stroke patients. Patients with acute or subacute ischemic and hemorrhagic stroke may require care in the intensive care unit (ICU). Several studies have shown the importance, benefit, and cost effectiveness of stroke patients being admitted to a stroke unit (grade IA). Stroke patients who receive care in a stroke unit have a 17% reduction in death, a 7% increase in ability to live at home, and 8% reduction in length of stay. This unit should be staffed by physicians with training in cerebrovascular disease and critical care.

Secondary Prevention

Secondary prevention is important for both transient ischemic attack (TIA) and ischemic stroke patients. TIA has been redefined as a brief episode of neurological dysfunction caused by a focal disturbance of the brain or retinal ischemia, with clinical symptoms typically lasting <1 hour and without imaging evidence of infarction. In previous practice, patients with TIA were worked up for etiology on an outpatient basis. A stroke team was rarely involved in their care and an outpatient workup took more than 2 weeks to complete. Recent data showed that in 55-year-olds the 90-day risk of stroke after TIA was 10.5%, with the greatest number occurring in the first week after the TIA. Large studies from the United Kingdom and California showed that half of the TIA patients had an acute stroke within 2 days of the TIA. It also showed that stroke was fatal in 21% of patients and was disabling in 64%. Patients with TIA and stroke should undergo an immediate evaluation for etiology and vascular risk factors. When patients with TIA are worked up by a stroke team urgently, stroke prevention techniques may be implemented earlier.

Role of Stroke Neurologist or Physician in Other Specialty in Secondary Prevention

Identification of modifiable risk factors for stroke that can be controlled should be discussed with the patient. Depending on the complexity of the case, a consulting physician may be asked to follow up the patient with stroke. Treatment decisions for comorbid conditions should follow current evidence-based guidelines from the ASA for secondary prevention.

Role of Director of Nursing and/or Advanced Practice Nurses

Stroke nurses participate in patient care and patient, staff, and community education; play an active role in stroke research; and maintain quality assurance and stroke registry entries (grade IIIC). The APNs also participate in the acute and inpatient hospital management of stroke patients. Their principal position duties are as follows:

1. Under the direction of the chief of vascular neurology, manage and supervise operations of the stroke program (e.g.,

create and update clinical pathways and order sets, and plan and implement patient education programs).
2. Participate in daily rounds in the hospital with other stroke team members.
3. Carry a stroke pager and take acute stroke calls.
4. Train all hospital staff on stroke signs and symptoms; develop and implement nursing education programs.
5. Facilitate interdisciplinary communication in the form of regular meetings or interdisciplinary rounds with ancillary staff (physical therapists, occupational therapists, SLPs, social workers, case managers, and nutritionists).
6. Train new members of the stroke team or new staff on the operations of the stroke team and their duties.
7. Maintain documentation on core compliance measures for stroke center certification
8. Maintain data on the Joint Commission on the Accreditation of Health care Organizations (JCAHO) measures for quality assurance. JCAHO performance measures include:
   a. Deep vein thombosis prophylaxis
   b. Discharged on antithrombotics
   c. Patients with atrial fibrillation receiving anticoagulation therapy
   d. tPA considered and tPA received—secondary rate
   e. Antithrombotic medication within 48 hours of hospitalization
   f. Lipid profile
   g. Screen for dysphagia
   h. Stroke education
   i. Smoking cessation
   j. The plan for rehabilitation considered
9. Organize and develop stroke center continuing medical education (CME) and continuing education unit (CEU) programs; be present at conferences and seminars; and work with administrators of the hospital, the National Stroke Association, the ASA, and the state health department for development of stroke center.
10. Manage or develop community events for stroke education, such as health fairs, lectures at community centers, worksites, and churches; acquire funding for educational programs and community events.
11. Provide education to stroke patients on their modifiable risk factors.

Interventional Neurologists, Interventional Neuroradiologists, and Vascular Neurosurgeons

Endovascular management of patients with ischemic stroke should follow the current guidelines for prevention of stroke:

1. For patients with recent TIA or ischemic stroke within the last 6 months and ipsilateral severe (70% to 99%) carotid artery stenosis, carotid endarterectomy (CEA) is recommended (grade IA). For ipsilateral moderate (50% to 69%) carotid stenosis, CEA is recommended depending on patient-specific factors such as age, gender, and comorbidities and severity of initial symptoms (grade IA). When CEA is indicated, surgery within 2 weeks is suggested rather than delaying the surgery (grade IIB).
2. In patients with symptomatic stenosis >70% in whom lesions are inaccessible by surgery or in whom other comorbidities increase their surgical risk, carotid artery stenting (CAS) is not inferior to CEA (grade IIB).
3. Extracranial–intracranial (EC/IC) bypass surgery is not routinely recommended (grade IIIA), but is currently under investigation as an option for revascularization.
4. Endovascular treatment may be considered for patients with symptomatic extracranial vertebral stenosis despite medical therapies (antithrombotics, statins, and antihypertensive medications) (grade IIC).
5. For patients with significant symptomatic intracranial stenosis despite medical therapy, the usefulness of endovascular therapy (angioplasty and/or stent placement) is uncertain and is considered investigational (grade IIC).

Rehabilitation

Rehabilitation may increase stroke patients' quality of life and reduce financial and physical burden on society (grade IA). All stroke team therapists, social workers, and case managers should meet requirements for state licensure.

1. Assessment by physical therapy, occupational therapy, and speech therapy should begin as soon as a patient is admitted and stabilized. Mobilization and resumption of self-care should begin as soon as possible. Strengthening and functional mobility should be included in the acute rehabilitation of patients with weakness after stroke (grade A).
2. An SLP has several important roles in caring for stroke patients. SLPs will perform initial and follow-up evaluations and treat dysphagia and speech, language, and cognitive deficits.
3. Nutritionists evaluate dietary needs and educate patients and their families on appropriate nutrition.
4. Discharge planner, social worker, or case manager services should begin on admission to shorten length of stay in the hospital and ensure that patients with stroke are discharged to an optimal destination for maximum long-term recovery.

Task Force and Quality Improvement Team

The American Heart Association launched a campaign entitled Metro Stroke Task Force (MSTF) in 1997. It consists of representatives from health care providers, hospital administrators, EMS, and civic and community leaders. The objectives of MSTF were to (a) educate the public about stroke risk factors and warning signs, (b) educate EMS personnel to recognize the symptoms of stroke and to treat it as an emergency, (c) coordinate the efficient transport of stroke patients to the nearest stroke center, and (d) encourage local hospitals/health care facilities to develop organized protocols for treatment of acute stroke. Meetings are scheduled regularly to identify specific problems and to improve the quality of patients' care. Ideally, multispecialty involvement includes a stroke neurologist as the team leader with emergency medicine physicians, primary care physicians, nurses, neuroradiologists, radiology technicians, neurosurgeons, cardiologists, rehabilitation personnel, and hospital administrators.

BUILDING A STROKE TEAM

The most important element in building a stroke team is obtaining a commitment from hospital leadership to develop the program. The financial commitment from the hospital includes funding personnel, facility, and technical support. Financing a stroke team may include salaries of personnel, such as stroke neurologists, hospitalists, APNs, data management personnel, and care coordinators dedicated to one hospital system, or it may include paying neurologists to take stroke call. Hospital organizations usually have imaging technicians, vascular lab personnel, case managers, and coordinators in place; however, duties and time commitment will expand once the system is in place. Therefore, additional staff may be needed for the coverage required.

After obtaining commitment from the hospital leadership the team must develop protocols with the EMS, ED, lab, pharmacy, radiology, ICU, and telemetry step-down units. With hospital support and protocols in place this multidisciplinary team may assemble whenever called to care for an acute stroke patient. The team's role has certainly expanded beyond that envisioned in 1970s.

SELECTED REFERENCES

Alberts MJ, Hademenos G, Latchaw RE, et al. Recommendations for the establishment of primary stroke centers. Brain Attack Coalition. *J Am Med Assoc* 2000;283(23):3102–3109.

Alberts MJ, Latchaw RE, Selman WR, et al. Recommendations for comprehensive stroke centers: a consensus statement from the Brain Attack Coalition. *Stroke* 2005;36(7): 1597-1616.

Alberts MJ. tPA in acute ischemic stroke: United States experience and issues for the future. *Neurology* 1998;51(3 Suppl 3): S53–S55.

Bates B, Choi JY, Duncan PW, et al. Veterans Affairs/Department of Defense Clinical Practice Guideline for the Management of Adult Stroke Rehabilitation Care: executive summary. *Stroke* 2005;36(9): 2049–2056.

Borhani NO. Stroke surveillance: the concept of stroke team in diagnosis, treatment and prevention. *Stroke* 1974;5(1):78–80.

Dion JE. Management of ischemic stroke in the next decade: stroke centers of excellence. *J Vasc Interv Radiol* 2004;15(1 Pt 2):S133–S141.

Douglas VC, Tong DC, Gillum LA, et al. Do the Brain Attack Coalition's criteria for stroke centers improve care for ischemic stroke? *Neurology* 2005;64(3):422–427.

Gobin YP, Starkman S, Duckwiler GR, et al. MERCI 1: a phase 1 study of Mechanical Embolus Removal in Cerebral Ischemia. *Stroke* 2004; 35(12):2848–2854.

Goldstein LB, Matchar DB, Hoff-Lindquist J, et al. VA Stroke Study: neurologist care is associated with increased testing but improved outcomes. *Neurology* 2003;61(6):792–796.

Hademenos G. Metro Stroke Task Force: first-year experience. *Stroke* 1999;30(11):2512.

Mitchell JB, Ballard DJ, Whisnant JP, et al. What role do neurologists play in determining the costs and outcomes of stroke patients? *Stroke* 1996;27(11):1937–1943.

Rothwell, PM, Warlow CP. Timing of TIAs preceding stroke: time window for prevention is very short. *Neurology* 2005;64(5):817–820.

Sacco RL, Adams R, Albers G, et al. Guidelines for prevention of stroke in patients with ischemic stroke or transient ischemic attack: a statement for healthcare professionals from the American Heart Association/American Stroke Association Council on Stroke: co-sponsored by the Council on Cardiovascular Radiology and Intervention: the American Academy of Neurology affirms the value of this guideline. *Circulation* 2006;113(10):e409–e449.

Schroeder EB, Wayne D, Morris D, et al. Determinants of use of emergency medical services in a population with stroke symptoms: the Second Delay in Accessing Stroke Healthcare (DASH II) Study. *Stroke* 2000;31(11):2591–2596.

Smith MA, Lioua J-I, Jennifer R, et al. 30-Day survival and rehospitalization for stroke patients according to physician specialty. *Cerebrovasc Dis* 2006;22(1):21–26.

Stroke Unit Trialists' Collaboration. Collaborative systematic review of the randomised trials of organised inpatient (stroke unit) care after stroke. *Br Med J* 1997;314(7088):1151–1159.

Tesman BL, Michela BJ. The stroke team concept as implemented in the area 8 regional medical program. *Stroke* 1970;1(1):19–22.

The National Institute of Neurological Disorders and Stroke rt-PA Stroke Study Group. Tissue plasminogen activator for acute ischemic stroke. *N Engl J Med* 1995;333(24):1581–1587.

Wojner-Alexandrov AW, Alexandrov AV, Rodriguez D, et al. Houston paramedic and emergency stroke treatment and outcomes study (HoPSTO). *Stroke* 2005;36(7):1512–1518.

CHAPTER

22

Neuroimaging in the Management of Stroke Patients

JAMES D. GEYER, DANIEL C. POTTS, STEPHENIE C. DILLARD, AND CAMILO R. GOMEZ

OBJECTIVES

- What is the importance of neuroimaging in stroke management?
- Which imaging modalities are most appropriate for each specific situation?
- How are the results of different imaging modalities to be integrated?
- What is the impact of neuroimaging on treatment protocols?

Advances in imaging technology have played a key role in the progress made over the last two decades in the treatment of stroke patients, facilitating the identification, classification, and documentation of the different pathologic processes that constitute the subspecialty field of *vascular neurology*. As such, neuroimaging is an integral part of both the training and practice of this specialty, with many specialists in vascular neurology also spending a considerable portion of their time in the application of imaging techniques for the diagnosis and treatment of their patients.

BACKGROUND AND RATIONALE

The importance of neuroimaging parallels both historically and practically to that of imaging in cardiovascular medicine. The utilization by cardiac specialists of echocardiography, nuclear cardiac imaging, magnetic resonance imaging (MRI) and magnetic resonance angiography (MRA) has been trailed by similar use of comparable imaging techniques by vascular neurologists. The present chapter addresses the most important concepts about imaging of stroke patients. We explore the rules that guide the selection of appropriate imaging modalities for specific clinical scenarios. We also discuss the most important characteristics of the techniques with greatest practical value, pointing out their advantages and disadvantages.

PURPOSE OF IMAGING: TASK-ORIENTED CHOICES

The most practical approach to a discussion of the application of neuroimaging techniques in stroke care is to first address the tasks, diagnostic or therapeutic, that require their use. From this perspective, the clinical scenarios in which imaging techniques are likely to be needed must be assessed along the following lines:

- What information is being sought, and how quickly is it needed?
- Which of the available imaging techniques is most likely to answer the question being asked?
- How will the information obtained by imaging affect further diagnostic algorithms, the treatment, and the prognosis of the patient?

On the basis of these considerations, the tasks that require the utilization of imaging during clinical care of patients with cerebrovascular disorders include initial diagnosis, categorization and therapeutic allocation, imaging of the brain blood vessels, characterization of the ischemic process, and assessment of prognosis.

Initial Diagnosis

Direct imaging of the brain is necessary to assess the status of the tissue, often documenting the damage caused by the stroke, and also to differentiate between the ischemic and the hemorrhagic ones. The techniques available to complete this task include computed tomography (CT) and MRI. As it will be discussed in the following sections, choosing between one and another involves considerations of speed, sensitivity, type of stroke, resource availability, and temporal profile of the event.

Categorization and Therapeutic Allocation

Once the diagnosis of stroke is made, a more precise definition of the condition has enormous therapeutic implications, both immediate and long term. The same technologic advances described in the preceding section have extended to improvements in image resolution, with better signal–noise ratios, and a superior definition of the pathologic processes. Furthermore, since the cerebral vasculature is so often implicated in the pathogenic process, imaging of the cerebral arteries and veins becomes an additional dimension in the categorization of these patients.

Imaging of the Brain Vessels

Imaging of the brain blood vessels is part of the standard risk stratification algorithm that every stroke patient must undergo. As such, documentation of vascular abnormalities causally associated with the stroke not only allows determination of the level of risk for subsequent stroke but also helps plan preventive therapy. In general, the tests that are available for the completion of this task are divided into two groups: (a) those that are noninvasive (i.e., ultrasonic, radiotomographic, and magnetic-based techniques) and (b) those that are invasive (catheterization and angiography). In addition to its diagnostic capabilities, the latter also allows the application of endovascular therapeutic techniques. Since we have already devoted an entire book chapter to catheterization and angiography, we will refrain from covering it in the present manuscript.

Characterization of the Ischemic Process

Although, as we noted earlier, documentation of the ischemic injury to tissue can be accomplished using CT and MRI, the possibility of visually demonstrating ischemic-yet-not-damaged tissue is gaining increasing popularity. At first, nuclear-based imaging techniques such as single photon emission computed tomography (SPECT) and positron emission tomography (PET) became the most studied methods for functional imaging of the brain. Then, a combination of nuclear and radiologic techniques (i.e., Xenon-CT) was introduced as a more practical tool for the assessment of emergency stroke situations. More recently, the use of more sophisticated magnetic-based techniques [diffusion-weighted MRI (DW-MRI) and perfusion-weighted MRI] promises to assist in the identification of ischemic tissue that may be salvageable, possibly having a role in the selection of patients for specific types of therapies, and even expanding the window of utilization of higher-than-average risk strategies (i.e., thrombolysis).

Assessment of Prognosis

Following identification and categorization of the stroke, it is possible to use the imaging information to "best fit" the potential outlook and final outcome of each patient. Furthermore, it is often possible to make predictions about the potential benefit of a specific treatment strategy. Clearly, this characteristic of imaging relates to the fact that the existing techniques represent the equivalent of bedside neuropathology and that they have direct correspondence with the natural history of every type of stroke.

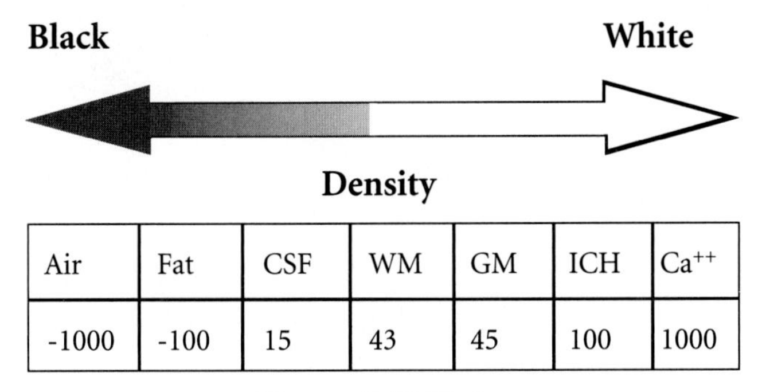

Air	Fat	CSF	WM	GM	ICH	Ca^{++}
-1000	-100	15	43	45	100	1000

FIGURE 22.1. Relationship between the various tissues and their corresponding Hounsfield Units (HU) in computed tomography (CT. Density increases as the HU increase. Note that the HU [and the density of intracranial hemorrhage (ICH)] is greater than white matter (WM) and of gray matter (GM).
CSF, cerebrospinal fluid.

THE AVAILABLE TOOLS: NEUROIMAGING TECHNIQUES

Computed Tomography: The Beginning of Contemporary Neuroimaging

Every discussion about imaging techniques in stroke must begin with CT. Its introduction in the 1970s changed the way all neurological diseases are diagnosed and treated. Suddenly, it was possible to directly look at the brain tissue and document the damage caused by either infarction or hemorrhage. Furthermore, CT allowed a rapid differentiation between these two different types of stroke and has ultimately made possible the application of aggressive treatment strategies such as thrombolysis. The principles of CT are relatively simple—narrow beams of X-rays are used to rotationally acquire tissue density information in one of several tomographic planes. The raw data acquired over a period of a few minutes is then entered into a computer that reconstructs the tissue sample in two-dimensional tomographic images. At present, fast helical scanning techniques and powerful reconstruction algorithms allow even three-dimensional reconstruction of the brain tissue and the brain blood vessels. The images obtained represent a map of the density of tissue in a scale of Hounsfield Units (HU, see Fig. 22.1) that spans between −1,000 (the *blackest of black* corresponding to air) and +1,000 (the *whitest of white* corresponding to calcium). The usefulness of CT in the evaluation of stroke is primarily related to the emergency assessment of acute patients. It is in this context that the technique allows the determination of hemorrhagic changes and the identification of early signs of ischemic tissue damage, and most recently, it has become a determining factor for the selection of patients for specific types of treatment (e.g., thrombolysis). Nevertheless, as we will describe in the following sections, CT is also quite important in the follow-up of the evolution of stroke in patients over time.

CT Angiography

CT angiography is a relatively noninvasive technique that couples helical CT scanning with contrast enhancement to obtain vascular images. It is performed by first obtaining a series of helical axial images following the injection of about 100 mL of iodinated contrast over approximately 20 minutes. These are then reconstructed using 1.25 mm thick slices and 0.5 to 1.0 mm increments. This protocol allows three-dimensional rendering of the angiographic images (see Fig. 22.2). The development of this technique required the introduction of a scanner that allowed the patients to be translated through a continuously rotating gantry, with very rapid data acquisition. The operator controls several variables that determine the protocol to be used for each region of interest to be imaged, including duration of the scan, speed of movement of the table, and collimation. As with any other technique, CT angiography has advantages and disadvantages. On one hand, it is not susceptible to flow perturbations and complex flow patterns like magnetic angiography. On the other hand, it utilizes ionizing radiation and iodinated contrast administration, which limit its use in patients with azotemia and contrast allergy, while resulting in a more lim-

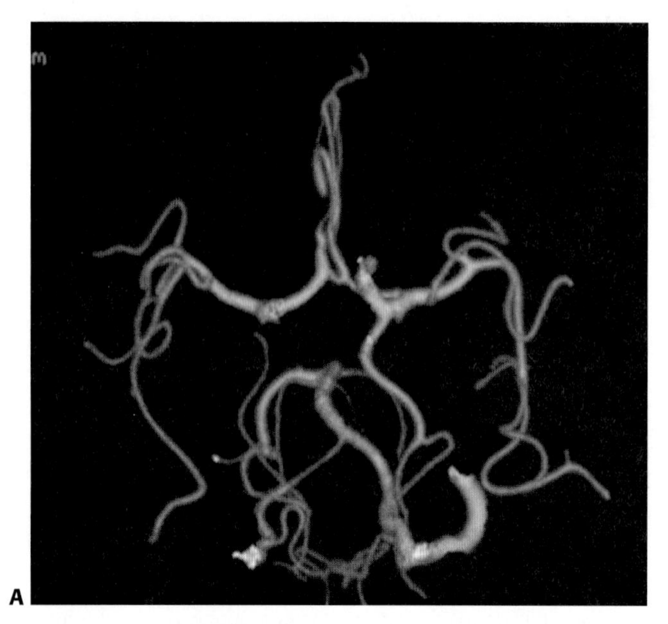

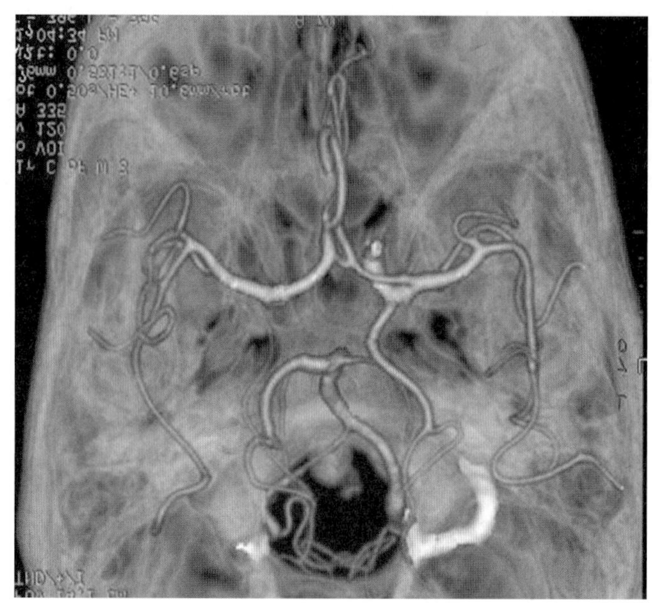

FIGURE 22.2. Three-dimensional rendering of the intracranial arteries using computed tomographic angiography (CTA). The arteries are displayed by themselves in the axial plane **(A)**. It is also possible to display them in the context of the surrounding bony environment **(B)**. *(See color insert.)*

ited field of view (FOV) per study. The latter is very important, for it requires that the planning and postprocessing of the study take into consideration the question being asked. Furthermore, post-processing and three-dimensional rendering typically involve sculpting out some of the tissue that surrounds the vessels on the basis of its density. This process, when not carefully carried out, can conceivably lead to the exclusion of important structures or pathologic findings. Several studies have compared CT angiography with conventional angiography, finding an agreement of 80% to 95% between the two techniques, when studying extracranial carotid atherosclerotic stenotic plaques. In our experience, however, it is often misleading, and its best application is the definition of intracranial aneurysms before their treatment (see Fig. 22.3).

MRI: Versatility in Action

The utilization of MRI in clinical medicine became widespread during the 1980s. The increased sensitivity of this technique, as compared with CT, for the detection of abnormalities in brain structure made it an immediate candidate for the imaging modality of choice in the demonstration of infarction of the brain parenchyma. Over the course of the years, MRI has allowed the documentation of ischemic brain lesions earlier and more precisely, particularly in regions that had remained relatively unavailable to previous imaging modalities, such as the brainstem. More recently, the introduction of additional MRI sequences has resulted in the ability to image the brain vessels, as well as to study the degree of ischemia and viability of the tissue.

Parenchymal abnormalities in patients with ischemic stroke respond to the accumulation of water within the ischemic cells, first producing cytotoxic edema secondary to cellular membrane incompetence, and later due to blood brain barrier (BBB) breakdown. Increased tissue signal on T2-weighted, proton density and fast low-angled inversion recovery (FLAIR) images, as well as a less-pronounced drop in signal on T1-weighted sequences, accompanies this pathophysiologic process. As opposed to the flow-related findings noted earlier, the parenchymal changes evolve over a period of hours to days. As time goes by, the changes observed on MRI give way to a picture most representative of encephalo-malacia, necrosis, and gliosis. Thus, in the chronic stages, infarcted tissue appears as an

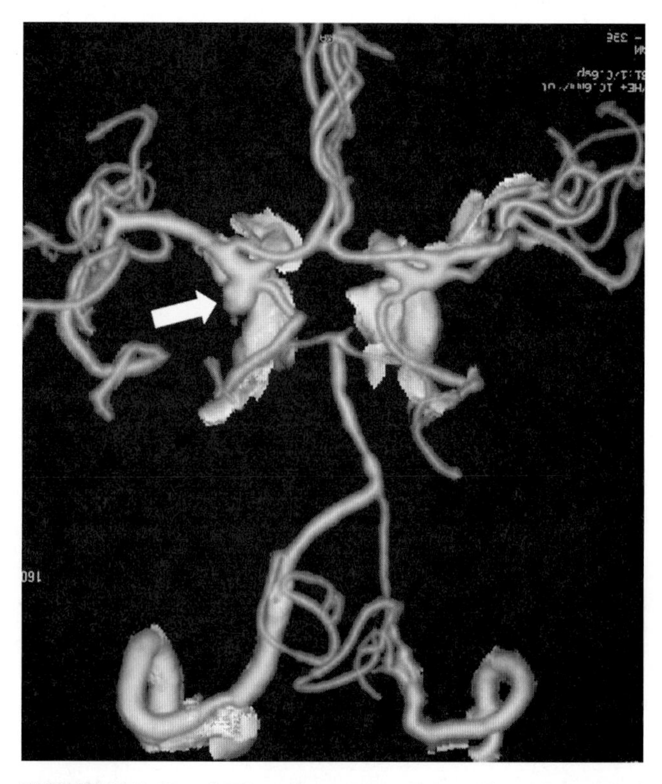

FIGURE 22.3. Use of CTA to diagnose aneurysms. Three-dimensional rendering of the CTA clearly identifies a left posterior communicating artery aneurysm (*arrow*). *(See color insert.)*

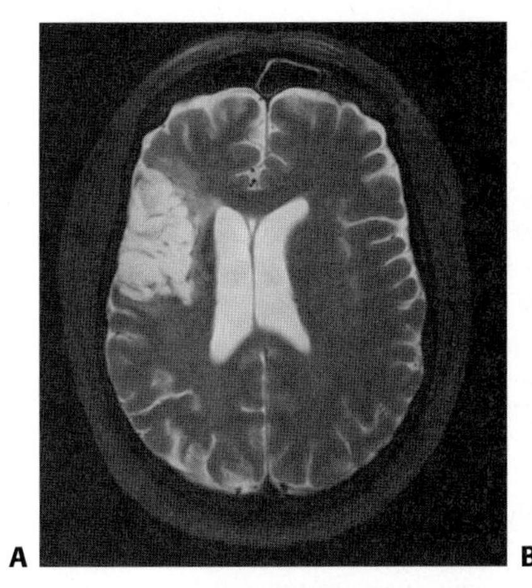

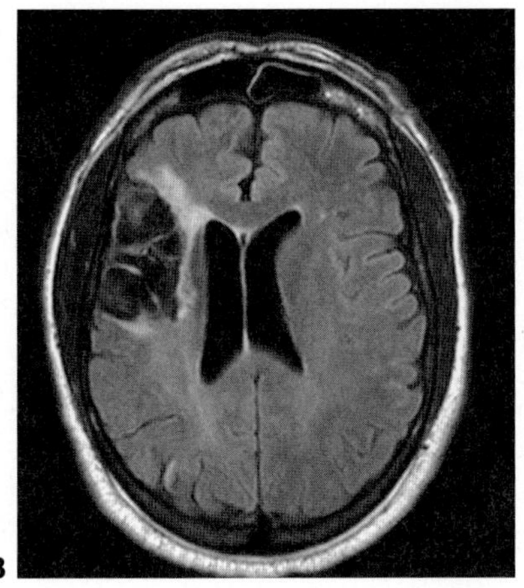

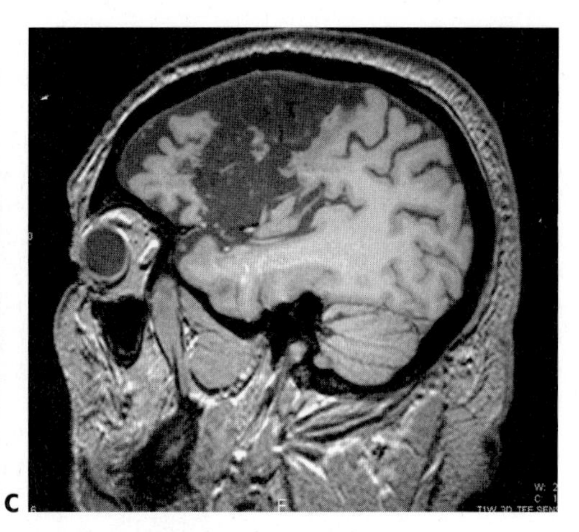

FIGURE 22.4. Appearance of a chronic infarction of a large portion of the right middle cerebral artery on magnetic resonance imaging, using SE sequences. T2-weighted imaging show the entire area of infarction as hyperintense **(A)**. FLAIR images display a core of low intensity with a margin of high intensity **(B)**. The cystic transformation of the damaged tissue can be greatly appreciated. T1-weighted images show the area as hypointense **(C)**.

area of high intensity on T2-weighted images, low intensity on T1-weighted images, moderate intensity on proton density images, and mixed intensity on FLAIR sequences (see Fig. 22.4).

The MRI appearance of intracranial hemorrhages over time is one of the most interesting subjects in neuroimaging, for it largely depends on the natural evolution of hemoglobin degradation within the tissue and the strength of the magnetic field (see Table 22.1 and Fig. 22.5). Typically, the sequence of conversion from oxyhemoglobin to deoxyhemoglobin, followed by that from deoxyhemoglobin to methemoglobin (first intracellular and then extracellular, as the erythrocytes disappear), and finally to hemosiderin, occurs as parts of a continuum that evolves over weeks to months. Hyperacute hemorrhage (i.e., a few hours), in the form the oxyhemoglobin, is isointense with the brain parenchyma on T1-weighted spin-echo (SE) images and hyperintense on T2-weighted SE images. After a few hours, the oxyhemoglobin evolves into deoxyhemoglobin within the hematoma (Fig. 22.5). The latter predominantly shortens T2, and this leads to low signal on T2-weighted images. After 3 to 4 days, deoxyhemoglobin is progressively converted to methemoglobin, which is a paramagnetic substance that shortens both T1 and T2, although its predominant effect is shortening T1 (Fig. 22.5). As a result, at this stage, hematomas display high signal in both T1- and T2-weighted images. Over the next few months, the methemoglobin is slowly broken down into hemichromes that produce only mild T1 shortening. Hematomas at this end stage have a slightly high signal on T1-weighted images but retain a high signal on the T2-weighted images. Finally, around the periphery of hematomas, macrophage activity results in degradation of the methemoglobin and conversion of the iron moiety to hemosiderin, which shortens T2 and produces a black ring around the hematoma on T2-weighted images. This can be observed within 2 weeks of hemorrhage, and it has a tendency to become thicker over time. In small hematomas (<1 cm), the low signal intensity from hemosiderin may essentially occupy the entire ultimate volume of the cavity. In our experience, the length of time for which the hemosiderin will remain in the area of a hematoma mimics autopsy findings many years after an intracerebral hemorrhage, and we suspect, using high-field MRI, it can be readily identified over the lifetime of the patient.

Gradient Refocused Echomagnetic Resonance Imaging Techniques

Our discussion in the previous section is largely applicable to SE techniques. However, over the last decade, as more knowledge has accumulated about the various methods of applying MRI to clinical practice, sequences that are more sensitive to intracranial hemorrhages have been introduced. In general, different materials vary in their ability to support magnetic fields within them. This property, known as magnetic susceptibility, is significantly different between some of the hemoglobin breakdown products (i.e., deoxyhemoglobin and methemoglobin) and the surrounding brain tissue. Such a difference exists because the substances in question have unpaired electrons that superimpose their own magnetic field on the external field. This creates field inhomogeneities that increase magnetic susceptibility artifacts and make these substances stand out against the background tissue.

TABLE 22.1 Imaging Characteristics of Intracranial Hemorrhages at Various Stages

Stage	Hgb	T1W	T2W	Time
Hyperacute	Oxy Hgb	Isointense	Hyperintense	<12 h
Acute	Deoxy Hgb	Isointense	Hypointense	1–3 d
Subacute (early)	Met Hgb (RBC)	Hyperintense	Hypointense	3–7 d
Subacute (late)	Met Hgb (Free)	Hyperintense	Hyperintense	>7 d
Chronic (rim)	Hemosiderin	Isointense	Hypointense	>14 d
Chronic (center)	Hemichromes	Isointense	Hyperintense	>14 d
Edema	Not applicable	Hypointense	Hyperintense	1–14 d

The presence of magnetic susceptibility artifacts can be emphasized by using techniques that are T2 Star (T2*) weighted. As an MRI parameter, T2* is the time constant that describes the decay of transverse magnetization, taking into account the inhomogeneities of the static magnetic field and the spin-spin relaxation in the human body. This interaction results in rapid loss of phase coherence and MRI signal. The T2* is always less than the T2 time, a characteristic that will be of benefit when studying intracranial hemorrhage. The gradient refocused echo (GRE) imaging sequences use a refocusing gradient in the phase encoding direction during the end module to maximize (refocus) the remaining transverse magnetization at the time when the next excitation pulse is due, while the other two gradients are balanced. These sequences can be identified by various acronyms used by the different companies to identify them (see Table 22.2), but fundamentally, all rely on the increased susceptibility artifact displayed by intracerebral hemorrhages at nearly any stage for their rapid detection due to their low signal appearance (see Fig. 22.6). Indeed, the literature describing the increased sensitivity of GRE techniques for detecting acute intracranial hemorrhages continues to grow, both in the acute and chronic care settings. The latter relates to the ability to detect microhemorrhages in patients with conditions that place them at risk for additional future hemorrhages (e.g., amyloid angiopathy).

Diffusion-Weighted MRI

Ischemia of brain tissue results in disruption of oxidative phosphorylation due to impaired oxygen delivery to tissue. The brain cells resort to anaerobic glycolysis, a more inefficient form of energy production. These changes lead to impaired function of the Na-K pump function of the cell membrane, with consequent accumulation of intracellular sodium. Other high-energy phosphates are depleted, with accumulation of inorganic phosphate and lactic acid within the tissue. The osmotic gradient created by the accumulation of intracellular sodium facilitates the influx of water into the cells with the production of cytotoxic edema.

The signal intensity on DW-MRI is related to the random microscopic motion of water protons (Brownian motion), while conventional MRI sequences depend on the accumulation of water within the tissue. It is thus possible to detect slower proton motion within the ischemic tissue, with lower diffusion coefficients, as early as minutes following the onset of ischemia. Regardless of the exact

TABLE 22.2 Techniques for T2 Star (T2*) Brain Imaging

Acronym	Sequence Name
FAST	Fourier Acquired Steady State
FFE	Fast Field Echo
FLASH	Fast Low Angle Shot
FISP	Fast Imaging with Steady State Precession
GRASS	Gradient Recalled Acquisition in Steady State
SSFP	Steady State Free Precession

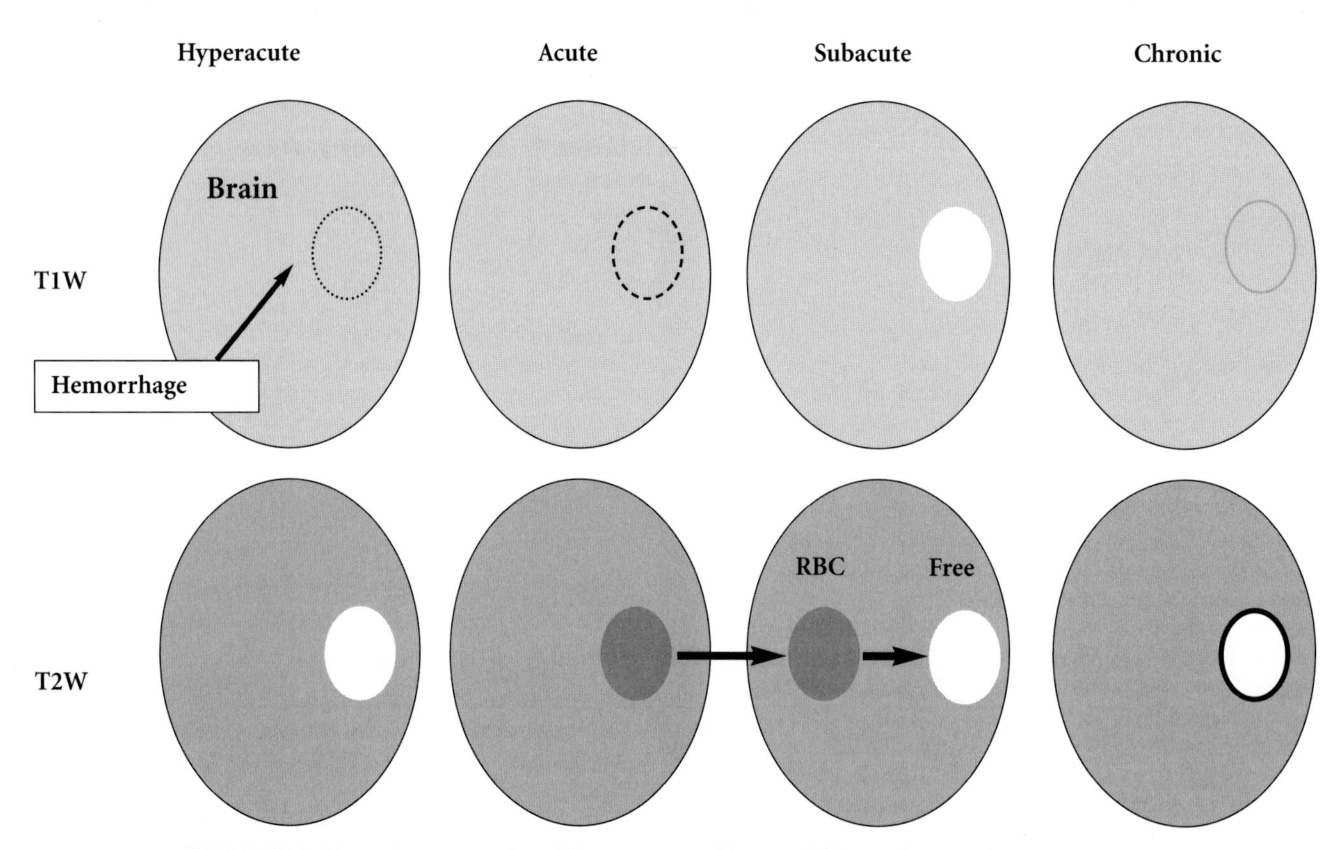

FIGURE 22.5. Schematic representation of the appearance of intracranial hemorrhages at their various stages (Table 22.1), when using SE MRI techniques, in terms of their intensity in the images. See the text for an explanation.
T1W, T1 weighted; T2W, T2 weighted; RBC, red blood cells; Hgb, hemoglobin

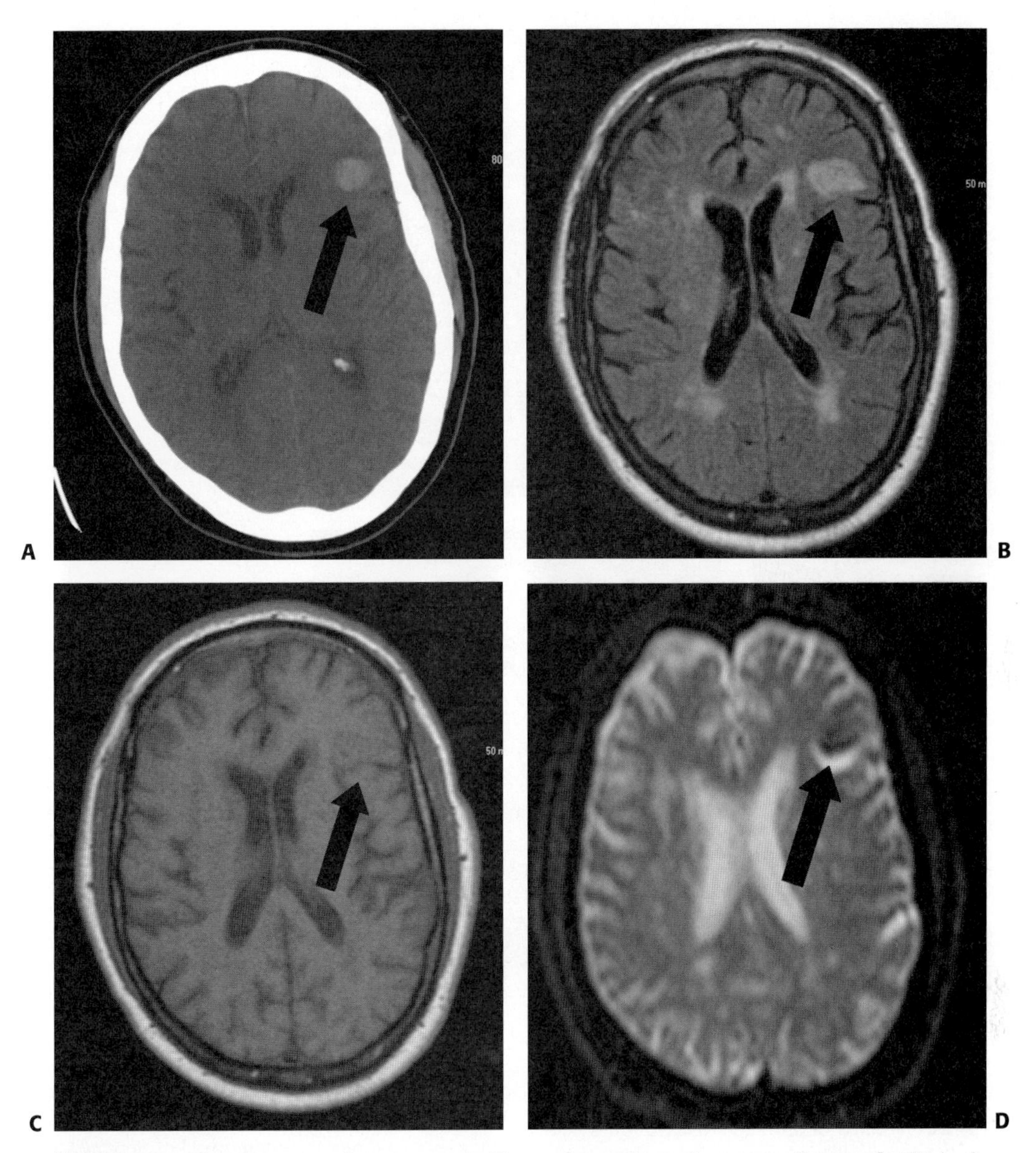

FIGURE 22.6. The appearance of an acute cortical hemorrhage using various types of images. **A:** CT clearly shows the hemorrhage as an area of increased density (*arrow*). **B:** MRI using SE a FLAIR sequences clearly shows the hemorrhage (*arrow*) but does not allow its differentiation from other chronic ischemic lesions. **C:** T1-weighted SE imaging does not clearly show the lesion, which is isointense (*arrow*). **D:** T2 Start (T2*) weighted sequence using GRE clearly shows the lesion as hypointense (*arrow*). CT, donputed tomography; MRI, magnetic resonance imaging; SE, secondary electron. FLAIR, fast, lw-angled inversion recovery, GRE, gradient refocused echo.

cause of these findings, it is apparent that DW-MRI findings represent the earliest sign of ischemic injury, perhaps at a stage in which the tissue can still be recovered. Regions of ischemia have a decreased apparent diffusion coefficient (ADC) and high signal intensity on DW-MRI, reflecting restricted diffusion of protons relative to normal brain (see Fig. 22.7). Further research is currently being conducted in this area, and the future utilization of this technique in the algorithms for imaging cerebrovascular disorders is yet to be uniformly defined.

Perfusion-Weighted MRI

The ability to induce enhancement of MRI with magnetic susceptibility agents that facilitate T2* relaxation provides a method for assessing cerebral blood volume and tissue perfusion. These agents, dysprosium or gadolinium DTPA-BMA (DyDTPA-BMA and GdDTPA-BMA, respectively), are confined to the intravascular space by the intact BBB. A field gradient is created at the capillary level, resulting in significant signal loss in regions with normal blood flow. In contrast, nonperfused areas appear relatively hyperintense. This technique has been shown to significantly advance the time of detection of focal brain ischemia and reveal small infarctions not shown by conventional MRI sequences. In addition, ultrafast MRI techniques (i.e., echo-planar and turbo FLASH) allow resolution of the passage of contrast through the vascular bed, with kinetic modeling of regional blood flow and volume (see Figs. 22.8 and 22.9).

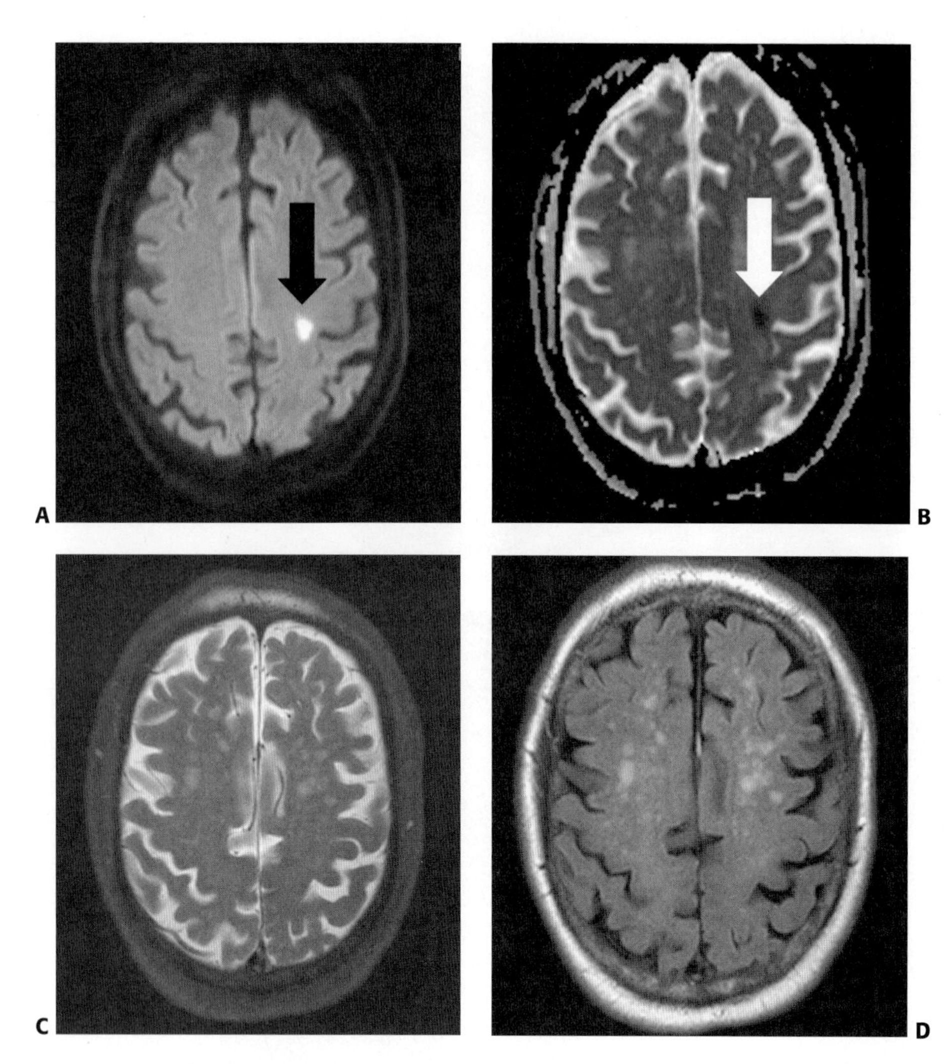

FIGURE 22.7. MRI appearance of an acute and small white matter infarction of the left hemisphere. The DWI sequence clearly shows the lesion as a hyperintense area (*black arrow,* **A**). The ADC is clearly reduced (*white arrow,* **B**). Note that neither the T2 weighted **(C)** nor FLAIR **(D)** images clearly display the infarction. MRI, magnetic resonance imaging; DWI, diffusion-weighted imaging; ADC, apparent diffusion coefficient.

Magnetic Resonance Spectroscopy

This is probably the least studied of all the MRI techniques currently being investigated. It is clear that ischemia causes a detectable decrease in intracellular pH concurrently with an increase in lactic acid concentration (Fig. 22.9). These findings are accompanied by depletion of adenosine triphosphate (ATP) and phosphocreatine and by increased inorganic phosphate concentration. With the development of better techniques for spectral editing and localization, it is possible to separate the tissue in question. This technique may be most useful in the assessment of the reversibility of ischemic brain damage. However, further studies will be necessary before a clear idea about its clinical role becomes available.

Magnetic Resonance Angiography

From the perspective of clinical practice, no discussion of the use of MRI for studying patients with stroke would be complete without describing the sequences that allow the assessment of the cerebral vasculature. In general, MRA adds to our ability to assess all aspects of stroke by helping us identify vascular anomalies, either congenital or acquired, that may be causally related to the cerebrovascular process (e.g., stenoses, vascular malformations). Originally, the use of SE MRI sequences produced images in which there was negative visualization of the cerebral blood vessels due to their characteristic signal-void relative to the speed of flowing blood. This was recognized early in the utilization of MRI but did not seem to provide a reliable method for studying the cerebral vasculature. The advent of fast-scanning MRI pulse sequencing, particularly GRE and bipolar flow-encoding gradient, has allowed direct vascular imaging and the widespread utilization of MRA.

At present, and specifically for imaging intracranial vessels, either time-of-flight (TOF) or phase-contrast (PC) techniques can be applied. The technique of TOF angiography is based on the phenomenon of flow-related enhancement, and it can be performed with either two-or three-dimensional volume acquisitions. It utilizes flip angles of <60 degrees and no refocusing 180-degree pulse (the echo is refocused by reversing the readout gradient). This type of MRA can be carried out using one of several GRE methods, including FLASH, FISP, and GRASS (Table 22.2). On the other hand, PC angiography is based on the detection f velocity-induced phase shifts to distinguish flowing blood from the surrounding stationary tissue. By using bipolar flow-sensitized gradients it is possible to subtract the two acquisitions of opposite polarity and no net phase (stationary tissue) from

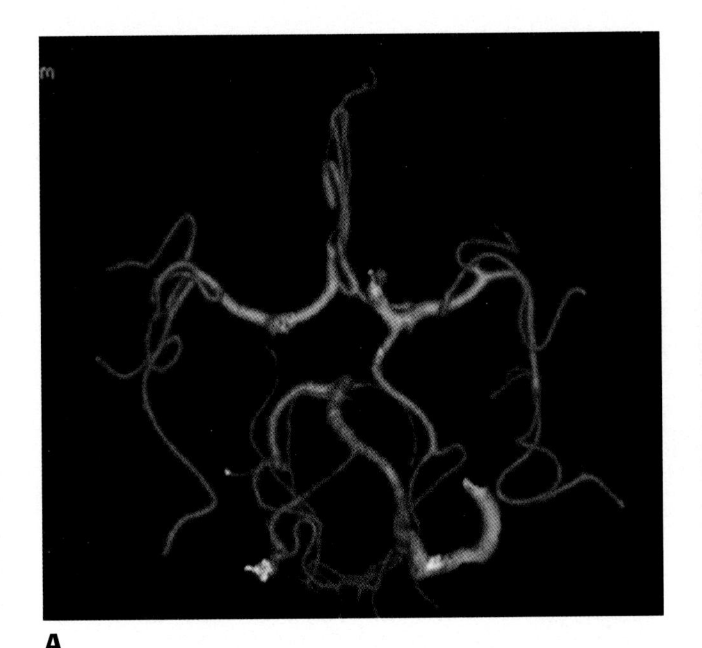

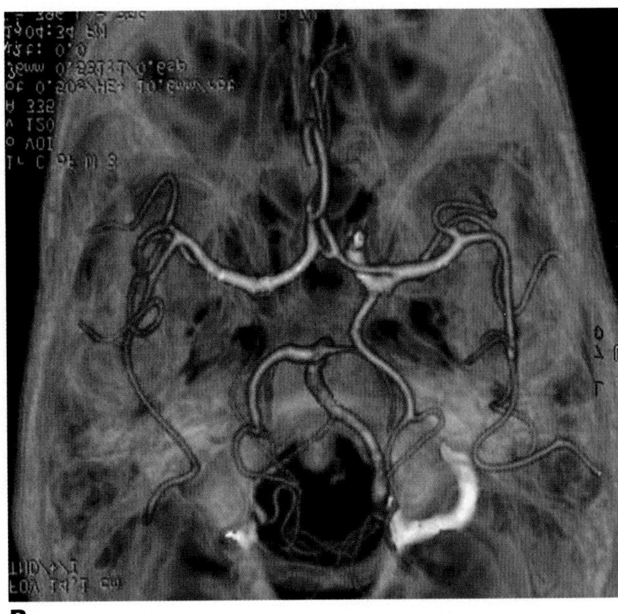

A B

FIGURE 22.2. Three-dimensional rendering of the intracranial arteries using computed tomographic angiography (CTA). The arteries are displayed by themselves in the axial plane **(A)**. It is also possible to display them in the context of the surrounding bony environment **(B)**.

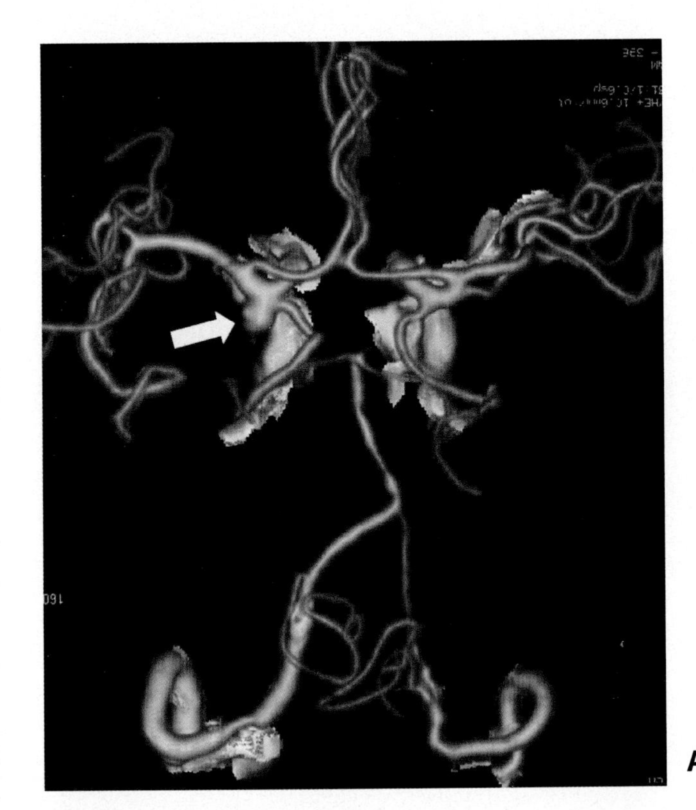

FIGURE 22.3. Use of CTA to diagnose aneurysms. Three-dimensional rendering of the CTA clearly identifies a left posterior communicating artery aneurysm (*arrow*).

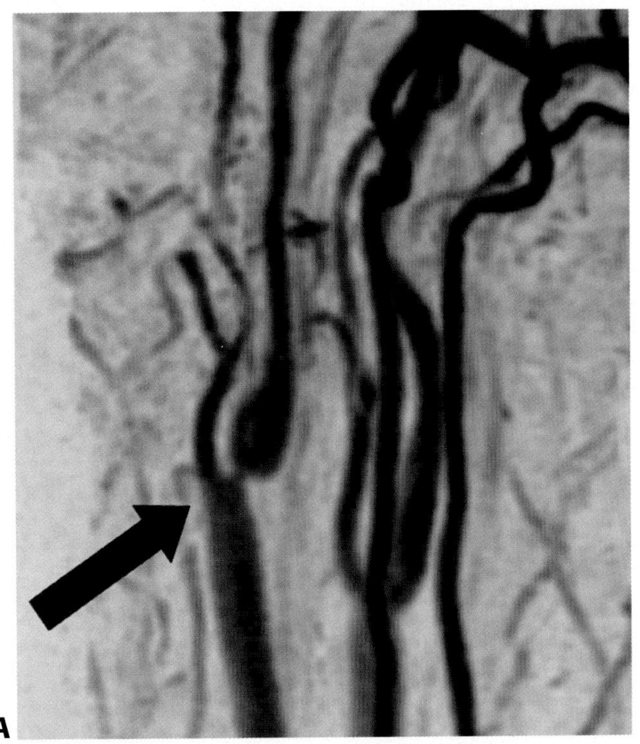

A

FIGURE 22.8. A–C. The hemodynamic effects of a moderate degree of internal carotid artery stenosis. The MRA shows a stenosis of the origin of the right internal carotid artery (*arrow*, **A**).

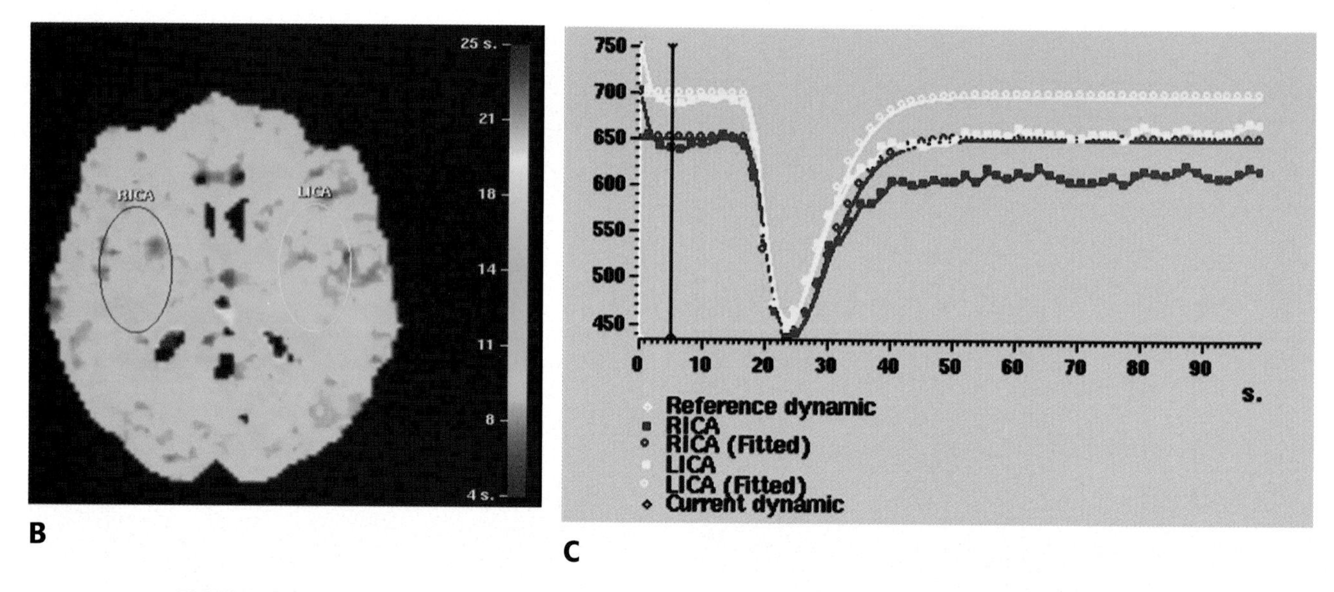

FIGURE 22.8. (*continued*) Perfusion MRI shows a graphic representation of the mean transit time (MTT) of the flow in both regions of interest **(B)**, as well as a direct measurement with graphic plot **(C)**. No significant side-to-side differences are found.

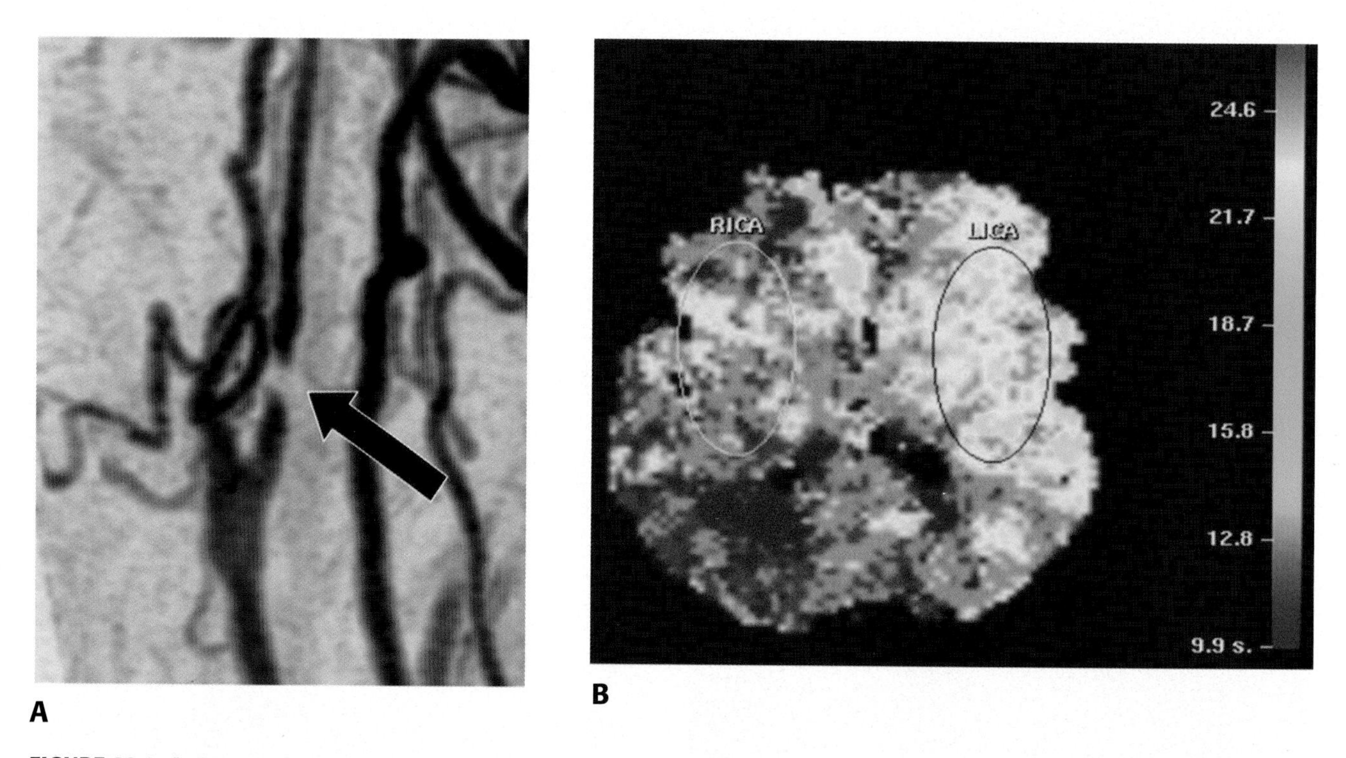

FIGURE 22.9. A–E. Hemodynamic and metabolic consequences of a severe internal carotid artery stenosis. The MRA shows a signal gap in the proximal right internal carotid artery (*arrow*, **A**). Perfusion MRI shows the imaging **(B)** representation of the mean transit time (MTT).

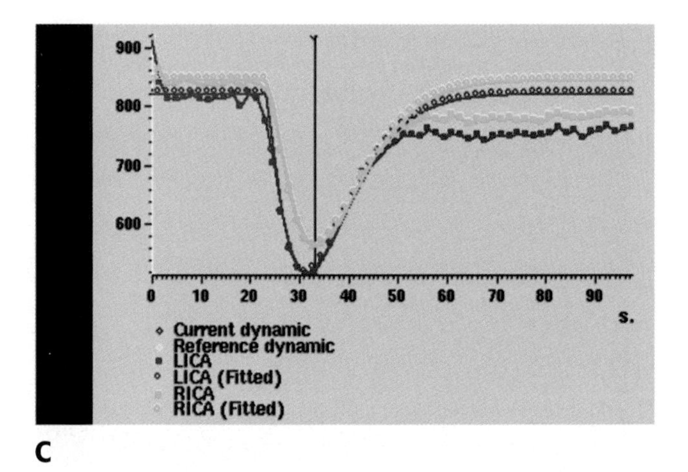

C

FIGURE 22.9. (*continued*) Perfusion MRI shows the mathematic/graphic **(C)** representation of the MTT of both regions of interest. There is clear delay in the right internal carotid artery territory. In addition, MR spectroscopy analysis of the arterial borderzones of the right **(D)** and left **(E)** internal carotid arteries also show a difference. On the right side, a tall peak consistent with lactate accumulation (*arrow*, **D**) is suggestive of ischemic metabolism.

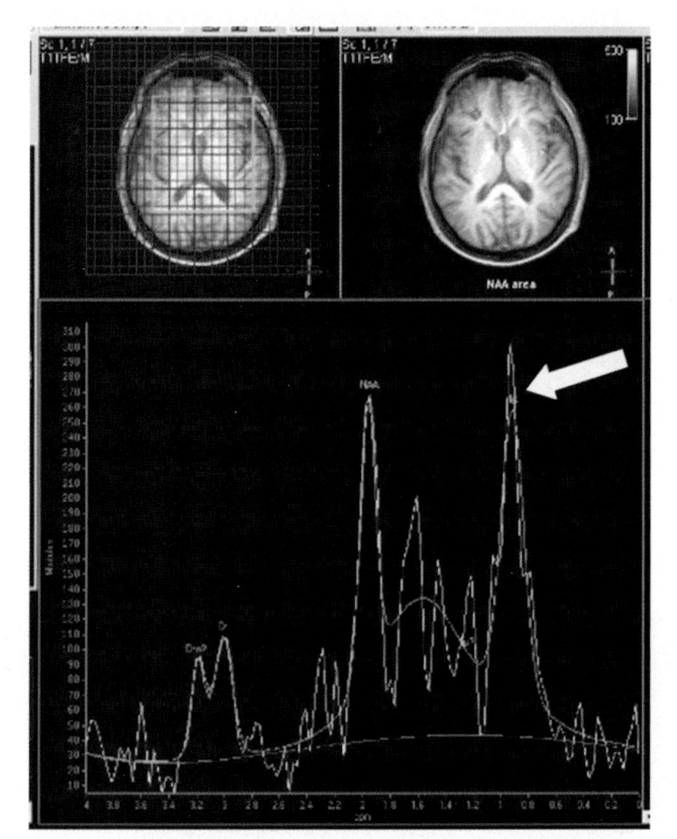

D

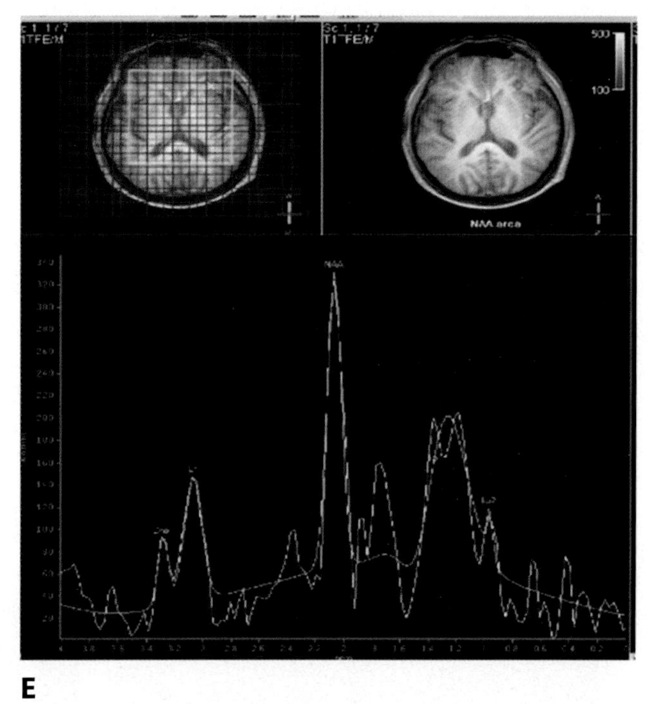

E

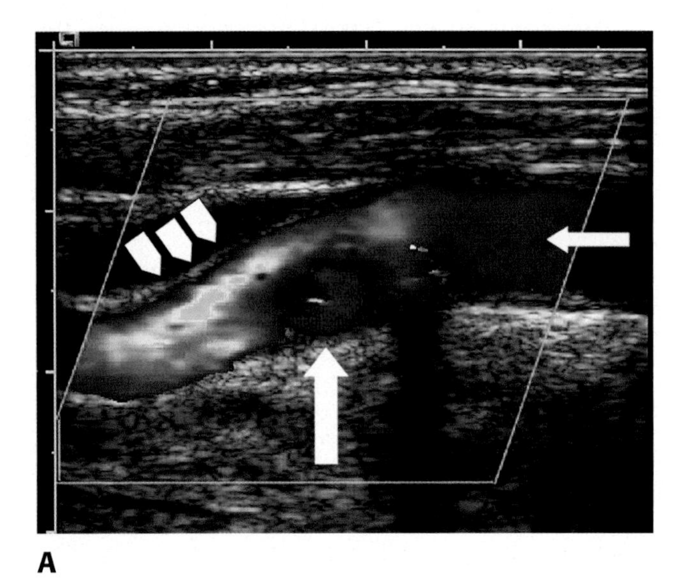

A

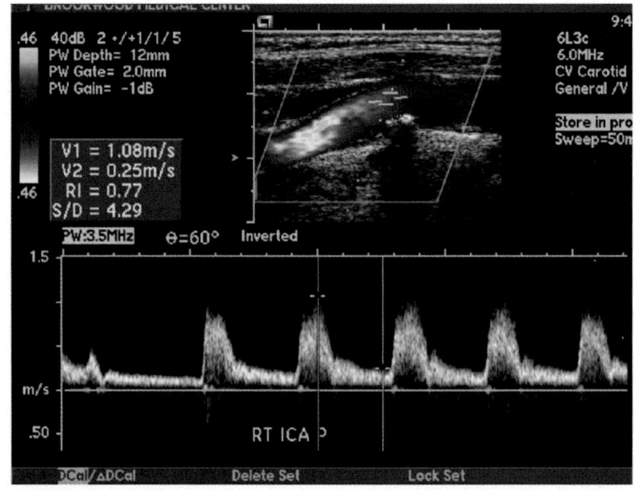

B

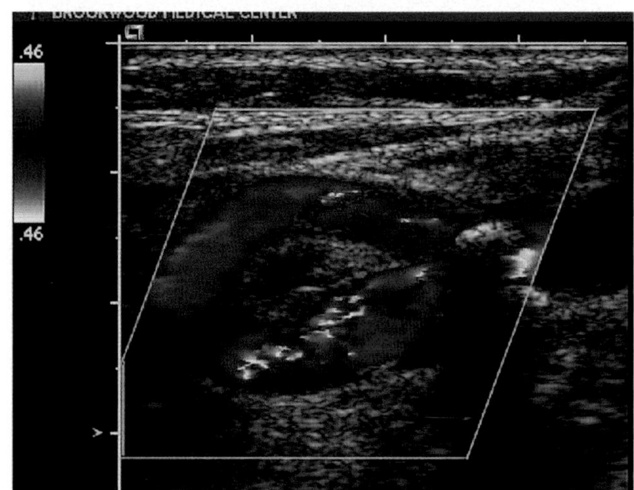

C

FIGURE 22.12. CDI superimposes a dynamic image of flow unto the B-mode image of tissue. Longitudinal view of the plaque shown in Figure 22.11C is characterized by a difference between laminar inflow (*small arrow*, **A**) and turbulent outflow (*arrowheads*, **A**). Flow reversal immediately distal to the plaque is also evident (*large arrow*, **A**). Clearly, CDI facilitates Doppler sampling **(B)**. Furthermore, it clarifies complex flow patterns in bifurcations **(C)**.

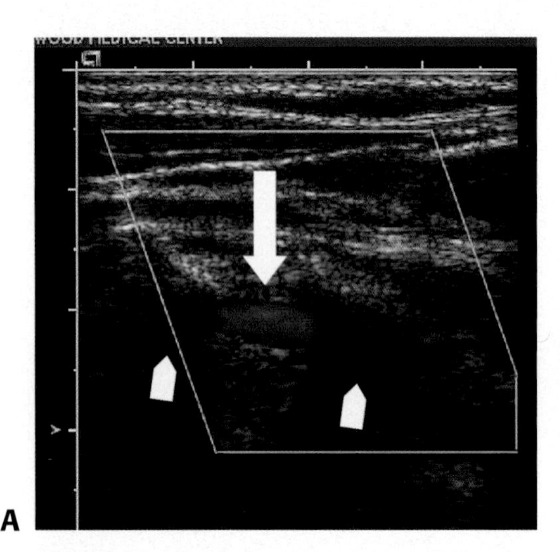

A

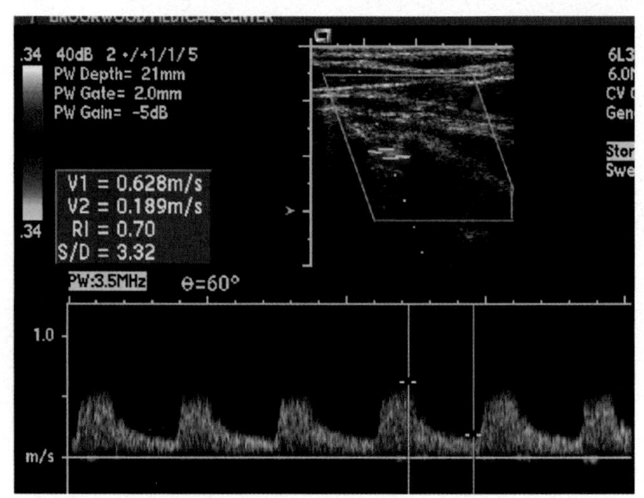

B

FIGURE 22.13. CDI allows examination of the extracranial vertebral arteries. Longitudinal views shows the vessel (*large arrow*, **A**) flowing within the vertebral canal. Visualization is intermittent due to the echogenic artifact of the vertebra (*arrowheads*, **A**). Doppler sampling of the vertebral artery is also possible **(B)**.

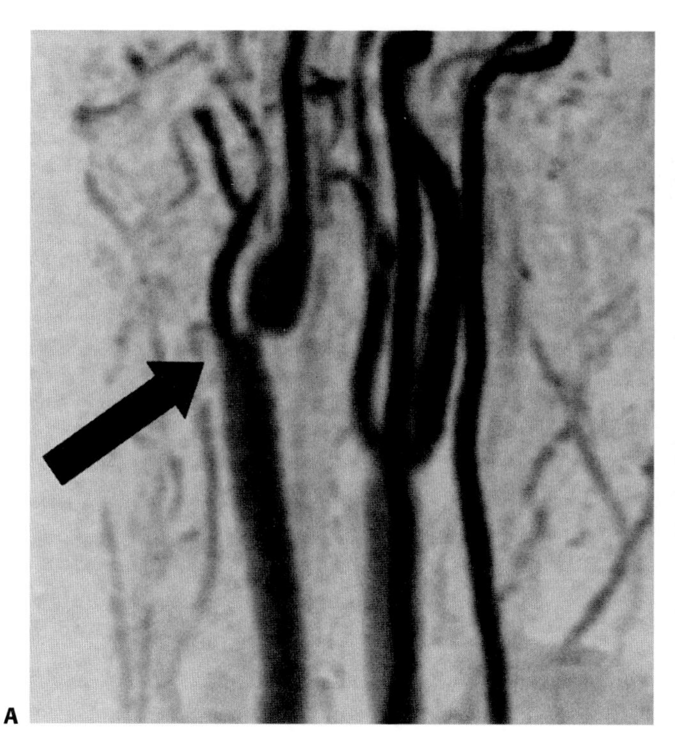

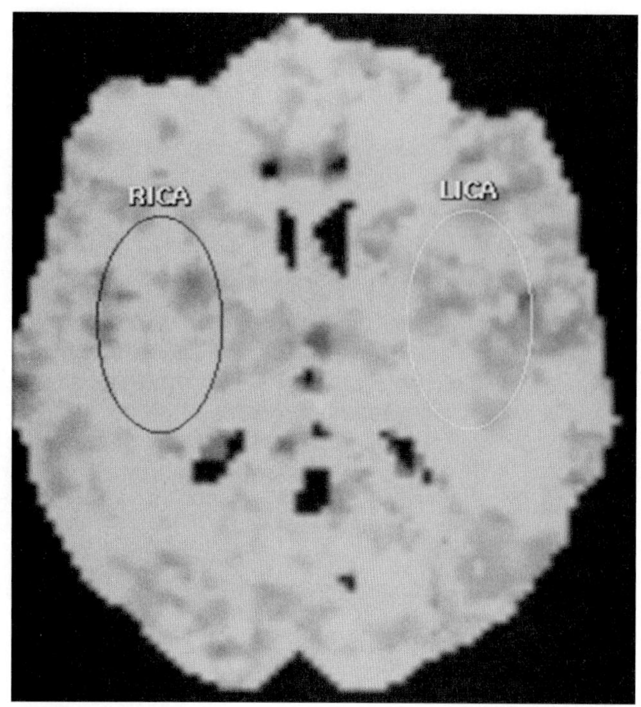

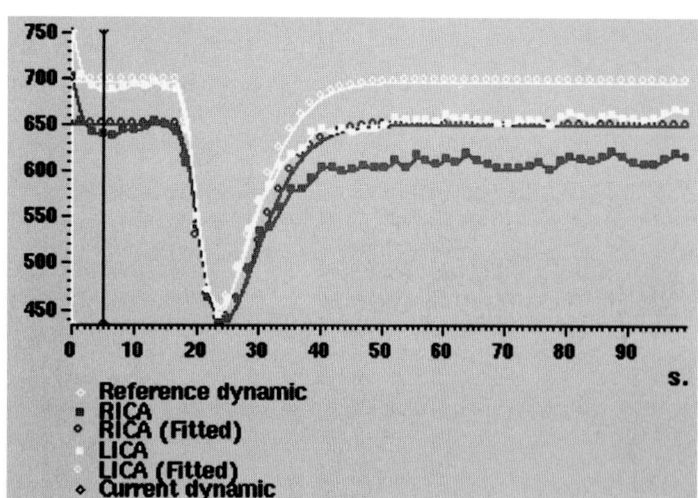

FIGURE 22.8. The hemodynamic effects of a moderate degree of internal carotid artery stenosis. The MRA shows a stenosis of the origin of the right internal carotid artery (*arrow*, **A**). Perfusion MRI shows a graphic representation of the mean transit time (MTT) of the flow in both regions of interest **(B)**, as well as a direct measurement with graphic plot **(C)**. No significant side-to-side differences are found. *(See color insert.)*

one another. The data that remain reflect the phase shift induced by flowing blood. The use of cardiac gating helps overcome the sensitivity of PC angiography to pulsatile and nonuniform flow.

The advantages of MRA are obvious; it can be carried out as part of the entire MRI evaluation of the patient, and for the intracranial circulation, it does not require contrast administration. Furthermore, in the context of using very high field (i.e., 3.0 Tesla) instruments, the vascular detail is simply exquisite, with an ability to resolve very small pathologic structures (see Fig. 22.10). The main disadvantage is the fact that it is not widely understood that MRA represents an anatomic rendering of flow dynamics, not vessel anatomy! This results in common misinterpretations of the images due to wrongful expectations and assumptions.

Neurovascular Ultrasonography: Noninvasive Flexibility

Ultrasound provides noninvasive methods by which it is possible to obtain diagnostic information, both anatomic and physiologic. All of these methods are based on the interaction of ultrasound waves transmitted into the tissues, and the echoes generated and returning from the tissues. The domain of vascular ultrasonography includes all the ultrasonic methods that are primarily used for the study of blood vessels and blood flow. It is possible to apply the principles of vascular ultrasonography to the evaluation of patients with disorders of the cerebral circulation.

In 1959, Satomura described the usefulness of Doppler ultrasound to evaluate arteries and veins. This was followed by the

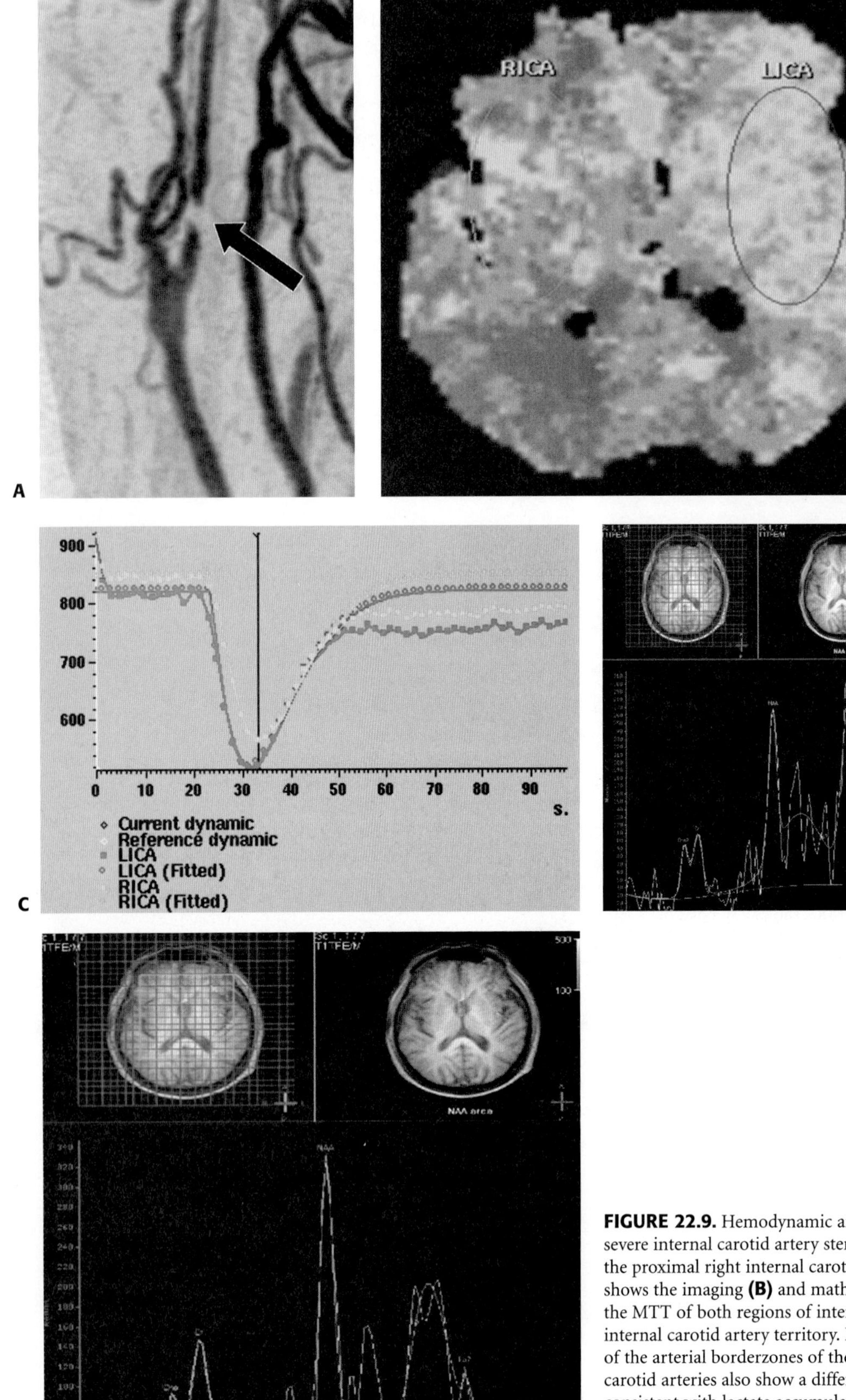

FIGURE 22.9. Hemodynamic and metabolic consequences of a severe internal carotid artery stenosis. The MRA shows a signal gap in the proximal right internal carotid artery (*arrow*, **A**). Perfusion MRI shows the imaging **(B)** and mathematic/graphic **(C)** representation of the MTT of both regions of interest. There is clear delay in the right internal carotid artery territory. In addition, MR spectroscopy analysis of the arterial borderzones of the right **(D)** and left **(E)** internal carotid arteries also show a difference. On the right side, a tall peak consistent with lactate accumulation (*arrow*, **D**) is suggestive of ischemic metabolism.*(See color insert.)*

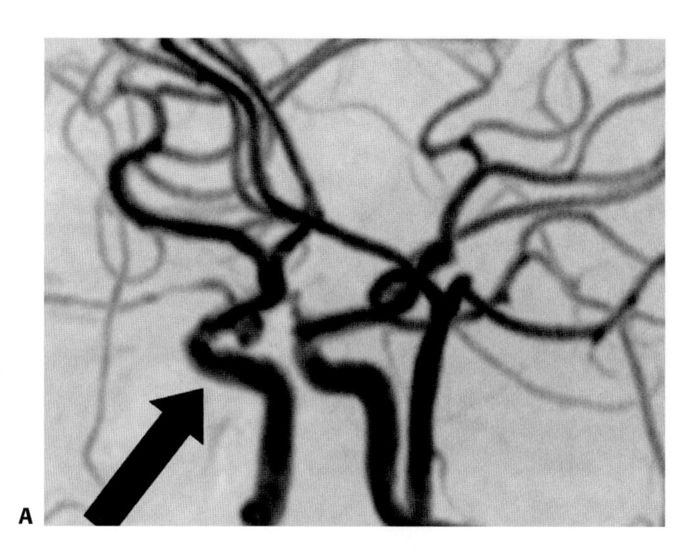

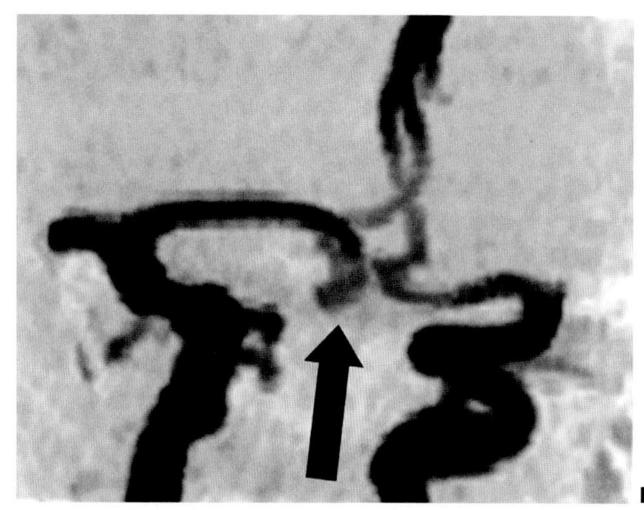

FIGURE 22.10. Ability of MRA to resolve small structures such as aneurysms. A right internal carotid artery wide neck clinoid aneurysm **(A)** is easily visualized. Three-dimensional postprocessing defines an anterior communicating artery aneurysm **(B)**.

development of Doppler instruments to study the peripheral vasculature and later the carotid arteries. In the assessment of carotid atherosclerosis, at first, Doppler techniques were utilized to document reversal of periorbital flow direction. This, at least theoretically, implicates high-grade internal carotid artery stenosis. Later, continuous wave (CW) Doppler transducers allowed the direct study of the extracranial carotid arteries and the detection of stenoses >50% by the flow acceleration they caused. Small plaques that had no hemodynamic effect, however, were commonly missed. Conversely, ultrasonic real-time B-mode imaging of the extracranial vessels, which resulted in the identification of smaller carotid artery plaques, failed to provide dynamic information about flow disturbances. The sensitivity and specificity of either of these ultrasonic techniques were still so low, which prevented their unconditional acceptance by many clinicians. In the late 1970s, the technique of real time imaging was combined with pulsed-wave Doppler and a new, more reliable system was introduced: Duplex ultrasound. This combined the sensitivity of high-resolution real time B-mode imaging for small plaques with the precision of pulsed-wave Doppler for assessing flow velocity characteristics at specific points within the blood vessels. The introduction of duplex ultrasound resulted in an immediate increase in the confidence with which noninvasive evaluation was considered, particularly in the outpatient setting. The technologic step that followed conventional duplex ultrasound was an imaginative yet improbable one: color Doppler imaging (CDI). Until 1982, the use of ultrasound to study the cerebral blood vessels was limited to their extracranial segments. The sonic barrier represented by the skull was first crossed by Aaslid and his collaborators when, using a low-frequency (2 MHz) pulsed Doppler ultrasonic transducer, they were able to noninvasively study the hemodynamic characteristics of the basal cerebral blood vessels. This marked the introduction of transcranial Doppler (TCD) as a research and later as a clinical tool.

Extracranial Ultrasound

The association between ischemic cerebrovascular events and atherosclerosis of the extracranial portion of the carotid arteries has been the main factor behind the development of neurovascular ultrasonography. In theory, carotid atheromatous plaques can be assessed in regard to (a) the degree of stenosis they cause, (b) their surface characteristics, and (c) their histomorphology. Using duplex ultrasound, plaques can be fully studied by direct visualization, both sagitally and transversely (see Fig. 22.11). This technique can assess the hemodynamic derangements caused by atheromatous plaques and help in the risk stratification of the patient.

The degree of stenosis caused by atheromatous plaques can be readily evaluated by duplex ultrasound, as follows: The B-mode image displays the spatial relationship between the plaque and the vessels, while the PW Doppler shows the turbulence and flow acceleration caused by it. This acceleration, accompanied by disruption of normal laminar flow, increases progressively as the lumen narrows and allows estimation of the degree of stenosis and hemodynamic impact of the plaque. The evaluation of plaque surface characteristics is geared toward the determination of whether the plaque is ulcerated, a factor that has been believed to contribute to the increased risk for stroke. Unfortunately, ulceration implies a disruption in the endothelium continuity, a characteristic not easily discernible by any of the available diagnostic techniques. From this perspective, ulcers would have to be differentiated from plaque surface irregularities (craters), which are probably more frequent and are associated with an intact endothelium. The ability of B-mode ultrasound to identify ulcers is not considered optimal, although it is similar to that of angiography. In regards to the assessment of plaque morphology, the literature suggests that soft plaques, as well as unstable plaques, represent a greater risk for the development of stroke. At present, plaque morphology can only be assessed ultrasonically, as follows: the B-mode images show whether the plaque is soft (fibrofatty), fibrous, or calcific depending on its echogenic characteristics (i.e., fibrofatty plaques are echolucent, while calcific plaques and echodense) (Fig. 22.11). Other characteristics, such as intraplaque hemorrhage, another finding believed to be a risk factor for stroke, can also be identified by B-mode ultrasound.

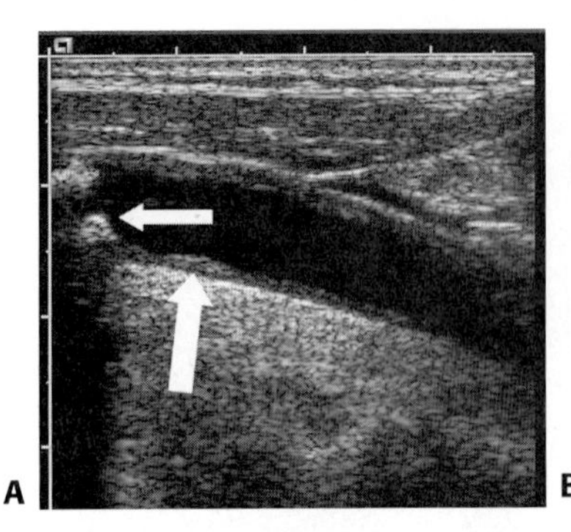

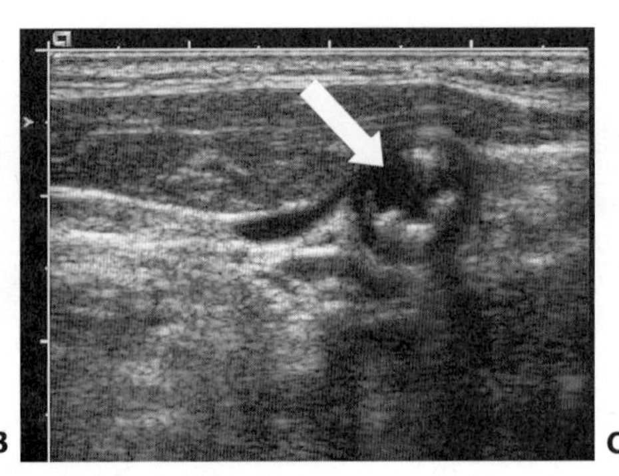

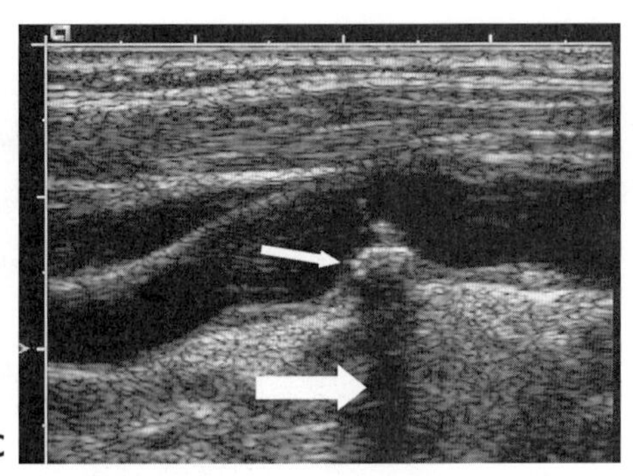

FIGURE 22.11. B-mode ultrasound examination of the extracranial carotid system. Sagittal imaging **(A)** allows identification of intimal thickening (*large arrow*) as well as a calcific plaque (*small arrow*). Transverse imaging **(B)** allows cross-sectional assessment of residual lumen (*arrow*). Calcific plaques (*small arrow*, **C**) are characterized by acoustic shadows (*large arrow*).

The main role of duplex ultrasound is the early assessment (screening) of patients at risk of ischemic stroke, and their follow-up. The recent results of multicenter studies designed to assess the effectiveness of carotid endarterectomy have placed significant pressure on clinicians because of the need for quick identification of patients with ischemic brain events resulting from atheromatous plaques that meet the criteria for surgical treatment. In spite of suggestions that these results (which are based on strict an often peculiar angiographic criteria) demand the absolute need for angiographic evaluation, clinical practice dictates that duplex ultrasound is a reliable tool that allows clinicians to plan further evaluation and care. Finally, the discussion so far has been centered on the ultrasonic evaluation of the carotid artery system. It must be noted, however, that the flow direction and velocity of the vertebral arteries within the vertebral canal of the cervical spine can also be assessed with duplex ultrasound.

Color Doppler Imaging

CDI presents two-dimensional cross-sectional Doppler shift information superimposed on grayscale anatomic images. It utilizes the pulse-echo imaging principle by which a pulse of ultrasound is emitted into the tissues and its echoes are then received and analyzed. Echoes returning from stationary tissues are detected and presented in grayscale in appropriate locations within the scan line. When a returning echo has a frequency different from when it was emitted, it implies the occurrence of a Doppler shift. Such Doppler shift can be detected along the scan line and its sign (positive or negative), magnitude, and variance can be recorded. These variables are utilized by the instrument to determine the hue, saturation, and luminance of the color pixel at its location on the display. Each pixel is then updated multiple times per second, creating dynamic images of the flowing blood (see Fig. 22.12). Recently, instrumentation capable of performing direct color velocity imaging (rather than frequency shift imaging) has also been introduced. Traditionally, CDI has been considered to have the following advantages over duplex.

1. It allows easier identification of vascular structures, leading to faster scanning time.
2. It is helpful in differentiating plaque stenoses from other problems, such as kinks.
3. It allows appreciation of flow disturbances, even in the absence of stenosis (Fig. 22.12).
4. It helps identify very small amounts of flow (e.g., critical stenosis or string sign).
5. It rapidly identifies echolucent plaques based on the absence of flow.
6. It allows better delineation of surface features.

In general, the application of CDI is quite similar to that of conventional duplex ultrasound. However, the sophisticated nature

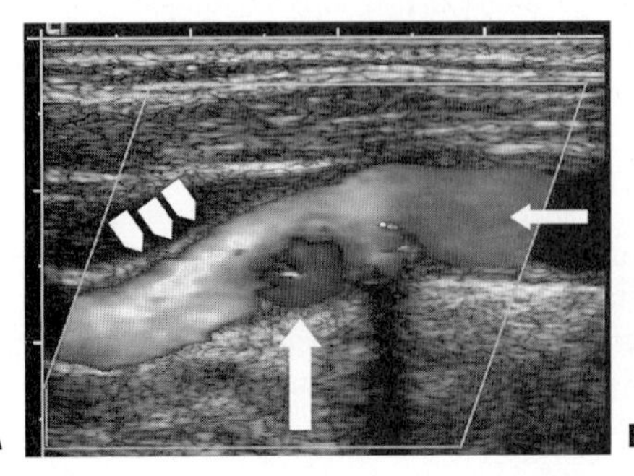

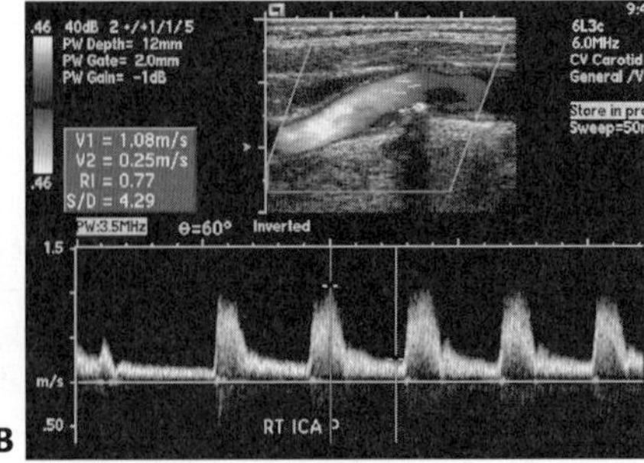

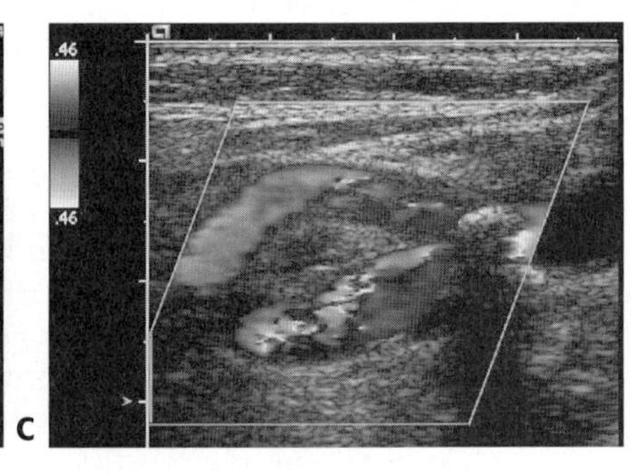

FIGURE 22.12. CDI superimposes a dynamic image of flow unto the B-mode image of tissue. Longitudinal view of the plaque shown in Figure 22.11C is characterized by a difference between laminar inflow (*small arrow*, **A**) and turbulent outflow (*arrowheads*, **A**). Flow reversal immediately distal to the plaque is also evident (*large arrow*, **A**). Clearly, CDI facilitates Doppler sampling **(B)**. Furthermore, it clarifies complex flow patterns in bifurcations **(C)**. *(See color insert.)*

of the images produced has resulted in its application in the evaluation of conditions other than carotid atherosclerosis, including carotid body tumors, intimal fibroplasia, and dissection. Finally, CDI has expanded the ability to evaluate the vertebral arteries as they course through the vertebral canal of the cervical spine extracranially (see Fig. 22.13).

Transcranial Doppler

TCD ultrasound is a diagnostic technique based on the use of a range-gated pulse-Doppler ultrasonic beam of 2 MHz frequency to assess the hemodynamic characteristics of the major cerebral arteries. The ultrasonic beam crosses the intact adult skull at points known as *windows*, bounces off the erythrocytes flowing within the basal brain arteries, and allows the determination of blood flow velocity, direction of flow, collateral patterns, and state of cerebral vasoreactivity. By sampling multiple cerebral blood vessels using TCD it is possible to identify patterns pointing to lesions localized intra- or extracranially, to follow up their natural history over time, and even to monitor the effects of therapeutic strategies. Although certainly having its own inherent limitations, TCD provides physiological information about the brain circulation, which cannot be obtained by any other means. In addition to the uniqueness of the information gathered by TCD, the other attractive characteristics of this technique are that it is noninvasive (i.e., safe), reproducible, versatile, and dynamic.

The utilization of TCD in clinical practice over the last decade has made us change to a limited extent our concept of the role that it plays. The technique, rather an ancillary procedure, is best conceived as a specialized stethoscope that allows clinicians to listen to the hemodynamic changes of the brain blood vessels and to compare the findings over time. Indeed, the best approach to TCD is to consider it as an extension of the clinical examination, analogous to the way in which electromyography has been regarded for many years. From the clinical point of view, TCD is an ideal tool not only for diagnosis but also for follow-up. Just as cardiologists have previously performed sequential auscultatory examinations of patients while looking for new murmurs that would alert the cardiologists to the development of valvular dysfunction, it is also possible to use TCD to alert us about the presence of hemodynamic disturbances representative of cerebrovascular pathology.

The clinical context in which TCD was introduced was the detection of vasospasm in patients with aneurysmal subarachnoid hemorrhage. Since then, however, there has been an explosion in its utilization in a variety of clinical and research scenarios. Time and time again the versatility of TCD has prevailed, and the technique has been able to show aspects of various clinical disorders, which were previously not fully understood.

APPLICATION SCENARIOS: DIMENSIONS OF PRACTICE

The tasks noted in the previous section must also be placed in the practical context of three distinct clinical scenarios: (a) the emergency care of a stroke victim, (b) monitoring of stroke evolution, and (c) the nonemergent risk stratification of patients at risk for stroke (for one or another reason). Depending on the scenario, the choice of imaging technique is then guided by the question being asked, the diagnostic characteristics inherent to each imaging modality, and the expectations of results based on the natural history of the process being investigated.

Imaging in Emergency Stroke Care

Most patients with acute stroke are initially evaluated in emergency departments by following algorithms with priorities that include answering specific questions with direct relevance to the management of the patient, both immediate and within the days that follow. At the bedside, the first set of clinical questions confronted by stroke specialists is as follows:

- Does the patient have a stroke?
- Is it an ischemic or a hemorrhagic stroke?
- What vascular territory has been compromised?

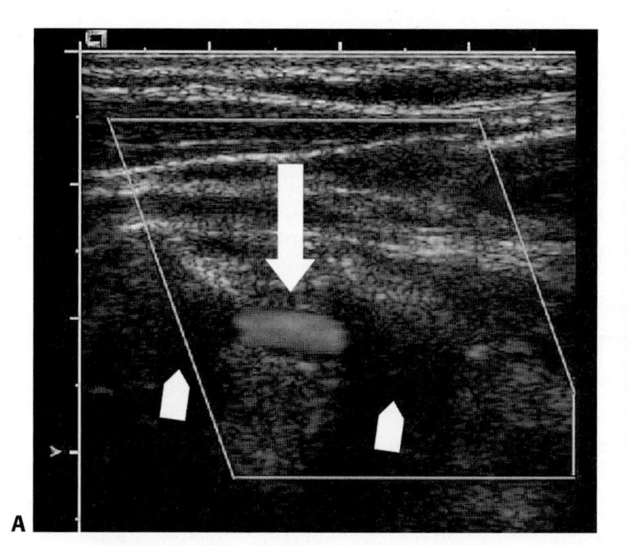

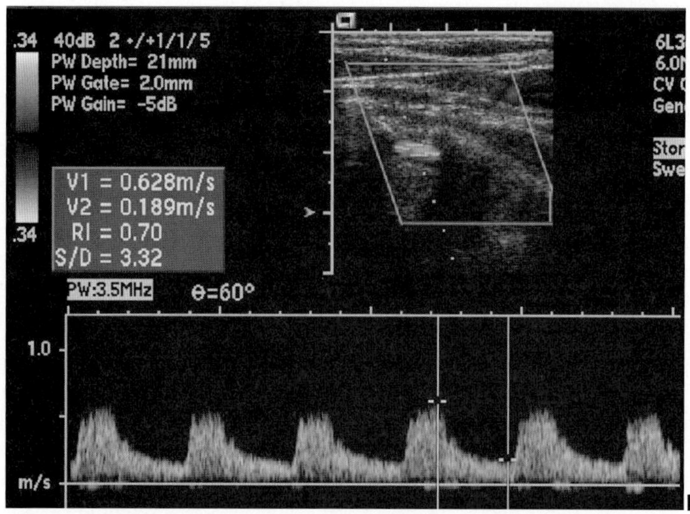

FIGURE 22.13. CDI allows examination of the extracranial vertebral arteries. Longitudinal views shows the vessel (*large arrow*, **A**) flowing within the vertebral canal. Visualization is intermittent due to the echogenic artifact of the vertebra (*arrowheads*, **A**). Doppler sampling of the vertebral artery is also possible **(B)**. *(See color insert.)*

- What is the risk of death or significant neurologic disability?
- What is the likelihood of neurologic deterioration?

Once the first set of questions is answered, and the presumptive diagnosis of stroke is made, imaging of the brain becomes an imminent necessity. It is important to know whether (a) the event is ischemic or hemorrhagic, (b) the brain has already undergone damage, and (c) there is any alternative diagnostic possibility. In the past, it was thought that astute clinicians could easily make the differentiation between hemorrhagic and ischemic stroke at the bedside. The introduction of CT in the 1970s, however, clearly showed the inaccuracies of clinical differentiation, while it provided an easy method for making this diagnostic distinction. In fact, at present, emergency CT imaging is of paramount importance in the early evaluation of patients with acute stroke, as well as a pivoting point in any emergency stroke treatment algorithm. Even more recently, MRI techniques have become more popular in the emergency assessment of stroke patients because of their versatility, thoroughness, and ability to provided significantly relevant ancillary information that has direct effect on the treatment protocols.

In the urgent evaluation of suspected stroke patients, all possible neuroimaging findings can be allocated into one of the following categories:

- *Normal brain tissue*: Many patients presenting early with acute or hyperacute ischemic brain processes have normal CT scans. This results from the low sensitivity of the test for the detection of ischemic tissue within the first few hours of evolution. A normal CT scan in the context of a patient with an acute focal neurologic deficit by no means excludes the diagnosis of ischemic stroke, and in fact, this should be considered a good sign. Indeed, the fact that the tissue is not shown as irreparably damaged should open numerous possibilities for therapeutic intervention. Clearly, for patients suspected of having hemorrhagic stroke, a normal CT scan almost completely excludes the diagnosis. In the case of MRI, on the other hand, the subject is quite different. In fact, it is very common to find evidence of acute ischemia (i.e., restricted diffusion) in patients whose symptoms may have completely cleared. This finding, which challenges the traditional definition of transient ischemic attack, has a corollary: A perfectly normal, high-quality DWI study almost unequivocally implies the absence of any type of stroke.
- *Abnormal, demonstrating the acute stroke*: The appearance of infarction on CT during the first few hours largely depends on the size and location of the affected tissue. Large territories supplied by the carotid artery system [e.g., middle cerebral artery (MCA)] have a tendency to be displayed earlier than smaller territories supplied by the vertebrobasilar system (e.g., penetrating pontine arteries). The early signs of infarction include changes of gray matter density with loss of gray–white matter differentiation, evolving into frank hypodensity and early signs of edema over the next 12 to 24 hours. Hemorrhagic strokes are displayed as hyperdense areas corresponding to the extravasated blood, for which CT is highly sensitive. The sensitivity of MRI for early ischemia, particularly due to the use of DWI sequences, is severalfold greater than that of CT. The ischemic lesions typically are displayed as areas of increased signal due to restricted diffusion. The use of MRI in the assessment of hemorrhagic stroke is a more recent topic, following the introduction of GRE techniques capable of sensitively displaying changes related to the magnetic characteristics of hemoglobin.
- *Abnormal, with findings related to the acute stroke*: Frequently, CT scans show abnormalities that bear a relationship with the ischemic stroke. For example, in patients with occlusion of the MCA, the hyperdense MCA signs have been described. This exemplifies the appearance of a vessel acutely occluded by a blood clot as a hyperdense structure within the Sylvian fissure. Also, a more common finding the calcification of the brain arteries (e.g., carotid or vertebral), implying the presence of atherosclerotic plaques that are capable of causing narrowing of these vessels. For patients with hemorrhagic strokes, it is sometimes possible to identify an aneurysm by its calcification and location. Using MRI, the same is true, but even to a greater extent since the MRI is much more informative because of the various other sequences that can be utilized concurrently.
- *Abnormal, displaying previous strokes*: Often, patients who present with acute stroke are found to have abnormal CT and MRI scans that demonstrate preexisting strokes. These represent the evidence of cerebrovascular abnormalities, either intrinsic or secondary to other processes, and they can help in the diagnostic process. For example, evidence of infarctions in multiple bilateral territories may represent evidence of a cardiogenic or aortogenic source of embolism. On the other hand, previous infarctions clustered within one hemisphere may represent the effect of unilateral severe carotid stenosis.
- *Abnormal, displaying an alternative diagnostic process*: Not every patient who presents with a clinical syndrome suggestive of stroke has one. CT and MRI are helpful in uncovering other conditions that mimic stroke and require alternative treatment (e.g., subdural hematoma).
- *Abnormal, showing a combination of the various above:* The routine utilization of contrast during CT examination of the emergency stroke patient is, in our opinion, unwarranted. The potential enhancement of any of the tissue in patients with acute ischemia serves no clinical purpose since it does not help guide treatment. Furthermore, there is at least some suggestion in the literature that contrast media are somewhat neurotoxic to ischemic tissue. For the patient with hemorrhagic stroke, it adds even less. Furthermore, in certain clinical scenarios, such a practice is dangerous. The intense nausea that can be produced by intravenous contrast administration, in fact, can jeopardize the fate of patients with ruptured aneurysms.

Monitoring of Stroke Evolution

Regardless of how the patient is being treated, the time continuum that follows initial evaluation and treatment demands that the clinical team follows the evolution of the patient to make on-the-fly decisions about which aspects of treatment to continue and which ones to change. In certain situations, such as in the intensive care unit (ICU), when clinical assessment may not be easy or feasible because of the need for deep sedation, imaging becomes of paramount importance to assess changes and guide therapy. In this context, currently portable CT scanners are available that allow the study of critically ill stroke patients without moving them out of the ICU, resulting in a significant advantage for the treatment team to follow up patients as they evolve, either positively or negatively. An example of the former is the resolution of hydrocephalus in a patient who requires a ventriculostomy following an intraventricular hemorrhage. On the other hand, the latter is best exemplified by the follow up of a patient with malignant brain edema secondary to a large hemispheric infarction.

As time elapses, the appearance of the two major forms of stroke on CT scanning changes. Infarcted tissue develops swelling and its margins become progressively better demarcated. Its density decreases progressively as the damaged tissue shrinks, producing ex vacuo enlargement of adjacent structures (i.e., ventricles). In the case of hemorrhages, on the other hand, the globin molecule of the blood breaks down, and the blood progressively loses its high-density appearance. This change occurs centripetally, and its speed depends largely on the size of the original hemorrhage. Subacute hemorrhages are typically isodense with the brain, while chronic ones present as remnant hypodensities that replace the injured tissue. The appearance of hemorrhagic strokes over time in MRI has been described in the preceding text.

Imaging and Risk Stratification Algorithms

The diagnostic perspective of patients with stroke revolves around defining the stroke subtype (i.e., identifying the cause and mechanism of the stroke). This leads to a somewhat educated prediction of the risk of subsequent strokes, while it allows the implementation of secondary prevention strategies tailored to the individual patient. In this context, the importance of imaging techniques cannot be overemphasized. Three categories of disorders are capable of leading to the production of stroke: (a) cardiac abnormalities, (b) neurovascular abnormalities per se, and (c) hematologic disorders. As noted earlier, cardiac imaging and hematologic disorders will not be covered in this chapter, since they are both addressed elsewhere in the book. Vascular imaging includes all techniques designed to display the cerebral vessels and their abnormalities. The techniques currently available for neurovascular diagnosis (excluding catheterization and angiography) include CTA, MRA, CDI, and TCD. The practical aspects of choosing one or another depend largely on the following variables: (a) the type of pathology being evaluated, (b) the timing of the evaluation, (c) the availability and technical quality of the diagnostic resources, and (d) the practitioners experience and judgment.

CONCLUSIONS

The utilization of imaging techniques for the evaluation of patients with stroke must be guided by the specific needs of the clinical situation. Newer tests being introduced will not necessarily replace the old ones but rather will provide additional dimensions to our ability to diagnose and treat different conditions capable of causing stroke. It is important to keep in mind that every one of these diagnostic techniques is operator dependent, even if to different degrees. As such, another aspect of choosing the appropriate diagnostic technique requires the recognition of the quality of the resources available.

SELECTED REFERENCES

Albers GW, Thijs VN, Wechsler L, et al. Magnetic resonance imaging profiles predict clinical response to early reperfusion: the diffusion and perfusion imaging evaluation for understanding stroke evolution (DEFUSE) study. *Ann Neurol* 2006;60(5):508–517.

Alexandrov AV, Molina CA, Grotta JC, et al. Ultrasound-enhanced systemic thrombolysis for acute ischemic stroke. *N Engl J Med* 2004;351(21): 2170–2178.

Alexandrov AV, Wojner AW, Grotta JC. CLOTBUST: design of a randomized trial of ultrasound-enhanced thrombolysis for acute ischemic stroke. *J Neuroimaging* 2004;14(2):108–112.

Alsop DC, Makovetskaya E, Kumar S, et al. Markedly reduced apparent blood volume on bolus contrast magnetic resonance imaging as a predictor of hemorrhage after thrombolytic therapy for acute ischemic stroke. *Stroke* 2005;36(4):746–750.

Aronen HJ, Laakso MP, Moser M, et al. Diffusion and perfusion-weighted magnetic resonance imaging techniques in stroke recovery. *Eura Medicophys* 2007;43(2):271–284.

Bilello M, Lao Z, Krejza J, et al. Statistical atlas of acute stroke from magnetic resonance diffusion-weighted-images of the brain. *Neuroinformatics* 2006;4(3):235–242.

Carstairs SD, Tanen DA, Duncan TD, et al. Computed tomographic angiography for the evaluation of aneurysmal subarachnoid hemorrhage. *Acad Emerg Med* 2006;13(5):486–492.

Chalela JA, Gomes J. Magnetic resonance imaging in the evaluation of intracranial hemorrhage. *Expert Rev Neurother* 2004;4(2):267–273.

Chalela JA, Kidwell CS, Nentwich LM, et al. Magnetic resonance imaging and computed tomography in emergency assessment of patients with suspected acute stroke: a prospective comparison. *Lancet* 2007;369(9558):293–298.

Chamorro A. Magnetic resonance perfusion diffusion mismatch, thrombolysis, and clinical outcome in acute stroke. *J Neurol Neurosurg Psychiatr* 2007;78(5):443.

Cheung RT. Differentiation between intracerebral hemorrhage and ischemic stroke by transcranial duplex sonography. *Stroke* 1999;30(8):1735–1736.

Davis DP, Robertson T, Imbesi SG. Diffusion-weighted magnetic resonance imaging versus computed tomography in the diagnosis of acute ischemic stroke. *J Emerg Med* 2006;31(3):269–277.

Demchuk AM, Hill MD, Barber PA, et al. Importance of early ischemic computed tomography changes using ASPECTS in NINDS rtPA Stroke Study. *Stroke* 2005;36(10):2110–2115.

Evans AL, Coley SC, Wilkinson ID, et al. First-line investigation of acute intracerebral hemorrhage using dynamic magnetic resonance angiography. *Acta Radiol* 2005;46(6):625–630.

Gahn G, von Kummer R. Ultrasound in acute stroke: a review. *Neuroradiology* 2001;43(9):702–711.

Greer DM, Koroshetz WJ, Cullen S, et al. Magnetic resonance imaging improves detection of intracerebral hemorrhage over computed tomography after intra-arterial thrombolysis. *Stroke* 2004;35(2):491–495.

Griffiths PD, Wilkinson ID. MR imaging of recent non-traumatic intracranial hemorrhage: early experience at 3 T. *Neuroradiology* 2006; 48(4):247–254.

Hunt KJ, Evans GW, Folsom AR, et al. Acoustic shadowing on B-mode ultrasound of the carotid artery predicts ischemic stroke: the Atherosclerosis Risk in Communities (ARIC) study. *Stroke* 2001;32(5):1120–1126.

Imaizumi T, Horita Y, Hashimoto Y, et al. Dotlike hemosiderin spots on T2*-weighted magnetic resonance imaging as a predictor of stroke recurrence: a prospective study. *J Neurosurg* 2004;101(6):915–920.

Joo SP, Kim TS, Kim YS, et al. Clinical utility of multislice computed tomographic angiography for detection of cerebral vasospasm in acute subarachnoid hemorrhage. *Minim Invasive Neurosurg* 2006;49(5):286–290.

Kosior RK, Wright CJ, Kosior JC, et al. 3-Tesla versus 1.5-Tesla magnetic resonance diffusion and perfusion imaging in hyperacute ischemic stroke. *Cerebrovasc Dis* 2007;24(4):361–368.

Kuwahara S, Fukuoka M, Koan Y, et al. Diffusion-weighted imaging of traumatic subdural hematoma in the subacute stage. *Neurol Med Chir (Tokyo)* 2005;45(9):464–469.

Kuwahara S, Fukuoka M, Koan Y, et al. Subdural hyperintense band on diffusion-weighted imaging of chronic subdural hematoma indicates bleeding from the outer membrane. *Neurol Med Chir (Tokyo)* 2005; 45(3):125–131.

Kuwahara S, Miyake H, Fukuoka M, et al. Diffusion-weighted magnetic resonance imaging of organized subdural hematoma—case report. *Neurol Med Chir (Tokyo)* 2004;44(7):376–379.

Lee SW, Choi SH, Hong Y, et al. Effects of magnetic resonance imaging diffusion gradient recalled echo on a patient with an intracranial hemorrhage presenting to the emergency department. *Eur J Emerg Med* 2006; 13(2):117–118.

Molina CA, Alexandrov AV. Transcranial ultrasound in acute stroke: from diagnosis to therapy. *Cerebrovasc Dis* 2007;24(Suppl 1):1–6.

Murphy BD, Fox AJ, Lee DH, et al. Identification of penumbra and infarct in acute ischemic stroke using computed tomography perfusion-derived blood flow and blood volume measurements. *Stroke* 2006; 37(7):1771–1777.

Nguyen BT, Mullins ME. Computed tomography follow-up imaging of stroke. *Semin Ultrasound CT MR* 2006;27(3):168–176.

Nijjar S, Patel B, McGinn G, et al. Computed tomographic angiography as the primary diagnostic study in spontaneous subarachnoid hemorrhage. *J Neuroimaging* 2007;17(4):295–299.

Okazaki S, Moriwaki H, Minematsu K, et al. Extremely early computed tomography signs in hyperacute ischemic stroke as a predictor of parenchymal hematoma. *Cerebrovasc Dis* 2008;25(3):241–246.

Perren F, Loulidi J, Poglia D, et al. Microbubble potentiated transcranial duplex ultrasound enhances IV thrombolysis in acute stroke. *J Thromb Thrombolysis* 2007;25:219–223.

Ringelstein EB. Echo-enhanced ultrasound for diagnosis and management in stroke patients. *Eur J Ultrasound* 1998;7(Suppl 3):S3–S15.

Ringelstein EB. Ultrafast magnetic resonance imaging protocols in stroke. *J Neurol Neurosurg Psychiatr* 2005;76(7):905.

Ringleb PA, Schwark Ch, Köhrmann M, et al. Thrombolytic therapy for acute ischaemic stroke in octogenarians: selection by magnetic resonance imaging improves safety but does not improve outcome. *J Neurol Neurosurg Psychiatr* 2007;78(7):690–693.

Rivers CS, Wardlaw J, Armitage P, et al. Acute ischemic stroke lesion measurement on diffusion weighted imaging—important considerations in designing acute stroke trials with magnetic resonance imaging. *J Stroke Cerebrovasc Dis* 2007;16(2):64–70.

Sato M. Nakano M, Sasanuma J, et al. Preoperative cerebral aneurysm assessment by three-dimensional magnetic resonance angiography: feasibility of surgery without conventional catheter angiography. *Neurosurgery* 2005;56(5):903–912; discussion 903–912.

Saverino A, Del Settea M, Contia M, et al. Hyperechoic plaque: an ultrasound marker for osteoporosis in acute stroke patients with carotid disease. *Eur Neurol* 2006;55(1):31–36.

Scaroni R, Tambasco N, Cardaloli G, et al. Multimodal use of computed tomography in early acute stroke, part 2. *Clin Exp Hypertens* 2006;28(3–4):427–431.

Schellinger PD, Fiebach JB. Intracranial hemorrhage: the role of magnetic resonance imaging. *Neurocrit Care* 2004;1(1):31–45.

Schuster R, Waxman K. Is repeated head computed tomography necessary for traumatic intracranial hemorrhage? *Am Surg* 2005;71(9):701–704.

Singhal AB, Ratai E, Benner T, et al. Magnetic resonance spectroscopy study of oxygen therapy in ischemic stroke. *Stroke* 2007;38(10):2851–2854.

Sitburana O, Koroshetz WJ. Magnetic resonance imaging: implication in acute ischemic stroke management. *Curr Atheroscler Rep* 2005;7(4): 305–312.

Smith JS, Chang EF, Rosenthal G, et al. The role of early follow-up computed tomography imaging in the management of traumatic brain injury patients with intracranial hemorrhage. *J Trauma* 2007;63(1):75–82.

Suarez JI, Tarr RW, Selman WR. Aneurysmal subarachnoid hemorrhage. *N Engl J Med* 2006;354(4):387–396.

Suzuki Y, Masateru N, Hisato I, et al. Perfusion computed tomography for the indication of percutaneous transluminal reconstruction for acute stroke. *J Stroke Cerebrovasc Dis* 2006;15(1):18–25.

Tambasco N, Scaroni R, Corea F, et al. Multimodal use of computed tomography in early acute stroke, part 1. *Clin Exp Hypertens* 2006; 28(3–4):421–426.

Tang S-C, Huang S-J, Jeng J-S, et al. Third ventricle midline shift due to spontaneous supratentorial intracerebral hemorrhage evaluated by transcranial color-coded sonography. *J Ultrasound Med* 2006;25(2): 203–209.

Tsivgoulis G, Alexandrov AV. Ultrasound-enhanced thrombolysis in acute ischemic stroke: potential, failures, and safety. *Neurotherapeutics* 2007; 4(3):420–427.

Walker DA, Broderick DF, Kotsenas AL, et al. Routine use of gradient-echo MRI to screen for cerebral amyloid angiopathy in elderly patients. *Am J Roentgenol* 2004;182(6):1547–1550.

Westerlaan HE, Gravendeel J, Fiore D, et al. Multislice CT angiography in the selection of patients with ruptured intracranial aneurysms suitable for clipping or coiling. *Neuroradiology* 2007;49(12):997–1007.

Westerlaan HE, van der Vliet AM, Hew JM, et al. Magnetic resonance angiography in the selection of patients suitable for neurosurgical intervention of ruptured intracranial aneurysms. *Neuroradiology* 2004;46(11):867–875.

Woydt M, Greiner K, Perez J, et al. Transcranial duplex-sonography in intracranial hemorrhage. Evaluation of transcranial duplex-sonography in the diagnosis of spontaneous and traumatic intracranial hemorrhage. *Zentralbl Neurochir* 1996;57(3):129–135.

Young RJ, Destian S. Imaging of traumatic intracranial hemorrhage. *Neuroimaging Clin N Am* 2002;12(2):189–204.

CRITICAL PATHWAY
Neuroimaging of the Stroke Patient

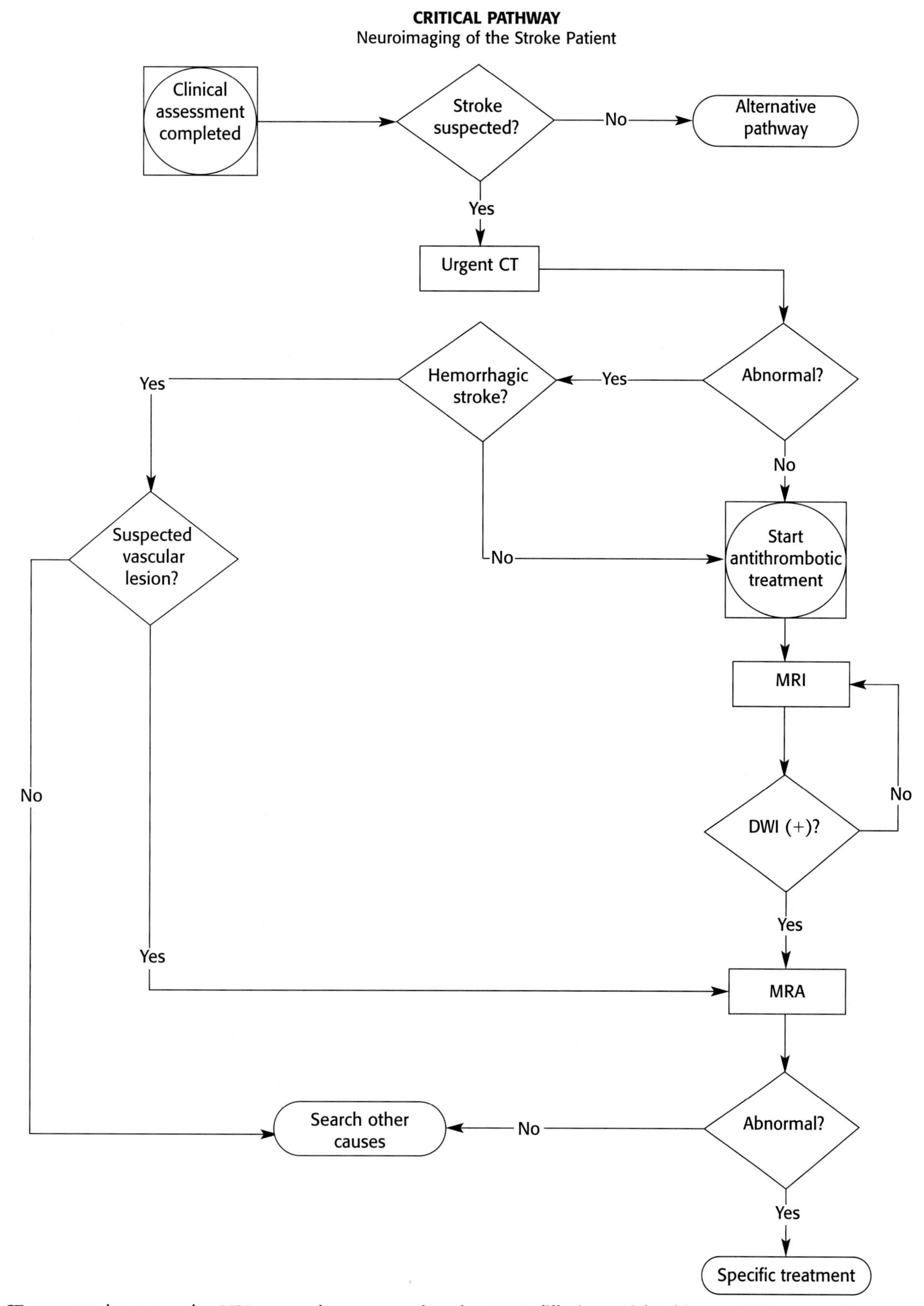

CT, computed tomography; MRI, magnetic resonance imaging; DWI, diffusion-weighted image; MRA, magnetic resonance angiography.

CHAPTER 23

Cardiology Evaluation of Ischemic Stroke

MICHAEL J. FOGLI AND EDWARD T. MARTIN

OBJECTIVES

- How are cardiovascular processes that can lead to embolization and clinical stroke identified?
- Which clinical scenarios require further diagnostic testing?
- What are the strengths and weaknesses of various diagnostic tests for cardiac evaluation of ischemic stroke?
- Which research studies have compared the effectiveness of diagnostic modalities?

BACKGROUND

Although the occurrence of an acute stroke justifiably triggers a rapid response from clinicians, once intracranial hemorrhage has been excluded, and once it has been determined that the patient is outside the time window to receive benefit from thrombolytic therapy, the emphasis quickly shifts to prevention of recurrent stroke. Since 15% to 20% of strokes derive from an intracardiac source, significant resources are frequently expended in search of embolic source, with the goal of instituting therapy that may prevent a recurrent ischemic embolic event.

Unfortunately, in many instances, the testing performed does not consider the clinical context in which the stroke has occurred or the effect of the potential result on subsequent management. In many cases, this may lead to an excessive expenditure of time as well as testing and financial resources. However, with a proper understanding of the different causes of cardioembolic stroke as well as the strengths and limitations of cardiac imaging modalities, a thorough, but cost effective evaluation can be performed.

ETIOLOGIES OF CARDIAC SOURCE OF EMBOLI

The differential diagnosis of intracardiac embolic source includes any mass structure that can attach to the endocardial surface of the heart, including thrombus, tumor, or vegetation (see Table 23.1). For a cerebrovascular ischemic event to occur, the embolic mass must originate from the left-sided cardiac structures (left atrium, mitral valve, left ventricle, aortic valve, or ascending aorta) or cross from the right side of the heart to the left side through an intracardiac communication, such as a patent foramen ovale (PFO) or an atrial septal defect.

By far the most common source of intracardiac mass leading to embolic stroke is thrombus in the left atrial appendage, accounting for nearly one half of all cases. Most of these cases are associated with atrial fibrillation or atrial flutter, since the lack of effective atrial contraction promotes stasis of blood in the atria, which results in thrombus formation. Importantly, any cardiac problem that leads to atrial dilation and low flow velocity increases the risk of thrombus formation, even in the absence of atrial fibrillation. In patients with rheumatic mitral stenosis, for example, the risk of thrombus formation can be very high, even when there is no evidence of atrial fibrillation or atrial flutter because of left atrial dilatation and stasis of atrial blood.

Stasis of blood flow not only occurs in the atria, but can also lead to thrombus formation in the left ventricle. In patients with acute or remote myocardial infarction involving the left ventricular apex or with apical akinesis due to a nonischemic cardiomyopathy, thrombus formation in the apex is common and serves as a substrate for ischemic stroke.

Interatrial communications that provide opportunity for passage of thrombotic material from the venous circulation to the arterial side constitute another important cause of an ischemic cerebrovascular accident (CVA). Most common among these is a PFO. The foramen ovale is a flap-like valve between the left and right atria that allows passage of oxygenated blood from the umbilical vein to the left atrium during fetal life, which normally closes early after birth. However, in 25% of adults, this flap remains patent and provides the opportunity for microemboli to move from the right atrium to left atrium. These microemboli usually originate from thrombi in the deep pelvic or leg veins and can dislodge and embolize during maneuvers that increase right atrial pressure, such as Valsalva or cough.

Valvular structures can also serve as the substrate for the attachment of pathologic masses that involve high embolic risk. Endocarditis is associated with an embolic event in 44% of cases; in one retrospective study, 18% of patients with endocarditis presented with an embolic stroke. Mechanical prosthetic heart valves are especially prone to thrombus deposition as well as infection. Valvular tumors, although uncommon, show a high propen-

TABLE 23.1 Sources of Cardioembolic Stroke

Left atrial appendage thrombus
Left ventricular apical thrombus
Patent foramen ovale with right-to-left shunting
Atrial septal defect
Aortic arch atheroma
Valvular vegetation
Cardiac tumor (myxoma, papillary fibroelastoma, etc.)

sity for embolization, and should be considered in the differential diagnosis of valve masses. Most of the valve tumors are benign. Papillary fibroelastoma is the most common valve tumor that is seen leading to an embolic stroke. It also requires surgical resection to prevent recurrent emboli and therefore requires accurate characterization.

Finally, atheromatous disease in the ascending aorta and aortic arch can serve as a substrate for thrombus formation and subsequent embolic phenomena, especially at the site of an ulcerated plaque. Available data from autopsy studies indicate that the risk of ischemic stroke is greatest in those subjects with atheroma thickness measuring at least 4 mm. Subsequent case–control and prospective cohort studies utilizing transesophageal echocardiography (TEE) support this hypothesis.

DIAGNOSTIC MODALITIES AND APPLICATIONS

The most basic and widely available cardiac imaging study is the transthoracic echocardiogram (TTE), which uses conventional real-time ultrasound imaging at 3.0 to 5.0 MHz. In addition to its wide availability, it has the advantage of being portable, completely free of complications, and relatively inexpensive. However, because image quality depends on the ability of ultrasound waves to penetrate tissue, factors such as obesity and hyperaerated lung can degrade image quality. Therefore, the utility of the study depends on the body habitus of the patient and the anatomic structure being imaged as well as the experience and the ability of the sonographer acquiring the images.

In general, structures closer to the chest wall, such as the right ventricular outflow tract and left ventricular apex, are seen the best, while posterior structures, such as the left atrium, the atrial septum, and the mitral valve, are less well seen. For instance, studies evaluating the test characteristics of TTE have shown that for the detection of thrombus in the left ventricular apex, the sensitivity and specificity are in the range of 86% to 95%, whereas for detection of left atrial appendage clot, the sensitivity is only 39% to 63%. Moreover, the sensitivity for detecting a PFO is not quite 50%, which is similar to the sensitivity for detection of endocarditis on native heart valves. Because of artifacts associated with poor ultrasound penetration of metal, finding vegetation or thrombus on mechanical valves with echocardiography is even more problematic, with a sensitivity of only 25%.

To overcome the diagnostic limitations of transthoracic imaging, TEE is usually performed to achieve greater accuracy in identifying cardioembolic sources. The procedure is considered minimally invasive and is performed using conscious sedation. After conscious sedation is achieved, an ultrasound-tipped probe is inserted into the esophagus and stomach. The juxtaposition of the esophagus to the posterior heart structures allows for use of higher frequency (lower depth penetration) ultrasound transducers, with frequencies in the range of 5.0 to 7.0 MHz. This provides greater spatial resolution and thus enhanced ability to visualize left atrial thrombus, PFO, valvular vegetations, and tumors. Published studies have demonstrated sensitivities and specificities approaching 100% for the detection of left atrial clot and PFO. For detection of endocarditis, sensitivities and specificities range from 90% to 95%. Since its inception over a decade ago, TEE has been shown repeatedly to be superior to TTE for detecting cardiac sources of emboli. The more pertinent issue remains whether the incremental diagnostic yield of the transesophageal approach in identifying patients who may benefit from anticoagulation or other intervention for stroke prevention justifies the additional time, cost, procedural risk, and patient discomfort involved with conscious sedation and esophageal intubation.

Transcranial Doppler imaging was developed in the early 1980s and uses ultrasound to assess changes in blood flow velocities in intracranial vessels. Its principal use in identifying cardiac source of embolus in the transient ischemic attack (TIA) or stroke patient is in the detection of a PFO or a small atrial septal defect (ASD). To detect a PFO, an intravenous agitated saline contrast bolus is injected while the patient performs a Valsalva maneuver, and flow signal from the middle cerebral artery is assessed. If a PFO is present, the microbubbles from the injected saline cross the defect, and an early appearance of microembolic signal occurs. Early studies have shown that the sensitivity of transcranial Doppler for the detection of a PFO is 68%, when using TEE as the gold standard. The sensitivity is low because the technique can fail to detect very small shunts, since the bubbles can dissipate before they are detected. Improved sensitivities have been achieved in more recent studies by refining the testing technique. Therefore, with a transcranial Doppler examination, one can achieve PFO detection rates similar to those with TEE without the potential discomfort and complications associated with the more invasive study.

Cardiac magnetic resonance imaging (MRI) has moved forward rapidly in recent years as a viable alternative for diagnosing a wide variety of cardiac problems. Its principal advantage over echocardiography for detection of PFO or other intracardiac communication is its wider field of view. The area of the heart visualized on transthoracic or transesophageal echocardiography is limited by the sampling and placement of the transducer. The wider field of view enables detection of defects which may be in unusual locations.

In addition, there are currently "real-time" MRI sequences available that allow for dynamic imaging of the heart. This dynamic imaging can be coupled with a first-pass gadolinium contrast injection such that contrast can be seen crossing from right atrium to left atrium. One pilot study has shown the ability of these real-time contrast-enhanced MRI sequences to correctly identify the presence or absence of a PFO in 20 consecutive patients when compared with TEE.

MRI can also be used to detect left atrial appendage thrombus. In one study of 50 patients with nonrheumatic atrial fibrillation who underwent both TEE and MRI, the MRI correctly identified thrombus in the 16 patients in whom it was detected by TEE. Finally, because of the versatility of MRI, it can also be used to evaluate the aorta for potential sources of embolic phenomena.

COMPARATIVE STUDIES AND PRACTICAL RECOMMENDATIONS

Several studies and clinical practice guidelines have been published to establish an effective clinical approach for the diagnosis of cardiac source of emboli. The major question addressed by these studies is whether TTE is sufficient to identify patients who may have an embolic source of their stroke, or whether TEE should be the test of choice for these patients.

An early single-center series found that of 106 consecutive subjects with stroke or TIA, 35% had a potential source of embolism by history. However, in this study, oral anticoagulation was considered definitely recommended only in those patients with either left atrial thrombus or spontaneous echocardiographic contrast in the left atrium. All but one patient with these findings had atrial fibrillation, such that anticoagulation would have been recommended anyway. Protruding aortic atheroma was found in 9% of patients, but details about atheroma thickness were not given. The authors concluded that TEE appeared not to be cost effective as a routine strategy in the evaluation of stroke patients, but recommended its use in selected patients.

Accordingly, a large single-center study of 824 consecutive patients with stroke or systemic embolism in whom both transthoracic and transesophageal echocardiograms were performed found that TEE had a very low yield in patients with a normal transthoracic study, since 95% of patients with left atrial thrombus, or spontaneous echocardiographic contrast, or complex aortic atheroma had an abnormal TTE and/or atrial fibrillation.

In contrast, a study from a single center in Germany examined 503 patients with acute brain ischemia in whom both transthoracic and transesophageal echocardiograms were performed. The investigators found that out of 212 anticoagulation-eligible subjects in whom no obvious source of stroke was found, TEE revealed a high-risk source of stroke in 8% of subjects in whom anticoagulation was indicated.

Another single-center study of 231 patients with stroke or TIA who underwent both TTE and TEE found that TEE detected a major stroke risk factor warranting anticoagulation in 16% of patients studied whereas TTE did so in only 3%. However, no mention was made of how many of these patients were in atrial fibrillation.

Therefore, among the studies with the largest number of stroke patients, there appears to be little benefit in performing TEE examination in patients with normal transthoracic studies. The smaller studies demonstrated improved detection of patients who would benefit from anticoagulation on the basis of finding intracardiac thrombus. However, the yield of diagnosing intracardiac thrombus in stroke patients with sinus rhythm was low—8% to 10% of patients with sinus rhythm had intracardiac thrombus on TEE that was missed on TTE. The principal weaknesses of these studies in making the broad recommendation of performing TEE in all stroke patients is that they were relatively small studies performed at a single center, thereby limiting their generalizability.

The most recently available clinical guideline on the subject from the Canadian Task Force on Preventive Health Care advocates performing a TEE initially in stroke patients with clinical evidence of cardiac disease by history, physical examination, ECG, or chest radiography. In patients without clinical cardiac disease in whom no preexisting indications or contraindications for anticoagulation exist, the committee members comment on the low yield of finding a significant embolic source in patients younger than 45 years but state that overall, insufficient evidence exists to recommend for or against echocardiography in this setting.

The most rigorous approach may be to determine the rate of intracardiac thrombus in stroke patients in one's own center to develop whether performing TEE in all stroke patients as a matter of protocol is cost effective. For most of the centers where this approach is not practical, the weight of the evidence favors screening all stroke or TIA patients with no obvious embolic source with a transthoracic study, preferably with saline bubbles to also screen for PFO. Then, if the TTE is abnormal, one would proceed with a TEE.

Also as a practical matter, TEE should be done on all patients in whom an aggressive approach to diagnosis and therapy will have a significant prognostic impact. For example, a young stroke patient without the usual stroke risk factors may benefit from an initial evaluation with a TEE.

On the basis of experience and review of the literature, a diagnostic algorithm is included that outlines a mechanistic approach to the workup of a patient with a stroke to rule out a cardioembolic source (see Critical Pathway on last page of this chapter).

CONCLUSION

Embolic stroke can result from diverse pathophysiologic processes including congenital defects, infectious vegetation, neoplastic disorders, and atherosclerosis. Integrating patient demographic factors with clinical variables can lead to the use of the appropriate imaging modality, providing an accurate diagnosis in an expeditious and cost-effective manner. Additionally, the wider availability and acceptance of newer imaging technologies will continue to add versatility and accuracy to the diagnostic process.

SELECTED REFERENCES

Agmon Y, Khandheria B, Gentile F, Seward JB. Clinical and echocardiographic characteristics of patients with left atrial thrombus and sinus rhythm: experience in 20 643 consecutive transesophageal echocardiographic examinations. *Circulation* 2002;105(1):27–31.

Amarenco P, Cohen A, Tzourio C, et al. Atherosclerotic disease of the aortic arch and the risk of ischemic stroke. *N Engl J Med* 1994;331:1474–1479.

Black IW, Hopkins AP, Lee LC, Jacobson BM, Walsh WF. Role of transesophageal echocardiography in evaluation of cardiogenic embolism. *Br Heart J* 1991;66:302–307.

Cheitlin MD, Armstrong WF, Aurigemma GP, et al. ACC/AHA/ASE 2003 Guideline update for the clinical application for echocardiography summary article. A report of the American College of Cardiology/American Heart Association Task Force on Practice Guidelines. *J Am Coll Cardiol* 2003;42:954–970.

Cramer SC. Patent foramen ovale and its relationship to stroke. *Cardiol Clin* 2005;23(1):7–11.

de Bruijn SF, Agema WR, Lammers GJ, et al. Transesophageal echocardiography is superior to transthoracic echocardiography in management of patients of any age with transient ischemic attack or stroke. *Stroke* 2006;37(10):2531–2534.

DeRook FA, Comess KA, Albers GW, Popp RL. Transesophageal echocardiography in the evaluation of stroke. *Ann Intern Med* 1992;117:922–932.

Di Tullio M, Sacco RL, Venketasubramanian N, Sherman D, Mohr JP, Homma S. Comparison of diagnostic techniques for the detection of a patent foramen ovale in stroke patients. *Stroke* 1993;24(7):1020–1024.

Leung DY, Black IW, Cranney GB, et al. Selection of patients for transesophageal echocardiography after stroke and systemic embolic events: role of transthoracic echocardiography. *Stroke* 1995;26: 1820–1824.

Droste DW, Kriete JU, Stypmann J, et al. Contrast transcranial Doppler ultrasound in the detection of right-to-left shunts: comparison of different procedures and different contrast agents. *StrokE* 1999; 30:1827–1832.

Droste DW, Lakemeier S, Wichter T, et al. Optimizing the technique of contrast transcranial Doppler ultrasound in the detection of right-to-left shunts. *Stroke* 2002;33:2211–2216.

Nemec JJ, Marwick TH, Lorig RJ, et al. Comparison of transcranial Doppler ultrasound and transesophageal contrast echocardiography in the detection of interatrial right-to-left shunts. *Am J Cardiol* 1991; 68: 1498–1502.

Gunter R, Michael F, Florentin A. Transesophageal echocardiography in patients with focal cerebral ischemia of unknown cause. *Stroke* 1996;27:691–694.

Harloff A, Handke M, Reinhard M, Geibel A, Hetzel A. Therapeutic strategies after examination by transesophageal echocardiography in 503 patients with ischemic stroke. *Stroke* 2006;37(3):859–864.

Hata JS, Ayres RW, Biller J, et al. Impact of transesophageal echocardiography on the anticoagulation management of patients admitted with focal cerebral ischemia. *Am J Cardiol* 1993;72:707–710.

Kapral MK, Silver FL. Preventive health care, 1999 update: 2. Echocardiography for the detection of a cardiac source of embolus in patients with stroke. Canadian Task Force on Preventive Health Care. *CMAJ* 1999;161(8):989–996.

Kizer JR, Devereux RB. Patent foramen ovale in young adults with unexplained stroke. *N Engl J Med* 2005;353:2361–2372.

Manning J. Echocardiography in detection of intracardiac sources of embolism. *Up To Date* 2006. Jan: www.utdol.com.

Manning WJ. Role of transesophageal echocardiography in the management of thromboembolic stroke. *Am J Cardiol* 1997;80(4C): 19D–28D.

Messe SR, Schwartz RS, Perloff JK. Atrial septal abnormalities and cerebral embolic in adults. *Up To Date* 2006. Jan: www.utdol.com.

Mohrs OK, Petersen SE, Erkapic D, et al. Diagnosis of patent foramen ovale using contrast-enhanced dynamic MRI: a pilot study. *Am J Roentgenol* 2005;184:234240.

Ohyama H, Hosomi N, Takahashi T, et al. Comparison of magnetic resonance imaging and transesophageal echocardiography in detection of thrombus in the left atrial appendage. *Stroke* 2003;34:24362439.

Oppenheimer SM, Lima J. Neurology and the heart. *J Neurol Neurosurg Psychiatry* 1998(3):289–297.

Pearson AC, Labovitz AJ, Tatineni S, Gomez CR. Superiority of transesophageal echocardiography in detecting cardiac source of embolism in patients with cerebral ischemia of uncertain etiology. *J Am Coll Cardiol* 1991;17:66–72.

Pinto FJ. When and how to diagnose patent foramen ovale. *Heart* 2005;91:438440.

Pop G, Sutherland GR, Koudstaal PJ, Sit TW, de Jong G, Roelandt JR. Transesophageal echocardiography in the detection of intracardiac embolic sources in patients with transient ischemic attacks. *Stroke* 1990;21:560–565.

Sastre-Garriga J, Molina C, Montaner J, et al. Mitral papillary fibroelastoma as a cause of cardiogenic embolic stroke: report two cases and review of the literature. *Eur J Neurol* 2000;7(4):449–453.

Sen S, Laowatana S, Lima J, Oppenheimer SM. Risk factors for intracardiac thrombus in patients with recent ischaemic cerebrovascular events. *J Neurol Neurosurg Psychiatry*. 2004;75(10):1421–1425.

Strandberg M, Marttila RJ, Helenius H. Transoesophageal echocardiography in selecting patients for anticoagulation after ischaemic stroke or transient ischaemic attack. *J Neurol Neurosurg Psychiatry* 2002;73(1):29–33.

The French Study of Aortic Plaques in Stroke Group. Atherosclerotic disease of the aortic arch is a risk factor for recurrent ischemic stroke. *N Engl J Med* 1996;334:1216.

Vitebskiy S, Fox K, Hoit BD. Routine transesophageal echocardiography for the evaluation of cerebral emboli in elderly patients. *Echocardiography* 2005;22(9):770–774.

Warner MF, Momah KI. Routine transesophageal echocardiography for cerebral ischemia. Is it really necessary? *Arch Intern Med* 1996;156: 17191723.

CRITICAL PATHWAY
Diagnostic Approach to Patients with Suspected Embolic Stroke

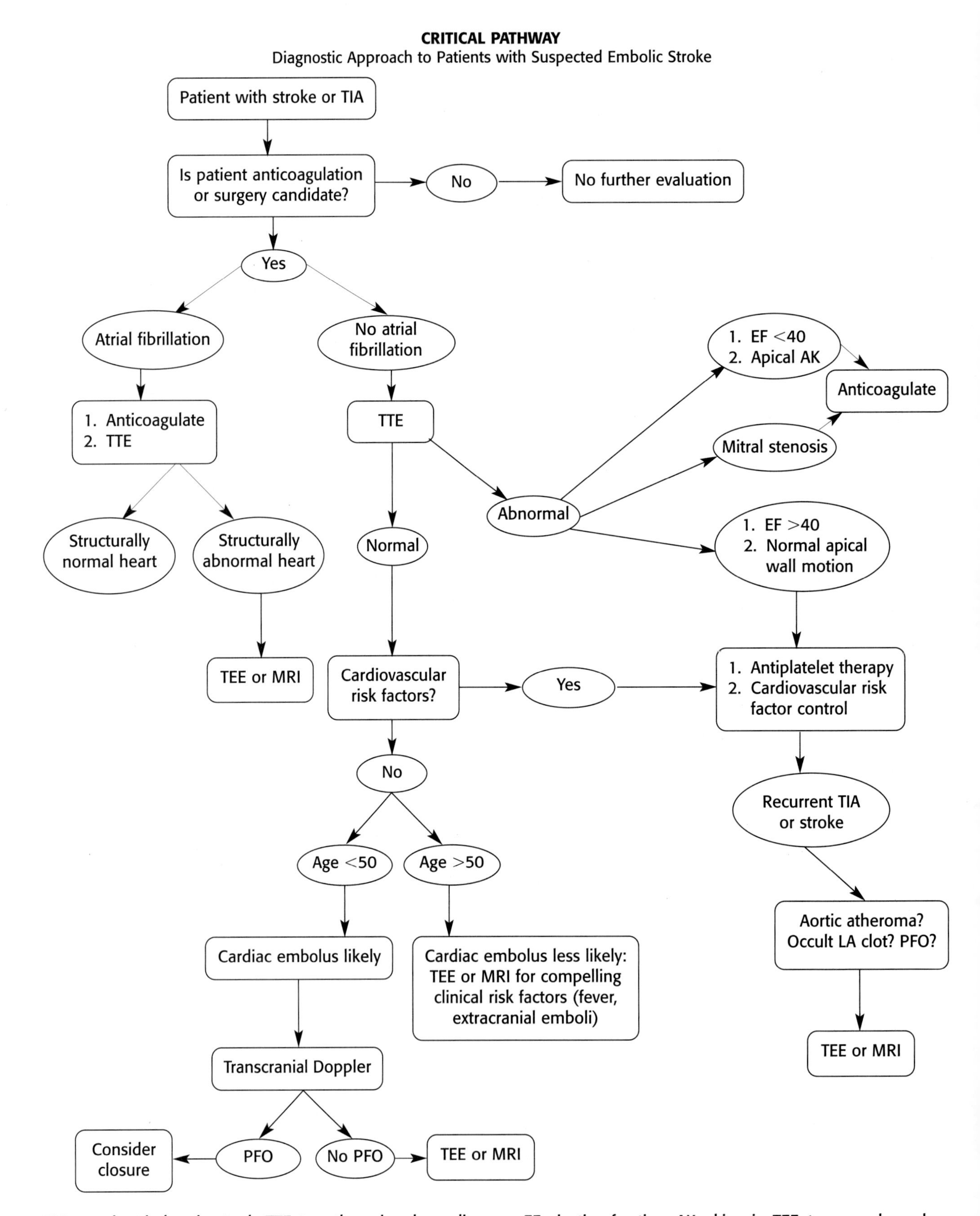

TIA, transient ischemic attack; TTE, transthoracic echocardiogram; EF, ejection fraction; AK, akinesis; TEE, transesophageal echocardiography; LA, left atrial; MRI, magnetic resonance imaging; PFO, patent foramen ovale.

CHAPTER

24 Antithrombotic Therapy for Ischemic Stroke Prevention

JAMES D. GEYER AND CAMILO R. GOMEZ

OBJECTIVES

- What antithrombotic medications are available for ischemic stroke prevention?
- What are the goals of therapy in using antithrombotic medications?
- When is antithrombotic therapy indicated?
- How is the most appropriate antithrombotic agent in each clinical circumstance to be chosen?
- What is the best approach to the asymptomatic patient?

The era of thrombolytic therapy has generated much needed excitement and publicity about ischemic stroke and its management. However, regardless of the effectiveness of ischemic stroke treatment, its prevention remains the most cost-effective approach to care. In fact, irrespective of the treatment received, all ischemic stroke patients need an aggressive secondary stroke prevention plan.

BACKGROUND AND RATIONALE

Ischemic stroke recurrence within 5 years varies between 25% and 42% according to different studies, with approximately one third occurring in the first 30 days and the noted variance being related to the root cause of the index event. Identifying this root cause for each patient via the application of comprehensive stroke evaluation and risk stratification protocols and subsequently managing all modifiable risk factors constitute the two components of secondary ischemic stroke prevention. A dimension of the prevention of ischemic stroke is the administration of pharmacologic agents whose primary objective is to reduce the risk of thromboembolic vascular occlusion by directly influencing one or several components of the natural coagulation mechanism. The following is a discussion of the mechanisms of action, indications, and practical utilization of the available antithrombotic agents in the prevention of ischemic stroke.

Mechanisms of Coagulation and Thrombosis

The term *hemostasis* refers to the complex interaction between blood vessels, platelets, coagulation factors, coagulation inhibitors, and fibrinolytic proteins to maintain the blood within the vascular compartments in a fluid state. As such, a delicate balance between the procoagulant and the anticoagulant properties of the blood and the circulatory system maintains hemostasis. Traditionally, the hemostatic process has been divided into two phases: primary and secondary. Primary hemostasis is initiated when platelets adhere, using a specific platelet collagen receptor glycoprotein Ia/IIa, to collagen fibers in the vascular endothelium. This adhesion is mediated by von Willebrand factor (vWF), which forms links between the platelet glycoprotein Ib/IX/V and collagen fibrils. The platelets are then activated and release the contents of their granules into the plasma, in turn activating other platelets and white blood cells. The platelets undergo a change in their shape, which exposes a phospholipid surface for those coagulation factors that require it. Fibrinogen links adjacent platelets by forming links via glycoprotein IIb/IIIa.

Secondary hemostasis is provided by the coagulation cascade (see Fig. 24.1). In turn, the coagulation cascade of secondary hemostasis has two pathways, the contact activation pathway (formally known as the intrinsic pathway) and the TF pathway (formally known as the extrinsic pathway), that lead to fibrin formation. It was previously thought that the coagulation cascade consisted of two pathways of equal importance joined to a common pathway. It is now known that the primary pathway for the initiation of blood coagulation is the tissue factor (TF) pathway. The pathways are a series of reactions in which a zymogen (i.e., an inactive enzyme precursor) of a serine protease and its glycoprotein cofactor are activated to become active components that then catalyze the next reaction in the cascade. The coagulation factors are serine proteases (enzymes) except for factor VIII and factor V, which are glycoproteins, and factor XIII, which is a transglutaminase. The coagulation cascade can be summarized as follows:

1. *TF pathway*: The main role of the TF pathway is to generate a thrombin burst. In turn, thrombin is the single most important constituent of the coagulation cascade in terms of its feedback activation roles. Following damage to the blood vessel endothelium, TF is released, which then forms a complex with factor VIIa (TF-FVIIa). This activates factor IX and factor X. Factor VII itself is activated by thrombin,

factor XIa, plasmin, factor XII, and factor Xa. The activation of factor Xa by TF-FVIIa is almost immediately inhibited by TF pathway inhibitor (TFPI). Factor Xa and its cofactor factor Va form the prothrombinase complex, which activates prothrombin to thrombin. Thrombin then activates other components of the coagulation cascade, including factors V and VII (which activate factor XI, which in turn activates factor IX), and activates and releases factor VIII from being bound to vWF. Factor VIIIa is the cofactor of factor IXa and together they form the tenase complex, which activates factor X, and so the cycle continues.

2. *Contact activation pathway*: The primary complex is formed on collagen by high-molecular-weight kininogen (HMWK), prekallikrein, and factor XII (Hageman factor). Prekallikrein is converted to kallikrein and factor XII becomes factor XIIa. Factor XIIa converts factor XI into factor XIa. Factor XIa activates factor IX, which with its cofactor factor VIIIa form the tenase complex that activates factor X to factor Xa.
3. *Thrombin*: Thrombin has a large array of functions. Its primary role is the conversion of fibrinogen to fibrin, the building block of a hemostatic plug. In addition, it activates factors VIII and V and their inhibitor protein C (in the presence of thrombomodulin), and it also activates factor XIII, which forms covalent bonds that crosslink the fibrin polymers that form from activated monomers.

Following activation by the contact factor or TF pathways the coagulation cascade is maintained in a prothrombotic state by the continued activation of factors VIII and IX to form the tenase complex until it is downregulated by the regulatory mechanisms.

The counterbalance of the procoagulative tendency of the cascade is provided by a variety of regulatory mechanisms, which serve two main purposes: (a) limit the amount of fibrin clot formed to avoid ischemia of tissues and (b) localize clot formation to the site of tissue or vessel injury, thereby preventing widespread thrombosis.

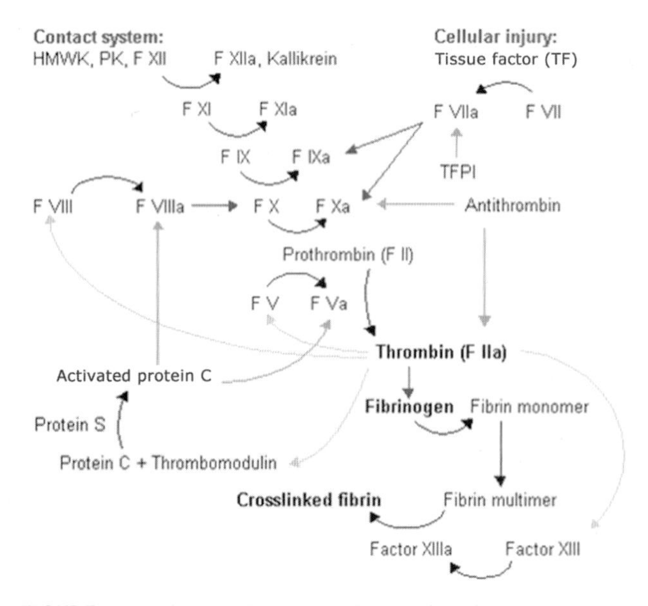

FIGURE 24.1. The coagulation cascade, including the contact system and the cellular injury system. HMWK, high molecular weight kininogen; PK, prekallikrein; F, factor.

1. *TF pathway inhibitor:* As discussed earlier, coagulation is initiated when vessel or tissue injury exposes circulating factor VII to TF. Through this interaction, a TF-VIIa complex is formed, and this can subsequently activate small amounts of factors IX and X, eventually resulting in limited quantities of thrombin. TFPI is a protein that mediates the feedback inhibition of the TF-FVIIa complex, resulting in decreased activation of both factors IX and X. Small amounts of factor Xa are required for TFPI to achieve its inhibition of the TF-VIIa complex. Therefore, on initiation of the cascade, TF-FVIIa complexes are formed and small amounts of factor Xa and thrombin are generated. The limited quantities of factor Xa will result in feedback inhibition of its own synthesis via TFPI. An important point to consider is that heparin increases the action of TFPI two- to fourfold. This occurs by virtue of two mechanisms. The first involves heparin binding TFPI and TF-FVIIa complex, bringing them closer together and hence increasing their interaction. In addition, heparin also causes the release of endothelial stores of TFPI.
2. *Antithrombin III (AT):* This is a protein synthesized by liver and endothelial cells, which binds and directly inactivates thrombin and the other serine proteases (factors IXa, Xa, and XIa). The uncatalyzed reaction between the serine proteases and AT is relatively slow. The serine proteases still have time to generate thrombin and fibrin before becoming inactivated. However, in the presence of heparin or similar sulfated glycosaminoglycans, the reaction between AT and the serine proteases is virtually instantaneous resulting in the immediate blockage of fibrin formation. Normal endothelial cells express heparan sulfate (a sulfated glycosaminoglycan). AT binds to this and is then able to inactivate any nearby serine proteases, thus preventing the formation of fibrin clot in undamaged areas. Note that in the presence of heparin, the primary target of AT is *thrombin*.
3. *Activated proteins C and S:* Proteins C and S are both vitamin K–dependent *inhibitors* of the procoagulant system. Together, they inactivate factors Va and VIIIa. Protein C circulates in the blood as a zymogen and is activated to a serine protease by the binding of thrombin to thrombomodulin. Protein S markedly enhances the activity of protein C. By inactivating factors Va and VIIa, proteins C and S significantly decrease the tempo of thrombin generation, thereby significantly dampening the cascade.
4. *Thrombomodulin:* This is an endothelial cell receptor that binds thrombin. When thrombomodulin and thrombin form a complex, the conformation of the thrombin molecule is changed. This altered thrombin molecule now readily activates protein C and loses its platelet-activating and protease activities. Therefore, the binding of thrombomodulin to thrombin converts thrombin from a tremendously potent procoagulant into an anticoagulant. This is important in the normal physiological state because normal endothelial cells produce thrombomodulin, which binds any circulating thrombin, thus preventing clot formation in undamaged vessels.

5. *The fibrinolytic system:* The continuous generation of cross-linked fibrin would create a clot capable of obstructing normal blood flow. The fibrinolytic system is present to keep clot formation in check by actually degrading the fibrin strands. Plasminogen is an inactive protein made in endothelial cells, liver cells, and eosinophils. It is activated to plasmin by an enzyme called *plasminogen activator.* Plasmin has this ability to degrade fibrin strands, preventing the build-up of excess clot.

The Practical Side: Virchow's Triad

Despite the apparent complexity of the processes described earlier, and from the *vascular neurology* point of view, it is more practical to consider that nearly all clinical conditions capable of producing ischemic stroke can be viewed as a function of Virchow's triad. In the 19th century, the Polish pathologist Rudolph Virchow described for the first time the mechanism for pulmonary thromboembolism (in fact, he coined the term *embolism*). More than a century later, he was credited (although arguably) with enumerating the three different conditions that are capable of inducing thromboembolism: blood flow stasis, injury to the vascular endothelium, and hypercoagulability (see Fig. 24.2).

Interestingly, even to this day the practical applications of the concepts in Virchow's triad cannot be overemphasized. In fact, nearly every clinical condition capable of resulting in ischemic stroke corresponds to one or more of the three components. The corollary of our last proposition is that by analyzing each clinical situation in the context of how it fits into the Venn diagram created by the different aspects of Virchow's triad (Fig. 24.2), it should be possible to choose the best antithrombotic strategy to be followed. This is emphasized later in the chapter, particularly as we combine the concepts exposed with theoretical considerations about the various types of thrombi and the existing clinical evidence pertaining to ischemic stroke prevention.

A thrombus is a blood clot that forms within the cardiovascular system and thrombosis is the general mechanism that leads to its formation. On the basis of what has been discussed earlier, it is easy to understand that one or another disturbance of the overall systemic procoagulant–anticoagulant balance always represents the root cause of every ischemic stroke. To expand further, we must consider the cardiovascular microenvironment where such disturbance takes place, as well as its impact on the type of thrombus and its management. It is generally understood that despite the uniformity of the various steps that constitute the coagulation cascade, thrombi that form under conditions of slow blood flow (i.e., stasis or stagnation) are morphologically different from those that form in areas of rapid blood flow (i.e., turbulence). Along these lines, the former are known as *red clots* because they are composed of numerous red cells trapped within large networks of fibrin (see Fig. 24.3A). The latter, on the other hand, are composed mainly of platelet aggregates linked together by fibrin strands (see Fig. 24.3B) and are known as *white clots.* As we will review later, ischemic stroke prevention requires an understanding of the vascular microenvironment and flow conditions of the root cause of the index event, as well as the predictable type of clot to be prevented by antithrombotic pharmacologic intervention.

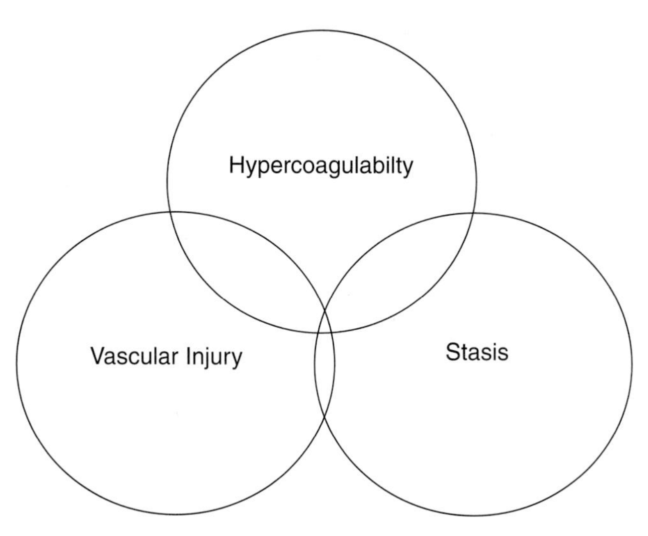

FIGURE 24.2. Virchow's triad, including the three components that promote intravascular coagulation.

CLINICAL APPLICATIONS AND METHODOLOGY

Aspirin: The Fundamental Antithrombotic Agent

Aspirin appears to have a number of effects but its primary antithrombotic effect is its ability to irreversibly inhibit the enzyme cyclooxygenase (COX), blocking the prostaglandin pathway of platelet activation (see Fig. 24.4). The activity of COX is the rate-limiting step in the synthesis of thromboxane A_2 (TXA_2), a powerful platelet activator. This results in a permanent defect in TXA_2-dependent platelet function via inhibition of COX-1. The activity of COX-2 is much less affected, and therefore, the production of endothelial prostacyclin (a vasodilator and platelet inhibitor), which is both COX-1 and COX-2 dependent, is inhibited to a lesser degree. Aspirin has a half-life of 15 to 20 minutes with peak plasma levels at 30 to 40 minutes. Inhibition of platelet function is evident within 1 hour. Enteric-coated aspirin delays the time to peak plasma level by 3 to 4 hours. COX-1 activity in megakaryocytes is also inhibited, resulting in the appearance of dysfunctional budding platelets. Since the effect on TXA_2 is irreversible, the effect of aspirin lasts for the lifespan of the platelets, which approximates 10 days.

Many trials have demonstrated the efficacy of aspirin in secondary stroke prevention. However, only four of the reported trials have shown a statistically significant benefit for the primary endpoint of the study, while reductions in various secondary endpoints reached significance in many others. This variability in outcomes highlights the challenges surrounding the study of stroke and the selection of a given treatment by the clinician. Perhaps the best summary of the current knowledge of the effect of aspirin in stroke prevention is illustrated by the meta-analysis published by the Antiplatelet Trialists Collaboration (APTC). It examined 197 randomized studies of antiplatelet agents versus control and 90 randomized comparisons between various antiplatelet agents. In short, the APTC concluded that the use of aspirin generally results in a 23% odds reduction in vascular events (stroke, myocardial infarction, and vascular death). Additional meta-analyses of trials that only studied the effect of aspirin in populations of stroke patients have in general suggested that, for this subset, aspirin reduces the

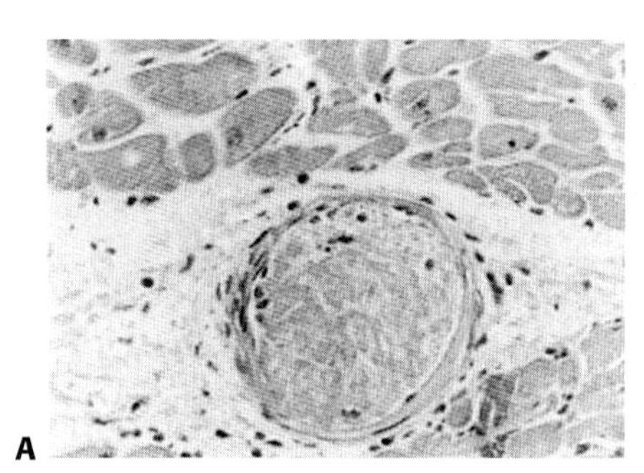

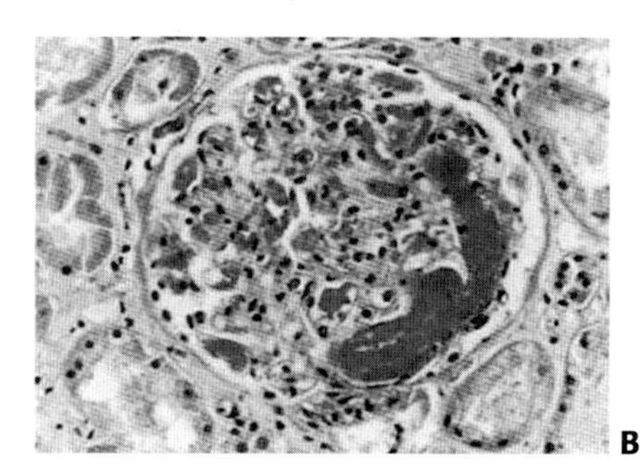

FIGURE 24.3. A: Myocardial arteriole contains one hyaline thrombus, composed predominantly of platelets and platelet-derived material, from a patient who died during an episode of thrombotic-thrombocytopenic purpura. **B:** Glomerular arteriolos with clots composed predominantly of fibrin and red blood cells from a patient who died with disseminated intravascular coagulation. (Courtesy of Dr. A Saleem).

risk of clinically important vascular events by approximately 15%. Furthermore, these meta-analyses support the notion that the benefit of aspirin in prevention of ischemic stroke is greater than its risk of leading to hemorrhagic complications.

The appropriate daily dose of aspirin for stroke prevention has been the subject of a heated controversy over the years. This controversy has been triggered by two important factors: (a) the variable results of the different randomized studies and (b) the theoretical considerations about a dose-dependent preferential effect of aspirin on COX-1 and COX-2. In general, early stroke prevention trials used higher doses of aspirin than more recent studies. This progressive change in dosing obeyed the idea that, by using smaller daily doses, it was possible to have a lesser inhibitory effect on the production of prostacyclin by the vascular wall, thereby taking advantage of the vasodilatory and antithrombotic effects of this compound. Whether this is the case or not, the various studies published have almost invariably shown that smaller doses of aspirin are quite effective in reducing the risk of ischemic stroke. This was also illustrated in the meta-analysis of the APTC, which demonstrated that doses >1,000 mg per day were no more effective for stroke prevention than smaller doses. This concept, compounded by the finding that the hemorrhagic side effects of aspirin become more frequent as the daily dose is increased, has resulted in a general trend to use smaller doses than we used a decade ago. In fact, in 1998, the Food and Drug Administration (FDA) changed its recommended aspirin dosage for ischemic stroke prevention to lower doses (50 to 325 mg per day).

Another aspect of the clinical use of aspirin involves the concept of aspirin resistance, defined as the presence of platelet activation and adhesion despite the administration of aspirin. This has been the subject of considerable study during the last few years and a source of potential improvement in our ability to reduce the risk of ischemic stroke further by manipulating this variable. The reported rate of aspirin resistance in the literature has been as high as 12% to 29% of cardiac patients, as determined by incomplete platelet inhibition measured using aggregometry, emphasizing the importance and effect of this problem. More important, the risk of death, myocardial infarction, and stroke has been reported in a magnitude of six- to ninefold higher in patients with partial platelet inhibition. However, it is important to consider that the whole concept of aspirin resistance may be fictitious and simply based the wrongful expectation that the dosing of aspirin must conform to a one-size-fits-all. Quite the contrary, we submit that these studies have demonstrated is that the biologic effect of aspirin varies between different individuals and that a single dose does not fit the entire population. This interpretation of the data is no different from the understanding that the same dose of warfarin is unlikely to lead to the same international normalized ratio (INR) in all individuals.

Finally, from the safety point of view, bleeding (major and minor) and gastrointestinal toxicity are the two most common side effects associated with aspirin treatment. However, the data from the various studies suggests that, particularly at lower doses, aspirin is a fairly safe compound.

Thienopyridines: Increasing the Advantage

Thienopyridines are selective, noncompetitive, and irreversible binders of the adenosine diphosphate (ADP) receptor on the platelet surface, mainly targeting the P2Y or P2T ADP receptor subtypes (see Fig. 24.4). Under normal circumstances, the ADP released from activated platelets at the thrombosis site is a powerful platelet activator. Therefore, these drugs induce blockage of the effect of ADP on platelet activation. The two drugs widely available in this class of compounds are ticlopidine and clopidogrel. Their effects, as well as their efficacy in the prevention of ischemic stroke, are similar in magnitude and profile. This will be evident later, when we discuss practical recommendations for the use of antiplatelet agents.

Two major trials evaluated ticlopidine in patients with stroke. The Canadian American Ticlopidine Study (CATS) was a randomized, double-blind, multicenter study comparing ticlopidine (250 mg twice daily) with placebo for the prevention of stroke, myocardial infarction, or vascular death. The Ticlopidine Aspirin Stroke Study (TASS) was a much larger, double-blind, multicenter trial that compared ticlopidine (250 mg twice daily) with aspirin (650 mg twice daily) in patients with recent transient ischemic attack, amaurosis fugax, reversible ischemic neurological deficit, or minor stroke. Following a subgroup analysis of the TASS study cohort that suggested a greater benefit of ticlopidine in blacks led to the African American Antiplatelet Stroke Prevention Study (AAASPS). This failed to demonstrate such a selective beneficial effect in reducing stroke, myocardial infarction, and vascular death. In fact, there was a slight benefit in favor of aspirin. The Clopidogrel and Aspirin Prevention in Recurrent Ischemic Events trial (CAPRIE) was a double-blind randomized study of aspirin (325 mg per day) versus clopidogrel (75 mg per day) in >19,000 patients with stroke, myocardial infarction, or peripheral arterial disease (PAD), evaluating the primary composite outcome of ischemic stroke, myocardial infarction, and vascular death. The results of these studies will be discussed later, when we compare all of the antiplatelet agents and their utilization in clinical practice.

Thienopyridines, ticlopidine and clopidogrel have been associated with a number of side effects, the most common being diarrhea. The occurrence of hemorrhagic complications with either drug has been comparable to that of aspirin. In addition, ticlopidine has also been associated with abnormal liver enzymes and neutropenia. Finally, thrombotic thrombocytopenic purpura (TTP) is a rare complication of ticlopidine therapy but is often fatal and difficult to predict.

Dipyridamole: A Final Twist

Dipyridamole is a pyrimidopyrimidine derivative from the papaverine family, which has antithrombotic properties and vasodilatory effects that are exerted on both cellular (red blood cells and platelets) and vascular structures (endothelium and smooth muscle cells). Dipyridamole inhibits phosphodiesterases (see Fig. 24.4) resulting in increased concentrations of cyclic adenosine monophosphate (cAMP) and cyclic guanosine monophosphate (cGMP) that act as inhibitors of platelet activation and adhesion. It also blocks adenosine uptake by erythrocytes. Adenosine stimulates platelet adenylate cyclase (resulting in increased cAMP levels) and is a powerful vasodilator. Other secondary mechanisms of action may also contribute.

Standard dipyridamole has a variable rate of absorption and subsequently a low bioavailability even when administered four times daily. This appears to be one of the reasons that initial studies with immediate-release dipyridamole proved unsuccessful. Extended-release dipyridamole (ER-DP), combined with aspirin, provides a more consistent plasma level at twice-daily dosing. The first European Stroke Prevention Study (ESPS) showed a clear benefit for the aspirin/dipyridamole combination over placebo, with a 38% relative reduction in the risk of fatal or nonfatal stroke. The ESPS-2 was a large, double-blind, multicenter study that was powered to detect significant benefits of low-dose aspirin and dipyridamole, both individually and in combination. The combination of low-dose aspirin (50 mg per day) combined with ER-DP administered at a higher dose (400 mg per day) resulted in a significant stroke risk reduction. Again, the specifics will be discussed later, as we make recommendations.

The combination use of aspirin and ER-DP is associated with a number of side effects the most important of which is headache, and in practice, this is an important cause of treatment discontinuation. Except for this, the safety profile of the combined aspirin and ER-DP is similar to that of aspirin alone.

Triflusal: The Little Drug That Couldn't

Triflusal was a different antiplatelet agent, structurally related to aspirin, that exerted its antithrombotic effect by acting on different targets involved in platelet aggregation. It was studied largely in Europe, in a randomized multicenter study involving >2,000 patients with transient ischemic attack or nondisabling stroke. The Triflusal versus Aspirin Cerebral Infarction Prevention (TACIP) followed up these patients for a mean period of 30 months. At the end, TACIP failed to show a significant difference between the two treatment groups but showed significantly greater hemorrhagic complications among patients treated with aspirin. These results were not surprising, considering the similarities between the two drugs.

Warfarin: A Different Dimension

Warfarin is a vitamin K antagonist that blocks the cyclic interconversion of vitamin K and its 2, 3-epoxide. Vitamin K is a cofactor for the post-translational carboxylation of glutamate on the *N*-terminal regions of vitamin K–dependent proteins. Coagulation factors II, VII, IX, and X require carboxylation for their biological activity. Coumarins, including warfarin, inhibit the vitamin K

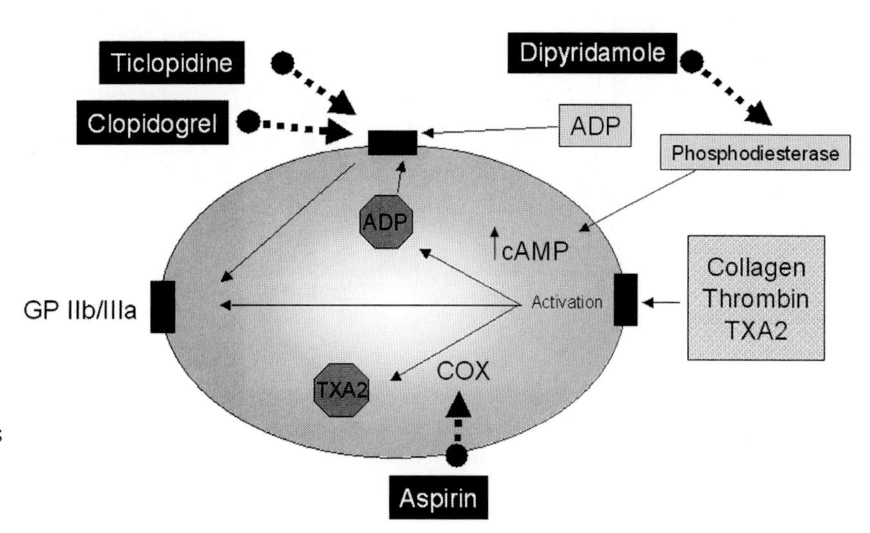

FIGURE 24.4. The platelet and the mechanism of action of the major antiplatelet agents. ADP, adenosine diphosphate; TXA2, thromboxane A2; COX, cyclooxygenase; cAMP, cyclic adenosine monophosphate; GP IIb/IIIa, glycoprotein IIb/IIIa.

conversion cycle as described earlier, thereby reducing procoagulant activity. Some anticoagulant proteins, such as proteins C and S, may also have temporary procoagulant effect in the presence of partial anticoagulation with warfarin. Warfarin has a narrow therapeutic window and a variable, somewhat unpredictable, dose–response relationship. A number of factors converge to cause these problems including dietary vitamin K intake, warfarin's variable affinity for its hepatic receptor, drug–drug interactions, and poor patient compliance among others.

The use of oral anticoagulation with warfarin has been shown to be very effective in patients with cardiogenic ischemic stroke secondary to atrial fibrillation or to acute myocardial infarction. Typically, these studies have shown a benefit that depends on maintaining the INR within a narrow range (i.e., 1.8–3.0). In addition, patients with prosthetic mechanical valves also benefit from treatment with warfarin, although they require higher INR (i.e., 2.5–3.5). Figure 24.5 demonstrates the beneficial effect of warfarin almost under any circumstance for the prevention of stroke in patients with atrial fibrillation, as evidenced by many different randomized studies.

The application of warfarin for ischemic stroke prevention in other clinical scenarios has not been as successfully demonstrated by randomized prospective studies. In fact, some of them have shown significantly high (although predictable) complication rates. For example, the Stroke Prevention in Reversible Ischemia Trial (SPIRIT) was a multicenter European study comparing the effectiveness of anticoagulation to a very low dose aspirin (30 mg) in secondary prevention of stroke in patients with transient ischemic attack or minor stroke of presumed arterial (i.e., noncardiac) origin. The trial was stopped after the first interim analysis because of safety concerns. There had been 53 major bleeding complications in the anticoagulation arm versus only 6 in the aspirin arm. However, the target INR had been set at 3.0 to 4.5, and therefore, such an outcome is not surprising.

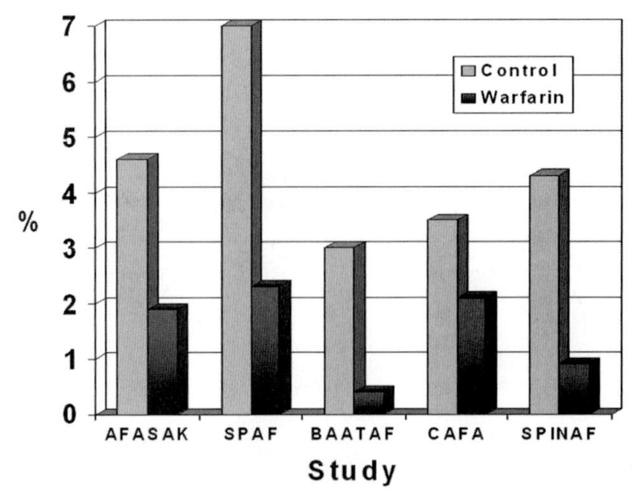

FIGURE 24.5. Event rates of the major randomized prospective studies of anticoagulation in atrial fibrillation. AFASAK, Atrial fibrillation, Aspirin, and Anticoagulant Therapy study; SPAF, Stroke Prevention in Atrial Fibrillation study; BAATAF, Boston Area Anticoagulation Trial for Atrial Fibrillation; CAFA, Canadian Atrial Fibrillation Anticoagulation study; SPINAF, Stroke Prevention in Nonrheumatic Atrial Fibrillation study.

Conversely, the Warfarin-Aspirin Recurrent Stroke Study (WARSS) was a multicenter, randomized study comparing dose-adjusted warfarin to produce an INR = 1.4 to 2.8 with that of aspirin (325 mg per day) on the composite primary endpoint of recurrent ischemic stroke or death from any cause within 2 years of follow-up. The population studied, again, was that of patients with noncardioembolic stroke. The study was designed to demonstrate a superiority of warfarin over aspirin, and after enrolling a total of 2,206 patients, it showed no statistically significant difference between the two treatment groups. Considering the unusually low target INR range, however, we do not find the results of this study surprising either. Our last comment extends to the WARSS results in specific subgroups of noncardiogenic stroke patients.

Finally, there is the issue of using warfarin in patients with hypercoagulability syndromes–related inherent or acquired imbalances of the coagulation cascade. The data on these scenarios are largely derived from empirical observation. However, in practice we have found a lot less argument about the use of anticoagulation in patients with thombophilic coagulopathies, despite the lack of randomized prospective data.

PRACTICAL RECOMMENDATIONS

Following our exposition of the various agents available, it is apparent that choosing one or another antithrombotic agent may not be easy, particularly when the results of the major trials often appear conflictive. In fact, one of the most important arguments against the unequivocal strength of reported prospective randomized trials is the extensive editorial controversies that typically follow the publication of any major study. This should underscore the fact that the data can be always interpreted in more than one way.

Before we share with the reader our most practical approach to the problem of antithrombotic therapy for ischemic stroke prevention, we must create the framework for our strategy. In general, the overwhelming majority of the studies published to date about this subject have significant fundamental flaws that should influence the applicability of their results to clinical practice. The first problem involves those studies in which the study population is said to comprise noncardiogenic stroke patients. The assumptions here are that, from the etiopathogenic point of view, ischemic stroke patients can be assigned to one or another group on the basis of presumed cardiogenicity of the index event. Furthermore, these studies assume that the noncardiogenic group of patients will require a uniform and homogeneous approach to antithrombotic therapy. We find the studies that suffer from this handicap commonly lead to negative results, without either the control or the treatment group showing a beneficial effect over the other. In fact, a closer look at each of these studies shows that the diagnostic evaluation of the patients enrolled has been haphazard and suboptimal, casting a long shadow of doubt as to what condition is being treated.

Another problem relates to the nonuniform definition of the study population, making any subsequent comparison between results very difficult and generating some doubt about the validity of some of the meta-analyses. This is particularly problematic when we consider the inherent limitations of such post hoc comparisons. Along these lines, the use of composite end-points that are not comparable also makes interstudy comparisons very difficult.

Finally, we have found it particularly difficult to believe data collected in studies with inaccurate definitions of the endpoints; for example, the use of a definition of transient ischemic attack that is irrespective of imaging findings that confirm the presence of infarction, and that takes into consideration only the fact that the symptoms lasted <24 hours. These practices—the lumping of patients, their improper diagnostic evaluation, and the mischaracterization of endpoints—represent a disservice to the vascular neurology community and do not advance science in any meaningful way.

Having said this, we are left with the need to provide each patient under our care with the best approach to secondary ischemic stroke prevention. We must emphasize, as we have done in other chapters, that antithrombotic agents are but just one of the dimensions of risk factor modifications and that the success of any of these medications is interdependent on additional strategies that include lipid management, diabetes control, and blood pressure reduction, among others. In this context, we submit that it is impossible to provide any patient with the most effective antithrombotic therapy strategy without having gained an understanding of the most likely root cause of the index event, its vascular microenvironment, and the most likely composition of the thrombus to be prevented. In general, patients who have conditions that are largely associated with flow stagnation should be offered correction of the anatomic abnormality that produces such stasis (e.g., severe arterial stenosis treated by revascularization) or, if not feasible, considered for treatment with warfarin, which is a superior drug for the prevention of red thrombi. We do not endorse the indiscriminate utilization of warfarin, even for cardiogenic stroke, since many cardiogenic sources of embolism do not require warfarin for management. The use of warfarin requires the following important considerations:

1. There must be a clear indication of pathology known to produce stagnation.
2. Coumadin, the brand name, should be used to ensure that the same product is being used and to avoid unpredictable fluctuations in the INR values.
3. Same daily dose should be used to avoid oscillations of the INR that result in unnecessary dose adjustments or excessive dosing.
4. No major contraindications for chronic anticoagulation must be present.

On the other hand, we propose that patients without obvious stagnation, whose vascular microenvironment is more likely to lead to the production of white thrombi, should be offered double antiplatelet therapy. Although at first this could be interpreted as a recommendation for using low-dose aspirin plus ER-DP, the usefulness of combining aspirin and clopidogrel should not be dismissed without some discussion. The first argument on our last suggestion is whether clopidogrel is as effective as aspirin plus ER-DP in stroke reduction. We think both strategies are just as effective as one another, probably not for the same subgroup of patients. In Table 24.1 we can see the stroke event rates reported by the three major studies comparing aspirin with the three other major antiplatelet agents. For the purpose of our comparison we only used the stroke subgroup of CAPRIE, since it is the only one that remotely compares to the populations of the other two studies. It is easy to see that although the relative risk reduction produced by clopidogrel seems the smallest, the major differences between the studies were noted among the groups treated with aspirin. In fact, the event rates of the three treatment drugs were almost identical. One could easily conclude from this comparison that too low or too high dose of aspirin is counterproductive, while the aspirin dose used in CAPRIE was the optimal.

TABLE 24.1 Stroke Event Rates for the Major Trials Comparing Aspirin and Other Antiplatelet Agents

	ASA	Study Drug	RRR
TASS	13%	10%	23%
CAPRIE	10.5%	9.7%	7.6%
ESPS-2	12.5%	9.5%	24%

ASA, acetylsalicylic acid/aspirin; RRR, relative risk reduction; TASS, Ticlopidine Aspirin Stroke Study = rates in 3,069 patients at 36 mo (ASA at 1,300 mg/d); CAPRIE, Clopidogrel and Aspirin Prevention in Recurrent Ischemic Events = rates in stroke subgroup of 3,233 patients on clopidogrel and 3,198 patients on ASA (325 mg/day) at 36 months; ESPS-2, second European Stroke Prevention Study = rates in 3,200 patients at 24 months.

The second argument about the suggestion of using aspirin and clopidogrel is based on the poor design of the Management of Atherothrombosis with Clopidogrel in High-Risk Patients with Recent Transient Ischemic Attack or Ischemic Stroke (MATCH) study, which in our view makes its results predictable, and poorly applicable to the population of patients we treat. This trial suffers from nearly every flaw in design that we described earlier. First of all, the study was said to categorize patients according to the Trial of Org 10172 in Acute Stroke Therapy (TOAST) classification, yet the investigators were not required to complete a standardized and comprehensive evaluation that renders the classification of patients suspect and prone to lumping artifact. In defining transient ischemic attack as one of the endpoints, the only criterion used was the presence of symptoms for <24 hours without any consideration of imaging results from additional evaluation. This renders the event adjudication also suspect and fraught with misallocations. Finally, the follow-up period of only 18 months was simply too short to detect a more modest yet meaningful benefit. This could easily explain the gently diverging Kaplan-Meier curves and the tendency for nearly every subgroup to show hazard ratios in favor of double antiplatelet therapy. We found the results of the MATCH study predictable and not sufficient to counterbalance the beneficial effect of double antiplatelet therapy shown in both the Clopidogrel in Unstable Angina to Prevent Recurrent Events (CURE) and Clopidogrel for the Reduction of Events During Observation (CREDO) studies.

One final intriguing concept that we feel compelled to place forward is that of triple antiplatelet therapy. As we noted earlier, although the effect of either clopidogrel or aspirin + ER-DP seems to be of similar magnitude, it is likely that these drugs do not cover the exact same segments of the population but rather overlapping ones (see Fig. 24.6). Indeed, ER-DP is a relative weak antiplatelet agent compared with clopidogrel. This is easily noted in the lack of complaints by the patients treated with ER-DP of bruising, one of the most common complaints about clopidogrel. However, ER-DP

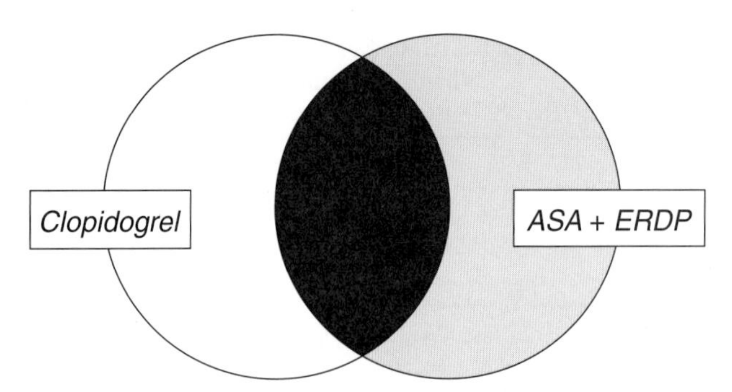

FIGURE 24.6. Venn diagram depicting the hypothetical overlap between clopidogrel and acetyl salicylic acid + extended-release dipyridamole (ASA + ERDP).

is a potent vasodilator, and this characteristic (likely to be responsible for the headaches it produces) may add considerably to the antithrombotic effects of low-dose aspirin and clopidogrel. Although still hypothetical, this concept may need to be investigated in the future. In any case, the complexity of the subject underscores the need for a standardized biological monitoring method to assess antiplatelet activity and *then* correlate this with clinical outcomes. In the meantime, our approach provides a systematic method for tailoring therapy to each patient base on the root cause of the index event.

SELECTED REFERENCES

Aronow WS. Antiplatelet therapy in the treatment of atherothrombotic disease: considering the evidence. *Geriatrics* 2007;62(4):12–24.

Aronow WS. Use of antiplatelet drugs in secondary prevention in older persons with atherothrombotic disease. *J Gerontol A Biol Sci Med Sci* 2007 ;62(5):518–524.

Ballew KA. Clopidogrel plus aspirin did not differ from aspirin alone for reducing MI, stroke, and CV death in high-risk atherothrombosis. *ACP J Club* 2006;145(2):33.

Bhatt DL, Fox KA, Hacke W, et al., CHARISMA Investigators. Clopidogrel and aspirin versus aspirin alone for the prevention of atherothrombotic events. *N Engl J Med* 2006;354(16):1706–1717.

Blann A. Antiplatelet therapy and the vascular tree. *Heart* 2006;92(1):3–4.

Brass LM. Strategies for primary and secondary stroke prevention. *Clin Cardiol* 2006;29(10 Suppl):II21–II27.

Chong JY, Mohr JP. Anticoagulation and platelet antiaggregation therapy in stroke prevention. *Curr Opin Neurol* 2005;18(1):53–57.

de Borst GJ, Hilgevoord AA, de Vries JP, et al. Influence of antiplatelet therapy on cerebral micro-emboli after carotid endarterectomy using postoperative transcranial Doppler monitoring. *Eur J Vasc Endovasc Surg* 2007;34(2):135–142.

Diener HC, Bogousslavsky J, Brass LM, et al. Management of atherothrombosis with clopidogrel in high-risk patients with recent transient ischaemic attack or ischaemic stroke (MATCH): study design and baseline data. *Cerebrovasc Dis* 2004;17(2–3):253–261.

Durand-Zaleski I, Bertrand M. The value of clopidogrel versus aspirin in reducing atherothrombotic events: the CAPRIE study. *Pharmacoeconomics* 2004;22(Suppl 4):19–27.

ESPRIT. Oral anticoagulation in patients after cerebral ischemia of arterial origin and risk of intracranial hemorrhage. *Stroke* 2003; 34(6):45–46.

Fontana P, Reny JL. New antiplatelet strategies in atherothrombosis and their indications. *Eur J Vasc Endovasc Surg* 2007;34(1):10–17.

Forbes CD. Secondary stroke prevention with low-dose aspirin, sustained release dipyridamole alone and in combination. ESPS Investigators. European Stroke Prevention Study. *Thromb Res* 1998;92(1 Suppl 1):S1–S6.

Hankey GJ. Antiplatelet therapy for the prevention of recurrent stroke and other serious vascular events: a review of the clinical trial data and guidelines. *Curr Med Res Opin* 2007;10:1453–1462.

Jacobson AK. Platelet ADP receptor antagonists: ticlopidine and clopidogrel. *Best Pract Res Clin Haematol* 2004;17(1):55–64.

Jamieson DG. Update on the use of antiplatelet agents in secondary stroke prevention. *J Natl Med Assoc* 2007;99(3):306.

Kikano GE, Brown MT. Antiplatelet therapy for atherothrombotic disease: an update for the primary care physician. *Mayo Clin Proc* 2007;82(5): 583–593.

Leonardi-Bee J, Bath PM, Bousser MG, et al. Dipyridamole in Stroke Collaboration (DISC). Dipyridamole for preventing recurrent ischemic stroke and other vascular events: a meta-analysis of individual patient data from randomized controlled trials. *Stroke* 2005;36(1): 162–168.

Liao JK. Secondary prevention of stroke and transient ischemic attack: is more platelet inhibition the answer? *Circulation* 2007;115(12): 1615–1621.

Markus HS, Droste DW, Kaps M, et al. Dual antiplatelet therapy with clopidogrel and aspirin in symptomatic carotid stenosis evaluated using doppler embolic signal detection: the Clopidogrel and Aspirin for Reduction of Emboli in Symptomatic Carotid Stenosis (CARESS) trial. *Circulation* 2005;111(17):2233–2240.

Massie BM, Krol WF, Ammon SE, et al. The Warfarin and Antiplatelet Therapy in Heart Failure trial (WATCH): rationale, design, and baseline patient characteristics. *J Card Fail* 2004;10(2):101–112.

Moussouttas M. Emerging therapies: ESPRIT. *Stroke* 2007;38(4):1142.

Plosker GL, Lyseng-Williamson KA. Clopidogrel: a review of its use in the prevention of thrombosis. *Drugs* 2007;67(4):613–646.

Redman AR, Allen LC. Warfarin versus aspirin in the secondary prevention of stroke: the WARSS study. *Curr Atheroscler Rep* 2002; 4(4): 319–325.

Redman AR, Ryan GJ. Aggrenox((R)) versus other pharmacotherapy in preventing recurrent stroke. *Expert Opin Pharmacother* 2004;5(1):117–123.

Sacco S, Carolei A. CHARISMA: the antiplatelet saga continues. *Stroke* 2007;38(3):854.

Sacco RL, Prabhakaran S, Thompson JL, et al. Comparison of warfarin versus aspirin for the prevention of recurrent stroke or death: subgroup analyses from the Warfarin-Aspirin Recurrent Stroke Study. *Cerebrovasc Dis* 2006;22(1):4–12.

Serebruany VL, Malinin AI, Atar D. Combination antiplatelet therapy with aspirin and clopidogrel: the role of antecedent and concomitant doses of aspirin. An analysis of 711 patients. *Cardiology* 2007; 107(4):307–312.

Sivenius J, Cunha L, Diener HC, et al. Antiplatelet treatment does not reduce the severity of subsequent stroke. European Stroke Prevention Study 2 Working Group. *Neurology* 1999;53(4):825–829.

Sivenius J, Cunha L, Diener HC, et al. Second European Stroke Prevention Study: antiplatelet therapy is effective regardless of age. ESPS2 Working Group. *Acta Neurol Scand* 1999;99(1):54–60.

Sudlow C. Dipyridamole with aspirin is better than aspirin alone in preventing vascular events after ischaemic stroke or TIA. *BMJ* 2007;334 (7599):901.

Testa L, Zoccai GB, Porto I, et al. Adjusted indirect meta-analysis of aspirin plus warfarin at international normalized ratios 2 to 3 versus aspirin plus clopidogrel after acute coronary syndromes. *Am J Cardiol* 2007; 99(12):1637–1642.

Wang TH, Bhatt DL, Topol EJ. Aspirin and clopidogrel resistance: an emerging clinical entity. *Eur Heart J* 2006;27(6):647–654.

Wilterdink JL, Easton JD. Dipyridamole plus aspirin in cerebrovascular disease. *Arch Neurol* 1999;56(9):1087–1092.

CRITICAL PATHWAY
Antithrombotic Therapy for Ischemic Stroke Prevention

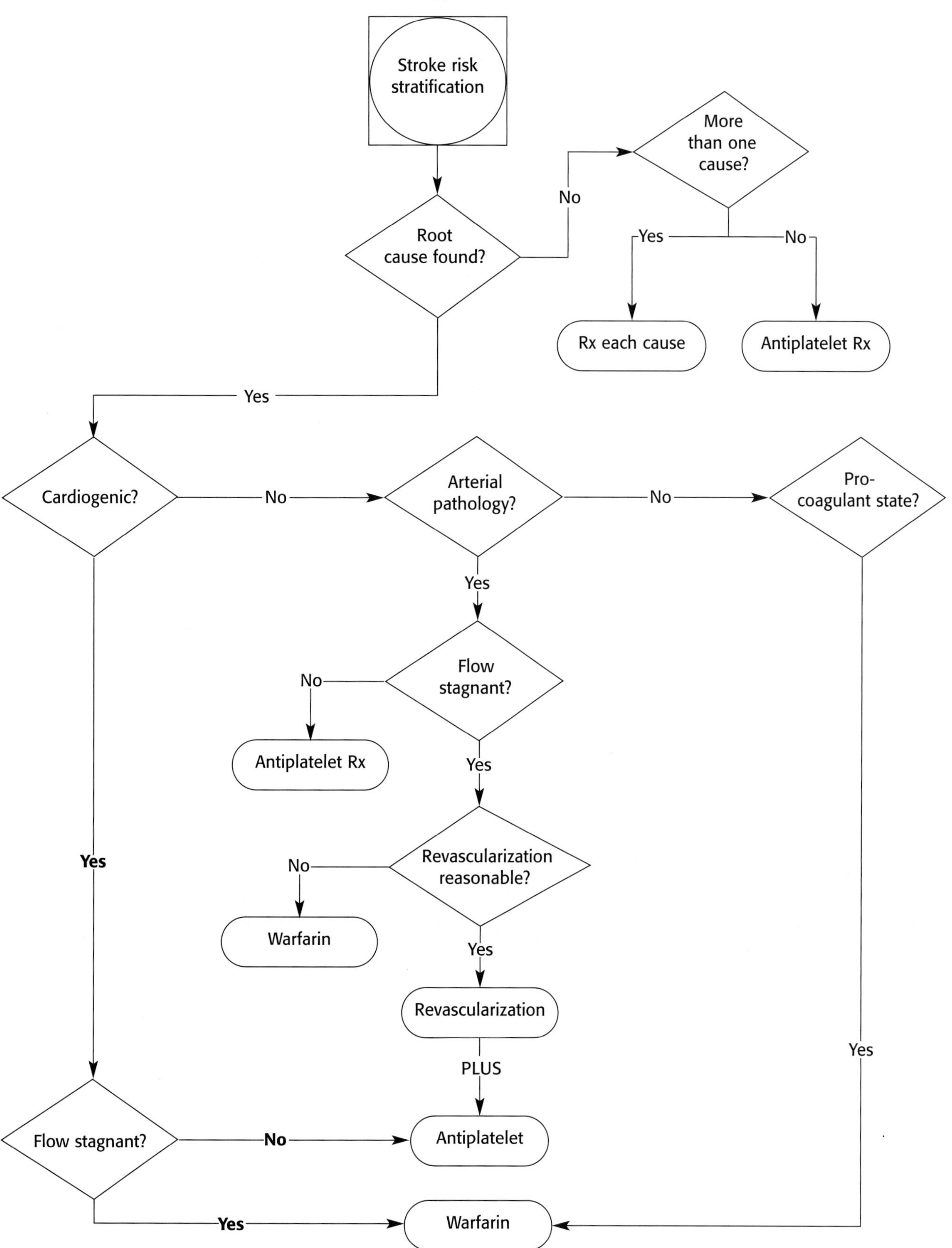

CHAPTER

25 Thrombolytic Therapy for Acute Ischemic Stroke

RIMA M. DAFER AND JOSÉ BILLER

OBJECTIVES

- What are the indications for intravenous thrombolysis?
- What are the indications for intra-arterial thrombolysis?
- What role can ultrasound play in thrombolysis?
- Can thombolysis be used during pregnancy?
- What is the treatment paradigm for venous sinus thrombosis?

Intravenous (IV) thrombolytic therapy with recombinant tissue plasminogen activator (rt-PA) remains the only Food and Drug Administration (FDA)–approved drug for hyperacute management of ischemic stroke. Recently, the mechanical thrombectomy device Mechanical Embolus Removal in Cerebral Ischemia (MERCI) has been approved to remove thrombi from the cerebral vasculature in selected patients with acute ischemic stroke. A number of new lytic agents and strategies are being pursued, including pharmacological or mechanical intra-arterial (IA) thrombolysis. The use of such therapies remains limited to specialized stroke centers where advanced imaging technologies and onsite interventional radiologists are available. In addition, new agents are being studied, including more selective thrombolytic agents. In this chapter, we present the available data on the use of IV and IA thrombolytic therapy in acute ischemic stroke.

Stroke remains the major cause of adult disability and the third leading cause of death, with approximately 750,000 new or recurrent strokes occurring annually in the United States. Ischemic stroke accounts for more than 80% of all strokes, with death occurring in 8% to 12% of patients within 30 days of the ischemic event. Management of hyperacute ischemic stroke relies mostly on vessel recanalization, with restoration or improvement of cerebral perfusion. The National Institute of Neurological Diseases and Stroke (NINDS) study of IV rt-PA in acute ischemic stroke was the first to prove beneficial, and this resulted in a paradigm shift in our approach to the stroke patients.

Despite much debate over the utility of IV rt-PA-based thrombolysis in the treatment of acute ischemic stroke within a 3-hour window of stroke symptoms, substantial data showed that IV rt-PA improves outcomes for patients with acute ischemic stroke with significant net reduction of death and dependence. However, the use of IV thrombolysis in ischemic stroke remains limited by the increased risk of intracerebral (ICH). To date, and >10 years after IV-based rt-PA approval for the treatment of ischemic stroke by the FDA, <5% of patients with acute ischemic stroke receive IV thrombolysis, mainly because of narrow treatment window of opportunities, and an apparent physicians' resistance.

INTRAVENOUS THROMBOLYSIS

IV thrombolytic therapy has been used in acute cerebral ischemia in attempts to restore vessel patency. Several thrombolytic agents have been tested in acute cerebral infarction including streptokinase (SK), urokinase (UK), and pro-urokinase (pro-UK), but rt-PA remains the only approved drug in the United States, Canada, Europe, Australia, South America, and Japan for the treatment of select patients with acute ischemic stroke.

The pivotal NINDS for IV thrombolysis with rt-PA trials randomized 624 subjects within 3 hours of stroke onset to 0.9 mg per kg of IV rt-PA or placebo. Patients receiving thrombolysis had a better chance of functional independence with minimal or no disability at 3 months follow-up in all four outcome measures [National Institute of Health Stroke Scale (NIHSS), Barthel Index (BI), modified Rankin Scale (mRS), and Glasgow Outcome Scale], with a 12% absolute improvement in the group receiving thrombolysis compared to placebo (minimal improvement of disability of 50% with rt-PA versus 38% with placebo) and a number needed to treat (NNT) of 6 for normal or near normal outcome and 3.1 for overall improved outcome. Despite the apparent substantial benefit for thrombolysis within the 3-hour window of treatment for all stroke subtypes, the data from the NINDS trial was cautiously received as the rate of bleeding complication, specifically symptomatic intraparenchymal hemorrhage (sICH), reached 6.4% inpatients receiving IV rt-PA compared to 0.6% for patients treated with placebo ($p < 0.001$).

However, European and Australian studies failed to reproduce such benefit for IV rt-PA, mainly because of heterogeneity of trials designs, use of different thrombolytic agents, and extended window for intervention. Similarly, the use of IV thrombolysis beyond 3 hours of the stroke symptoms onset showed limited benefit in acute ischemic stroke with a significant increase in the risk of ICH.

Three randomized placebo-controlled trials of IV SK were conducted in the mid-1990s. In the Australian Streptokinase Trial (ASK), patients were randomized to receive 1.5 million units of IV SK and aspirin versus placebo within 4 hours of onset of stroke symptoms. Similarly, the Multicenter Acute Stroke Trial–Italy (MAST-I) and the Multicenter Acute Stroke Trial–Europe (MAST-E) randomized subjects to receive 1.5 million units of IV SK or placebo within an extended time window of 6 hours from symptoms onset. These trials were prematurely terminated because of increased risk of deaths and sICH among patients who received SK.

As such, the European Cooperative Acute Stroke Studies (ECASS) failed to show a distinct benefit for rt-PA when used within 6 hours of ischemic stroke onset. In ECASS I, patients were randomized to 1.1 mg per kg or placebo, while in ECASS II the dose of rt-PA was comparable to that in the NINDS trial. Despite the negative results, and after excluding patients with protocol violation due to evidence of extended infarct signs on baseline computed tomography (CT) scan, improvement in functional outcome was noticeable at 3 months follow-up in the thrombolysis group.

The Thrombolytic Therapy in Acute Ischemic Stroke Study randomized patients with acute ischemic stroke into the thrombolysis arm with 0.9 mg per kg IV rt-PA or placebo in patients presenting within <6 hours of symptoms; the time window was then changed to 0 to 5 hours. This study found no significant rt-PA benefit with an increased risk of sICH in patients receiving thrombolyis >3 hours from onset of symptoms.

The Alteplase Thrombolysis for Acute Non-interventional Therapy in Ischemic Stroke (ATLANTIS) trials found no significant difference in functional outcome at 90 days between patients receiving 0.9 mg per kg rt-PA at 3 to 5 hours after stroke onset and placebo groups with increased risk of sICH in the rt-PA group.

A Cochrane review of pooled analysis of 2,775 patients enrolled in the six IV rt-PA (up to 6 hours of stroke onset) provided a clear evidence of a time-dependent benefit of thrombolytic therapy, with odds of a favorable outcome increased by 2.8-fold in patients treated within the first 90 minutes of symptom onset, compared to 1.6-fold in the 91- to 180-minute window and 1.4-fold within 181- to 270-minute window; treatment at 271 to 360 minutes did not improve outcome. Overall, the odds ratios (OR) for fatal ICH and sICH with rt-PA were 3.60 and 3.13, respectively.

The favorable results of the NINDS rt-PA trials have been duplicated in phase IV studies examining the use of IV rt-PA in routine clinical practice, with similar rates of sICH. The Safe Implementation of Thrombolysis in Stroke–Monitoring Study (SITS-MOST) evaluated the safety and efficacy of alteplase in a 3-hour time-window in a phase IV trial. A total of 6,483 patients were included in 285 European centers. Symptomatic ICH occurred in 7.3% of patients (1.7% observed within 24 hours after treatment). The 3-month mortality rate was 11.3%, and the rate of good clinical outcome defined as mRS of 0 to 2 was 55%.

In summary, treatment with IV thrombolysis within 3 hours of onset of stroke symptoms is associated with substantial benefit in functional outcome, despite an increased rate of sICH. In contrast, the use of IV thrombolysis beyond 3 hours of symptom onset is associated with significant increased risk of bleeding with a less substantial benefit from therapy. Accordingly, current guidelines recommend the use of IV rt-PA at dose of 0.9 mg per kg, with a maximum dose of 90 mg within 3 hours of ischemic stroke onset in carefully selected patients.

With the advent of neuroimaging, efforts are constantly made to attempt extending the narrow and rigid 3-hour window for IV thrombolysis with careful patient selection for treatment algorithms by the potential applications of modern CT techniques such as CT angiography, perfusion CT, and magnetic resonance imaging (MRI) diffusion/perfusion thrombolysis.

Interventional Procedures

Because IV rt-PA can only be administered to carefully selected patients within a 3-hour time window, and with an overall <5% of acute ischemic stroke patients receiving thrombolytic therapy, IA thrombolysis has been pursued as an alternative strategy to treat patients with large vessel arterial occlusion strokes with longer time windows (<6 hours in the carotid artery territory or <12 to 24 hours in the basilar artery territory) and a contraindication for IV thrombolysis.

INTRA-ARTERIAL THROMBOLYSIS

IA thrombolysis has been shown to offer advantages over IV thrombolysis in patients with large vessel occlusive disease and in those presenting with symptoms beyond 3 hours of the treatment window for rt-PA.

In the Prolyse in Acute Cerebral Thromboembolism (PROACT) study, 36 patients with angiographically demonstrated arterial occlusions were treated with UK or rt-PA within 3 hours of stroke onset. Nearly half the patients treated showed no or little disability at 1 to 3 months (mRS of 0 or 1), and vessel recanalization was achieved in 75%. The rate of sICH was 11% and the mortality rate was 22%.

The PROACT II study, a phase-III double-blind trial, randomized 180 subjects with acute ischemic stroke within 6 hours of stroke onset with documented middle cerebral artery (MCA) occlusion to IA thrombolysis with pro-UK at a dose of 9 mg (pro-UK group) and heparin or IV heparin alone (control group). Good outcome defined at mRS of 2 or less was achieved in 40% of patients receiving pro-UK compared to 25% of control ($p = 0.04$). Similarly, the group receiving IA thrombolysis showed a recanalization rate of 66% versus 18% for the control group ($p < 0.001$). Symptomatic ICH occurred in 10% of pro-UK treated patients and in only 2% of the control group ($p = 0.06$), while the overall rate of ICH was 40%. Because of the small size of the study and the high rate of ICH, pro-UK was not approved by the FDA for the hyperacute management of ischemic stroke. Other thrombolytic agents including UK, reteplase, and rt-PA have been used intra-arterially in postoperative patients, and those receiving therapeutic anticoagulation.

In summary, IA thrombolysis may prove beneficial in carefully selected patients with acute ischemic stroke postoperatively, those receiving active warfarin treatment, or those with large arterial strokes with suspected MCA or intracranial internal carotid artery (ICA) occlusion who are likely to fail treatment with IV thrombolysis. However, the off-label use of IA thrombolysis within 6 hours of carotid territory stroke symptoms remains limited to well-equipped tertiary stroke centers with experienced interventional neuroradiology team. The window for vertebrobasilar circulation territory arterial occlusions is unknown and could potentially extend beyond 6 and up to 24 hours.

INTRAVENOUS AND INTRA-ARTERIAL THROMBOLYSIS

Because of concerns that IA thrombolysis may deny patients presenting within 3 hours of symptom onset from receiving IV thrombolysis due to time delay associated with diagnostic angiography, the feasibility and safety of a combined IV and IA thrombolysis approach to recanalization in patients with ischemic stroke have been studied in proof-of-concept trials.

In a pilot double-blinded, randomized, placebo-controlled multicenter phase-I study of 35 patients, subjects were randomized to IV rt-PA or IV placebo followed by local IA administration of rt-PA when angiographic large arterial occlusion was documented. Seventeen patients received combined IV/IA thrombolysis and 18 were enrolled in the placebo/IA arm. A higher recanalization rate was achieved in the IV/IA group compared to placebo/IA (6 of 11 versus 1 of 10, $p = 0.03$). Life-threatening bleeding complications occurred in two patients in the IV/IA group, while sICH occurred in one placebo/IA patient and only in two IV/IA patients.

The Interventional Management Study (IMS) enrolled 80 subjects with large ischemic stroke with median baseline NIHSS of 18. Patients received IV rt-PA at dose of 0.6 mg per kg, 60 mg maximum over 30 minutes within 3 hours of stroke onset. Additional rt-PA was administered via a microcatheter at the site of the thrombus in the appropriate intracranial artery up to a total dose of 22 mg over 2 hours of infusion or until thrombolysis was achieved. The 3-month mortality in IMS subjects (16%) was numerically lower, but not statistically different from the mortality of the placebo- (24%) and the rt-PA-treated subjects (21%) in the NINDS rt-PA stroke trial. The rate of sICH was similar to IV rt-PA–treated patients in the NINDS rt-PA stroke trial, but significantly higher than that in the placebo group (6.3% versus 1%, $p = 0.018$).

Similarly, the IMS II compared combined IV/IA approach to placebo for recanalization for ischemic stroke. Subjects received IV rt-PA (0.6 mg per kg over 30 minutes) within 3 hours of onset, followed by additional IA rt-PA when arterial occlusion was documented on angiography, via the EKOS synography microinfusion catheter or a standard microcatheter at the site of the thrombus up to a total dose of 22 mg over 2 hours of infusion or until thrombolysis. Bridging treatment was associated with a lower 3-month mortality rate compared to placebo and rt-PA-treated subjects in the NINDS rt-PA stroke trial (16% versus 24% versus 21%). Symptomatic ICH occurred in 9.9% of patients.

A recent review of the off-label use of bridging IV/IA thrombolysis in 273 patients reports a sICH rate of 6.95%. Overall, the combined bridging IV and IA approach to recanalization appears safe and potentially efficacious, and is the subject of intensive ongoing research in large multicenter randomized clinical trials.

INTRA-ARTERIAL MECHANICAL THROMBOLYSIS

Despite the significant rate of vessel recanalization, the increased risk of sICH remains a limiting factor for the use of pharmacological IA thrombolysis in acute ischemic stroke. Mechanical endovascular embolectomy has been pursued as an alternate strategy in attempts to limit the risk of systemic and cerebral bleeding complications. A number of devices have been tried including laser devices, suction creating saline (Angiojet) catheters, and intravascular ultrasound devices. The MERCI device has been approved for mechanical extraction of clots after a stroke based on a pilot study that showed efficacy of the MERCI retriever for opening intracranial vessels in patients ineligible for IV rt-PA.

The MERCI trial demonstrated a recanalization rate in 46% (69/151) patients compared with the 18% historical control of the PROACT-II study. There was sICH in 7.8% of cases. Mortality occurred in 32% of recanalized patients versus 54% of unrecanalized patients ($p = 0.01$), with a good outcome defined as mRS <2 in 46% of recanalized patients versus 10% of unrecanalized patients ($p < 0.001$). By contrast, however, there was only a 27% mortality in the placebo control arm of the PROACT-II study used as a comparison for the MERCI trial and the MCA recanalization rate of 45% in MERCI compared unfavorably with the 66% recanalization rate in the pro-UK arm of PROACT-II.

In the multi-MERCI prospective, single-arm trial, patients with large vessel ischemic stroke who received IV rt-PA but did not recanalize, or those who were ineligible for IV thrombolysis, were treated within 8 hours of stroke symptom onset. One hundred and eleven patients with significant large vessel stroke (mean NIHSS 19 $\pm$ 6.3) underwent the thrombectomy procedure. Thirty patients (27%) received IV tPA before intervention. Treatment with the MERCI device alone resulted in successful recanalization in 60 of 111 (54%) treatable vessels and in 77 of 111 (69%) after adjunctive therapy with IA rt-PA or mechanical manipulation. Symptomatic ICH occurred in 9.0% of patients.

Further analysis of the MERCI and multi-MERCI trials assessed the success rate of the MERCI retriever mechanical thrombectomy device in recanalization of ICA occlusions and stroke outcome. Of the 80 patients with ICA occlusion, 53% had successful recanalization with the MERCI retriever alone and 63% with the device combined with endovascular treatment. The rate of sICH was not significantly different between recanalized and unrecanalized group. Good clinical outcome was observed in 39% of patients with ICA recanalization and in 3% of patients without recanalization ($p < 0.001$). The 90-day mortality was significantly lower in the recanalized group compared to the unrecanalized group (30% versus 73%, $p < 0.001$).

Currently, however, only two endovascular devices are approved for removal of clot from the cerebral vasculature to reduce clot burden in acute stroke due to large-vessel occlusive disease, as opposed the treatment of stroke. These devices should be used as adjuvant to thrombolysis. Active clinical trials to confirm their efficacy in stroke patients are underway.

THROMBOLYSIS AND ULTRASONOGRAPHY

The use of transcranial Doppler (TCD) with rt-PA is thought to safely enhance the effectiveness of thrombolysis in restoring vessel patency and to improve clinical outcome and accelerate clinical recovery within 2 hours of initiation of drug therapy. The exact mechanism of TCD use is unclear, perhaps involving heat generated by ultrasound or direction agitation of blood by ultrasound pressure waves or microbubbles.

In the Combined Lysis of Thrombus in Brain ischemia using transcranial Ultrasound and Systemic tPA (CLOTBUST) trial, clinical recovery with complete vessel recanalization within 2 hours was observed in patients receiving rt-PA combined with ultrasound energy administration via a continuous 2 MHz TCD probe compared to thrombolysis alone ($p = 0.02$). However, different results were achieved in smaller studies where transcranial color-coded duplex (TCCD) sonography showed a trend toward a higher risk of hemorrhagic transformation following exposure to multifrequency, multielement duplex ultrasound.

EMERGING PHARMACOLOGICAL THERAPIES

Tenectoplase (TNK) is a third-generation thrombolytic agent with a longer half-life, improved fibrin specificity, and increased resistance to plasminogen activator inhibitor 1 (PAI-1) as compared to rt-PA. In an open-label dose-escalation study of patients with ischemic stroke, TNK given as IV bolus infusion within 3 hours of stroke onset was shown to be safe at doses of 0.1 to 0.4 mg per kg. Future studies are needed to compare the efficacy and safety of TNK versus rt-PA.

Desmoteplase is a promising genetically engineered version of a clot-dissolving protein derived from vampire-bat saliva, thought to be a potential alternative to rt-PA in the treatment of acute ischemic stroke. It has an extended half-life allowing for single bolus administration with the prospect of a lower risk of systemic or intracranial bleeding complications. In two independent phase II randomized, double-blinded, placebo-controlled, dose-escalation studies in acute ischemic stroke, desmoteplase was shown to be safe at doses of 90 and 125 μg per kg when given as single-bolus IV infusion dose in the time window of 3 to 9 hours. The Desmoteplase in Acute Ischemic Stroke (DIAS) in Europe, Asia, and Australia and Dose Escalation study of Desmoteplase in Acute Ischemic Stroke (DEDAS) in the Unites States and Germany were largely identical in design and methodology, and were conducted using MRI-measured diffusion/perfusion mismatch of ≥20% as a key inclusion criterion. Overall, greater improvement in reperfusion was observed in the desmoteplase-treated patients compared to the placebo group, and favorable clinical outcome was observed at 90 days. The rate of sICH was low at doses of 90 and 125 μg per kg compared to the higher doses studied.

Preliminary results of DIAS-2 trial were presented at the 16th European Stroke Conference in Glascow, which showed no benefit with either 90- or 125-μg per kg dose. Mortality rate was higher in the treatment group compared with the placebo group, although death was thought to be due to causes unrelated to the treatment. ICH at 72 hours was observed in 4% of patients receiving the study drug.

Thrombolysis in Children

Ischemic stroke in children is uncommon with a rate estimated at 2 to 3 per 100,000 children aged 1 to 14 years. Unlike adults, ischemic stroke in children is predominantly secondary to cardiac embolism or hypercoagulable states. Because of its rarity and various causative factors, pediatric stroke is rarely diagnosed within an early time frame. In one hospital database, the mean time to diagnosis was 35.7 hours. In the absence of evidence-based treatment guidelines, the role of thrombolytic therapy in pediatric ischemic stroke remains anecdotal and limited to isolated case reports of adolescents. Despite a high reported recanalization rate, major bleeding complications were observed in 40% of children. In a recent data analysis from the Nationwide Inpatient Sample, which included 2,904 children between 1 and 17 years of age who experienced a stroke from 2000 to 2003, only a very small percentage of children with ischemic stroke (1.6%) received thrombolytic therapy. The mean age of thrombolysis-treated patients was 11.1 ± 4.1; all of the children who were given thrombolytic agents were boys. The study showed a higher risk of death and dependency from a stroke in children treated with thrombolytic therapy, with prolonged hospital stay and ventilator dependence. However, the study did not have information on stroke severity, functional or outcome scales. The use of rt-PA and other thrombolytic agents in pediatric stroke has not been endorsed by the American Stroke Association.

Thrombolysis in Pregnancy

Pregnancy is a procoagulant state, which could potentially increase the risk of arterial and venous strokes. Pregnant subjects have historically been excluded from clinical trials, and in the absence of clinical guidelines, pregnancy is considered a relative contraindication for thrombolysis despite evidence that rt-PA does not cross the placenta. A total of 28 cases describing the use of rt-PA in pregnancy has been reported in the literature so far; ten of those were in patients with ischemic stroke. In these case reports, the thrombolysis complication rates were similar to those in nonpregnant women, with an estimated fetal fatality of 8%. Taking into account that the complication rate did not exceed those of large randomized controlled trials, the use of thrombolytic therapy should be carefully considered among carefully selected pregnant patients with life-threatening or potentially debilitating ischemic stroke.

THROMBOLYSIS IN CEREBRAL VENOUS DURAL SINUS THROMBOSIS

Despite the lack of safety and efficacy data from randomized controlled clinical trials, local thrombolysis with or without rheolytic mechanical thrombectomy has recently gained popularity in the management of cerebral venous dural sinus thrombosis (CVDST). More than 30 cases have been reported in the literature describing the use of thrombolysis for patients with CVDST and rapidly deteriorating clinical course despite anticoagulation therapy in attempts to restore rapid recanalization of the occluded venous sinus, with favorable outcome.

THROMBOLYSIS IN CERVICOCEPHALIC ARTERIAL DISSECTION

Despite its potential feasibility, the experience of thrombolysis in cervicocephalic arterial dissection (CCAD) is limited to case reports. The diagnosis of CCAD was not a contraindication for enrollment in acute ischemic stroke thrombolytic trials, although the safety and efficacy of thrombolysis in such circumstances have not been determined. Both IV- and IA thrombolysis have been used in CCAD, with good outcomes ranging from 40% to 60%, and a mortality rate of 6% to 13%, in the absence of intracranial hemorrhagic complications.

THROMBOLYSIS IN CENTRAL RETINAL ARTERY OCCLUSION

Acute central retinal artery occlusion (CRAO) is a major neuro-ophthalmological emergency associated with sudden painless and acute painless loss. The extent of visual loss depends on the segment of retina that has been affected. While spontaneous improvement occurs in <15% of cases, conventional management provides limited benefit for visual recovery. Several case series implicated that either IV- or IA thrombolysis is a potentially efficacious and safe treatment for CRAO or branch retinal artery occlusion (BRAO). In a retrospective chart review of 80 patients with retinal artery occlusion, treatment with IA rt-PA within 6 to 18 hours of symptom onset was associated with limited benefit compared to the rate of spontaneous improvement and conventional forms of therapy. When given within 6 hours of onset symptoms, IA UK enhanced the chance of visual improvement especially when compared to younger patients.

In the absence of randomized controlled trials, and based on retrospective studies and case reports, it is prudent to say that thrombolysis may be potentially safe with a trend for visual improvement in CRAO when used within 6 hours of symptom onset.

DIAGNOSTIC WORKUP

All patients with acute ischemic stroke should undergo extensive and thorough general and neurological assessment. The NIHSS is a standardized useful tool to evaluate many of the domains of neurological deficits, including motor, sensory, and visual impairments, and thereby to determine the severity of neurological impairment. An immediate unenhanced cranial CT scan is imperative in excluding other causes for the focal neurological deficit, preferably with CT perfusion and CT angiography to assess the intracranial circulation and to determine the absence or presence of large vessel arterial occlusive disease. Alternatively, MRI of the brain with diffusion and perfusion studies, together with magnetic resonance angiography (MRA) is helpful in outlining the core of the infarct and the penumbra size, and in determining the extent of arterial occlusion. Laboratory studies to be obtained include complete blood count (CBC), platelet count, prothrombin time (PT), international normalized ratio (INR) activated partial thromboplastin time (aPTT), blood glucose, and in women of childbearing age, a pregnancy test. Blood should be screened for type- and cross-match. An electrocardiogram (ECG) and cardiac enzymes are obtained to exclude cardiac etiologies (see Table 25.1). A Foley catheter or nasogastric tube if necessary should be placed before initiation of thrombolytic therapy.

TABLE 25.1 Initial Prethrombolysis Acute Ischemic Stroke Workup

Determine exact time of onset of symptoms
Assess using NIHSS
Insert two large peripheral IV lines
Blood for CBC and platelets
CK and troponins
PT (INR), aPTT
Serum glucose, serum lytes, BUN, creatinine
Blood type and screen
CT or MRI/DWI
CT perfusion or MRI/DWI/PWI
Perform CTA or MRA
12-lead ECG
Urine β-hCG for women of childbearing age

NIHSS, National Institute of Health Stroke Scale; CBC, complete blood count; CK, creatine kinase; PT, prothrombin time; INR, international normalized ratio;aPTT, activated partial thromboplastin time; BUN, blood urea nitrogen; CT, computed tomography; MRI, magnetic resonance imaging; DWI, diffusion-weighted DWI; PWI, perfusion weighted imaging; CTA, computed tomography angiography; CTA,; MRA, magnetic resonance angiography; ECG, electrocardiogram; hCG, human chorionic gonadotropin.

DOSAGE

Treatment is administered as soon as the imaging studies and laboratory results are reviewed, and after all contraindications for thrombolytic therapy have been excluded (see Tables 25.2 and 25.3).

The recommended dose of IV rt-PA in acute ischemic stroke is 0.9 mg per kg, to a maximum of 90 mg. Ten percent of the total dose is given as an initial bolus over 1 minute, and the rest as an infusion over 1 hour. In patients with symptoms and signs consistent with large artery occlusion, bridging between IV- and IA thrombolysis may be considered. The suggested dose is 0.6 mg per kg of IV rt-PA initially, and if neuroimaging testing confirms the findings of large vessel disease, IA thrombolysis with repeated boluses of 5 mg, to a maximum of 20 mg, is used. Mechanical thrombectomy may be considered as adjuvant therapy in patients who fail to recanalize with pharmacological thrombolysis.

PERITHROMBOLYSIS MANAGEMENT

All patients should be monitored in designated units with well-trained staff.

Insertion of Foley catheter or nasogastric tube should be avoided. Antiplatelet agents or anticoagulants should not be given within the first 24 hours of treatment. Once infusion of rt-PA begins, vital signs are monitored every 15 minutes for 2 hours, then every 30 minutes for 6 hours, and then every 60 minutes for the next 16 hours. Patients should be monitored in an intensive clinical setting for symptoms or signs of ICH. Hypertension (>180/105 mm Hg) should be avoided (see Table 25.4). Patients should be monitored for signs of intracerebral hemorrhage (mental status changes, clinical deterioration, headache, nausea, and vomiting). If ICH is suspected, thrombolytic therapy should be stopped immediately and emergency unenhanced CT scan of brain obtained. CBC with platelet count, PT, INR, aPTT, and fibrinogen levels are checked. In the event of intracranial hemorrhage, patients should be transfused with six to eight units of cryoprecipitate containing factor VIII and six to eight units of platelets. Neurosurgical consultation should be called. Clinical deterioration with extension of the initial infarction has been reported after administration of rt-PA.

SIDE EFFECTS

The main adverse effects of thrombolysis include systemic bleeding or ICH, the latter occurring in 6% to 7% of acute ischemic strokes patients receiving IV thrombolysis, with higher rates reported with IA or combined IV/IA thrombolysis.

Hemorrhagic transformation post thrombolysis has been classified by using clinical and radiological criteria as follows: hemorrhagic infarction (HI), parenchymal hemorrhage (PH), and sICH. Hemorrhagic transformation has been associated with the presence of hypodensity on baseline CT scan. Higher rates of PH and sICH have also been reported in patients with parenchymal hypoattenuation on baseline CT. A higher risk of bleeding has been observed in patients with congestive heart failure, elevated baseline

TABLE 25.2 Exclusion Criteria for Intravenous Thrombolytic Therapy

Rapidly improving or minor stroke symptoms
Onset of symptoms beyond 3 h[a]
History of head trauma or stroke during the preceding 3 mo
History of ICH or symptoms at presentation suggestive of SAH
Known history of cerebral aneurysm or other CNS vascular malformation
Major surgery during the preceding 14 d
Arterial puncture or invasive procedures (including lumbar puncture) at a noncompressible site within the preceding 7 d
Gastrointestinal or urinary tract hemorrhage within the previous 21 d
Seizure at onset of stroke symptoms[b]
Uncontrolled systolic blood pressure >185 mm Hg and diastolic pressure >110 mm Hg[c]
Blood glucose concentrations <50 mg/dL
Platelet count ≤100,000/mm^3 or history of acquired or hereditary coagulopathies
Anticoagulant or heparin used within preceding 48 h with elevated aPTT or INR >1.7
Presumed septic embolism
Suspected life expectancy <3 mo
CT scan or MRI showing intracranial bleeding, intracranial mass lesions, or early evidence of acute stroke including early infarct signs such as sulcal edema involving more than one third of a cerebral lobar territory

ICH, intracerebral hemorrhage; SAH, subarachnoid hemorrhage; CNS, central nervous system; aPTT, activated partial thromboplastin time; INR, international normalized ratio; CT, computed tomography; MRI, magnetic resonance imaging.

[a] Symptom onset defined from when patient first seen abnormal. Patients who awaken with symptoms are ineligible for thrombolysis unless they were seen to be normal within the 3 h before awakening from sleep.

[b] In patients with history of seizures, careful consideration is required regarding whether presentation could reflect a postictal state.

[c] Antihypertensive medication to bring the blood pressure within an acceptable range before thrombolysis is permitted but aggressive measures with agents that could result in relative hypotension should be avoided. Acceptable medications include intravenous labetalol or nicardipine.

systolic blood pressure, advanced age, and in patients treated with aspirin before thrombolysis. Additional risk factors for HT include high NIHSS score, elevated serum glucose level, large lesion volume of initial DWI lesion, and sizable abnormalities on acute diffusion coefficient (ADC) analysis. The risk of sICH in patients with microbleeds receiving thrombolytic therapy remains unclear.

Other rare side effects include orolingual angioedema, anaphylactoid reactions, and other allergic reactions and febrile illness.

Complications associated with IA thrombolysis (pharmacological or mechanical) include ICH, subarachnoid hemorrhage (SAH), groin complications related to catheterization, vessel perforations, intramural arterial dissection or embolization in other uninvolved arteries, reaction to contrast material, and potential heparin-related specific complications including heparin-induced thrombocytopenia.

TABLE 25.3 Contraindications for Intra-arterial Thrombolysis

As per IV thrombolysis[a]
Symptoms of stroke >6 h[a,b]
Suspected lacunar stroke
Sensitivity to radiographic contrast dye or other contraindication to cerebral angiography
Arterial stenosis proximal to the clot preventing passage of a microcatheter

[a] Except for onset of symptoms, which may be extended for up to 6 h for chemical IA thrombolysis, and [b] up to 8 h with mechanical thrombolysis. Window of treatment is variable in basilar artery occlusion, and may be extended up to 24 h in carefully selected patients.

TABLE 25.4 Management of Blood Pressure after Thrombolytic Therapy

BP measurement every 15 min for the first 2 h, every 30 min for the next 6 h, and then every 1 h until 16 h from treatment
If diastolic BP 105–120 mm Hg or systolic BP 180–230 mm Hg, labetolol 10 mg IV over 1–2 min; may repeat or double the dosage every 10–20 min to a maximum dose of 300 mg or labetalol 10 mg IV bolus followed by continuous infusion at a rate of 2–8 mg/min
If diastolic BP 121–140 mm Hg or systolic BP >230 mm Hg, labetolol 10 mg IV over 1–2 min; may repeat or double the dosage every 10–20 min to a maximum dose of 300 mg or labetalol 10 mg IV bolus, followed by continuous infusion at a rate of 2–8 mg/min or nicardipine 5 mg/h IV infusion as initial dose, titrate by increasing 2.5 mg/h every 5 min to maximum of 15 mg/h
If diastolic BP >140 mm Hg, sodium nitroprusside infusion of at a rate of 0.5 μm/kg/min and titrate to desired BP

BP, blood pressure.

CONCLUSION

Early and rapid diagnosis and aggressive management are standard of care and the key to salvage ischemic brain tissue in acute ischemic stroke. The benefits of thrombolytic therapy with rt-PA in acute ischemic stroke over placebo in carefully selected patients have been well documented. Data from thrombolytic trials suggests that IV rt-PA may be associated with less hazard (3 out of 100 patients harmed mainly secondary to sICH) and more benefit (32 out of 100 patients) with thrombolysis, with decreased death or dependence. The evaluation of patients with acute ischemic stroke for thrombolysis requires extensive clinical expertise combined with modern neuroimaging to determine the best treatment modality for carefully selected patients.

SELECTED REFERENCES

Adams HP, Jr, Adams RJ, Brott T, et al. Guidelines for the early management of patients with ischemic stroke: a scientific statement from the Stroke Council of the American Stroke Association. *Stroke* 2003;34(4):1056–1083.

Adams HP, Jr, del Zoppo G, Alberts MJ, et al. Guidelines for the early management of adults with ischemic stroke: a guideline from the American Heart Association/American Stroke Association Stroke Council, Clinical Cardiology Council, Cardiovascular Radiology and Intervention Council, and the Atherosclerotic Peripheral Vascular Disease and Quality of Care Outcomes in Research Interdisciplinary Working Groups: the American Academy of Neurology affirms the value of this guideline as an educational tool for neurologists. *Stroke* 2007;38(5):1655–1711.

Aleu A, Mellado P, Lichy C, et al. Hemorrhagic complications after off-label thrombolysis for ischemic stroke. *Stroke* 2007;38(2):417–422.

Alexandrov AV, Molina CA, Grotta JC, et al. Ultrasound-enhanced systemic thrombolysis for acute ischemic stroke. *N Engl J Med* 2004;351(21):2170–2178.

Arnold M, Koerner U, Remonda L, et al. Comparison of intra-arterial thrombolysis with conventional treatment in patients with acute central retinal artery occlusion. *J Neurol Neurosurg Psychiatr* 2005;76(2):196–199.

Arnold M, Nedeltchev K, Schroth G, et al. Clinical and radiological predictors of recanalisation and outcome of 40 patients with acute basilar artery occlusion treated with intra-arterial thrombolysis. *J Neurol Neurosurg Psychiatr* 2004;75(6):857–862.

Arnold M, Nedeltchev K, Sturzenegger M, et al. Thrombolysis in patients with acute stroke caused by cervical artery dissection: analysis of 9 patients and review of the literature. *Arch Neurol* 2002;59(4):549–553.

Baker MD, Opatowsky MJ, Wilson JA, et al. Rheolytic catheter and thrombolysis of dural venous sinus thrombosis: a case series. *Neurosurgery* 2001;48(3):487–493; discussion 93–94.

Barnwell SL, Higashida RT, Halbach VV, et al. Direct endovascular thrombolytic therapy for dural sinus thrombosis. *Neurosurgery* 1991;28(1):135–142.

Becker KJ, Brott TG. Approval of the MERCI clot retriever: a critical view. *Stroke* 2005;36(2):400–403.

Benedict SL, Ni OK, Schloesser P, et al. Intra-arterial thrombolysis in a 2-year-old with cardioembolic stroke. *J Child Neurol* 2007;22(2):225–227.

Bourekas EC, Slivka AP, Casavant MJ. Intra-arterial thrombolysis of a distal internal carotid artery occlusion in an adolescent. *Neurocrit Care* 2005;2(2):179–182.

Bourekas EC, Slivka AP, Shah R, et al. Intraarterial thrombolytic therapy within 3 hours of the onset of stroke. *Neurosurgery* 2004;54(1):39–44.

Chalela JA, Katzan I, Liebeskind DS, et al. Safety of intra-arterial thrombolysis in the postoperative period. *Stroke* 2001;32(6):1365–1369.

Chaloupka JC, Mangla S, Huddle DC. Use of mechanical thrombolysis via microballoon percutaneous transluminal angioplasty for the treatment of acute dural sinus thrombosis: case presentation and technical report. *Neurosurgery* 1999;45(3):650–656.

Chow K, Gobin YP, Saver J, et al. Endovascular treatment of dural sinus thrombosis with rheolytic thrombectomy and intra-arterial thrombolysis. *Stroke* 2000;31(6):1420–1425.

Clark WM, Albers GW, Madden KP, et al. The rtPA (alteplase) 0- to 6-hour acute stroke trial, part A (A0276g): results of a double-blind, placebo-controlled, multicenter study. Thromblytic therapy in acute ischemic stroke study investigators. *Stroke* 2000;31(4):811–816.

Clark WM, Wissman S, Albers GW, et al. Recombinant tissue-type plasminogen activator (Alteplase) for ischemic stroke 3 to 5 hours after symptom onset. The ATLANTIS Study: a randomized controlled trial. Alteplase Thrombolysis for Acute Noninterventional Therapy in Ischemic Stroke. *JAMA* 1999;282(21):2019–2026.

Combined intravenous and intra-arterial recanalization for acute ischemic stroke: the Interventional Management of Stroke Study. *Stroke* 2004;35(4):904–911.

Curtin KR, Shaibani A, Resnick SA, et al. Rheolytic catheter thrombectomy, balloon angioplasty, and direct recombinant tissue plasminogen activator thrombolysis of dural sinus thrombosis with preexisting hemorrhagic infarctions. *Am J Neuroradiol* 2004;25(10):1807–1811.

Dafer RM, Biller J. Desmoteplase in the treatment of acute ischemic stroke. *Expert Rev Neurother* 2007;7(4):333–337.

D'Alise MD, Fichtel F, Horowitz M. Sagittal sinus thrombosis following minor head injury treated with continuous urokinase infusion. *Surg Neurol* 1998;49(4):430–435.

Davalos A. Thrombolysis in acute ischemic stroke: successes, failures, and new hopes. *Cerebrovasc Dis* 2005;20(suppl 2):135–139.

Derex L, Hermier M, Adeleine P, et al. Clinical and imaging predictors of intracerebral haemorrhage in stroke patients treated with intravenous tissue plasminogen activator. *J Neurol Neurosurg Psychiatr* 2005;76(1):70–75.

Derex L, Nighoghossian N, Turjman F, et al. Intravenous tPA in acute ischemic stroke related to internal carotid artery dissection. *Neurology* 2000;54(11):2159–2161.

Di Rocco C, Iannelli A, Leone G, et al. Heparin-urokinase treatment in aseptic dural sinus thrombosis. *Arch Neurol* 1981;38(7):431–435.

Elford K, Leader A, Wee R, et al. Stroke in ovarian hyperstimulation syndrome in early pregnancy treated with intra-arterial rt-PA. *Neurology* 2002;59(8):1270–1272.

Eskridge JM, Wessbecher FW. Thrombolysis for superior sagittal sinus thrombosis. *J Vasc Interv Radiol* 1991;2(1):89–93.

Fiehler J, Albers GW, Boulanger JM, et al. Bleeding Risk Analysis in Stroke Imaging before ThromboLysis (BRASIL). Pooled analysis of T2*-weighted magnetic resonance imaging data from 570 patients. *Stroke* 2007;38:2738.

Flint AC, Duckwiler GR, Budzik RF, et al. Mechanical thrombectomy of intracranial internal carotid occlusion: pooled results of the MERCI and Multi MERCI Part I trials. *Stroke* 2007;38(4):1274–1280.

Furlan AJ, Eyding D, Albers GW, et al. Dose Escalation of Desmoteplase for Acute Ischemic Stroke (DEDAS): evidence of safety and efficacy 3 to 9 hours after stroke onset. *Stroke* 2006;37(5):1227–1231.

Gabis LV, Yangala R, Lenn NJ. Time lag to diagnosis of stroke in children. *Pediatrics* 2002;110(5):924–928.

Georgiadis D, Baumgartner RW. Thrombolysis in cervical artery dissection. *Front Neurol Neurosci* 2005;20:140–146.

Georgiadis D, Lanczik O, Schwab S, et al. IV thrombolysis in patients with acute stroke due to spontaneous carotid dissection. *Neurology* 2005;64(9):1612–1614.

Gerszten PC, Welch WC, Spearman MP, et al. Isolated deep cerebral venous thrombosis treated by direct endovascular thrombolysis. *Surg Neurol* 1997;48(3):261–266.

Gruber A, Nasel C, Lang W, et al. Intra-arterial thrombolysis for the treatment of perioperative childhood cardioembolic stroke. *Neurology* 2000;54(8):1684–1686.

Gurley MB, King TS, Tsai FY. Sigmoid sinus thrombosis associated with internal jugular venous occlusion: direct thrombolytic treatment. *J Endovasc Surg* 1996;3(3):306–314.

Hacke W, Albers G, Al-Rawi Y, et al. The Desmoteplase in Acute Ischemic Stroke Trial (DIAS): a phase II MRI-based 9-hour window acute stroke thrombolysis trial with intravenous desmoteplase. *Stroke* 2005;36(1): 66–73.

Hacke W, Donnan G, Fieschi C, et al. Association of outcome with early stroke treatment: pooled analysis of ATLANTIS, ECASS, and NINDS rt-PA stroke trials. *Lancet* 2004;363(9411):768–774.

Hacke W, Furlan A. The Phase II Study of Desmoteplase in Acute Ischemic Stroke Trial 2. 16th European Stroke Conference. May 29-June 1, 2007. Abstract.

Hacke W, Kaste M, Fieschi C, et al. Intravenous thrombolysis with recombinant tissue plasminogen activator for acute hemispheric stroke. The European Cooperative Acute Stroke Study (ECASS). *JAMA* 1995, 274(13):1017–1025.

Hacke W, Kaste M, Fieschi C, et al. Randomised double-blind placebo-controlled trial of thrombolytic therapy with intravenous alteplase in acute ischaemic stroke (ECASS II). Second European-Australasian Acute Stroke Study Investigators. *Lancet* 1998;352(9136):1245–1251.

Haley EC, Jr, Lyden PD, Johnston KC, et al. A pilot dose-escalation safety study of tenecteplase in acute ischemic stroke. *Stroke* 2005;36(3): 607–612.

Holder CA, Bell DA, Lundell AL, et al. Isolated straight sinus and deep cerebral venous thrombosis: successful treatment with local infusion of urokinase. Case report. *J Neurosurg* 1997;86(4):704–707.

Horowitz M, Purdy P, Unwin H, et al. Treatment of dural sinus thrombosis using selective catheterization and urokinase. *Ann Neurol* 1995;38 (1):58–67.

IMS II Trial Investigators. The Interventional Management of Stroke (IMS) II Study. *Stroke* 2007;38(7):2127–2135.

Ingall TJ, O'Fallon WM, Asplund K, et al. Findings from the reanalysis of the NINDS tissue plasminogen activator for acute ischemic stroke treatment trial. *Stroke* 2004;35(10):2418–2424.

Janjua N, Alkawi A, Georgiadis A, et al. Feasibility of IA thrombolysis for acute ischemic stroke among anticoagulated patients. *Neurocrit Care* 2007;7:152–155.

Janjua N, Nasar A, Lynch JK, et al. Thrombolysis for ischemic stroke in children: data from the nationwide inpatient sample. *Stroke* 2007;38(6): 1850–1854.

Kasner SE, Gurian JH, Grotta JC. Urokinase treatment of sagittal sinus thrombosis with venous hemorrhagic infarctions. *J Stroke Cerebrovasc Dis* 1998;7:421–425.

Kattah JC, Wang DZ, Reddy C. Intravenous recombinant tissue-type plasminogen activator thrombolysis in treatment of central retinal artery occlusion. *Arch Ophthalmol* 2002;120(9):1234–1236.

Kermode AG, Ives FJ, Taylor B, Davis SJ, Carroll WM. Progressive dural venous sinus thrombosis treated with local streptokinase infusion. *J Neurol Neurosurg Psychiatr* 1995;58(1):107–108.

Khoo KB, Long FL, Tuck RR, Allen RJ, Tymms KE. Cerebral venous sinus thrombosis associated with the primary antiphospholipid syndrome. Resolution with local thrombolytic therapy. *Med J Aust* 1995; 162(1):30–32.

Kim SY, Suh JH. Direct endovascular thrombolytic therapy for dural sinus thrombosis: infusion of alteplase. *Am J Neuroradiol* 1997; 18(4):639–645.

Kirton A, Wong JH, Mah J, et al. Successful endovascular therapy for acute basilar thrombosis in an adolescent. *Pediatrics* 2003;112(3 Pt 1): e248–e251.

Klijn CJ, Hankey GJ. Management of acute ischaemic stroke: new guidelines from the American Stroke Association and European Stroke Initiative. *Lancet Neurol* 2003;2(11):698–701.

Kohrmann M, Juttler E, Huttner HB, Nowe T, Schellinger PD. Acute stroke imaging for thrombolytic therapy—an update. *Cerebrovasc Dis* 2007; 24(2–3):161–169.

Kuether TA, O'Neill O, Nesbit GM. Endovascular treatment of traumatic dural sinus thrombosis: case report. *Neurosurgery* 1998;42:1163–1167.

Larrue V, von Kummer RR, Muller A, Bluhmki E. Risk factors for severe hemorrhagic transformation in ischemic stroke patients treated with recombinant tissue plasminogen activator: a secondary analysis of the European-Australasian Acute Stroke Study (ECASS II). *Stroke* 2001;32(2):438–441.

Leonhardt G, Gaul C, Nietsch HH, Buerke M, Schleussner E. Thrombolytic therapy in pregnancy. *J Thromb Thrombolys* 2006;21(3):271–276.

Lewandowski CA, Frankel M, Tomsick TA, et al. Combined intravenous and intra-arterial r-TPA versus intra-arterial therapy of acute ischemic stroke: Emergency Management of Stroke (EMS) Bridging Trial. *Stroke* 1999;30(12):2598–2605.

Manthous CA, Chen H. Case report: treatment of superior sagittal sinus thrombosis with urokinase. *Conn Med* 1992;56(10):529–530.

Manzione J, Newman GC, Shapiro A, Santo-Ocampo R. Diffusion- and perfusion-weighted MR imaging of dural sinus thrombosis. *A J Neuroradiol* 2000;21(1):68–73.

Ming S, Qi Z, Wang L, Zhu K. Deep cerebral venous thrombosis in adults. *Chin Med J (Engl)* 2002;115(3):395–397.

Molina CA, Ribo M, Rubiera M, et al. Microbubble administration accelerates clot lysis during continuous 2-MHz ultrasound monitoring in stroke patients treated with intravenous tissue plasminogen activator. *Stroke* 2006;37(2):425–429.

National Institute of Neurological Disorders. Tissue plasminogen activator for acute ischemic stroke. The National Institute of Neurological Disorders and Stroke rt-PA Stroke Study Group. *N Engl J Med* 1995;333(24): 1581–1587.

Nighoghossian N, Hermier M, Adeleine P, et al. Old microbleeds are a potential risk factor for cerebral bleeding after ischemic stroke: a gradient-echo T2*-weighted brain MRI study. *Stroke* 2002;33(3):735–742.

Niwa J, Ohyama H, Matumura S, Maeda Y, Shimizu T. Treatment of acute superior sagittal sinus thrombosis by t-PA infusion via venography—direct thrombolytic therapy in the acute phase. *Surg Neurol* 1998;49(4):425–429.

Novak Z, Coldwell DM, Brega KE. Selective infusion of urokinase and thrombectomy in the treatment of acute cerebral sinus thrombosis. *A J Neuroradiol* 2000;21(1):143–145.

Ogiwara H, Maeda K, Hara T, Kimura T, Abe H. Spontaneous intracranial internal carotid artery dissection treated by intra-arterial thrombolysis and superficial temporal artery-middle cerebral artery anastomosis in the acute stage—case report. *Neurol Med Chir (Tokyo)* 2005;45(3): 148–151.

Ortiz GA, Koch S, Wallace DM, Lopez-Alberola R. Successful intravenous thrombolysis for acute stroke in a child. *J Child Neurol* 2007; 22(6):749–752.

Pettersen JA, Hill MD, Demchuk AM, et al. Intra-arterial thrombolysis for retinal artery occlusion: the Calgary experience. *Can J Neurol Sci* 2005;32(4):507–511.

Phan TG, Wijdicks EF. Intra-arterial thrombolysis for vertebrobasilar circulation ischemia. *Crit Care Clin* 1999;15(4):719–742, vi.

Philips MF, Bagley LJ, Sinson GP, et al. Endovascular thrombolysis for symptomatic cerebral venous thrombosis. *J Neurosurg* 1999;90(1):65–71.

Polak JF. Ultrasound energy and the dissolution of thrombus. *N Engl J Med* 2004;351(21):2154–2155.

Qureshi AI, Ali Z, Suri MF, et al. Intra-arterial third-generation recombinant tissue plasminogen activator (reteplase) for acute ischemic stroke. *Neurosurgery* 2001;49(1):41–48; discussion 8–50.

Rael JR, Orrison WW, Jr, Baldwin N, Sell J. Direct thrombolysis of superior sagittal sinus thrombosis with coexisting intracranial hemorrhage. *A J Neuroradiol* 1997;18(7):1238–1242.

Renowden SA, Oxbury J, Molyneux AJ. Case report: venous sinus thrombosis: the use of thrombolysis. *Clin Radiol* 1997;52(5):396–369.

Rosamond W, Flegal K, Friday G, et al. Heart disease and stroke statistics—2007 update: a report from the American Heart Association Statistics Committee and Stroke Statistics Subcommittee. *Circulation* 2007;115(5):e69–e171.

Sampognaro G, Turgut T, Conners JJ, III, White C, Collins T, Ramee SR. Intra-arterial thrombolysis in a patient presenting with an ischemic stroke due to spontaneous internal carotid artery dissection. *Catheter Cardiovasc Interv* 1999;48(3):312–315.

Schellinger PD, Thomalla G, Fiehler J, et al. MRI-based and CT -based thrombolytic therapy in acute stroke within and beyond established time windows. An Analysis of 1210 Patients. *Stroke* 2007;38: 26450–2650.

Selim M, Fink JN, Kumar S, et al. Predictors of hemorrhagic transformation after intravenous recombinant tissue plasminogen activator: prognostic value of the initial apparent diffusion coefficient and diffusion-weighted lesion volume. *Stroke* 2002;33(8):2047–2052.

Smith TP, Higashida RT, Barnwell SL, et al. Treatment of dural sinus thrombosis by urokinase infusion. *A J Neuroradiol* 1994;15(5): 801–807.

Smith WS, Sung G, Starkman S, et al. Safety and efficacy of mechanical embolectomy in acute ischemic stroke: results of the MERCI trial. *Stroke* 2005;36(7):1432–1438.

Smith WS. Safety of mechanical thrombectomy and intravenous tissue plasminogen activator in acute ischemic stroke. Results of the Multi Mechanical Embolus Removal in Cerebral Ischemia (MERCI) trial, part I. *AJNR Am J Neuroradiol* 2006;27(6):1177–1182.

Spearman MP, Jungreis CA, Wehner JJ, Gerszten PC, Welch WC. Endovascular thrombolysis in deep cerebral venous thrombosis. *A J Neuroradiol* 1997;18(3):502–506.

Tsai FY, Higashida RT, Matovich V, et al. Acute thrombosis of the intracranial dural sinus: direct thrombolytic treatment. *A J Neuroradiol* 1992;13(4):1137–1141.

Tsivgoulis G, Alexandrov AV. Ultrasound-enhanced thrombolysis in acute ischemic stroke: potential, failures, and safety. *Neurotherapeutics* 2007;4(3):420–427.

Vines FS, Davis DO. Clinical-radiological correlation in cerebral venous occlusive disease. *Radiology* 1971;98(1):9–22.

Wahlgren N, Ahmed N, Davalos A, et al. Thrombolysis with alteplase for acute ischaemic stroke in the Safe Implementation of Thrombolysis in Stroke-Monitoring Study (SITS-MOST): an observational study. *Lancet* 2007;369(9558):275–282.

Wardlaw JM, Zoppo G, Yamaguchi T, Berge E. Thrombolysis for acute ischaemic stroke. *Cochrane Database Syst Rev* 2003(3):CD000213.

Wasay M, Bakshi R, Kojan S, Bobustuc G, Dubey N, Unwin DH. Nonrandomized comparison of local urokinase thrombolysis versus systemic heparin anticoagulation for superior sagittal sinus thrombosis. *Stroke* 2001;32(10):2310–2317.

Weatherby SJ, Edwards NC, West R, Heafield MT. Good outcome in early pregnancy following direct thrombolysis for cerebral venous sinus thrombosis. *J Neurol* 2003;250(11):1372–1373.

Weber J, Remonda L, Mattle HP, et al. Selective intra-arterial fibrinolysis of acute central retinal artery occlusion. *Stroke* 1998;29(10):2076–2079.

Wiese KM, Talkad A, Mathews M, Wang D. Intravenous recombinant tissue plasminogen activator in a pregnant woman with cardioembolic stroke. *Stroke* 2006;37(8):2168–2169.

Yamini B, Loch Macdonald R, Rosenblum J. Treatment of deep cerebral venous thrombosis by local infusion of tissue plasminogen activator. *Surg Neurol* 2001;55(6):340–346.

CHAPTER

26 Endovascular Treatment of Acute Ischemic Stroke

CAMILO R. GOMEZ AND JAMES D. GEYER

OBJECTIVES

- When is endovascular treatment (i.e., endovascular rescue) of acute ischemic stroke indicated?
- What are the goals of applying endovascular techniques to the treatment of acute ischemic stroke?
- Which ischemic stroke patients should be considered for endovascular treatment?
- What approaches are available for the application of endovascular techniques in the treatment of ischemic stroke?
- How can the perioperative management of patients undergoing endovascular rescue optimize outcomes?

Stroke continues to be the third leading cause of death and the most important cause of disability in the United States. The treatment of acute ischemic stroke has changed significantly in the last decade, primarily because of the successful application of strategies for early management, including thrombolysis.

BACKGROUND AND RATIONALE

General Considerations

In 1996 the Food and Drug Administration (FDA) approved the of tissue plasminogen activator (tPA) for intravenous (IV) use in ischemic stroke. This has rekindled the interest in using aggressive therapeutic approaches to the management of stroke patients. The concept that early, rapid, and decisive intervention improves the chances of outcome is the common denominator of all effective stroke therapies. Conversely, unnecessary delays decrease the chances of successful treatment, regardless of the therapeutic approach.

However, some of us have been puzzled by the general expectation (by practitioners, regulating agencies, and pharmaceutical companies) that, following the approval of tPA, the overwhelming majority of ischemic stroke patients would be treated with this medication. Current estimates show that no more than 10% of all stroke patients receive IV tPA, and this is constantly portrayed as an implication that many candidates who are to receive this therapy are being deprived of what could constitute a life-saving treatment. In our opinion, the issue has a somewhat different interpretation and is not such a big surprise. Let us start by considering that only a minority of all patients screened for treatment in the National Institute of Neurologic Disorders and Stroke (NINDS) tPA study (i.e., the pivotal trial that led to the approval of tPA for current use) were actually enrolled. Thus, should it really surprise us that, if the same criteria are used for selecting patients for IV tPA treatment in everyday practice, only a similarly small proportion of them will be candidates for treatment? In this context lies the problem of what to do with the remaining 90% of stroke patients, especially those with large artery occlusion, whose prognosis for survival and recovery is poor following conventional treatment. Moreover, if *all* the literature on the use of IV tPA for ischemic stroke is examined, earlier studies that included angiographic monitoring invariably showed that its effectiveness was reduced in the setting of large artery occlusion (i.e., large clot burden).

Thus, for over 20 years there has been a worldwide interest in the application of endovascular techniques in the treatment of acute ischemic stroke. The present chapter is a discussion of the most important aspects of what is now referred to as neuroendovascular rescue, a concept that encompasses all endovascular (i.e., intra-arterial) procedures used to restore flow to a cerebral arterial territory compromised by acute closure with ongoing ischemia. Although the concept originally referred to the intra-arterial (IA) administration of thrombolytic agents, it presently includes a variety of other techniques that can be applied under similar clinical circumstances. In fact, endovascular techniques designed to recanalize acutely occluded brain arteries without the use of thrombolytic drugs are becoming increasingly popular, since they seem to expand the applicability of this type of treatment, without significantly increasing the risk of complications. In particular, the risk of hemorrhagic cerebral complications seems to be dramatically reduced when thrombolytic medications are not used.

Once the concept of neuroendovascular rescue is expanded beyond the IA administration of thrombolytic drugs, a new horizon of possibilities becomes evident: for example, the treatment of individuals who present beyond 6 hours of onset or of those who are fully anticoagulated with warfarin at the time of the stroke or even of those who have recently undergone major surgical procedures. In these patients, the use of thrombolytic therapy is somewhat hazardous and other techniques may need to be considered to restore flow to territories supplied by occluded large arteries (see Table 26.1). The present is a review of the most important concepts surrounding the use of endovascular techniques for the treatment of acute ischemic stroke.

Fundamental Concepts of Brain Ischemia

Brain ischemia leading to infarction (ischemic stroke) typically results from acute thrombotic or embolic occlusion of a cerebral artery. The interrupted delivery of needed metabolites, especially oxygen and glucose, halts the electrophysiologic and biochemical activity of the neural cells in the compromised vascular territory. Knowledge about the temporal sequence of events surrounding cerebral ischemia is mainly drawn from observations of global ischemic events. Graded reductions of regional cerebral blood flow (rCBF) have provided further insights into the pathophysiology of ischemia. For a matter of seconds following the onset of ischemia, cellular function persists and then stops because of the very high metabolic requirement for continued repolarization of neural membranes. A reduction in rCBF of up to 50% is well tolerated by a compensatory increase in oxygen and metabolite extraction from the more slowly moving column of blood. Further reductions, however, typically produce ischemic dysfunction and can lead to neuronal damage.

The exact mechanism of cell death is not known. Among the most important factors appear to be the rapid exhaustion of energy stores (i.e., ATP), the dysfunction of electrolytic membrane pumps, the extracellular accumulation of potassium, the intracellular accu mulation of free calcium, the liberation of arachidonic acid with production of free oxygen radicals, and the rise in hydrogen ion concentration. Lactic acid accumulation invariably contributes to the latter. In addition, experimental evidence suggests that the accumulation of certain neurotransmitters that are essentially neurotoxic (e.g., glutamate) also contributes to the cellular damage.

There are several important factors that differentiate regional alterations in CBF compared to the effects of global brain ischemia. First, the focal derangement in the circulation is variable in degree. Often, the obstruction to regional flow is incomplete rather than total (i.e., a thrombus or an embolus does not block flow completely), and adjacent collateral vessels often compensate focal alterations in the circulation. In addition, there is currently no adequate bedside means for determining whether the clinical neurological dysfunction is due to an arrest of cellular function from a rCBF <20 mL/100 g/minute or due to cell death from a rCBF <10 mL/l00 g/minute. This challenges the existence of a dichotomy involving completed and evolving stroke (or stroke in evolution). In fact, many patients with ischemic deficits experience variable degrees of recovery during the days or weeks following the insult, suggesting a prolonged but reversible metabolic arrest of neuronal function. Finally, the focally ischemic area is not homogeneous, and different zones with variable severity can be recognized within the affected vascular territory:

1. A central ischemic zone (i.e., the ischemic core) probably destined to progress to infarction. This zone has minimal flow, usually <10 cm^3/100 g brain/minute.
2. A bordering zone in which flow and metabolism fluctuate between conditions adverse or favorable for tissue viability. This is also known as the *ischemic penumbra* and has CBF values between l0 and l5 cm^3/l00 g brain/minute.
3. A collateral zone, where tissue is viable and frequently hyperemic. This is an important zone since it lends itself useful during early treatment.

The issues just described emphasize the cornerstone concept of the emergency treatment of cerebral ischemia: *the preservation and recovery of the ischemic penumbra.* Indeed, every strategy for ischemic stroke intervention (accepted or under investigation) is based on the premise that, by limiting the amount of neural tissue damaged by the ischemic process, it is possible to positively influence the outcome of the patient (i.e., lowering mortality and neurological disability). From this point of view, the currently available methods to achieve this goal include (a) flow restoration, (b) collateral optimization, (c) arrest of clot propagation, and (d) neuronal protection. It will quickly become clear how they all interact as part of neuroendovascular rescue protocols.

TABLE 26.1 Different Procedures Available for Endovascular Treatment of Stroke

Pharmacological
Thrombolytic drugs
Alteplase (Activase)
Reteplase (Retavase)
Tenecteplase (TNKase)
Glycoprotein IIb/IIIa inhibitors
Abciximab (Reopro)
Tirofiban (Aggrastat)
Eptifibatide (Integrilin)
Vasoactive drugs
Nicardipine
Verapamil
Nitroglycerin
Nitroprusside
Nonpharmacological
Mechanical disruption
Balloon angioplasty
Stenting
Embolectomy
Aspiration
Augmentative

Basic Principles of Neuroendovascular Rescue

The primary goal of neuroendovascular rescue is restoration of flow to the occluded artery's territory. In fact, the entire subject rests on the concept that without restoring flow it will be nearly impossible to achieve a good outcome. The use of the techniques described in this chapter requires consideration of the following assumptions:

1. During the first 12 to 24 hours of onset, at least part of the ischemic deficit is potentially recoverable.
2. Flow restoration is necessary for having the best opportunity for a good outcome.
3. Avoidance or minimization of the use of thrombolytic pharmacological agents limits the risk of reperfusion hemorrhage and expands the potential therapeutic window.

TABLE 26.2 Major Series of Intra-arterial Thrombolysis in the Carotid Circulation before the Year 2000

Study	Points	Agent	Success (%)	Outcome (%)	Sx ICH (%)
Zeumer (1983)	5	SK	60	60	0
Hacke (1988)	43	UK/SK	44	23	9
Masumoto (1991)	10	UK	40	40	N/A
Barnwell (1994)	3	UK	100	100	0
Sasaki (1995)	9	UK/tPA	78	52	0
Becker (1996)	12	UK	83	25	17
Casto (1996)	4	UK	75	25	0
Brandt (1996)	51	UK/tPA	51	20	14
Cross (1997)	20	UK	50	20	15
Wijdicks (1997)	9	UK	78	56	11
Gonner (1998)	10	UK	50	50	10
Totals and average	**176**		**64.5**	**42.8**	**7.6**

Sx ICH, symptomatic intracerebral hemorrhage; SK, streptokinase; UK, urokinase; tPA, tissue plasminogen activator.

4. Patients with optimal cardiovascular (i.e., cardiac function) and cerebrovascular (i.e., collateral arterial system) status tolerate and respond better to rescue techniques.

In addition, once the patient has undergone endovascular treatment, care must continue to be meticulous to avoid an unexpected complication that would turn a successful treatment into a catastrophe. These issues underscore the need for practitioners of neuroendovascular therapy and neurointensive care to interact closely to maximize the chances of each patient to survive the ictus in the best neurological condition possible.

Intra-arterial Thrombolysis

Local administration of thrombolytic pharmacological agents via a microcatheter placed in close proximity of (or within) the arterial clot has been in use for many years and has been the de facto technique for endovascular management of acute ischemic stroke. By the turn of the last century, there were 26 series, published between 1983 and 1999, with a total of 550 patients (374 in the carotid system and 176 in the vertebrobasilar system) treated using a variety of thrombolytic agents, primarily urokinase and tPA (see Tables 26.2 and 26.3). The recanalization rates approximated 75% in the carotid system and 65% in the vertebrobasilar system. Favorable neurological outcomes approximated 65% of the cases in the carotid system and 45% in the vertebrobasilar system, with symptomatic hemorrhagic transformation rates of 6% to 7%. Most of the reported patients had been treated between 3 and 6 hours following onset of the ischemic syndrome, although there is some notion that longer therapeutic windows can be used in the treatment of vertebrobasilar occlusions. The Prolyse in Acute Cerebral Thromboembolism (PROACT I and II) trials were perhaps the most important stroke IA thrombolysis studies of that era. They included only patients with middle cerebral artery (MCA) occlusion randomized for treatment or placebo IA injection within 6 hours of onset. The incipient success of PROACT I was followed by the second trial (PROACT II), generally considered positive with good outcomes in 40% of patients treated with IA prourokinase, as opposed to only 25% in the control group. Recanalization rates

TABLE 26.3 Major Series of Intra-arterial Thrombolysis in the Vertebrobasilar Circulation before the Year 2000

Study	Points	Agent	Success (%)	Outcome (%)	Sx ICH (%)
Zeumer (1983)	5	SK	60	60	0
Hacke (1988)	43	UK/SK	44	23	9
Masumoto (1991)	10	UK	40	40	N/A
Barnwell (1994)	3	UK	100	100	0
Sasaki (1995)	9	UK/tPA	78	52	0
Becker (1996)	12	UK	83	25	17
Casto (1996)	4	UK	75	25	0
Brandt (1996)	51	UK/tPA	51	20	14
Cross (1997)	20	UK	50	20	15
Wijdicks (1997)	9	UK	78	56	11
Gonner (1998)	10	UK	50	50	10
Totals and average	**176**		**64.5**	**42.8**	**7.6**

Sx ICH, symptomatic intracerebral hemorrhage; SK, streptokinase; UK, urokinase; tPA, tissue plasminogen activator.

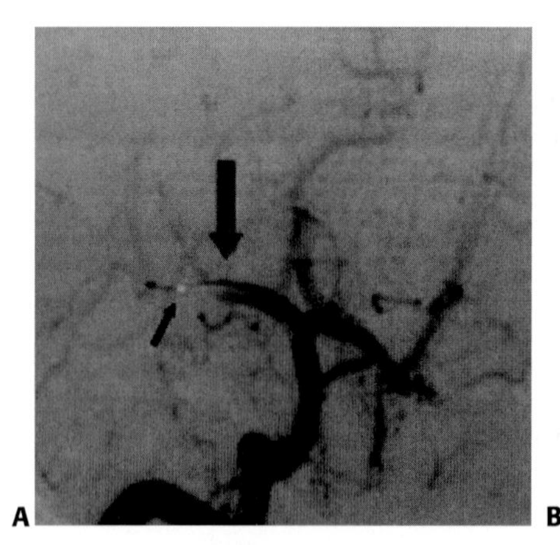

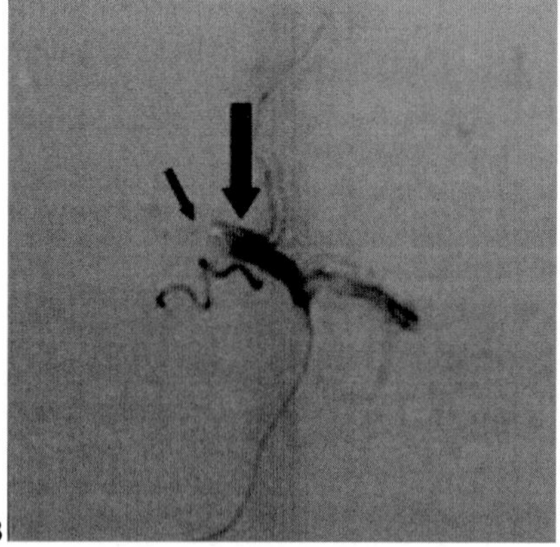

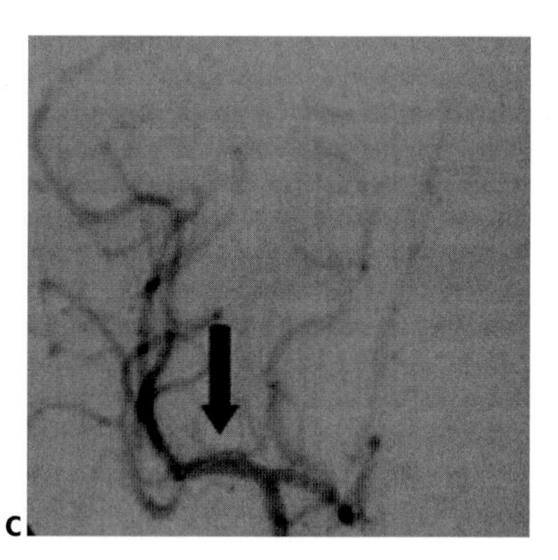

FIGURE 26.1. Intra-arterial administration of tPA in a patient with an occluded right MCA. **A:** The point of occlusion is marked (*large arrow*), as it is the tip of the microcatheter embedded into the clot (*small arrow*). **B:** Injection of contrast directly through the microcatheter allows better definition of the clot. The point of occlusion and the tip of the microcatheter are identified just as before. **C:** Complete recanalization with reperfusion is achieved. The point where the vessel was occluded is identified.

with IA therapy were greater than those reported for IV treatment, particularly in large artery occlusions. Unfortunately, the results were not sufficiently robust to convince the FDA to approve the drug for this indication.

Currently, the only type of thrombolytic agent available for use in clinical practice is tPA, which activates tissue plasminogen conversion to plasmin. Subsequently, plasmin breaks up the fibrin in the thrombus. Three different forms of it are currently available in the market: alteplase (Activase), reteplase (Retavase, and tenecteplase (TNKase), and various authors have expressed their own preference for one or another of these medications. The authors have recently favored the use of reteplase, because of its effectiveness and ease of use. The drug is typically administered directly into the occluding clot, preferably using a microcatheter with side holes (see Fig. 26.1) in increments of 2 to 4 units each, as opposed to 8 units of reteplase, which almost invariably result in arterial recanalization. Eight units is the maximum, as the complications reported in the literature exceeding this amount are counterproductive. In addition, if the vessel has not recanalized following the administration of 6 to 8 units of reteplase, the composition of the occluding material comes into question, and an alternative rescue strategy is often considered.

Finally, there has also been significant interest in the use of a combination of IV-tPA at a lower dose (0.6 mg per kg) followed by IA-tPA. This technique has been reported to be successful in prospective clinical trials, showing outcomes at 3 months that compared favorably with those of the placebo arm of the Neurological Disorders and Stroke (NINDS) IV-tPA trial (see Table 26.4). However, the authors favor the use of full-dose IV-tPA in all patients who qualify, followed by taking those who are clinically suspected of having a large arterial occlusion to the catheterization laboratory immediately. This allows confirmation of the recanalization of the vessel as well as the opportunity to apply additional nonpharmacological measures if necessary. The importance of this strategy is underscored by the high rates of reocclusion of vessels treated with IA-tPA.

Intra-arterial Antithrombotic Therapy

Another group of medications that has been shown to be useful in the endovascular management of patients with acute ischemic stroke is the glycoprotein IIb/IIIa (GpIIbIIIa) inhibitors. These drugs block the final step in the aggregation of platelets, the binding of platelets to fibrinogen via the GpIIbIIIa surface receptors. There are three commercially available GpIIbIIIa inhibitors: abciximab (Reopro), tirofiban (Aggrastat), and eptifibatide (Integrilin). These medications have been studied both alone and as adjuvant to thrombolytic agents. The latter concept is based on the principles

TABLE 26.4 Comparison between the Use of Limited Dose Intravenous Tissue Plasminogen Activator *PLUS* Intra-arterial Tissue Plasminogen Activator and the Controls in the NINDS Intravenous Tissue Plasminogen Activator Study

	IMS Study (n = 80)	NINDS Placebo (n = 211)	Odds Ratio (95% CI)
Rankin 0-1	30%	18%	2.29 (1.2, 4.4)
Rankin 0-2	43%	28%	2.04 (1.2, 3.6)
NIHSS ≤1	25%	15%	2.24 (1.1, 4.5)

IMS, Interventional Management Study; NINDS, National Institute of Neurologic Disorders and Stroke; CI, confidence interval; NIHSS, National Institute of Health Stroke Scale.

of facilitating recanalization, reducing the amount of thrombolytic agent used, and preventing reocclusion due to platelet activation. In addition, the authors have found the GpIIbIIIa inhibitors to be useful during endovascular therapy, when the window is simply too long for thrombolysis or when other techniques such as balloon angioplasty and stenting are required. The latter are also capable of inducing very strong platelet activation, thereby promoting reocclusion. Dosing of these agents for IA use requires thoughtful consideration. The authors commonly administered between half to a full loading dose and reserve the subsequent continued drip for select circumstances. Just as with the tPA agents available, the reader must understand that none of these drugs is currently approved by the FDA for this indication.

Direct Mechanical Disruption

Mechanical clot disruption has been successfully applied to the treatment of acute ischemic stroke by various authors. This approach, in its simplest form, is quite practical as it allows the operator to limit the amount of thrombolytic agent used, as well as in the treatment of patients who are not candidates for pharmacological thrombolysis. The technique involves restoring flow to van occluded arterial bed by disrupting the occluding particle using the microwire and microcatheter complex (see Fig. 26.2). Although not effective in every instance, it can be very rewarding when patients who are on chronic anticoagulants develop acute embolic occlusions. Procedurally, although apparently simple, mechanical disruption carries with it a certain amount of complexity since it requires the operator to gently manipulate the microwire–microcatheter complex across the point of occlusion. This often necessitates a back-and-forth pattern of movement and in our experience has the best result when accompanied by concurrent administration of different pharmacological agents, such as vasodilating or antithrombotic drugs.

Balloon Angioplasty and Stenting

The technique of balloon angioplasty with or without stenting for neuroendovascular rescue, in principle, is similar to that used in elective cases. Patients are premedicated with aspirin (325 mg) and clopidogrel (375 mg loading dose) in the emergency department before the procedure, via nasogastric tube if necessary. Online quantitative angiography of the lesion and the adjacent arterial segments is performed using the contrast-filled guiding catheter for calibration. Although the balloons used are also a matter of preference, the authors have been partial to the use of coronary balloons (e.g., Cross-Sail, Guidant, Inc. or Quantum, Boston Scientific, Inc.) because of their efficiency, security, and effectiveness. For extracranial occlusions, the lesion is crossed using floppy-tipped microwires and microcatheters. One of the critical aspects of urgent angioplasty and stenting of large arterial extracranial occlusions is the need to assess the clot burden distal to the point of occlusion, to determine whether distal clot aspiration to decrease the risk of further embolization will be necessary (see Fig. 26.3). Once the proximal occlusion is crossed, injection through the microcatheter often demonstrates the extent of the occlusive process. If a distal protection device is considered necessary, the authors favor the use of the SpiderFX (ev3, Inc.), largely because it can be deployed over any microwire of our choice. The point of focal occlusion is then predilated with a low profile moderately compliant coronary balloon. In cases where there is extensive intraluminal clot, if aspiration or embolectomy is not an option, sequential dilation of the arterial segment with the balloon is carried out, often in conjunction with IA administration of GpIIbIIIa inhibitors. One or more stents are then deployed across the lesion, as necessary, and they are further dilated to firmly embed them into the vessel wall (see Fig. 26.3).The technique of intracranial angioplasty and stenting is slightly different. The authors have found it more practical to approach the lesion with a floppy-tipped 0.014″ microwire and a microcatheter, after the guide catheter has been placed as close to the segment to be treated as possible. For lesions in the intracranial carotid artery, the MCA, or one of its branches, the guide catheter (6 Fr) can be advanced to the distal cervical internal carotid artery before its entrance into the petrous bone (see Fig. 26.4). For distal vertebral and basilar angioplasty, the guide catheter should be advanced, if possible, to the distal V2 segment of the vertebral artery. Once the lesion is crossed with the microwire and the microcatheter, these are advanced distally to some of the

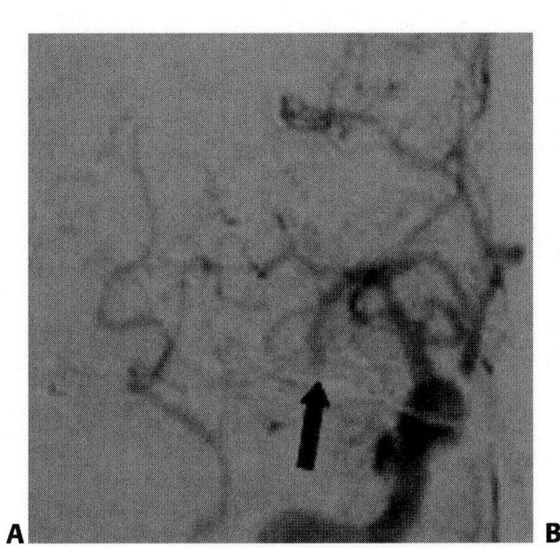

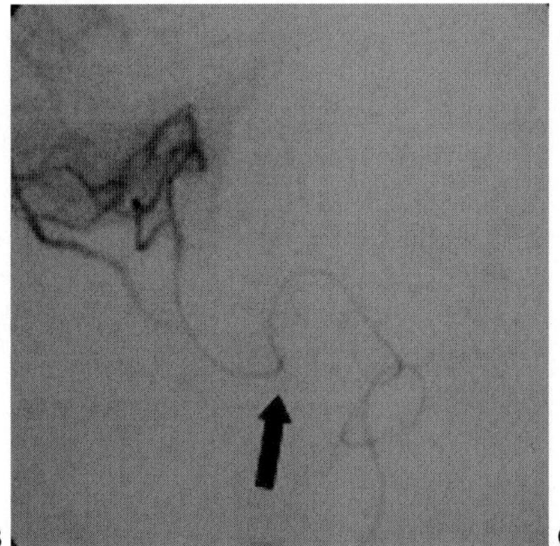

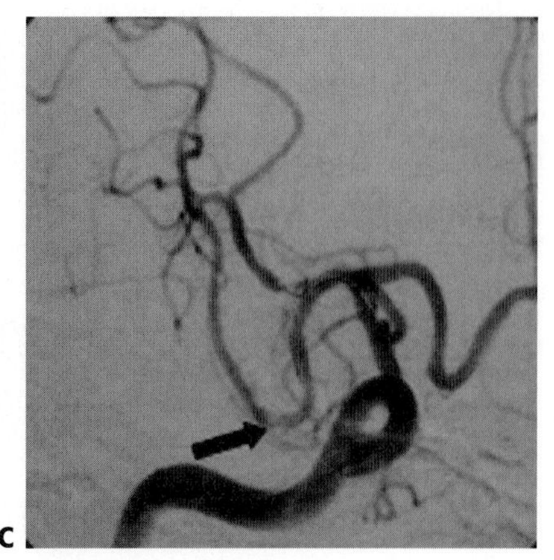

FIGURE 26.2. Mechanical disruption of a right middle cerebral artery occlusion in a patient with atrial fibrillation and International Normalized Ratio = 2.75. **A:** The occlusive particle is identified (*large arrow*). **B:** The microcatheter is advanced distal to the occlusion point (*large arrow*), and contrast injection demonstrates the distal vasculature. **C:** Withdrawing the microcatheter while leaving the microwire in place demonstrates the immediate recanalization (*large arrow*). No thrombolytic pharmacological agents were used.

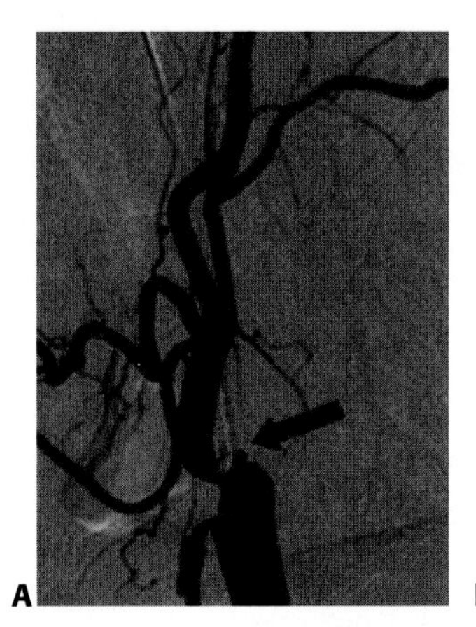

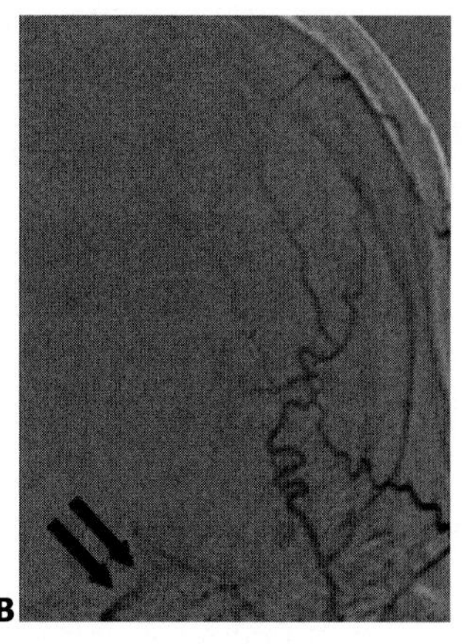

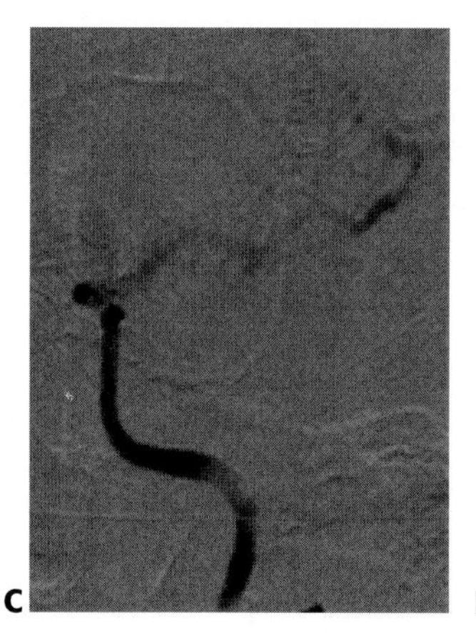

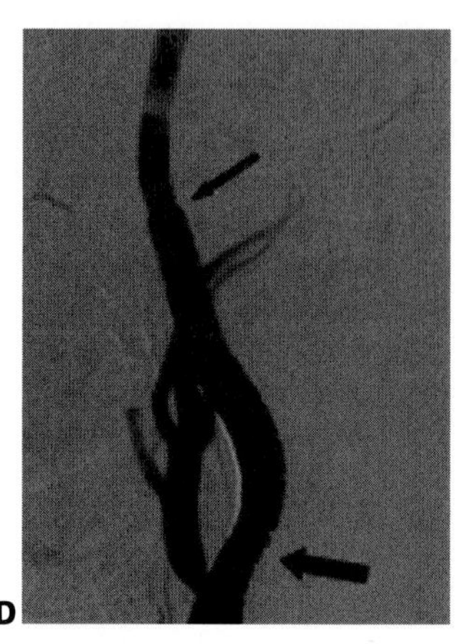

FIGURE 26.3. Angioplasty and stenting of an occluded internal carotid artery at its origin. **A:** The point of occlusion (*arrow*) is almost certain to be secondary to a local plaque thrombosis. **B:** Contrast injection proximal to the occlusion faintly demonstrates the terminal internal carotid artery (*arrows*). **C:** Contrast injection through a microcatheter crossing the occlusion point (*arrow*) demonstrates the patency of the distal vessel. **D:** The final image demonstrates correction of the occlusion following stent deployment. The previously occluded point (*large arrow*) and the distal end of the stents (*small arrow*) are demonstrated.

cortical branches of the middle or posterior cerebral arteries, depending on the lesion is being treated. Again, injection through the microcatheter displays the status of the distal circulation and the extent of the occlusive process. At this point, the microwire is substituted for another with similar tip characteristics but sufficiently long (i.e., 300 cm) to allow the exchange of devices over it, and sufficiently stiff to allow tracking of balloons and stents. The microcatheter is removed and the balloons are introduced over the exchange microwire. The balloon is inflated at low pressures (only until the waist is lost) for several minutes (i.e., 5 to 10 minutes) (see Fig. 26.4). The effectiveness of this technique seems to be enhanced by the concurrent IA administration of antithrombotic or thrombolytic agents. Deployment of stents intracranially is a more complex problem, and one that requires careful consideration. Certainly, if the procedure uncovers an underlying stenotic lesion that threatens reocclusion, stenting is justified (see Fig. 26.5). However, in most cases of embolism, this may not be necessary.

Embolectomy and Clot Aspiration

Mechanical embolectomy can be helpful in situations when the occlusive particle does not yield to simple balloon angioplasty or a primary rescue technique. Originally, it involved the use of a microsnare to secure the occluding particle, pulling it back and outside of the body (see Fig. 26.6). This can be accomplished either totally or partially and, as with the other techniques described, even partial restoration of flow may be sufficient to improve the neurological outcome of the patient. More recently, however, the FDA has approved the use of the Mechanical Embolus Removal in Cerebral Ischemia (MERCI) device (Concentric Medical, Inc.) based on the results of a multicenter study that showed recanalization rates of approximately 48% using the device by itself and of approximately 60% with adjuvant therapy. The device, shaped as a corkscrew, allows the operator to capture the occluding particle and remove it from most large arteries of the brain.

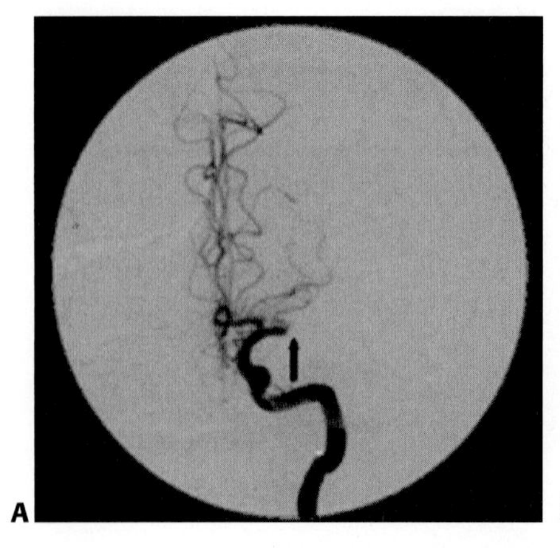

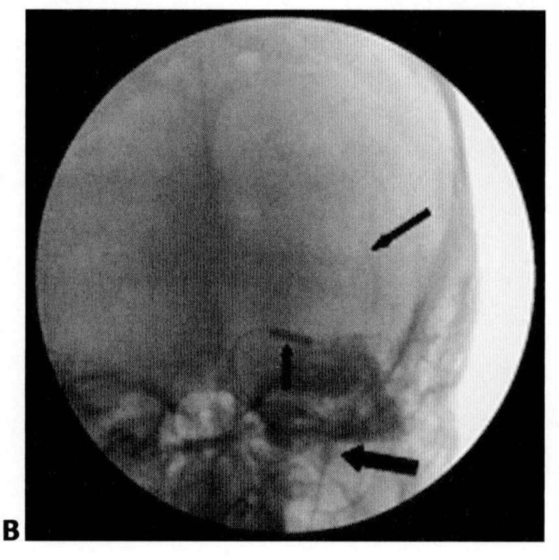

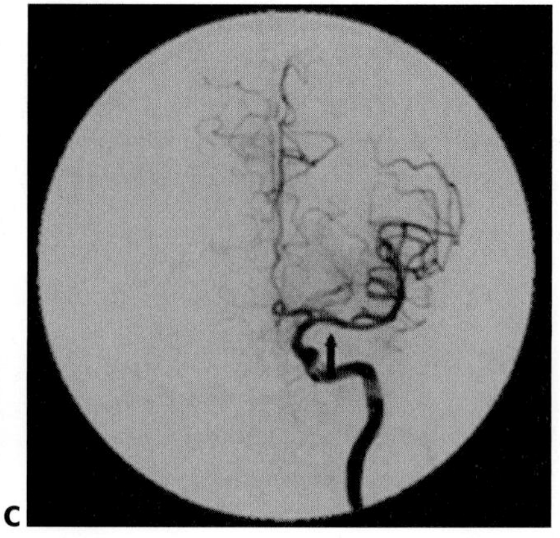

FIGURE 26.4. Balloon angioplasty of an acutely occluded left middle cerebral artery. **A:** The point of occlusion is clearly identified (*arrow*). **B:** Balloon inflation is clearly demonstrated (*small short arrow*). Note how the guide catheter's tip is in the distal cervical internal carotid artery (*large arrow*), and the microwire is in the distal circulation (*small long arrow*). **C:** The final result is that of vascular recanalization. The previously occluded point is demonstrated (*arrow*).

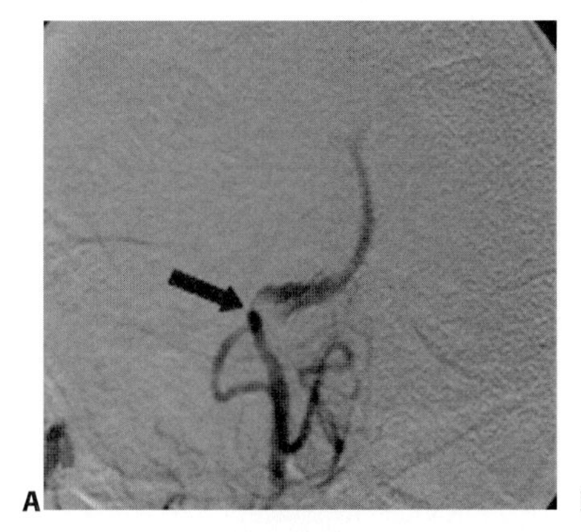
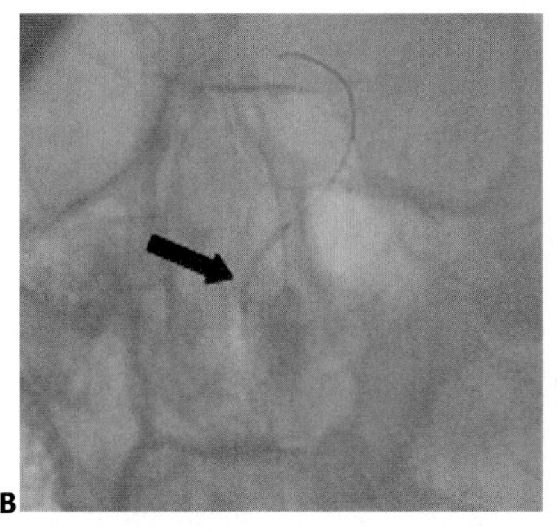
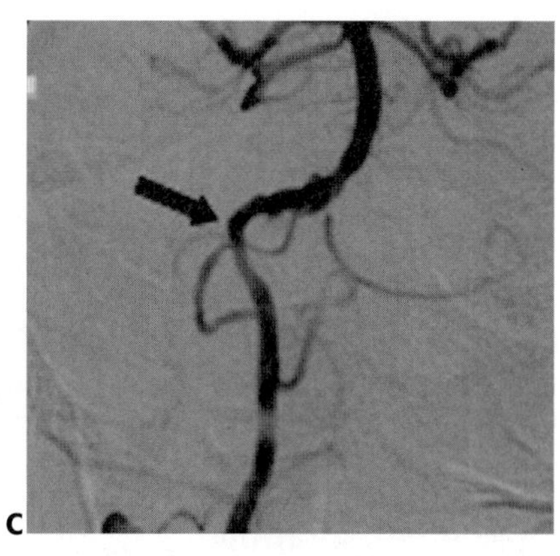

FIGURE 26.5. Urgent stenting of a proximal basilar artery in a patient with progressive brainstem ischemia. **A:** The flow-compromising lesion is a near-occlusion of the proximal basilar artery (*arrow*). **B:** The lesion is predilated and further treated by deploying a coronary stent (*arrow*). **C:** The final result is restoration of flow to the basilar artery. The location of the original lesion is marked (*arrow*).

Over the past few years, technological advances have allowed the introduction of devices designed to allow aspiration of the intraluminal clot and its removal with the consequent decrement in clot burden. The most important of the available devices is the Angiojet (Possis, Inc.), originally introduced for clot debulking in the coronary and peripheral vascular beds. The device consists of a catheter connected to an external pump capable of delivering pressures of up to 10,000 psi. The saline jets delivered to the tip of the catheter create a Bernoulli effect that allows rapid removal of large amounts of thrombus. There are several available models of catheters approved for coronary and peripheral use, and the one previously designed for intracranial is not likely to become available because of the excessive complications during clinical trials, specifically arterial perforation. In any case, of the catheters available, the authors favor the use of the XMI-RX because of its trackability and ease of use. It is effective in vessels with a minimum

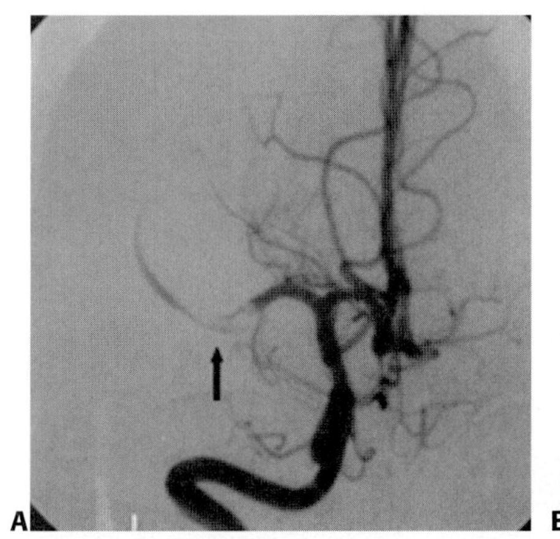
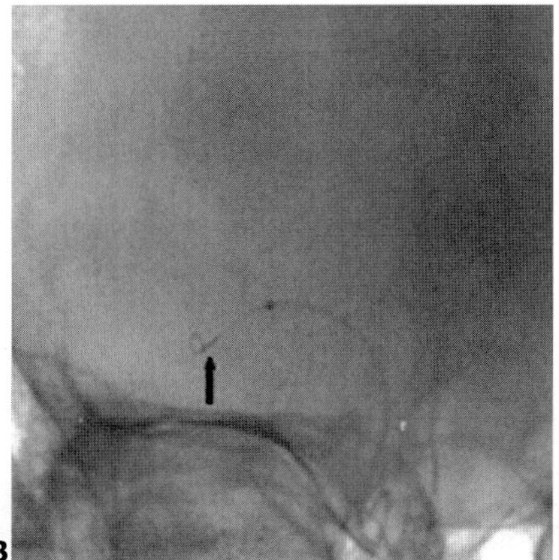
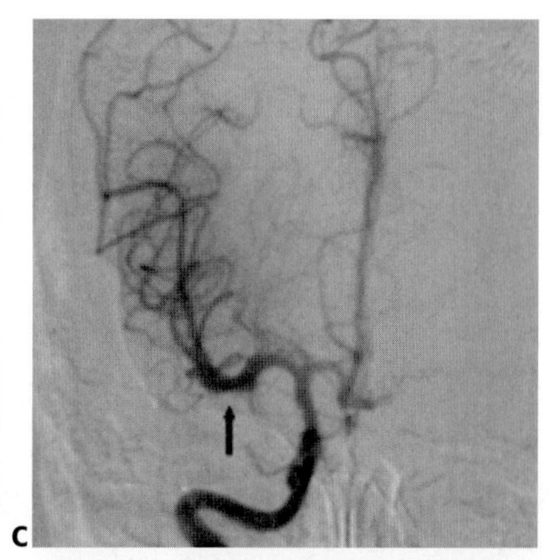
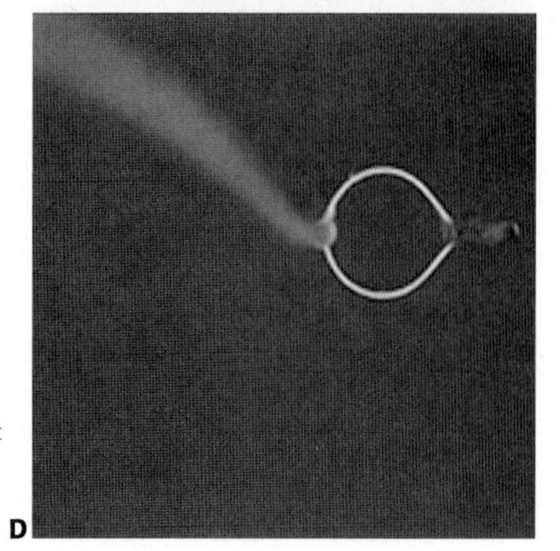

FIGURE 26.6. Embolectomy using an off-the-shelf microsnare. **A:** The occlusion of the right MCA is evident (*arrow*) in this patient with a cardiomyopathy and at the time connected to a left ventricular assist device (LVAD). **B:** The microsnare is advanced slightly beyond the point of occlusion (*arrow*). **C:** The result is complete recanalization of the vessel (*arrow*). **D:** The clot removed is seen in the microsnare.

diameter of 2 mm, is compatible with microwires and rapid exchange systems, and has enough of a working length to be used in neurological procedures. It has been used successfully to aspirate clots that extend into the petrous and precavernous portions of the internal carotid artery. Moreover, it is effective in the treatment of sino-venous thrombosis. Another available off-the-shelf device is the X-Sizer (ev3, Inc.), which works on a similar principle.

Other devices based on different technology (e.g., laser) have been unsuccessfully studied, primarily because of safety considerations. Finally, also it must be emphasized that the simplest method for aspiration involves the use of a syringe and the generation negative pressure on the guide catheter.

Flow Augmentation

One last word is necessary about a different type of endovascular procedure designed to improve the outcome of stroke patients: endovascular flow augmentation by controlled aortic occlusion. The cardiovascular system, being a closed loop, maintains a certain amount of circulating blood volume at any point of time. This amount, equal to the cardiac output, is shared by all organs, with the brain receiving approximately 20% of the entire amount. Theoretically, it is possible to increase brain perfusion by diverting blood volume from other regions of the body. This theory led to the introduction of an abdominal aorta controlled occlusion catheter that has been under investigation for the past few years. The device consists of two balloons that are inflated in the abdominal aorta above and below the renal arteries (see Fig. 26.7), increasing resistance to flow to the lower portions of the body and thus diverting blood volume to the brain. The objective is for the diverted blood volume to optimize collateral circulation, expanding the therapeutic window and giving other therapeutic strategies an opportunity. The preliminary results have been encouraging, even as a freestanding technique.

Vasoactive Pharmacological Intervention

An inherent part of our using all these techniques has been the concurrent administration of drugs that have potentially beneficial vasoactive and possibly neuroprotective effects. It has now been our practice to routinely cross the point of occlusion with a microcatheter and perform supraselective injection of contrast, documenting the localization of both the occlusion and the microcatheter, as well as the magnitude of the distal clot burden (see Fig. 26.8). This is followed with an injection of nicardipine (200 to 300 μg), nitroglycerin (200 to 300 μg), verapamil (200 to 300 μg), or nitroprusside (100 to 200 μg), alone or in combination. These agents, all of which are potent vasodilators, are capable of relieving the distal spasm created by the occlusive particle, reducing the resistance to flow in the distal microcirculation, and at least theoretically, helping flush debris into the venous system. It is important to be sure that one is prepared to deal with the possible systemic hypotensive effect of any of these medications once they cross into the systemic circulation. Otherwise, there is much to gain and little to lose with their use. Another hypothetical benefit of this approach is that, if one were to administer a drug with a potentially neuroprotective effect (e.g., nicardipine), it would be delivered to the tissue that needs it rather than being wasted into adjacent territories. Thus, at a time when the overwhelming majority of the studies addressing the use of neuroprotective agents for acute stroke treatment have turned out to be negative, one possible future avenue of research is to include this strategy among those used in neuroendovascular rescue.

CLINICAL APPLICATIONS AND METHODOLOGY

General Considerations

Neuroendovascular rescue is not appropriate for every stroke patient. It is imperative that the reader understands that without optimal patient selection and preparation, the endovascular procedure is destined to fail. Furthermore, without optimal postoperative care, technically successful procedures are likely to become catastrophes, an even more troublesome scenario since the possibility of recanalization has already been realized. These admonishments are meant to underscore the importance of seamless care through the emergency department, the catheterization laboratory, and the intensive care unit. Such a care requires dedication, knowledge, teamwork, and predetermined protocols. In essence, the endovascular procedure is only but *a part* of the entire treatment

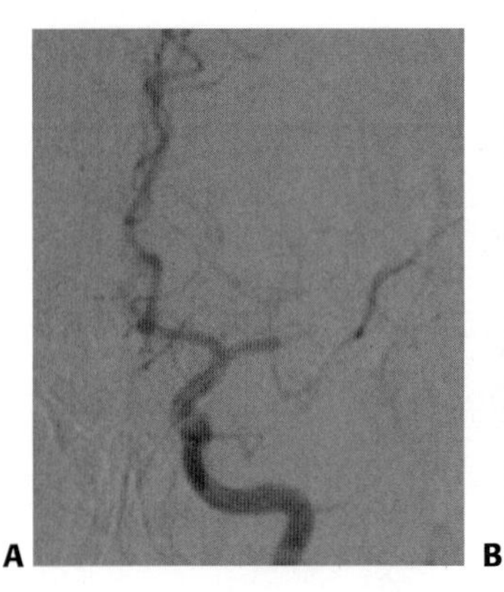
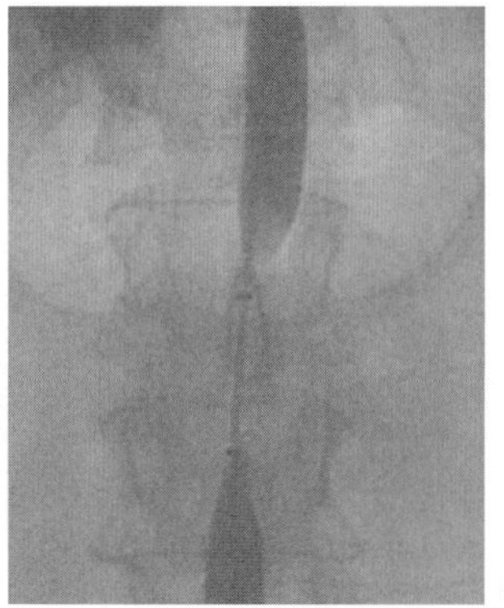
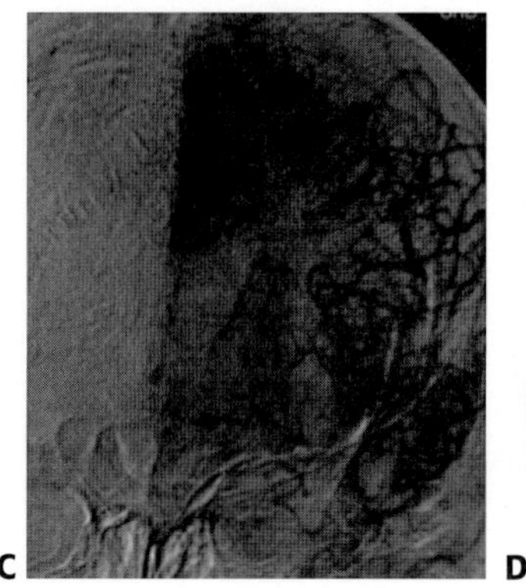
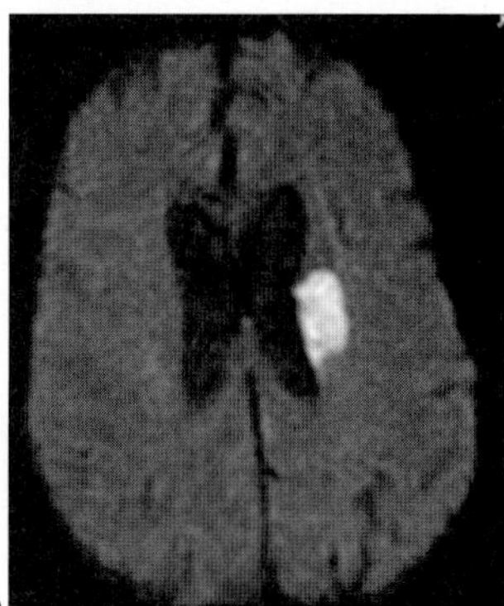

FIGURE 26.7. Cerebral flow augmentation in a patient with left middle cerebral artery occlusion. **A:** The occluded vessel is demonstrated. **B:** The two balloons (supra- and infrarenal) of the aortic occlusion catheter are demonstrated. **C:** Angiography demonstrates the large amount of collaterals optimized by the diversion of blood volume. **D:** Diffusion-weighted imaging demonstrates the final lesion, with a large portion of the hemisphere being spared.

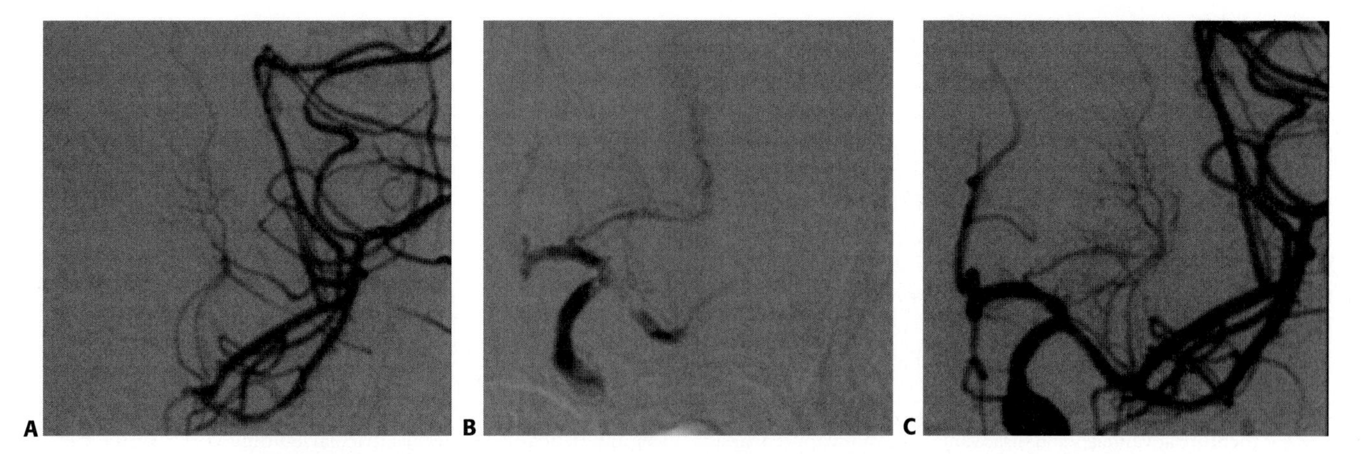

FIGURE 26.8. A: Occlusion of the terminal left internal carotid artery is demonstrated. **B:** Contrast injection of the distal circulation is followed by instillation of vasoactive agents. **C:** The final result of the intervention is demonstrated.

and its application must be contextual with the entire clinical scenario. It is useful to illustrate these concepts by placing the care of these patients in the context of the cerebral hemodynamic continuum (see Fig. 26.9). This process begins with the acute arterial occlusion, and its outcome is largely dependent on how quickly reperfusion is achieved, as well as how the cerebral circulation is supported before and after reperfusion.

Patient Selection and Preparation for Intervention

Patients who present to the emergency department should only be considered for neuroendovascular rescue *after* basic emergency measures of stroke treatment are implemented, they have undergone computed tomography (CT), and they have been evaluated by a neurovascular specialist. The former step is geared toward optimizing the cardiovascular and cerebrovascular status of the patient, often promoting rapid neurological improvement. This improvement, when it follows simple treatment measures, is important since it will have an effect on the benefit–risk assessment of the patient being considered for the intervention. In our institution, every patient is immediately placed in the supine position, and this is followed by the administration of supplemental oxygen (to achieve an O_2 saturation of 100%), aspirin (325 mg preferable chewed or by nasogastric tube), and an IV bolus of 10 to 15 cm^3 per kg of isotonic crystalloid (e.g., 0.9% NaCl). These steps are all parts of what is described as code stroke (see Chapter 20). Then, emergency CT allows the identification of hemorrhagic changes, the presence of early signs of infarction, and at times, the documentation of an occluded cerebral artery (i.e., hyperdense sign).

Once the emergency steps of stroke care have been carried out, and a neurovascular specialist has examined the patient, a benefit–risk analysis of the clinical situation is imperative. The importance of this assessment and the degree of expertise required for its accomplishment cannot be overemphasized. If neuroendovascular rescue is considered to bethe best therapeutic option, the patient must immediately be taken to the catheterization laboratory for angiography and intervention. Conversely, to bring every single stroke patient for emergency angiography would be not only impractical and wasteful, but also probably inordinately dangerous in some cases. Ideally, the best candidate for neuroendovascular rescue is someone who has clinical evidence of a large artery occlusion (i.e., internal carotid, middle cerebral, or basilar arteries) The reasons are obvious: (a) these are the most readily accessible vessels by endovascular means, (b) these are the easiest clinical syndromes to identify, and (c) these are the patients with the most to lose if their arteries are not recanalized (i.e., best benefit –risk ratio).

The literature of the last decade suggests that specific neuroimaging techniques can be used to select patients who are likely to benefit from procedures directed at restoring blood flow within the affected arterial territory. In particular, magnetic resonance

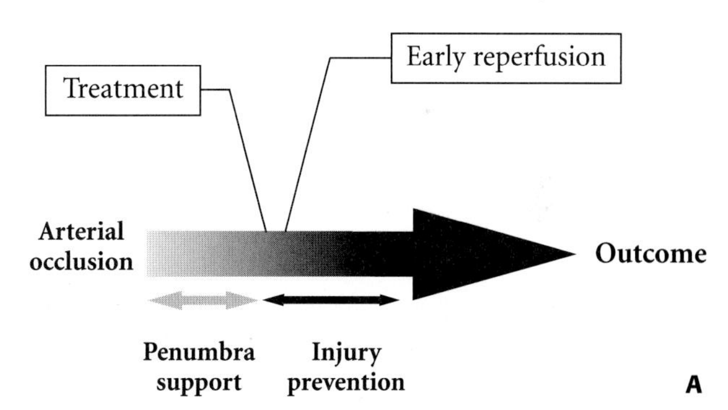

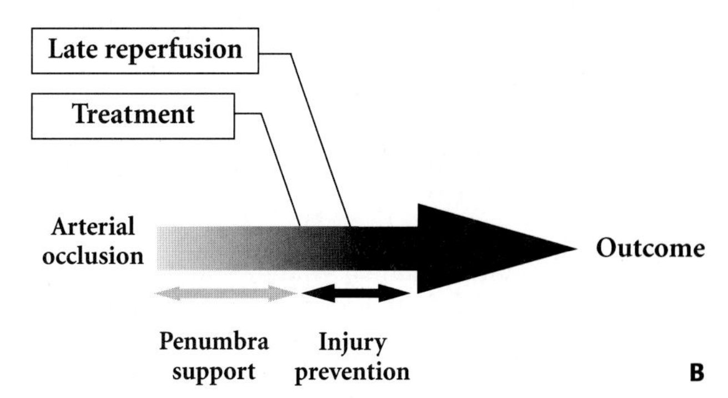

FIGURE 26.9. The cerebral hemodynamic continuum illustrates how penumbra support is the concept behind prereperfusion treatment (i.e., hypervolemia, hypertension), while injury prevention must guide management after reperfusion. The differences in emphasis between early **(A)** and late **(B)** reperfusion, even after treatment administered at the same point, are demonstrated.

imaging (MRI) techniques [i.e., magnetic resonance angiography (MRA), diffusion-weighted imaging (DWI), and perfusion-weighted imaging (PWI)], are actively being investigated as possible screening tools for the selection of acute stroke patients for different types of intervention. Other techniques worth mentioning from the perspective of patient selection for intervention are transcranial Doppler (TCD) and Xenon-CT. The former has been reported as being useful not only in diagnosing large arterial occlusions but also in monitoring the progression of the recanalization, and even enhancing the effect of the thrombolytic agent. The latter has been shown to allow discrimination of areas of no flow versus those with some residual flow and potentially salvageable.

Another issue that must be considered prior to the procedure is whether the patients should be electively intubated or not. Clearly, there are advantages and disadvantages to both approaches, but the authors currently prefer to electively intubate the patient, since this allows sedation (with or without neuromuscular paralysis), making for an easier and faster procedure. The authors typically use propofol (Diprivan) for sedation and vecuronium (Norcuron) for temporary neuromuscular blockade. The downside of this approach is that these patients do not get extubated as promptly as is preferred, and there is an increased risk of pneumonia once they are intubated. Finally, it is important to understand that intubation and paralysis limit the possibility of clinically monitoring the patient during the procedure.

Intraprocedural Management

During the procedure, the care of the patient changes as the brain flow is restored (Fig. 26.9). Before recanalization, the goal is to maintain a state of slight hypervolemia, as well as some degree of hypertension, to optimize the collateral circulation. However, once the vessel is successfully recanalized (i.e., improvement of flow from TIMI = 0 to TIMI = 2 to 3), the hemodynamic need change. The authors recommend maintenance of euvolemia and control of the systolic blood pressure (SBP) [not the mean arterial blood pressure (MABP)] at approximately 150 torr, to limit the risk of reperfusion hemorrhage. Special consideration is given to the patient who requires angioplasty and stenting of the common carotid bifurcation region, and who is prone to develop hypotension from stimulation of the baroreceptors. This patient may require vasopressor support, particularly if the hemodynamic compromise occurs at a time when he is sedated and paralyzed.

Postprocedural Care and Avoidance of Complications

Following successful recanalization of the occluded vessel, the goal is to maintain euvolemia. Fluid management is best guided by plotting the patient's own left ventricular Starling curve. In the past, this had required the use of a pulmonary artery (PA) catheter. At present, there are several less invasive techniques for accomplishing this, including devices for transesophageal aortic Doppler (TEAD) monitoring and central venous oximetry catheters In the case of a successful rescue procedure, (i.e., final flow of TIMI = 2 to 3) the SBP should be maintained at 150 torr or so. On the other hand, if flow restoration is unsuccessful, the MABP should be kept at approximately 100 to 110 torr to optimize collateral flow. The access femoral arterial sheath can be sutured in place at the end of the procedure and used to transduce the arterial blood pressure readings. However, the authors prefer to close the arteriotomy site and place a conventional arterial line if necessary. Sedation and neuromuscular blocking agents are discontinued as soon as possible, allowing better clinical assessment of the patient, and facilitating early extubation and rehabilitation.

Another aspect of postprocedural care is that of antithrombotic therapy following intervention. Aspirin and clopidogrel (Plavix) *must* be continued in patients who have had stents deployed. The issue of whether to maintain heparinization or not depends on various factors: (a) degree of flow restored, (2) concurrent presence of an indication for long-term warfarin (Coumadin) therapy, and (3) use of thrombolytic agents during the procedure. For patients whose flow is restored to TIMI = 2 to 3 levels, and no other concurrent reason for anticoagulation, heparin is generally not necessary in the short term. Those who have either suboptimal flow restoration or another indication for warfarin (Coumadin) must be kept on heparin. It is important to understand that heparin increases the risk of reperfusion hemorrhages, and that its use must be carefully weighted against potential problems that it may cause.

TABLE 26.5 Treatment Window and Concerns for the Use of Thrombolysis in Our Uncontrolled Series of 55 Patients

Treatment window: 1 to >24 h (mean = 11.2)
Concerns for thrombolysis:
- Prolonged window (*n* = 40)
- Recent surgery (*n* = 6)
- Active anticoagulation (*n* = 7)
- Recent major trauma (*n* = 3)

TABLE 26.6 Procedures Performed and Complications in Uncontrolled Series of 55 Patients

Procedures performed:
- Balloon angioplasty = 50
- Stenting = 33
- Adjuvant thrombolysis = 9
- Embolectomy = 3

Complications (*n* = 6; 10.9%)
- Neurological (*n* = 4):
  - Perforation (2); reocclusion (1); hemorrhage (1)
- Other (*n* = 2): access-related hematomas

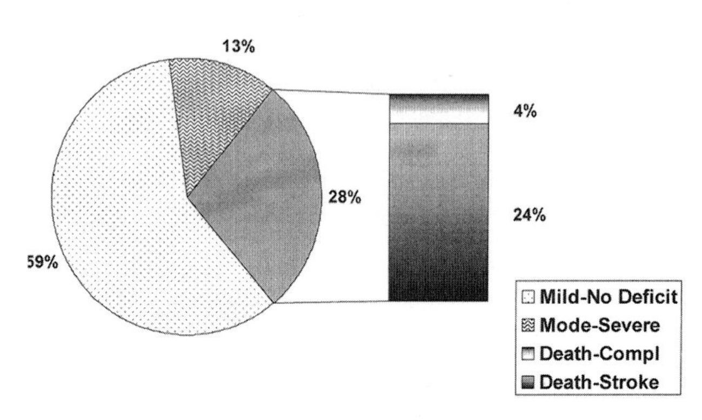

FIGURE 26.10. Neurological outcomes of uncontrolled series of 55 patients.

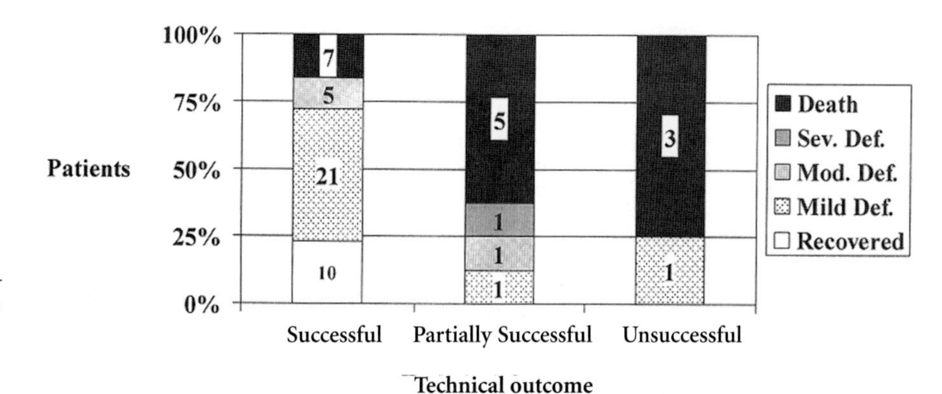

FIGURE 26.11. A comparison of the ultimate clinical outcome as a function of the success of the interventional procedure in an uncontrolled series of 55 patients. def, deficit.

This is particularly true if thrombolytic or parenteral antithrombotic agents (i.e., GpIIbIIIa antagonists) are administered during the intervention. Finally, as noted earlier, a special circumstance is that of the period during which the arterial sheath is left in place. A continuous infusion of IV heparin, at doses of 400 to 500 units per hour is usually sufficient to prevent thrombosis and limb ischemia. In general, once the dust settles following the restoration of flow, the care of the patient is not very different than any other stroke patient, emphasizing secondary prevention and rehabilitation.

CONCLUSION

On the basis of the principles outlined, the authors have implemented treatment protocols. An uncontrolled single-center series, accumulated over a period of approximately 5 years, included 55 patients (35 men; 44 whites; mean age = 56.1 years) with large artery occlusions. All patients presented with characteristics that imposed concerns for the use of thrombolytic agents in standard fashion (see Table 26.5). The procedures used varied according to the angiographic findings and the clinical scenario, and the procedural complications were small (see Table 26.6). However, the results of the interventions were competitive, with almost 60% of the patients showing minimal or no deficit on discharge (see Fig. 26.10). In fact, the overwhelming majority of the deaths were the result of the original stroke, and this was particularly associated with unsuccessful recanalization at the end of the procedure (see Fig. 26.11). These results are similar to those of published series. Of further interest is that, at 3-months follow-up, the National Institute of Health Stroke Scales of the survivors varied between 0 and 13 (mean = 5), comparing favorably with those obtained prior to treatment (18 and 28, respectively; mean = 22). These results illustrate the importance of considering neuroendovascular rescue in patients who qualify for such treatment.

SELECTED REFERENCES

Callahan AS, III, Berger BL. Intra-arterial thrombolysis in acute ischemic stroke. *Tenn Med* 1997;90(2):61–64.

Casto, L., Caverni L, Camerlingo M, et al. Intra-arterial thrombolysis in acute ischaemic stroke: experience with a superselective catheter embedded in the clot. *J Neurol Neurosurg Psychiatr* 1996;60(6):667–670.

del Zoppo GJ, Ferbert A, Otis S, et al. Local intra-arterial fibrinolytic therapy in acute carotid territory stroke. A pilot study. *Stroke* 1988;19(3): 307–313.

Eckert B, Koch C, Thomalla G, et al. Aggressive therapy with intravenous abciximab and intra-arterial rtPA and additional PTA/stenting improves clinical outcome in acute vertebrobasilar occlusion: combined local fibrinolysis and intravenous abciximab in acute vertebrobasilar stroke treatment (FAST): results of a multicenter study. *Stroke* 2005; 36(6):1160–1165.

Ernst R, Pancioli A, Tomsick T, et al. Combined intravenous and intra-arterial recombinant tissue plasminogen activator in acute ischemic stroke. *Stroke* 2000;31(11):2552–2557.

Flaherty ML, Woo D, Kissela B, et al. Combined IV and intra-arterial thrombolysis for acute ischemic stroke. *Neurology* 2005; 64(2):386–388.

Furlan A, Higashida R, Wechsler L, et al. Intra-arterial prourokinase for acute ischemic stroke. The PROACT II study: a randomized controlled trial. Prolyse in Acute Cerebral Thromboembolism. *JAMA* 1999;282(21): 2003–2011.

Furlan AJ, Abou-Chebi A. The role of recombinant pro-urokinase (r-pro-UK) and intra-arterial thrombolysis in acute ischaemic stroke: the PROACT trials. Prolyse in Acute Cerebral Thromboembolism. *Curr Med Res Opin* 2002;18(Suppl 2):s44–s47.

Gurewich V, Liu JN. Intra-arterial pro-urokinase in ischemic stroke. *Stroke* 1998;29(6):1255–1256.

Kase CS, Furlan AJ, Wechsler LR, et al. Cerebral hemorrhage after intra-arterial thrombolysis for ischemic stroke: the PROACT II trial. *Neurology* 2001;57(9):1603–1610.

Kim, D.J., Kim DI, Kim SH, et al. Rescue localized intra-arterial thrombolysis for hyperacute MCA ischemic stroke patients after early non-responsive intravenous tissue plasminogen activator therapy. *Neuroradiology* 2005;47(8):616–621.

Lansberg MG, Tong DC, Norbash AM, et al. Intra-arterial rtPA treatment of stroke assessed by diffusion- and perfusion-weighted MRI. *Stroke* 1999;30(3):678–680.

Lewandowski CA, Frankel M, Tomsick TA, et al. Combined intravenous and intra-arterial r-TPA versus intra-arterial therapy of acute ischemic stroke: Emergency Management of Stroke (EMS) Bridging Trial. *Stroke* 1999;30(12):2598–2605.

Pettersen JA, Hudon ME, Hill MD. Intra-arterial thrombolysis in acute ischemic stroke: a review of pharmacologic approaches. *Expert Rev Cardiovasc Ther* 2004;2(2):285–299.

Qureshi AI, Siddiqui AM, Suri MF, et al. Aggressive mechanical clot disruption and low-dose intra-arterial third-generation thrombolytic agent for ischemic stroke: a prospective study. *Neurosurgery* 2002;51(5): 1319–1327; discussion 1327–1329.

Qureshi AI, Ali Z, Suri MF, et al. Intra-arterial third-generation recombinant tissue plasminogen activator (reteplase) for acute ischemic stroke. *Neurosurgery* 2001;49(1):41–48; discussion 48–50.

Qureshi AI, Siddiquib AM, Kima SH, et al. Reocclusion of recanalized arteries during intra-arterial thrombolysis for acute ischemic stroke. *Am J Neuroradiol* 2004;25(2):322–328.

Shah QA, Georgiadis A, Suri MF, et al. Preliminary experience with intra-arterial nicardipine in patients with acute ischemic stroke. *Neurocrit Care* 2007;7(1):53–57.

Shaltoni HM, Albright KC, Gonzales NR, et al. Is intra-arterial thrombolysis safe after full-dose intravenous recombinant tissue plasminogen activator for acute ischemic stroke? *Stroke* 2007;38(1):80–84.

Suarez JI, Sunshine JL, Tarr R, et al. Predictors of clinical improvement, angiographic recanalization, and intracranial hemorrhage after intra-arterial thrombolysis for acute ischemic stroke. *Stroke* 1999;30(10): 2094–2100.

Zeumer H, Freitag HJ, Zanella F, et al. Local intra-arterial fibrinolytic therapy in patients with stroke: urokinase versus recombinant tissue plasminogen activator (r-TPA). *Neuroradiology* 1993;35(2): 159–162.

Zhang L, Zhang ZG, Zhang C, et al. Intravenous administration of a GPIIb/IIIa receptor antagonist extends the therapeutic window of intra-arterial tenecteplase-tissue plasminogen activator in a rat stroke model. *Stroke* 2004;35(12):2890–2895.

CRITICAL PATHWAY
Endovascular Treatment of Acute Ischemic Stroke Pathway

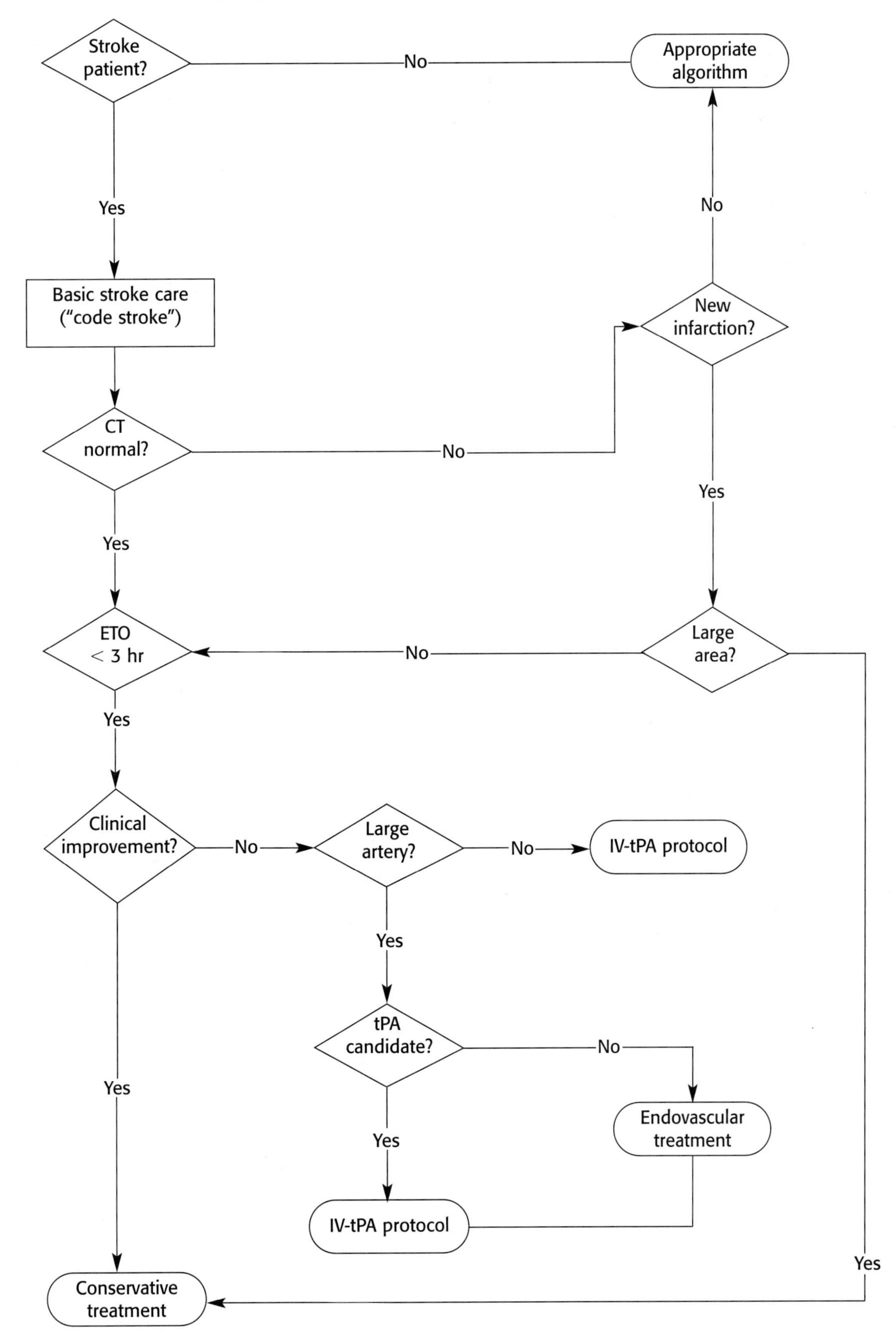

tPA, tissue plasminogen activator.

CHAPTER

27 Management of Spontaneous Intracerebral Hemorrhage

FRED RINCON AND STEPHAN A. MAYER

OBJECTIVES

- What are the risk factors for intracerebral hemorrhage (ICH)?
- How can the prognosis after ICH be accurately determined?
- When is cerebral angiography indicated in the patient with ICH?
- What is the optimal blood pressure management approach after ICH?
- How should elevated intracranial pressure and symptomatic intracranial mass effect be treated after ICH?
- What is the evidence for ultra-early hemostatic therapy after spontaneous ICH?
- When can anticoagulation be safely started after ICH?
- What are the indications for intraventricular thrombolysis after ICH?
- When is surgery indicated for the management of ICH?

Spontaneous intracerebral hemorrhage (ICH) is caused by the rupture of small vessels and arterioles damaged by chronic hypertension (HTN) in 50% to 70% of cases or by cerebral amyloid angiopathy (CAA) in approximately 15% of cases. Secondary causes of ICH include abnormal coagulation, vascular anomalies, conversion from embolic or ischemic strokes, tumors, and trauma. Occasionally, blood may extend into the ventricular system [intraventricular hemorrhage (IVH)] or the subarachnoid space [subarachnoid hemorrhage (SAH)].

ICH produces devastating neurological disability and is by far the most untreatable form of stroke. Thus, ICH continues to be a serious health problem worldwide. ICH has a prevalence of approximately 37,000 to 52,000 cases per year in the United States, and in a recent population-based study the overall incidence of ICH was estimated to be between 12 and 15 cases per 100,000 population. ICH is accompanied by a different risk factor profile than ischemic stroke. Hypertension, particularly if untreated, is the most important risk factor for ICH. Other risk factors include advanced age, male gender, black and Japanese race/ethnicity, hypocholesterolemia, high alcohol intake, and cocaine use.

Although often asymptomatic, CAA is an important risk factor for primary ICH in the elderly. CAA is characterized by the deposition of β-amyloid protein in small- to medium-sized blood vessels of the brain and leptomeninges, which may undergo fibrinoid necrosis as seen in chronic HTN. It can occur as a sporadic disorder, in association with Alzheimer disease, or with certain familial syndromes (apolipoprotein E_2 and apolipoprotein E_4 allele).

BACKGROUND AND RATIONALE

Disease Mechanisms

Formerly considered a monophasic event, ICH is rather a complex process that involves several pathological phases. The mechanisms by which the hematoma grows after ICH are still unclear but different theories may help explain its pathogenesis. Chronic sustained HTN or CAA lead to small vessel (100 to 600 μm in diameter) fragmentation and degeneration, and the generation of Charcot-Bouchard microaneurysms. These microvascular changes reduce vascular compliance and increase the likelihood of spontaneous arterial rupture. The most commonly affected sites in the brain are the basal ganglia (putamen, thalamus, caudate) (50%), the lobar regions (33%), and the pons and cerebellum (17%).

Spontaneous arterial rupture due to chronic vascular damage is followed by rapid high-pressure accumulation of blood within the brain tissue. Rapid increases in local tissue pressure and disruption of the normal cerebral anatomy lead to mass effect causing herniation of brain structures. The destructive forces of the rapidly expanding hematoma can generate severe reflex hypertension, which may exacerbate this process.

Ongoing bleeding or rebleeding into the hematoma is associated with early neurological deterioration and worst clinical outcomes. Brott et al demonstrated that increase in volume of >33% is detectable on follow-up computed tomography (CT) in approximately 38% of patients initially scanned within 3 hours and in two thirds of those scanned within 1 hour of onset. Early hematoma growth may occur in the absence of a coagulation disorder and appears to be from ongoing bleeding at multiple sites within the first few hours of onset. Earlier reports suggested that early hematoma growth was secondary to rebleeding into an ischemic penumbra zone. However, magnetic resonance imaging (MRI) studies using diffusion- and perfusion-weighted images (DWI/PWI) have found no evidence of such peri-ICH ischemic zone. Similarly, Zazulia et al. suggested that this region is not ischemic on the basis of a normal oxygen extraction ratio obtained from positron emission tomography (PET) studies. An overwhelming hematoma-induced inflammatory response has been evidenced by different animal and human studies. Activation of cytotoxic and humoral responses; induction of proteases such as thrombin, fibrinogen, and tissue plasminogen activator (tPA), and the effects of coagulation and blood products have recently been implicated in the pathogenesis of hematoma expansion and surrounding edema.

The only consistently identified predictor of early hematoma growth is the interval from the onset of symptoms to CT: The earlier the first scan is obtained, the more likely subsequent bleeding will be detected on a follow-up scan. As a corollary, hematoma growth occurs in only 5% of patients who are initially scanned beyond 6 hours of symptom onset.

Prognosis

The mortality of ICH approaches 50% at 1 year. Half of all deaths occur within the first 2 days of symptom onset, whereas most fatalities that occur after the first month are the result of secondary medical complications. Independent predictors for 30-day and 1-year mortality include large ICH volume, coma, older age, IVH, and infratentorial location. A useful clinical grading scale (the ICH score) that incorporates these five elements allows rapid estimation of 30-day mortality on admission (see Table 27.1). Except in the most severe cases, however, caution is warranted when communicating a very poor prognosis after ICH. It has become increasingly evident that physicians tend to underestimate the chances of a good outcome and that poor outcomes often arise from self-fulfilling prophecies: In one study, the implementation of a do-not-resuscitate order within the first 24 hours was the single most important determinant of survival after ICH. Several studies have shown that mortality after ICH is reduced in patients cared for in a specialty neurological intensive care unit. This is presumably the result of adherence to best medical practices, early transition to rehabilitation, and being cared for by a team of health care professionals that takes an active interest in promoting recovery.

CLINICAL APPLICATIONS AND METHODOLOGY

A simplified algorithm for the diagnosis and management of ICH is described in Figure 27.1.

Diagnosis

The diagnosis of ICH is suggested by the rapid onset of neurological dysfunction and signs of increased intracranial pressure (ICP), such as headache, vomiting, and decreased level of consciousness. The symptoms of ICH are related primarily to the etiology, anatomical location, and extension of the expanding hematoma. Abnormalities in the vital signs such as hypertension, tachycardia or bradycardia (Cushing's response), and abnormal respiratory patterns are common effects of elevated ICP and brainstem compression. Approximately 90% of patients have systolic blood pressure (SBP) ≥160 mm Hg and/or diastolic blood pressure (DBP) ≥100 mm Hg at the onset. Confirmation of ICH cannot rely solely on the clinical exam and requires the use of emergent CT scan or MRI.

Widespread use of nonenhancing CT scan of the brain has dramatically changed the diagnostic approach of this disease, becoming the method of choice to evaluate the presence of ICH. CT scan evaluates the size and location of the hematoma, extension into the ventricular system, degree of surrounding edema, and anatomical disruption. Hematoma volume may be easily calculated from CT

TABLE 27.1 The Intracranial Hemorrhage Score

Component	Points	Total Points	30-d Mortality (%)
Glasgow Coma Scale score			
3–4	2	5+	100
5–12	1	4	97
13–15	0		
ICH volume (mL)			
≥30	1	3	72
<30	0		
Intraventricular hemorrhage			
Yes	1	2	26
No	0	1	13
Age (y)			
≥80	1	0	0
<80	0		
Infratentorial origin			
Yes	1		
No	0		

ICH, intracranial hemorrhage.

Adapted from Hemphill JC, III, Bonovich DC, Besmertis L, et al. The ICH score: a simple, reliable grading scale for intracerebral hemorrhage(ICH). *Stroke* 2001;32(4):891–897.

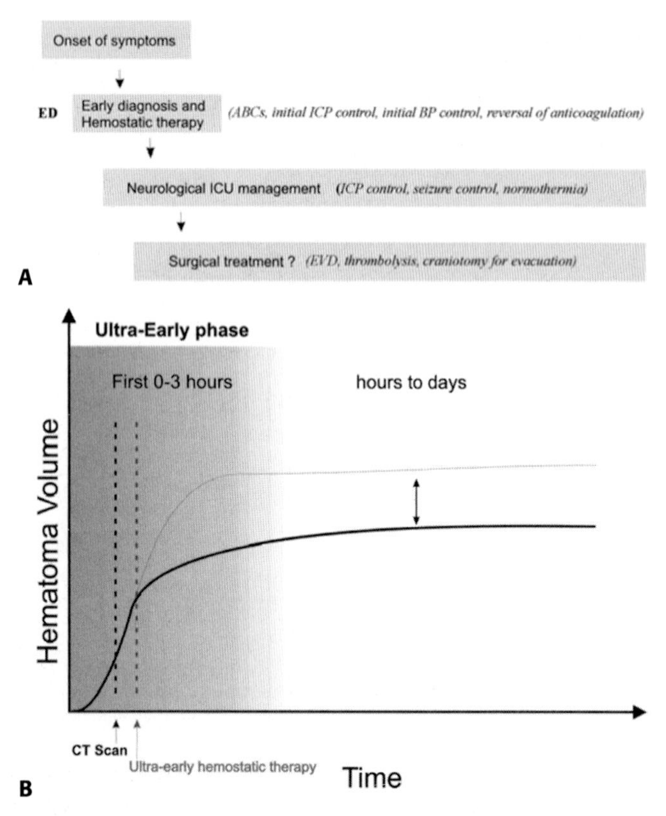

FIGURE 27.1. A: Simplified algorithm of management during intra cerebral hemorrhage (ICH). The cornerstone for success in treatment of ICH is to diagnose it as early as possible and to institute therapy within 3 hours of the onset of symptoms. This approach known as ultra-early hemostatic therapy requires rapid diagnostic workup, administration of effective hemostatic agents (e.g., recombinant factor VIIa), and if possible, close specialized management in the neuro-intensive care unit for assessment of possible neurological deterioration and complications. **B:** Ultra-early hemostatic therapy with recombinant factor VII (rFVIIa) has been shown to slow hematoma growth. If instituted soon after the diagnosis (*left dotted line*) intravenous infusion of rFVIIa (*right dotted line*) leads to an absolute decrease in expansion of hemorrhage (*double vertical arrow*) or may prevent early rebleeding. (Diagram courtesy of Manuel Buitrago, MD, PhD.)

scan images by use of the ABC÷2 method. Contrast-enhanced CT scan is not done routinely in most centers, but it may prove helpful in predicting hematoma expansion and outcomes. MRI techniques such as gradient echo (GRE, T2*) are highly sensitive for the diagnosis of ICH. Sensitivity of MRI for ICH is 100%. In the Hemorrhage and Early MRI Evaluation (HEME) study, MRI and CT were equivalent for the detection of acute ICH but MRI was significantly more accurate than CT for the detection of chronic ICH.

Catheter angiography is the diagnostic test of choice for detecting a vascular cause of secondary ICH. In one study, the yield of angiography for detecting a vascular malformation, aneurysm, venous sinus thrombosis, or vasculitis was zero in hypertensive patients older than 45 years and as high as 65% in patients with primary IVH and in nonhypertensive patients with lobar hemorrhage. Angiography should always be considered in younger nonhypertensive patients with ICH who have no obvious explanation for their hemorrhage. When an arteriovenous malformation (AVM) is diagnosed, there is no particular urgency to performing surgery or embolization, since the risk of major rebleeding is as low as 4% per year.

Emergency Department Management

Airway

Rapid neurological decline and depressed level of consciousness leads to loss of normal reflexes that maintain a patent airway and mandates immediate endotracheal intubation and mechanical ventilation. Failure to recognize imminent airway loss may result in aspiration, hypoxemia, or hypercapnia, which in turn can lead to cerebral vasodilatation and increased ICP. In general, many practitioners prefer to use sedative agents and nondepolarizing neuromuscular paralytic agents that do not have effects on ICP such as propofol, etomidate, atracurium, and vecuronium for rapid sequence intubation. Initially the respiratory rate and tidal volume should be set to maintain a pCO_2 of approximately 35 mm Hg. Aggressive early hyperventilation to pCO_2 levels <28 mm Hg should be avoided because of the potential to cause excessive vasoconstriction and exacerbation of ischemia.

Blood Pressure

Single center studies and a systematic review have reported an increased risk of deterioration, death, or dependency with increased BP after ICH. Extremes of BP should be corrected immediately to minimize the potential for hematoma expansion and to maintain adequate cerebral perfusion pressure (CPP), which is calculated as the difference between mean arterial pressure (MAP) and ICP. Extreme hypertension within the first 6 hours is common and should be aggressively but carefully treated to avoid excessive reduction of the CPP, which might precipitate ischemia in the perihematomal zone.

American Stroke Association guidelines recommend that MAP be maintained ≤130 mm Hg for ICH patients with a history of hypertension. In patients who have undergone craniotomy, MAP should be maintained ≤100 mm Hg. In all cases, SBP should be maintained >90 mm Hg, and in patients with an ICP monitor, cerebral CPP should be maintained >70 mm Hg. In the emergency department, hypertension can be initially treated with repeated intravenous (IV) boluses of labetalol every 10 minutes, with doses escalating from 20 to 80 mg. In the intensive care unit, BP is best controlled with continuous infusions of labetalol, esmolol, or nicardipine (see Table 27.2). Sodium nitroprusside should be avoided because of the tendency of this agent to cause cerebral vasodilation and elevated ICP.

Controversy exists about the initial treatment of BP in patients with ICH. Two studies have demonstrated that controlled BP reduction by approximately 20% has no adverse effects on cerebral blood flow in humans or animals, and as mentioned earlier, MR and PET studies have failed to demonstrate perihematomal ischemia in ICH patients imaged as early as 6 hours after onset. Given that this approach appears to be safe, a recent National Institutes of Health consensus panel gave its highest priority to a trial of aggressive BP control (MAP 100 to 120 mm Hg) within the first 3 hours of ICH onset.

Emergency Intracranial Pressure Therapy

Emergency measures for ICP control are appropriate for stuporous or comatose patients, or for those who present acutely with clinical signs of brainstem herniation. The head should be elevated to 30 degrees, 1.0 to 1.5 g per kg of 20% mannitol should be administered by a rapid infusion, and the patient should be hyperventilated to a pCO_2 of 28 to 33 mm Hg. These measures are designed to

TABLE 27.2 Intravenous Antihypertensive Agents for Acute Intracranial Hemorrhage

Drug	Mechanism	Dose	Cautions
Labetalol	α_1, β_1, β_2 receptor antagonist	20–80 mg bolus every 10 min, up to 300 mg; 0.5–2.0 mg/min infusion	Bradycardia, congestive heart failure, bronchospasm
Esmolol	β_1 receptor antagonist	0.5 mg/kg bolus; 50–300 μg/kg/min	Bradycardia, congestive heart failure, bronchospasm
Nicardipine	L-type calcium channel blocker (dihydropyridine)	5–15 mg/h infusion	Severe aortic stenosis, myocardial ischemia
Enalaprilat	ACE inhibitor	0.625 mg bolus; 1.25–5 mg every 6 h	Variable response, precipitous fall in BP with high renin states
Fenoldopam	Dopamine-1 receptor agonist	0.1–0.3 μg/kg/min	Tachycardia, headache, nausea, flushing, glaucoma, portal hypertension
Nitroprusside[a]	Nitrovasodilator (arterial and venous)	0.25–10 μg/kg/min	Increased ICP, variable response, myocardial ischemia, thiocyanate and cyanide toxicity

ACE, angiotensin-converting enzyme; BP, blood pressure; ICP, intracranial pressure.
[a] Nitroprusside is not recommended for use in acute ICH because of its tendency to increase ICP.
From Mayer SA, Rincon F. Management of intracerebral hemorrhage. *Lancet Neurol* 2005;4:662–672, with permission.

lower ICP as quickly and effectively as possible, to buy time before a definitive neurosurgical procedure (craniotomy, ventriculostomy, or placement of an ICP monitor) can be performed.

Hemostatic Therapy

Recombinant factor VII (rFVIIa, Novoseven, Novo Nordisk) is a powerful initiator of hemostasis that is currently approved for the treatment of bleeding in patients with hemophilia who are resistant to factor VIII replacement therapy. However, considerable evidence also exists suggesting that rFVIIa may enhance hemostasis in patients with normal coagulation systems as well.

In a randomized, double-blind, placebo-controlled phase II trial, treatment with rFVIIa at doses of 40, 80, or 160 μg per kg within 4 hours of ICH onset limited growth of the hematoma by approximately 50%. This was associated with a 38% reduction in mortality and significantly improved functional outcomes at 90 days, despite a 5% increase in the frequency of arterial thromboembolic adverse events. A follow-up phase III trial, however, failed to show a clinical benefit despite the fact that rFVIIa demonstrated a similar hemostatic effect and safety profile with the 80-μg-per-kg dose. Although ultra-early hemostatic therapy still holds promise as an emergency treatment for spontaneous ICH, further studies directed at treatment of patients at increased risk for active bleeding (i.e., scanned and treated within earlier time window, or with evidence of contrast extravasation on CT angiography) are needed.

Reversal of Anticoagulation

Warfarin anticoagulation increases the risk of ICH by 5- to 10-fold in the general population, and approximately 15% of ICH cases are associated with warfarin use. Among ICH patients, warfarin doubles the risk of mortality and dramatically increases the risk and time window for progressive bleeding and clinical deterioration. Failure to rapidly normalize the international normalized ratio (INR) to <1.4 further increases these risks. ICH patients receiving warfarin should be reversed immediately with fresh frozen plasma (FFP) or prothrombin complex concentrates (PCC), and vitamin K (see Table 27.3). Treatment should never be delayed to check coagulation tests. Unfortunately, normalization of the INR with this approach usually takes several hours, and clinical results are often poor. The associated volume load with FFP may also cause congestive heat failure in the setting of cardiac or renal disease. PCC, a concentrate of the vitamin K–dependent coagulation factors II, VII, IX, and X, normalizes the INR more rapidly than FFP, and can be given in smaller volumes but is not widely available in some countries.

Recent reports have described the use of rFVIIa to speed the reversal of warfarin anticoagulation in ICH patients. A single IV dose of rFVIIa can normalize the INR within minutes, with larger doses producing a longer duration of effect. Recombinant factor VIIa in doses ranging from 10 to 90 μg per kg has been used to reverse the effects of warfarin in acute ICH—primarily to expedite neurosurgical intervention—with good clinical results. When this approach is used, rFVIIa should be used as an adjunct to coagulation factor replacement and vitamin K, since its effect will only last several hours. ICH patients who have been anticoagulated with unfractionated or low-molecular-weight heparin should be reversed with protamine sulfate, and patients with thrombocytopenia or platelet dysfunction [i.e., antiplatelet use—aspirin, adenosine diphosphate (ADP)-receptor blocker or glycoprotein IIb/IIIa (GIIb/IIIa) receptor blocker] can be treated with a single dose of DDAVP, platelet transfusions, or both (see Table 27.3). Restarting anticoagulation in those patients with strong indication, such as in patients with prosthetic valve replacement, can be safely implemented in most cases approximately after 10 days after ICH.

Intensive Care Unit Management

Patient Positioning

To minimize ICP and reduce the risk of ventilator-associated pneumonia in mechanically ventilated patients, the head should be elevated 30 degrees.

Fluids

Isotonic fluids such as 0.9% saline (approximately 1 mL/kg/hour) should be given as the standard IV replacement fluid for patients with ICH. Free water given in the form of 0.45% saline or 5% dex-

TABLE 27.3 Emergency Management of the Coagulopathic Intracranial Hemorrhage Patient

Scenario	Agent	Dose	Comments	Level of Evidence[a]
Warfarin	FFP	15 mL/kg	Usually 4–6 units (200 mL) each are given; risk of volume overload	B
	Or PPC	15–30 U/kg	Works faster than FFP, but carries risk of DIC	B
	And Vitamin K (IV)	10 mg	Can take up to 24 h to normalize INR	B
	Optional IV rFVIIa	20–80μg/kg	Normalizes INR within 15 min; risk of adverse thromboembolic events; contraindicated in acute thromboembolic disease	C
Warfarin and emergency neurosurgical intervention	*Above plus* rFVIIa	20–80 μg/kg	Contraindicated in acute thromboembolic disease	C
UFH or LMWH	Protamine sulfate[b]	1 mg/100 units of heparin, or 1 mg of enoxaparin	Can cause flushing, bradycardia, or hypotension	C
	And DDAVP	0.3 μg/kg	Single dose required	C
Thrombolytic	Cryoprecipitate	6 units	Preferred	C
	Or FFP	15 mL/kg		C
	Plus Platelet transfusion	1 unit	Single unit required	C
	and optional DDAVP	0.3 μg/kg	Single dose required	C
Platelet dysfunction (ASA, ADP-R blocker), and/or thrombocytopenia	Platelet transfusion	6 units	Range 4–8 units based on size; transfuse to >100,000	C
	And DDAVP	0.3 μg/kg	Single dose required	C
Or GPIIb/IIIa blocker	Platelet transfusion	6 units	Range 4–8 units based on size; transfuse to >100,000	C
	And Cryoprecipitates	6 units		C
	And DDAVP	0.3 μg/kg	Single dose required	C

[a] Level of evidence A, based on one or more high quality randomized controlled trials; Level of evidence B, based on two or more high quality prospective or retrospective cohort studies; Level of evidence C, case reports and series, expert opinion.
[b] Protamine has minimal efficacy against danaparoid or fondaparinux.
FFP, fresh frozen plasma; PPC, prothrombin complex concentrate; DIC, disseminated intravascular coagulation; IV, intravenous; INR, international normalized ratio; rFVIIa, recombinant factor VII activated; UFH, unfractionated heparin; LMWH, low-molecular weight heparin; DDAVP, desmopressin; ASA, acetyl salicilic acid; ADP-R, adenosine phosphate receptor blocker; GPIIb/IIIa, platelet glycoprotein IIb/IIIa.
Adapted from Mayer SA, Rincon F. Management of intracerebral hemorrhage. *Lancet Neurolog* 2005;4:662–672, with permission.

trose in water can exacerbate cerebral edema and increase ICP because it flows down its osmotic gradient into injured brain tissue. Dextrose-containing solutions should generally be avoided unless hypoglycemia is present, since hyperglycemia may be detrimental to the injured brain. Systemic hypo-osmolality (<280 mOsm per L) should be aggressively treated with mannitol or 3% hypertonic saline. A state of euvolemia should be maintained by monitoring fluid balance, central venous pressure, and body weight.

Some centers are increasingly using hypertonic saline in the form of a 3% sodium chloride-acetate solutions (1 mL/kg/hour) as an alternative to normal saline in patients with significant perihematomal edema and mass effect. The goal is to establish and maintain a baseline state of hyperosmolality (300 to 320 mOsm per L) and hypernatremia (150 to 155 mEq per L), which may reduce cellular swelling and the number of ICP crises. When discontinuing treatment, care should be taken to taper the infusion slowly to avoid sharp reductions in osmolality, which might lead to rebound edema and ICP elevations. The serum sodium level should never be allowed to drop more than 8 to 12 mEq per L over 24 hours.

Anticonvulsant Therapy

The 30-day risk of clinically evident seizures after ICH is approximately 8%. Convulsive status epilepticus may be seen in 1% to 2% of patients, and the risk of long-term epilepsy ranges from 5% to 20%. Lobar location is an independent predictor of early seizures. Acute seizures should be treated with IV lorazepam (0.05 to 0.1 mg per kg) followed by an IV loading dose of phenytoin or fosphenytoin (20 mg per kg). Critically ill patients with ICH may benefit from prophylactic antiepileptic therapy, but no randomized trial has addressed the efficacy of this approach. Some centers prophylactically treat ICH patients with large supratentorial hemorrhages and depressed level of consciousness during the first week on the basis of evidence that this practice reduces the frequency of seizures from 14% to 4% during the first 7 days after severe traumatic brain injury. The American Heart Association (AHA) guidelines recommend antiepileptic medication for up to 1 month, after which therapy should be discontinued in the absence of seizures. This recommendation is supported by the results of a recent study that showed that the risk of early seizures was reduced by prophylactic antiepileptic drug (AED) therapy.

Electroencephalogram Monitoring

Continuous electroencephalographic (cEEG) monitoring has been shown to detect nonconvulsive seizures or status epilepticus in 28% of stuporous or comatose ICH patients, a finding consistent with studies of patients with other types of severe acute brain injury. Moreover, ictal activity detected by cEEG after ICH is associated with neurological deterioration and increased midline shift. It is our practice to perform surveillance cEEG monitoring for at least 48 hours in all comatose ICH patients and to treat nonconvulsive seizures and status with midazolam starting at 0.2 mg/kg/hour. However, the management of nonconvulsive status epilepticus is controversial.

Fever Control

Fever after ICH is common, particularly after IVH, and should be treated aggressively. Sustained fever after ICH has been shown to be independently associated with poor outcome, and even small temperature elevations have been shown to exacerbate neuronal injury and death in experimental models of ischemia. As a general standard, acetaminophen and cooling blankets should be given to all patients with sustained fever >38.3°C (101.0°F), but evidence for the efficacy of these interventions in neurological patients is meager. Newer adhesive surface cooling systems (Arctic Sun, Medivance, Inc.) and endovascular heat exchange catheters (Cool Line System, Alsius, Inc.) have been shown to be much more effective for maintaining normothermia. However, clinical trials are needed to determine whether these measures improve clinical outcome.

Nutrition

As is the case with all critically ill neurological patients, enteral feeding should be started within 48 hours to avoid protein catabolism and malnutrition. A small-bore nasoduodenal feeding tube may reduce the risk of aspiration events.

Deep Venous Thrombosis Prophylaxis

The ICH patients are at high risk for deep vein thrombosis and pulmonary embolism, a potentially fatal complication, because of limb paresis and their prolonged immobilized state. Dynamic compression stockings should be placed on admission.

A small prospective trial has shown that low-dose subcutaneous heparin (5,000 IU BID) started on the second day significantly reduces the frequency of venous thromboembolism with no increase in intracranial bleeding. Treatment with low-molecular-weight heparin (i.e., enoxaparin 40 mg daily) is a reasonable alternative.

Management of Intracranial Pressure

Large-volume ICH is often associated with increased ICP and brain tissue shifts related to ICP gradients and compartmentalized mass effect. This problem can be exacerbated by IVH, which leads to acute obstructive hydrocephalus. As a general rule, an ICP monitor or external ventricular drain (EVD) should be placed in all comatose ICH patients (Glasgow Coma Scale score of 8 or less) with the goal of maintaining ICP <20 mm Hg and CPP >70 mm Hg, unless their condition is so dismal that aggressive ICU care is not warranted (see Table 27.4). Placement of an EVD can be lifesaving in IVH patients with acute brainstem herniation. Compared to parenchymal monitors EVDs carry the therapeutic advantage of allowing CSF drainage and the disadvantage of a substantial risk of infection (approximately 10% during the first 10 days). A small retrospective study failed to show any relationship between changes in ventricular size and level of consciousness in ICH patients treated with EVDs.

Intraventricular administration of the thrombolytic agents urokinase (dose that ranged from 5,000 to 25,000 IU) and tissue plasminogen activator (1 mg every 8 hours) after EVD placement has been hypothesized to speed clot resolution, minimize the risk of catheter occlusion and chronic hydrocephalus, and potentially

TABLE 27.4 Stepwise Treatment Protocol for Elevated Intracranial Pressure in a Monitored Patient

1. *Surgical decompression*. Consider repeat CT scanning, and definitive surgical intervention or ventricular drainage
2. *Sedation*. Intravenous sedation to attain a motionless, quiet state
3. *CPP optimization*. Pressor infusion if CPP is <70 mm Hg, or reduction of blood pressure if CPP is >110 mm Hg
4. *Osmotherapy*. Mannitol 0.25–1.5 g/kg IV or 23.4% hypertonic saline 0.5–2.0 mL/kg (repeat every 1–6 h as needed)
5. *Hyperventilation*. Target pCO_2 levels of 26–30 mm Hg
6. *High-dose pentobarbital therapy*. Load with 5–20 mg/kg, infuse 1–4 mg/kg/h
7. *Hypothermia*. Cool core body temperature to 32°C –33°C

CT, computed tomography; CPP, cerebral perfusion pressure.

Adapted from Mayer SA, Chong J. Critical care management of increased intracranial pressure. *J Int Care Med* 2002;17:55–67, wirh permission.

improve outcome. However, these benefits may be counterbalanced by an increased risk of intracranial bleeding. Indications for IV thrombolytics include presence of blood >30% in any of the lateral ventricles, third or fourth ventricle. Contraindications to its use include craniotomy or untreated AVM or aneurysm. Trials are currently in progress to better define the risks and benefits of intraventricular thrombolytic therapy.

When ICP is monitored, use of a standard management algorithm results in better control, fewer interventions, and reduced duration of therapy. In general, CPP should never be allowed to fall below 70 mm Hg, and interventions to reduce ICP should be escalated or initiated whenever ICP remains above 20 mm Hg for more than 10 minutes.

An acute and sustained increase in ICP should prompt a repeat CT to assess the need for a definitive neurosurgical procedure. If the patient is agitated or fighting the ventilator, an IV sedative agent such as propofol (0.6 to 6 mg/kg/hour) or fentanyl (0.5 to 3.0 μg/kg/hour) should be given to enable the patient to attain a quiet, motionless state. Thereafter, if the CPP is low (generally <70 mm Hg), vasopressors such as dopamine (5 to 30 μg/kg/minute) or phenylephrine (2 to 10 μg/kg/minute) can lead to ICP reduction by decreasing the cerebral vasodilation that sometimes occurs in response to inadequate perfusion. Alternately, if CPP is elevated (generally >110 mm Hg) and has overwhelmed the brain's capacity to autoregulate, BP reduction with IV labetalol, nicardipine, or a similar agent (Table 27.2) can sometimes lead to a parallel reduction in ICP.

Mannitol and hyperventilation should be used after sedation and CPP optimization fail to normalize ICP. The initial dose of mannitol is 1 to 1.5 g per kg of a 20% solution, followed by bolus doses of 0.25 to 1.0 g per kg as needed. Additional doses can be given as frequently as once an hour, based on the initial response to therapy. Hypertonic saline, such as 23.4% saline solution, can be used as an alternative to mannitol, particularly when CPP augmentation is desirable. However, care should be taken to avoid fluid overload in the setting of heart or kidney failure. Hyperventilation is generally used sparingly and for brief periods in monitored patients, because its effect on ICP tends to last for only a few hours. Good long-term outcomes can occur when the combination of osmotherapy and hyperventilation is successfully used to reverse transtentorial herniation. Hemorrhages that are massive enough to lead to intracranial hypertension refractory to these measures are usually fatal. Corticosteroids such as dexamethasone are not indicated in the management of ICH, based on the results of randomized trials that have failed to demonstrate their efficacy. Steroids have the potential to cause hyperglycemia, immunosupression, impaired wound healing, and protein catabolism.

Surgical Management

The Surgical Treatment of Intracerebral Hemorrhage (STICH) trial, a landmark trial of >1,000 ICH patients, showed that emergent surgical hematoma evacuation within 72 hours of onset fails to improve outcome compared to a policy of initial medical management. These results are consistent with the results of a meta-analysis of all prior trials of surgical intervention for supratentorial ICH, which failed to demonstrate benefit. Although the STICH trial has rightfully dampened the enthusiasm of neurosurgeons for performing surgery, it must be remembered that the trial was based on the principle of clinical equipoise: Patients who the local investigator felt would most likely benefit from emergency surgery were not enrolled in the study. Thus, the results of the STICH trial may not be applicable to certain subsets of patients who have traditionally been felt to be good candidates for surgery, particularly younger individuals with large lobar hemorrhages and a rapidly deteriorating course due to mass effect. A small retrospective study showed the best results with emergency craniotomy in exactly this subset of patients.

One small minimally invasive endoscopic surgery trial showed better outcomes with this intervention than with medical management. A variety of other minimally invasive surgical approaches has also been shown to be feasible. Clinical trials will be needed to determine whether these interventions can improve outcome. In contrast to supratentorial ICH, there is much better evidence that cerebellar hemorrhages >3 cm in diameter benefit from emergent surgical evacuation. Abrupt and dramatic deterioration to coma can occur within the first 24 hours of onset in these patients. For this reason, it is generally unwise to defer surgery in these patients until further clinical deterioration occurs.

PRACTICAL RECOMMENDATIONS

Acute severe hypertension should be carefully controlled with IV labetalol or nicardipine to maintain MAP <130 mm Hg, which corresponds to an approximate BP of 180/105 mm Hg. More aggressive BP reduction may be preferable and is currently under study.

The use of rFVIIa within 4 hours of symptom onset of ICH is an attractive approach to minimize active bleeding. Whether this treatment should be adopted as a standard of care for noncoagulopathic ICH will depend on the result of the ongoing phase III trials.

For patients with coagulopathic ICH, particularly from warfarin use, FFP (15 mL/kg) and IV vitamin K (10 mg) should be given as soon as possible. Doses of rFVIIa ranging from 20 to 90 μg per kg can be given as an adjunct to expedite the reversal of anticoagulation as a treatment option.

Suspected ICP elevations and symptomatic intracranial mass effect (i.e., posturing, pupillary changes) should be treated emergently with head elevation, a large dose of 20% mannitol solution (1.0 to 1.5 g per kg), and moderate hyperventilation (pCO_2 28 to 32 mm Hg).

An EVD or ICP monitor should be placed in all patients in coma with evidence of intracranial mass effect or substantial IVH on CT, as long as their prognosis is such that aggressive ICU management is warranted.

ICU and especially stroke patients are at high risk for thromboembolic disease. In addition to dynamic compression stockings, low-dose heparin (5,000 U SC q12H) or enoxaparin (40 mg SC qd) can be safely started on day 2 after ictus.

SELECTED REFERENCES

Ananthasubramaniam K, Beattie JN, Rosman HS, et al. How safely and for how long can warfarin therapy be withheld in prosthetic heart valve patients hospitalized with a major hemorrhage? *Chest* 2001;119(2): 478–484.

Becker KJ, Baxter AB, Bybee HM, et al. Extravasation of radiographic contrast is an independent predictor of death in primary intracerebral hemorrhage. *Stroke* 1999;30(10):2025–2032.

Boeer A, Voth E, Henze T, et al. Early heparin therapy in patients with spontaneous intracerebral haemorrhage. *J Neurol Neurosurg Psychiatr* 1991; 54(5):466–467.

Broderick JP, Adams HP, Jr, Barsan W, et al. Guidelines for the management of spontaneous intracerebral hemorrhage: a statement for healthcare professionals from a special writing group of the Stroke Council, American Heart Association. *Stroke* 1999;30(4):905–915.

Broderick JP, Brott TG, Duldner JE, et al. Volume of intracerebral hemorrhage. A powerful and easy-to-use predictor of 30-day mortality. *Stroke* 1993;24(7):987–993.

Brott T, Broderick J, Kothari R, et al. Early hemorrhage growth in patients with intracerebral hemorrhage. *Stroke* 1997;28(1):1–5.

Brott T, Thalinger K, Hertzberg V. Hypertension as a risk factor for spontaneous intracerebral hemorrhage. *Stroke* 1986;17(6):1078–1083.

Claassen J, Mayer SA, Kowalski RG, et al. Detection of electrographic seizures with continuous EEG monitoring in critically ill patients. *Neurology* 2004;62(10):1743–1748.

Erhardtsen E, Nony P, Dechavanne M, et al. The effect of recombinant factor VIIa (NovoSeven) in healthy volunteers receiving acenocoumarol to an International Normalized Ratio above 2.0. *Blood Coagul Fibrinolysis* 1998;9(8):741–748.

Fogelholm R, Avikainen S, Murros K. Prognostic value and determinants of first-day mean arterial pressure in spontaneous supratentorial intracerebral hemorrhage. *Stroke* 1997;28(7):1396–1400.

Gebel JM, Jr, Jauch EC, Brott TG, et al. Relative edema volume is a predictor of outcome in patients with hyperacute spontaneous intracerebral hemorrhage. *Stroke* 2002;33(11):2636–2641.

Hemphill JC, III, Bonovich DC, Besmertis L, et al. The ICH score: a simple, reliable grading scale for intracerebral hemorrhage. *Stroke* 2001;32 (4):891–897.

Hemphill JC, III, Newman J, Zhao S, et al. Hospital usage of early do-not-resuscitate orders and outcome after intracerebral hemorrhage. *Stroke* 2004;35(5):1130–1134.

Kothari RU, Brott T, Broderick JP, et al. The ABCs of measuring intracerebral hemorrhage volumes. *Stroke* 1996;27(8):1304–1305.

Mayer SA, Brun NC, Begtrup K, et al. Recombinant activated factor VII for acute intracerebral hemorrhage. *N Engl J Med* 2005;352(8):777–785.

Mayer SA, Brun NC, Begtrup K, et al. Efficacy and safety of recombinant activated factor VII for acute intracerebral hemorrhage. *New Engl J Med* 2008;in press.

Mendelow AD, Gregson BA, Fernandes HM, et al. Early surgery versus initial conservative treatment in patients with spontaneous supratentorial intracerebral haematomas in the International Surgical Trial in Intracerebral Haemorrhage (STICH): a randomised trial. *Lancet* 2005; 365(9457):387–397.

Naff NJ, Carhuapoma JR, Williams MA, et al. Treatment of intraventricular hemorrhage with urokinase: effects on 30-Day survival. *Stroke* 2000;31 (4):841–847.

Passero S, Ciacci G, Ulivelli M. The influence of diabetes and hyperglycemia on clinical course after intracerebral hemorrhage. *Neurology* 2003; 61(10):1351–1356.

Passero S, Rocchi R, Rossi S, et al. Seizures after spontaneous supratentorial intracerebral hemorrhage. *Epilepsia* 2002;43(10):1175–1180.

Powers WJ, Adams RE, Yundt KD. Acute pharmacological hypotension after intracerebral hemorrhage does not change cerebral blood flow. *Stroke* 1999;30:242.

Qureshi AI, Wilson DA, Hanley DF, et al. Pharmacologic reduction of mean arterial pressure does not adversely affect regional cerebral blood flow and intracranial pressure in experimental intracerebral hemorrhage. *Crit Care Med* 1999;27(5):965–971.

Rincon F, Mayer SA. Novel therapies for intracerebral hemorrhage. *Curr Opin Crit Care* 2004;10(2):94–100.

Schellinger PD, Fiebach JB, Hoffmann K, et al. Stroke MRI in intracerebral hemorrhage: is there a perihemorrhagic penumbra? *Stroke* 2003;34 (7):1674–1679.

Sorensen B, Johansen P, Nielsen GL, et al. Reversal of the International Normalized Ratio with recombinant activated factor VII in central nervous system bleeding during warfarin thromboprophylaxis: clinical and biochemical aspects. *Blood Coagul Fibrinolysis* 2003;14(5): 469–477.

Vespa PM, O'Phelan K, Shah M, et al. Acute seizures after intracerebral hemorrhage: a factor in progressive midline shift and outcome. *Neurology* 2003;60(9):1441–1446.

Willmot M, Leonardi-Bee J, Bath PM. High blood pressure in acute stroke and subsequent outcome: a systematic review. *Hypertension* 2004;43 (1):18–24.

Zazulia AR, Diringer MN, Videen TO, et al. Hypoperfusion without ischemia surrounding acute intracerebral hemorrhage. *J Cereb Blood Flow Metab* 2001;21(7):804–810.

Zhu XL, Chan MS, Poon WS. Spontaneous intracranial hemorrhage: which patients need diagnostic cerebral angiography? A prospective study of 206 cases and review of the literature. *Stroke* 1997;28 (7):1406–1409.

CHAPTER

28 Management of Subarachnoid Hemorrhage

AZADEH FARIN, STEVEN L. GIANNOTTA, AND GENE SUNG

OBJECTIVES

- What are the pathophysiology and most common location for aneurysm formation?
- What are the risk factors for and outcomes of aneurysmal subarachnoid hemorrhage?
- What is the major cause of morbidity and mortality in the survivors? What are the other causes of neurological deterioration after aneurysmal subarachnoid hemorrhage?
- What are the key steps in the initial management of aneurysmal subarachnoid hemorrhage? What is the highest priority in initial management?
- How is acute hydrocephalus after aneurysmal subarachnoid hemorrhage treated?
- How are fluids and blood pressure managed in aneurysmal subarachnoid hemorrhage?

While the most common cause of subarachnoid hemorrhage (SAH) is trauma, ruptured intracranial aneurysms account for 75% to 80% of nontraumatic SAH cases. Other causes of spontaneous SAH include ruptured cerebral or spinal arteriovenous malformations, central nervous system vasculitides, cerebral artery dissection, perimesencephalic nonaneurysmal SAH, rupture of an arterial infundibulum, hemorrhagic tumor, coagulation disorders, dural sinus thrombosis, sickle cell disease, cocaine use, and pituitary apoplexy. In 7% to 20% of SAH cases, etiology is unknown. This chapter addresses the management of patients with aneurysmal SAH.

Incidence, Demographics, and Location

It is estimated that 1 in 17 Americans will develop a brain aneurysm during their lifetime. Approximately 28,000 intracranial aneurysms rupture each year in North America, reflecting an estimated annual incidence rate of 6 to 28 per 100,000. The range of autopsy prevalence of aneurysms is 0.2% to 7.9%; half are believed to rupture and only 2% of aneurysms are believed to present during childhood. The peak age for aneurysmal SAH is 55 to 60 years, however, approximately 20% of patients fall between the age of 15 and 45 years. Patients older than 70 have a greater risk of presenting with a poorer neurological examination and fare worse for each neurological grade. Aneurysms may arise from a defect in the muscular layer of the arterial wall or secondary to atherosclerotic or hypertensive vascular disease (see Fig. 28.1). Saccular or berry aneurysms are usually located on major vessels at the apex of branch points, which is the site of maximum hemodynamic stress in a vessel. Approximately 85% to 95% of saccular aneurysms are located in the anterior circulation [anterior communicating artery (ACA) 30%, posterior communicating artery (PCA) 25%, and middle cerebral artery (MCA) 20%]; 5% to 15% exist in the posterior circulation [10% on the basilar artery, usually basilar tip; 5% on the vertebral artery, with the posterior inferior cerebellar artery (PICA) junction as the most common site]. Multiple aneurysms are present in 20% to 30% of patients. Conditions associated with aneurysms include polycystic kidney disease, fibromuscular dysplasia, arteriovenous malformations, Ehlers-Danlos type IV, Marfan syndrome, pseudoxanthoma elasticum, coarctation of the aorta, Osler-Weber-Rendu syndrome, atherosclerosis, bacterial endocarditis, and family members with intracranial aneurysms.

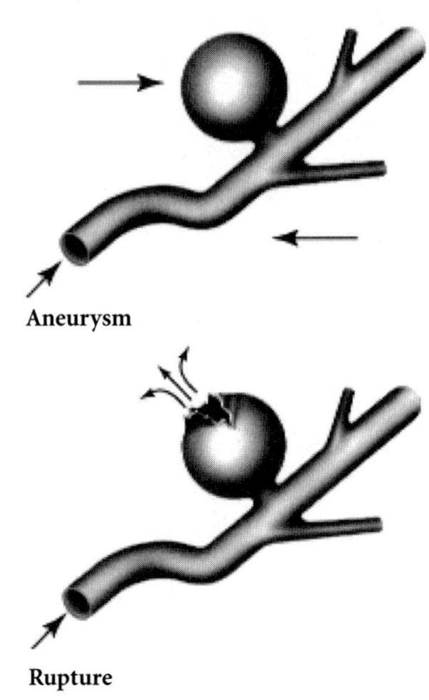

FIGURE 28.1. Diagram of aneurysm formation and rupture.

Risk Factors

Risk factors for aneurysmal SAH include hypertension, substance abuse (alcohol, tobacco, cocaine), oral contraceptive use, pregnancy and parturition, lumbar puncture (LP) or cerebral angiography in patients with unruptured aneurysms, and advanced age.

Outcome

Unfortunately, 10% to 15% of patients die before reaching the hospital. Rehemorrhage is a major cause of morbidity and mortality in the remaining survivors and occurs in 15% to 20% within the first 2 weeks of the initial hemorrhage. Therefore, the first priority is securing the aneurysm. Neurological deterioration resulting from the initial hemorrhage is responsible for 8% of deaths. Vasospasm, another feared consequence of aneurysmal SAH, is believed to be responsible for deaths in 7% and neurological deficit in another 7%. Overall, approximately half of aneurysmal SAH patients die within the first month; another study found that more than half the patients die within 2 weeks of their initial SAH. Overall mortality rate ranges from 32% to 67%. Only one third of survivors do well, one third have moderate to severe disability, and two thirds of those who undergo successful craniotomy for aneurysm clipping never return to their original quality of life.

CLINICAL APPLICATIONS AND PRACTICAL RECOMMENDATIONS

Signs and Symptoms

About half of patients with aneurysms have warning symptoms, usually 1 to 3 weeks before the main hemorrhage. One third of hemorrhages are believed to occur during sleep.

Headache is present in up to 97% of cases; the classic description is the "sudden onset of the worst headache of my life." Occasionally, the headache resolves within 1 day, and the patient is considered to have suffered a *sentinel headache or hemorrhage* or *warning headache* (30% to 60% of patients with SAH). In these cases, blood may appear on computed tomography (CT) or LP; however, warning headaches may also reflect aneurysmal enlargement or hemorrhage confined within the aneurysmal wall, and therefore, not demonstrate hemorrhage on LP or CT. One third of patients describe a lateralized headache, generally to the side of the aneurysm rupture. Among patients who present with sudden-onset severe headache, 25% have SAH; however, the differential diagnosis also includes benign thunderclap headaches (migranous vascular headaches though without SAH) and benign orgasmic cephalgia (severe headache accompanying orgasm).

Headache may be accompanied with hypertension, vomiting, syncopy, apoplexy, photophobia, loss of consciousness (may be temporary), focal neurological deficit (third nerve compression may cause diplopia or ptosis; hemiparesis), and low back pain secondary to irritation of lumbar nerve roots by SAH.

Meningismus (nuchal rigidity and neck pain especially to flexion) can be experienced in the first 6 to 24 hours. Patients may exhibit Brudzinski's sign (flexing the patient's neck is accompanied with involuntary hip flexion) or Kernig's sign (flexing the thigh to 90 degrees with the knee bent, then straightening the knee results in hamstring pain).

A comatose state may result from increased intracranial pressure (ICP), intraparenchymal hemorrhage, hydrocephalus, decreased cerebral blood flow (possibly due to intracranial hypertension or low cardiac output), and seizure.

Three types of ocular hemorrhages (OH) may accompany 20% to 40% of SAH. OH may be secondary to compression of the central retinal vein and the retinochoroidal anastamoses by intracranial hypertension causing venous hypertension and disruption of retinal veins. Subhyaloid (preretinal) hemorrhage is viewed as blood near the optic disc and may be associated with a higher mortality rate. Intraretinal hemorrhage may surround the fovea. Terson's syndrome, or hemorrhage within the vitreous humor, causes vitreous opacity and may be associated with a higher mortality rate. Patients should be followed up for elevated intraocular pressure and retinal detachment. Most cases clear spontaneously, but vitrectomy should be considered in some.

Evaluation and Diagnosis

For patients with suspected SAH based on history and examination, a noncontrast head CT is first obtained. If the head CT does not reveal SAH, a LP may be performed. Subsequently, a four-vessel cerebral angiogram is performed for confirmed cases of SAH or if a high degree of suspicion exists for a vascular etiology as the cause of the SAH.

SAH is detected in >95% of cases within 48 hours of hemorrhage by a good-quality noncontrast high-resolution fourth-generation CT, where it appears as high density within subarachnoid spaces (see Fig. 28.2). About 20% to 40% of cases additionally demonstrate intraparenchymal hemorrhage, 13% to 28% show intraventricular hemorrhage, and 2% to 5% exhibit subdural hemorrhage. Emergent evacuation may be required if mass effect is

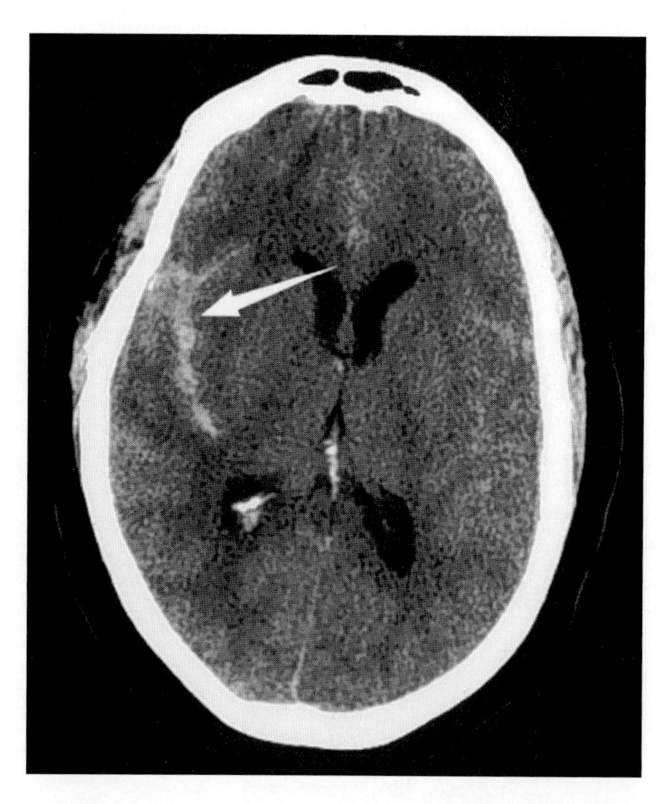

FIGURE 28.2. Computed tomography scan showing subarachnoid hemorrhage after the rupture of a right posterior communicating artery aneurysm.

present. Other notable features include hydrocephalus, which occurs acutely in 21% of aneurysmal ruptures and infarct. The quantity of blood within cisterns and fissures is a significant prognosticator for vasospasm. The location and pattern of bleeding may suggest aneurysm location in approximately 70% of cases; sylvian fissure hemorrhage is consistent with rupture of a PCA or MCA aneurysm; ACA aneurysms often exhibit hemorrhage in the anterior interhemispheric fissure; third and fourth intraventricular hemorrhage may reflect PICA aneurysm rupture or vertebral artery dissection. The Fisher scale is commonly used to summarize the CT scan appearance of SAH and correlate the imaging findings with the risk of vasospasm:

- Group 1: no blood detected
- Group 2: Diffuse deposition of subarachnoid blood; no clots or layers of blood >1 mm
- Group 3: localized clots and/or vertical layers of blood 1 mm or greater in thickness
- Group 4: diffuse or no subarachnoid blood, but intracerebral or intraventricular clots are present

LP remains the most sensitive test for SAH; however, the possibility of a traumatic puncture increases the false-positive rate. When this procedure is performed [and during placement of an external ventricular drain(EVD)], there is an increased risk of aneurysmal rupture/rerupture if more than several milliliters of cerebrospinal fluid (CSF) are removed and a large spinal needle (18 gauge and larger) is used, as the transmural pressure across the aneurysm wall may be increased by lowering the CSF pressure. Findings consistent with SAH include an elevated opening pressure, nonclotting bloody fluid that does not clear with sequential tubes, xanthochromia (may develop as early as 6 hours post hemorrhage; xanthochromia identified in a spun sample in the supernatant fluid via spectrophotometry is more accurate than visual inspection), usually >100,000 red blood cells per mm^3 (the number of red cells in the last tube should not be much lower than the number in the first tube), elevated protein levels due to blood degradation products, and normal or reduced glucose level, as red cells may consume some glucose.

Magnetic resonance imaging (MRI) is more sensitive 4 to 7 days and excellent >10 days after hemorrhage, as too little methemoglobin in the acute phase post rupture makes this modality insensitive during the initial 24 to 48 hours.

Cerebral angiography is considered the gold standard for diagnosis of cerebral aneurysms (see Fig. 28.3). This modality reveals the source of SAH in 80% to 85% of all cases and shows radiographical vasospasm (although clinical vasospasm rarely occurs before postbleed day 3). Unstable or premorbid patients are not typically good candidates; if early surgery or coiling is a possibility, angiography is performed as soon as possible. The most promising vessel based on initial head CT is injected first so that diagnosis is more likely to be obtained early during the procedure in case it must be terminated because of patient deterioration. If the patient remains stable, the procedure is continued until all four cerebral vessels have been injected to determine whether multiple aneurysms exist and to delineate collateral circulation. Once an aneurysm is revealed, additional views are obtained to further characterize the neck and orientation of the aneurysm. In the event no aneurysm is observed, the study is considered negative only if both PICA origins are visualized (1% to 2% of aneurysms occur at this location) and contrast is visualized to flow through the ACA.

Magnetic resonance angiography (MRA) has a sensitivity of approximately 86% to 95% for detecting aneurysms >3 mm in diameter, with a false-positive rate of 16% (compared to cerebral angiography). Ability to detect aneurysms is affected by size, rate, and direction of blood flow in the aneurysm relative to the magnetic field and direction of thrombosis and calcification. Currently, MRA is accepted as a screening test in patients who are at high risk for harboring intracranial aneurysms.

CT angiography (CTA) has a sensitivity of 95% and specificity of 83% in detecting aneurysms ≥2.2 mm. CTA is superior to cerebral angiography in that it shows a three-dimensional image of the aneurysm and its relation to adjacent bony structures, which can be helpful for treatment purposes.

Grading SAH

The Hunt and Hess Classification of SAH is commonly used to grade patients according to their presenting neurological examination. The grading system is summarized as follows:

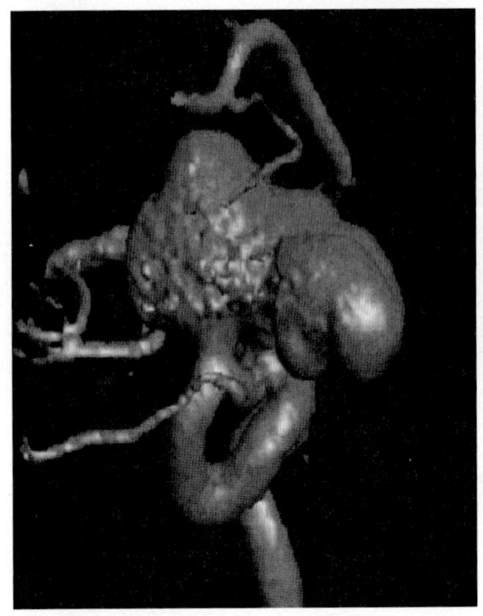

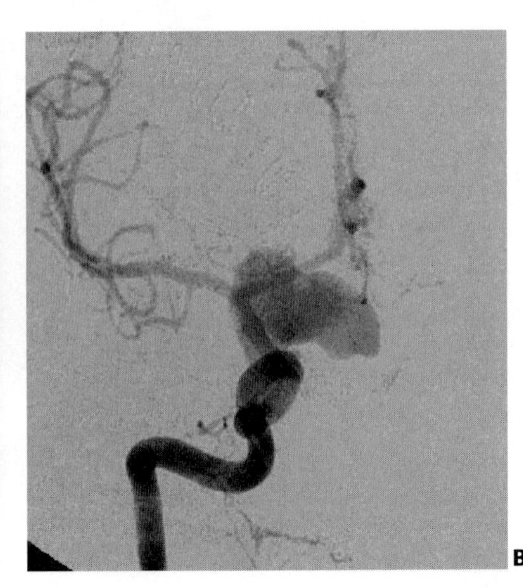

FIGURE 28.3 A: Three-dimensional rotational angiogram of a large multilobular aneurysm. **B:** Digital subtraction cerebral angiogram of a large multilobular aneurysm.

1. Asymptomatic, minimal headache, or slight nuchal rigidity
2. Moderate to severe headache, or nuchal rigidity; no neurological deficit except cranial nerve palsy
3. Drowsy, or minimal neurological deficit
4. Stuporous; moderate to severe hemiparesis; possibly early decerebrate or vegetative state
5. Deep coma; decerebrate rigidity; moribund appearance

In this analysis, patients falling into Grades 1 and 2 underwent surgery as soon as they were diagnosed. Grade ≥ 3 patients were conservatively managed until they improved to Grades 1 or 2, unless they exhibited life-threatening hematomas, in which case they proceeded to surgery regardless of grade. Patients falling into Grades 1 or 2 upon admission had a mortality rate of 20% but only 14% if they were taken to surgery for any procedure at Grades 1 or 2. The major cause of death in Grade 1 or 2 was found to be rehemorrhaging.

The World Federation of Neurologic Surgeons (WFNS) SAH Grading Scale is summarized as follows:

- Grade 1: Glasgow Coma Score (GCS) of 15, motor deficit absent
- Grade 2: GCS of 13-to 14, motor deficit absent
- Grade 3: GCS of 13 to 14, motor deficit present
- Grade 4: GCS of 7 to 12, motor deficit absent or present
- Grade 5: GCS of 3 to 6, motor deficit absent or present

This system uses GCS to evaluate level of consciousness and uses the presence of major focal neurological deficit to distinguish Grade 2 from Grade 3.

Clinical Management of Subarachnoid Hemorrhage

Initial Management

Prevention of rehemorrhage is the highest priority after establishing patient stability, as a subsequent hemorrhage may be neurologically devastating and life threatening. It is believed that 3,000 North Americans have a life-terminating rehemorrhage of a ruptured aneurysm each year. The risk of rebleeding is 4% on day 1 and then 1.5% each day up to 13 days. Up to 20% will rebleed within 2 weeks and half will rebleed within 6 months. After the initial 6 months, the risk is 3% per year with a mortality rate of 2% per year. One study found the highest risks of rebleeding to be in the first 6 hours after SAH and in patients with higher Hunt and Hess grades. For patients who are considered salvageable and for good operative or endovascular candidates based on their presenting neurological examination and other comorbidities, early aneurysm clipping or coiling is the only way to help prevent rehemorrhage and is discussed in a subsequent chapter. Though controversial, a loading dose of Amicar (ϵ-aminocaproic acid, 10 g IV, followed by 48 g per day of continuous drip) has been advocated by some clinicians for patients whose operative or endovascular treatment is delayed. This antifibrinolytic agent competitively inhibits the activation of plasminogen to plasmin, thereby reducing the risk of rehemorrhage. However, an increased risk of hydrocephalus, coronary artery thrombus, deep venous thrombus, and pulmonary embolus may also be observed. Some cite the increased rate of cerebral infarction secondary to vasospasm and the consequent failure to reduce early mortality in the setting of aneurysmal SAH as a contraindication to its use. One nonrandomized study including Grades 1 to 3 patients suggested limiting its use to only the period of delay before aneurysm clipping or coiling.

An additional life-threatening complication following SAH is hydrocephalus—acutely obstructive because of hematoma obstruction of CSF flow and CSF reabsorption at the level of arachnoid granulations, then subsequently communicating in the case of chronic hydrocephalus due to blood degradation products and pia-arachnoid adhesions impairing arachnoid granulation function. While the literature quotes a wide range of frequency of hydrocephalus on initial CT after SAH, acute hydrocephalus may not always lead to chronic hydrocephalus. Approximately 8% to 45% of all ruptured aneurysm patients and about half of those with acute hydrocephalus after SAH require shunts. Some patients may acutely deteriorate, while others may show no change in level of consciousness when hydrocephalus does ensue. Acute hydrocephalus is associated with increasing age, intraventricular blood, diffuse or thick focal accumulation of subarachnoid blood, hypertension, ruptured posterior circulation aneurysms (compared with MCA aneurysms which have a lower incidence of hydrocephalus), hyponatremia, poor initial neurological examination, and use of Amicar. Interestingly, half of all patents with acute hydrocephalus affecting level of consciousness in one study improved spontaneously. However, acute hydrocephalus can be life threatening, and the same study found approximately 80% of patients improved after EVD. LP and EVD carry an increased risk of aneurysmal rehemorrhage, especially if ICP is dramatically reduced acutely by aggressive CSF withdrawal resulting in a large differential between aneurysm intraluminal pressure compared with ICP, unless declining neurological status warrants further reduction of ICP. EVDs for acute hydrocephalus may increase or decrease the future need for a shunt.

Other issues of concern throughout the treatment period include vasospasm-attributed delayed ischemic neurological deficit (DIND), hyponatremia with hypovolemia, deep venous thrombosis and pulmonary embolism, and seizures. Any patient with a deteriorating neurological examination, whether before or after securing the aneurysm, deserves an immediate noncontrast head CT that may reveal rehemorrhage, hydrocephalus, ischemia secondary to vasospasm and venous infarct, retraction injury secondary to operative technique, or edema. Sodium level to rule out hyponatremia, as well as prothrombin time, partial thromboplastin time, and platelet count to rule out a bleeding tendency, should be checked acutely if there is a change in neurological examination and frequently if the values are consistently abnormal. A complete blood count can help assess rheology and the possibility of sepsis or anemia. An arterial blood gas should be performed to rule out hypoxemia or hypercarbia. If signs and symptoms point to intracranial hypertension, an ICP monitor or EVD may be inserted. Conservative CSF drainage, if needed before institution of hyperdynamic therapy, is advised over diuresis with mannitol, which works against hyperdynamic therapy. A transcranial Doppler (TCD) can be performed to detect or follow possible vasospasm. If this workup does not prove helpful in determining the etiology of neurological deterioration, a four-vessel cerebral angiogram may be indicated to assess for acute vasospasm. Even in the absence of Doppler findings or if angiography is unavailable, when the above workup and management do not reveal the cause of the deteriorating examination or result in an improved clinical picture, vasospasm may be suspected and hyperdynamic therapy is indicated.

Initial orders should include admission to the intensive care unit with vital signs and neurological examination checks every hour. Patients should be placed on bedrest with the head of bed elevated at 30 degrees with SAH precautions (low level of external stimulation, restricted visitation) and seizure precautions. Nursing orders should include strict input and output measurements, daily weights, knee-high TED hose and pneumatic compression boots, and Foley catheter if the patient is lethargic, incontinent, or unable to void in a bedpan or urinal. Preoperative or lethargic patients should be on NPO status and lethargic patients should have a nasogastric tube placed to suction except when medications are administered. Aggressive intravenous fluid hydration is critical to help prevent cerebral salt wasting and the possible sequelae of vasospasm. Therefore, patients typically are started on normal saline with 20 mEq of potassium chloride per L at 150 mL per hour. In fact, for patients with Fisher Grade 3 or worse, maintaining a positive fluid balance is even more important to prevent the devastating consequences of vasospasm, so supplemental fluid boluses are administered every 8 hours with this objective. Recently, high serum levels of magnesium were found to be possibly associated with a decreased risk of vasospasm, and supplementing each bag of intravenous fluid with 2 g of magnesium sulfate may be considered to achieve a serum level of almost 4.0. If the admission hematocrit is >40%, 500 mL of 5% albumin over 4 hours is administered upon admission. An arterial line is placed for hemodynamically unstable or stuporous patients or for those requiring frequent blood draws (ventilator-dependent patients who cannot protect their airways independently). A Swan-Ganz catheter is indicated for patients in vasospasm, those with possible cerebral salt wasting or syndrome of inappropriate antidiuretic hormone (SIADH) secretion, hemodynamically unstable patients, or those with Hunt and Hess Grade ≥ 3 to monitor pulmonary capillary wedge pressure (PCWP) and cardiac output; a central line can be used to monitor central venous pressure (CVP) when a pulmonary artery catheter is not possible. Continuous cardiac rhythm monitoring is critical, as arrhythmias may occur following SAH. An EVD is indicated in patients developing acute hydrocephalus or in those with a significant amount of intraventricular hemorrhage for measurement of ICP and drainage of bloody CSF. EVD placement causes symptomatic improvement in almost two thirds of patients, but may increase the risk of rehemorrhage. Some clinicians place EVDs in patients graded Hunt and Hess 3 or worse, hoping for clinical improvement so that overall prognosis may be improved. Serial LPs, though not common, can be used as an alternative to carefully lower the ICP. Intracranial hypertension must be treated immediately, and if CSF drainage does not suffice, other measures must be taken. Mannitol and furosemide (Lasix) have great clinical validity, but their use in lowering ICP in aneurysmal SAH is controversial at best, since these patients typically must be fluid overloaded to prevent vasospasm and to maintain perfusion, especially after the aneurysm is secured. Three percent hypertonic saline is an alternative that may lower ICP without causing hypovolemia.

Systolic blood pressure (SBP) should be maintained at 120 to 150 mm Hg by cuff for unsecured aneurysms to avoid rerupture. Once the aneurysm is secured and if the patient exhibits clinical vasospasm, blood pressure can be elevated. In the case of an unsecured aneurysm with accompanying vasopasm, slight volume expansion and hypertension with some hemodilution may help minimize the effects of vasospasm and cerebral salt wasting. For excessive hypertension, especially before the aneurysm is secured, labetalol (10 mg IV q10min PRN SBP >150 mm Hg) (contraindicated in cases of heart block or bradycardia) or hydralazine (10 mg IV q10min PRN SBP >150 mm Hg) (hold if heart rate >110) can be given. If repeated doses of these drugs are required, a nicardipine drip can be administered for longer term control (5 mg per hour IV, increase by 2.5 mg per hour q5-15min to a maximum of 15 mg per hour; at goal blood pressure, decrease to 3 mg per hour). Traditionally, nitroprusside has been used to lower blood pressure; however, as a vasodilator it may increase the possibility of rerupturing an unsecured aneurysm and hypotension may cause cerebral ischemia.

Oxygenation can be maintained with nasal cannula PRN based on arterial blood gas; intubated patients should have a pO2 >100 mm Hg with normocarbia. Hypercarbia (pCO2 >42 mm Hg) can result in vascular dilatation and intracranial hypertension; hypocarbia (pCO2 <30 mm Hg units) can result in vasoconstriction and cerebral ischemia.

Admission laboratories should include arterial blood gas, electrolytes, complete blood count, prothrombin time, and partial thromboplastin time. Daily laboratories should include arterial blood gas for intubated patients, electrolytes, and complete blood count. If hyponatremia develops, more frequent sodium checks are recommended. Serum and urine electrolytes and osmolalities q12hs should be checked if urine output is excessive (>250 mL per hour) or too low (<0.5 mL/kg/hour). Hematocrit and fibrinogen may be followed up to determine whether blood flow may be impaired by a high viscosity state during vasospasm. A chest X-ray is taken daily until the patient is clinically and hemodynamically stable, as SAH patients are at risk for developing neurogenic pulmonary edema. Also, in cases where cardiac function is already compromised when the patient presents, cardiogenic pulmonary edema can be detected on X-ray in patients who are given aggressive fluid hydration to ward off vasospasm. Continuous cardiac rhythm monitoring is indicated to detect life-threatening arrhythmias.

Intramuscularly administered medications are avoided to prevent pain. Prophylactic anticonvulsants are administered by many, since a seizure in the setting of an unsecured aneurysm may be neurologically devastating. Recognizing this fact, most clinicians administer anticonvulsants for at least 1 week postoperatively. Approximately 3% of patients with SAH have seizures during their acute illness not including seizures accompanying the initial hemorrhage; 5% have seizures postoperatively with or without SAH, and 10.5% have seizures in the 5 years following (20% of patients with MCA aneurysms, followed in frequency by those with PCA aneurysms, and then those with ACA aneurysms). Generally, phenytoin is used for this purpose. The intravenous form is painful when administered and can cause phlebosclerosis, but the similar fosphenytoin is advantageous in these dimensions. The loading dose is 17 mg per kg, followed by a maintenance dose of 300 mg qhs or whatever is required to maintain a therapeutic range of 10 to 20 mg. During craniotomy for aneurysmal clip ligation, after the dura is opened, phenobarbital may be administered to achieve burst suppression for cerebral protection should the aneurysm rupture or during prolonged periods of temporary clip time; this agent can also exert an anticonvulsant effect.

Sedation may be necessary in some patients who are agitated; otherwise hypertension and aneurysm rerupture may occur. Generally, short-acting agents, such as morphine, fentanyl, versed, and propofol, are administered in small quantities to allow frequent neurological examinations so that deterioration secondary to rerupture, vasospasm, or hydrocephalus can be detected immediately on clinical examination. Uncontrolled pain should be avoided, as it can lead to hypertension. Morphine and fentanyl also aid with analgesic effect for headache; in less severe cases codeine 30 to 60 mg by mouth (PO) q2-3h can be effective. Meperidine (Demerol) should not be used, as it lowers the seizure threshold. Dexamethasone 6 mg IV/PO q6h is also used by some to possibly mitigate edema from the aneurysm rupture itself and to help with neck and head pain as well as postcraniotomy retraction edema. Docusate 100 mg PO twice a day (BID) is used in patients who can take oral medications or down the gastric tube for stool-softening purposes to avoid increases in ICP. Antiemetics (except phenothiazines, which may lower the seizure threshold) may be administered, including trimethobenzamide 200 mg PR q4-6h, metoclopramide 10 mg IV q6h, and droperidol 0.625 mg IV q4h. Emesis should not be treated without examining the patient first, as it may indicate concerning hydrocephalus. Nimodipine, a calcium cannel blocker, may aid in neuroprotection and mitigation of vasospasm. It is administered as 60 mg PO/NG q4h initiated within 96 hours of initial SAH, for 21 days or until the patient is discharged home in good condition; the dose should be halved for liver failure. Blood pressure should be monitored continuously during nimodipine administration, as hypotension may ensue. H_2 blockers are administered to reduce the risk of stress ulcers. Any agent that impairs platelet aggregation or coagulation is contraindicated before the ruptured aneurysm is secured and for several days postcraniotomy. These agents include aspirin, dextran, heparin, and hetastarch.

Additional Considerations

Natriuresis and diuresis are often observed in conjunction with SAH, leading to hypovolemia and hyponatremia. Urinary loss of sodium, or cerebral salt wasting, has been demonstrated to be the cause of hyponatremia in most SAH patients; atrial natriuretic factor as the cause is still controversial. What is known is that a rise in atrial natriuretic factor and brain natriuretic peptide after SAH is associated with hypovolemia and sometimes hyponatremia. Hyponatremia, whether a consequence of cerebral salt wasting or SIADH, is of particular concern in the setting of aneurysmal SAH because hyponatremic patients have approximately three times the rate of infarction compared with normonatremic patients, and clinically, hyponatremic patients may behave similar to vasospastic patients with ischemic neurological deficits. Most laboratory values are similar between the two main causes of hyponatremia following aneurysmal SAH; however, SIADH patients tend to be fluid overloaded, whereas cerebral salt-wasting patients tend to be hypovolemic. In addition, patients with a history of diabetes, congestive heart failure, cirrhosis, or adrenal insufficiency, and those taking nonsteroidal anti-inflammatory drugs, acetaminophen, narcotics, or thiazides, have a higher risk of developing hyponatremia after SAH. Fluid restriction is not advised as treatment for hyponatremia in the setting of SAH, for if the cause were the more commonly occurring salt wasting, hemoconcentration would worsen ischemia from vasospasm. A Swan-Ganz catheter may be placed to check a full line of data every 4 hours to assess fluid status via such parameters as CVP (can also be measured with a simple subclavian line), cardiac output, and cardiac index. Where hypovolemia is suspected, normal saline, packed red blood cells, or 5% albumin may be administered as appropriate. If hyponatremia with salt wasting is suspected, options include salt tablets [2 g PO BID/three times a day], 0.9% normal saline (150 mL per hour) or 3% hypertonic saline (10 to 30 mL per hour; note that achieving normonatremia too quickly may result in central pontine myelinolysis), or fludrocortisone acetate 0.2 mg IV or PO BID with possible side affects including pulmonary edema, hypokalemia, and hypertension. To maintain euvolemia, some clinicians have also used Urea (Ureaphil) 0.5 g per kg; dissolve 40 g in 150 mL normal saline, IV over 60 minutes q8h with normal saline as maintenance fluid and supplemental boluses of 5% albumin.

Over half of SAH patients experience cardiac arrhythmias and electrocardiogram (ECG) changes, such as T-wave abnormalities, QT prolongation, ST segment elevation or depression, U-waves, premature atrial or ventricular contraction, supraventricular tachycardia, ventricular flutter, or ventricular fibrillation. Some ECG patterns observed in the setting of SAH resemble acute myocardial infarction. This may be a consequence of hypothalamic ischemia causing increased sympathetic tone and a catecholamine surge resulting in subendocardial ischemia or coronary artery vasospasm. Myocardial hypokinesis may also accompany SAH, believed to be secondary to a defect in troponin-I and resembling myocardial infarction on echocardiography, but with negative cardiac enzymes and complete reversibility in most cases in less than a week. Approximately 10% of these patients may have true myocardial infarction. In the event hypotension ensues secondary to cardiac arrhythmia causing decreased cardiac output, dopamine may be indicated to enable an adequate blood pressure during burst suppression or during hyperdynamic therapy for vasospasm.

Clinical vasospasm, or DIND, is a neurological deficit following SAH that can be attributed to ischemic changes in particular vascular territories (see Fig. 28.4). It is the most significant cause of morbidity and mortality in patients surviving SAH who reach the hospital; some consider it to be more dangerous than even aneurysm rupture and rerupture itself. Vasospasm may result in reversible deficits, but it is fatal in 7% of SAH cases. It is believed to be a consequence of inflammatory mediators resulting in muscle necrosis, vessel thickening, opening of interendothelial tight junctions, and proliferation of smooth muscle cells. It is rarely seen before postbleed day 3; the more likely time point for vasospasm is postbleed days 6 to 8, but it can occur as late as postbleed day 17. Clinical vasospasm is almost always resolved by postbleed day 12; however, radiographical vasospasm may take up to 1 month to resolve. Patients in vasospasm may appear confused or exhibit headache, meningismus, or decreased level of consciousness with neurological deficit. In the early stages, angiography may be required for diagnosis, as CT scan would not typically show ischemic consequences of acute vasospasm until at least 24 hours. Diagnosis of vasospasm requires eliminating other potential causes of neurological deterioration, including hydrocephalus, cerebral edema, seizure, hyponatremia, hypoxia, and sepsis. Adequate hydration and blood transfusion can help prevent vasospasm by correcting post-SAH hypovolemia and anemia.

The anterior cerebral artery is more likely to become vasospastic than the MCA. In anterior cerebral artery syndrome, frontal lobe functions are compromised secondary to vasospasm, resulting in abulia, presence of grasp and suck reflexes, urinary incontinence, lethargy, confusion, and whispering. ACA aneurysmal rupture can result in bilateral anterior cerebral artery distribution infarcts stemming from vasospasm. MCA syndrome manifests as hemiparesis, aphasia, or apractagnosia.

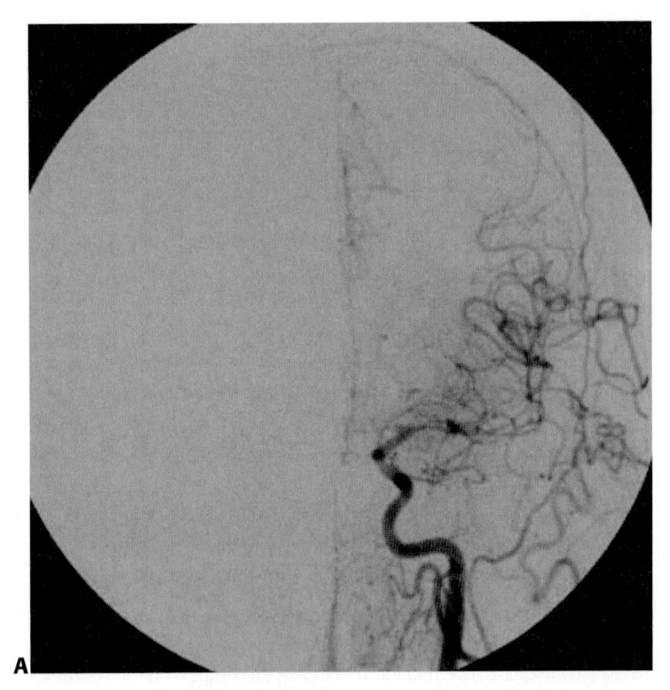

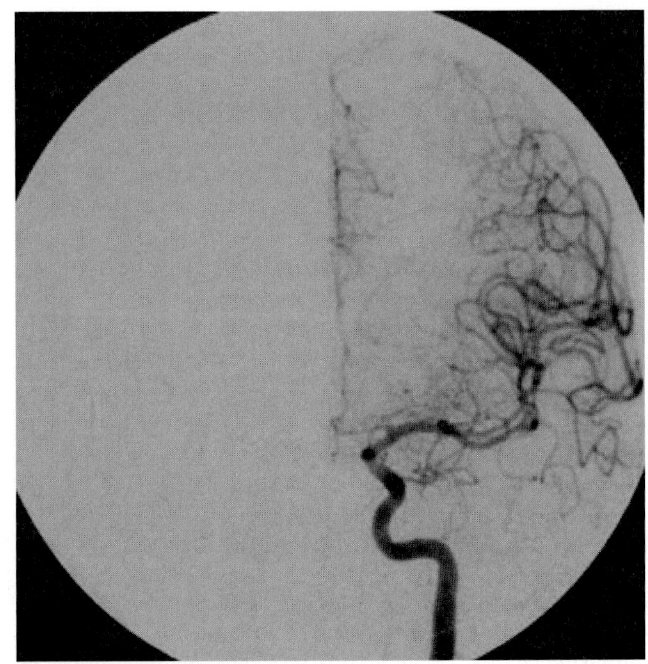

FIGURE 28.4 A: Left carotid angiogram showing severe vasospasm with narrowing of the left middle cerebral artery (MCA) and anterior cerebral artery (ACA) on day 8 following subarachnoid hemorrhage from aneurysm rupture. **B:** Repeat left carotid angiogram following 8 mg of intra-arterial nicardipine, which shows improvement in the caliber and flow through the left ACA and MCA.

Vasospasm can be defined radiographically on angiography as vessel narrowing with slowing of contrast filling, especially when compared with previous angiograms showing a normal caliber vessel in question. Radiographical vasospasm is observed in 30% to 70% of angiograms completed 1 week after SAH, whereas symptomatic vasospasm occurs in only 20% to 30% of SAH patients. There is not always perfect correlation between neurological deficit and radiographical spasm. Other methods of detecting vasospasm include electroencephalography (a reduced percentage of a activity from a mean of 0.45 to 0.17 predicts the onset of vasospasm before it is detected via angiography or via TCD; reduced amplitude was exquisitely sensitive for predicting vasospasm), xenon cerebral blood flow studies (which detect large changes in blood flow), positron emission tomography, and single-photon emission computed tomography. Commonly, TCD is used daily or every other day to help detect vasospasm, because a narrowed vessel lumen results in elevated blood flow velocity. A mean MCA velocity of <120 cm per second is consistent with a normal vessel; mild vasospasm is suspected at velocities of 120 to 200 cm per second and severe vasospasm is diagnosed at vessel velocities of >200 cm per second. Daily increases of >50 cm per second may also indicate vasospasm. The Lindegaard ratio, or ratio of MCA to ICA velocity, helps remove hyperemia as a confounding factor. A ratio of 3 to 6 is consistent with mild vasospasm and a ratio >6 is consistent with severe vasospasm.

Hematomas in direct contact with the proximal ACA and MCA are especially concerning for contributing to vasospasm. Other risk factors for vasospasm include increasing age, history of cigarette smoking, history of hypertension, pial enhancement on head CT with contrast 3 days after SAH as a refection of increased blood–brain barrier permeability, antifibrinolytic therapy, and use of angiographic dye. The patient's presenting Hunt and Hess grade, as well as Fisher grade (an indicator of amount and pattern of bleeding), correlates with vasospasm risk, as indicated in Table 28.1.

Calcium channel blockers antagonize the slow channel of calcium influx, thereby decreasing contraction of vascular smooth muscle and possibly preventing vasospasm. These agents also have a neuroprotective role because of their effects on increasing red

TABLE 28.1 Correlation of Clinical Vasospasm with Hunt and Hess Grade and of Fisher Grade with Angiographic and Clinical Vasospasm

Correlation of Clinical Vasospasm with Hunt and Hess Grade

Hunt and Hess Grade	% Patients with Clinical Vasospasm
1	22
2	33
3	52
4	53
5	74

Correlation of Fisher Grade with Angiographic and Clinical Vasospasm

Fisher Group	Number of Patients	Angiographic Spasm	Clinical Spasm
1	11	4	0
2	7	3	0
3	24	24	23
4	5	2	0

cell deformability (which improves blood rheology), blocking calcium entry into ischemic cells that may contribute to injury from infarction, antiplatelet aggregation effect, and dilatation of collateral leptomeningeal arteries. Nimodipine is lipophilic, and therefore, crosses the blood–brain barrier to block dihydropyridine-sensitive or L-type calcium channels. Although this agent does not improve radiographical vasospasm or mortality, it has been shown in four randomized, double-blind placebo-controlled trials to reduce the incidence and severity of ischemic deficits due to vasospasm in patients with SAH from ruptured intracranial aneurysms regardless of the postictus neurological condition or Hunt and Hess Grade, resulting in improvement of neurological outcome. Adverse effects include systemic hypotension, renal failure, and pulmonary edema.

Standard management of patients in vasospasm includes hyperdynamic therapy, or triple H therapy (hypervolemia, hypertension, hemodilution), which is believed to result in indirect arterial dilatation and enhanced perfusion of ischemic areas of the brain by alteration of the rheologic properties of blood. Iatrogenic hypertension by expansion of blood volume has been shown to be beneficial in this population, but may not reduce overall mortality. Of note, hypertension in a patient with an unsecured ruptured aneurysm may provoke a devastating rehemorrhage. It is felt that the optimal hematocrit is approximately 30% to 35% so that the lower viscosity enables unobstructed passage of red cells through vessels without compromising oxygen-carrying capacity. There is some evidence that initiating triple H therapy before onset of vasospasm may mitigate the neurological deterioration from vasospasm, since these patients are often hypovolemic early after their initial rupture, and by the time vasospasm is obvious, its effects may already be irreversible. Hyperdynamic therapy may be dangerous in patients with massive cerebral edema or large ischemic infarcts, as edema may become exacerbated or hemorrhagic conversion of the infarct may ensue, respectively. Normal saline at 150 mL per hour maintenance, along with normal saline or albumin boluses 250 to 500 mL q6-8h, as well as dopamine, dobutamine (β-agonist, start at 5 μg/kg/minute and titrate to maximize cardiac output), or phenylephrine (a-agonist to be started at 2 μg/kg/minute if clinical examination does not improve after 1 hour), should be used to increase SBP in 15% increments until the patient shows neurological improvement or until CVP reaches 8 to 12 cm H_2O, PCWP reaches 16 to 20 mm Hg (the goal CVP or PCWP is that which maximizes the patient's cardiac output and index), SBP in cases in which the aneurysm is secured reaches 160 to 230 mm Hg and for unsecured aneurysms SBP $<$160 mm Hg to reverse ischemic symptoms in the absence of ischemic cardiac disease, TCD velocities reach baseline, and cardiac index becomes $>$4.0. Once the neurological examination improves, blood pressure may be decreased gradually as long as the patients retain their neurological status. Different clinicians prioritize optimizing several but not necessarily all of the aforementioned parameters; the endpoint is to improve neurological examination, or without this, to meet the aforementioned parameters. Furthermore, achieving these parameters may be influenced by the patient's premorbid cardiac and pulmonary function, in particular conditions such as heart failure and pulmonary edema. Patients undergoing hyperdynamic therapy should have a pulmonary artery catheter placed. Some catheters have a packing port, which can be used to counteract reflex vagal bradycardia (can also be treated with atropine 1 mg IV q3-4h to keep the pulse at 80 to 120), and some enable continuous cardiac output measurement.

The objective of maintaining the volume status in vasospasm is to achieve euvolemia or slight hypervolemia. An isotonic crystalloid such as normal saline is generally used. Whole blood or packed red cells are transfused if hematocrit drops $<$35%. Five percent albumin at 100 mL per hour to maintain 35%to 40% hematocrit can be used for less dilutional effect than crystalloid; if hematocrit is $>$35% to 40%, crystalloid can be used. Some advocate 20% mannitol at 0.25 g/kg/hour drip to improve rheological properties of blood in the microcirculation, but hypovolemia can precipitate ischemia. Urinary output can be replaced with crystalloid to maintain volume status; if the hematocrit is $<$40%, 5% albumin at 20 mL per hour can be used. Excess diuresis may be treated with vasopressin (aqueous vasopressin 5 units SQ or vasopressin IV drip, start at 0.2 units per minute and titrate to 0.5 units per minute to keep urine output $<$200 mL per hour), but hyponatremia may result from this therapy. If hypovolemia continues, fludrocortisone 2 mg per day or desoxycortisone 20 mg per day in divided doses can be administered. Digitalis may be useful in the setting of cardiac failure. Complications of hyperdynamic therapy include pulmonary edema, rehemorrhage, dilutional hyponatremia, myocardial infarction, and pulmonary artery catheter complications (sepsis, subclavian vein thrombosis, pneumothorax, hemothorax). This protocol was used in 58 patients with vasospasm, including 22 patients with unsecured aneurysms. Neurological improvement was noted in 81%; no change was observed in 16% and 10% deteriorated. Failure of hyperdynamic therapy warrants consideration of endovascular techniques if vasospasm persists.

Although surgical manipulation of vessels during vessel clipping may increase the risk of vasospasm, a secured aneurysm enables hyperdynamic therapy to be instituted without fear of aneurysm rerupture; in addition, hematoma evacuation may reduce the incidence of vasospasm. Other treatments for vasospasm include pharmacologic dilatation with smooth muscle relaxants including endothelin receptor antagonists, sympatholytics, intra-arterial papaverine, and the still experimental a-ICAM-1 inhibition (antibody to intracellular adhesion molecule). A recent manuscript was the first to show clinical benefits with immediate statin therapy in this setting. Specifically, treatment with pravastatin after aneurysmal SAH was shown to ameliorate vasospasm, improve cerebral autoregulation, and reduce vasospasm-related ischemia. Unfavorable outcome at discharge was reduced primarily because of a reduction in overall mortality.

Catheter-directed balloon angioplasty of vasospastic vessels by interventional neuroradiologists can result in clinical improvement in 60% to 70% of patients, but this form of vasodilatation, which is limited only to large accessible vessels, carries risks of arterial occlusion, arterial rupture, migration of the aneurysm clip or coil, and arterial dissection. Candidates must have failed hyperdynamic therapy, have undergone aneurysm clipping or coiling, and be free of infarction on head CT before angioplasty is considered. Intra-arterial papaverine (200 to 300 mg IV over 30 minutes) can cause vasodilatation, but it is considered a suboptimal agent, for its effects are transient and less pronounced compared with direct mechanical dilatation; in addition, it can worsen vasospasm, result in thrombocytopenia, and cause intracranial hypertension. It may be used to dilate vessels to enable passage of the angioplasty balloon.

Vasospasm may also be mitigated but not completely prevented through the evacuation of spasmogenic material. Hematoma evacuation or subarachnoid irrigation with thrombolytic agents during craniotomy or postoperatively through a catheter or intrathecally is

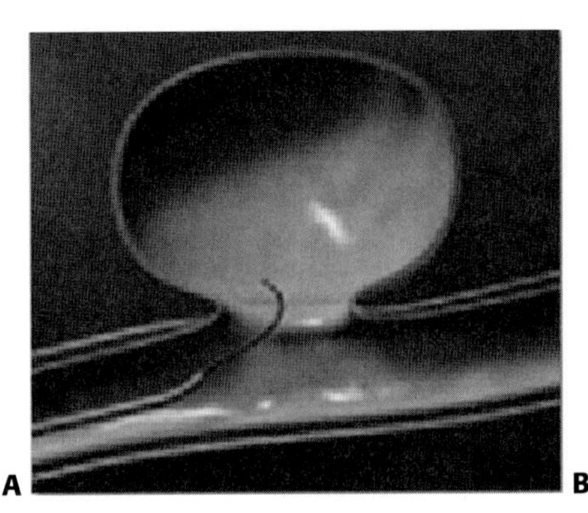
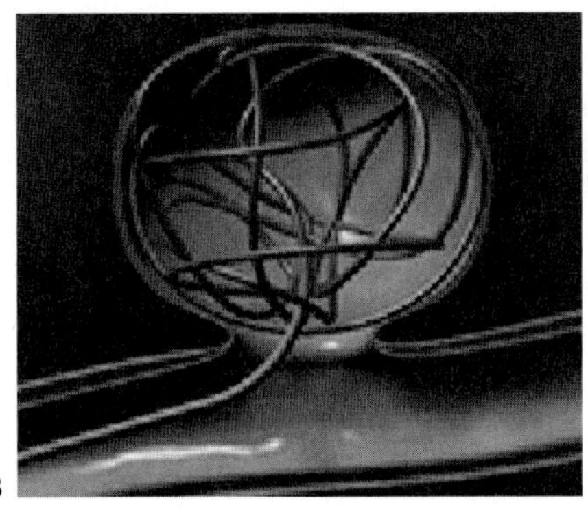
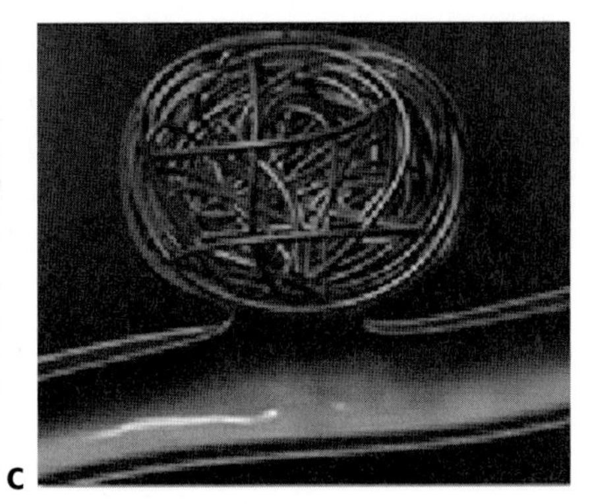

FIGURE 28.5. Treatment of a brain aneurysm with detachable platinum coils. **A:** Tiny platinum coils are threaded through a microcatheter and pushed into the aneurysm. The coils are flexible enough to conform to the aneurysm shape. **B:** The aneurysm is filled in with coils, obstructing the flow of blood into the aneurysm. Each coil is attached to a delivery wire, allowing the physician to reposition or withdraw the coil to ensure ideal placement. **C:** Once properly positioned within the aneurysm, the coil is detached from the delivery wire using an electrolytic detachment process (electrical charge).

still considered experimental and must be performed in the setting of a secured aneurysm. Lumbar drainage and EVD can also help evacuate the spasmogenic blood products.

In extreme cases, extracranial–intracranial bypass around the vasospastic region may be considered.

Treatment of Aneurysms

Not all aneurysms merit treatment on diagnosis. Patients with extremely poor neurological status or poor premorbid medical conditions may not tolerate craniotomy or endovascular treatment. Additional considerations in these patients include the risk of the aneurysm rerupturing, the size and location of the aneurysm, the patient's age, family history, and the risks associated with treatment.

Until recently, optimal treatment of intracranial aneurysms was considered to be craniotomy with microsurgical clip ligation. During this procedure, the aneurysm is ideally approached proximally so that its neck is accessible to the surgeon. The patient may be placed under burst suppression to minimize ischemic damage in case of intraoperative rupture or while a temporary vascular occlusion clip is placed on the feeding vessel. At this point, a permanent clip is placed across the neck of the aneurysm, blocking blood flow from entering the aneurysm lumen and causing rupture, without obstructing blood flow into nearby normal vessels. In some cases involving fusiform aneurysms or aneurysms with critical branches originating from the dome, clipping may not be possible; therefore, wrapping the aneurysm with Teflon and fibrin glue may be indicated.

A recently published landmark multicenter prospective randomized clinical trial, the International Subarachnoid Aneurysm Trial (ISAT), compared clipping and endovascular treatment of ruptured aneurysms and demonstrated that endovascular coil embolization had superior outcomes compared with craniotomy for clip ligation in certain patients. Aneurysm coiling will be covered in greater detail in a subsequent chapter (see Figs. 28.5, 28.6, 28.7, 28.8, and 28.9).

Microsurgical clipping and endovascular coiling are the most common methods employed to treat aneurysms; however, other options exist. Trapping of the aneurysm may also be considered, during which proximal and distal arterial occlusion are carried out surgically or with balloons, followed by extracranial–intracranial bypass to continue flow distally. Proximal or hunterian ligation may be performed for giant aneurysms; however, there is an increased risk of developing contralateral aneurysms with this procedure. Balloon embolization has also been effective in some cases, during which a balloon is placed inside the lumen using endovascular techniques. Risks include possible aneurysm growth and embolization of thrombus.

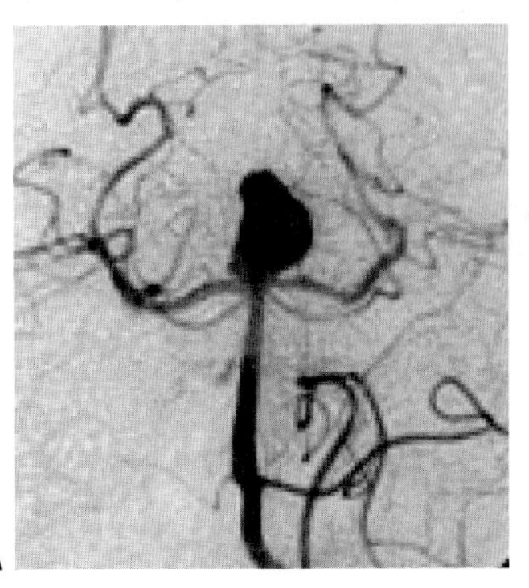
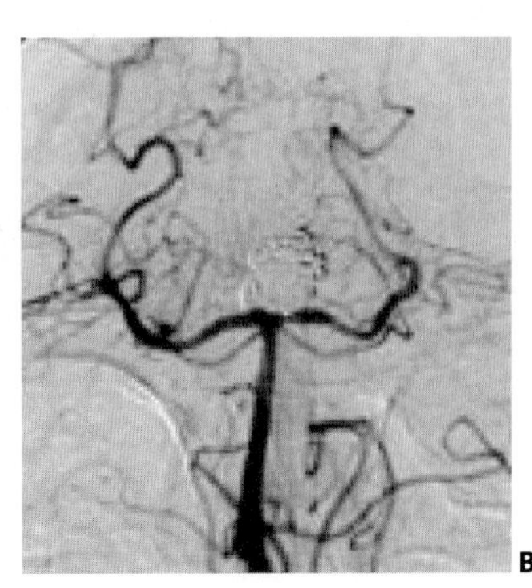

FIGURE 28.6 A: Angiogram of an aneurysm before treatment. The aneurysm is the dark bulge on the vessel. **B:** Angiogram of an aneurysm after endovascular coiling treatment. The aneurysm has been filled in with coils, so blood can no longer flow into the aneurysm. The aneurysm now appears as a silver bulge on the angiogram.

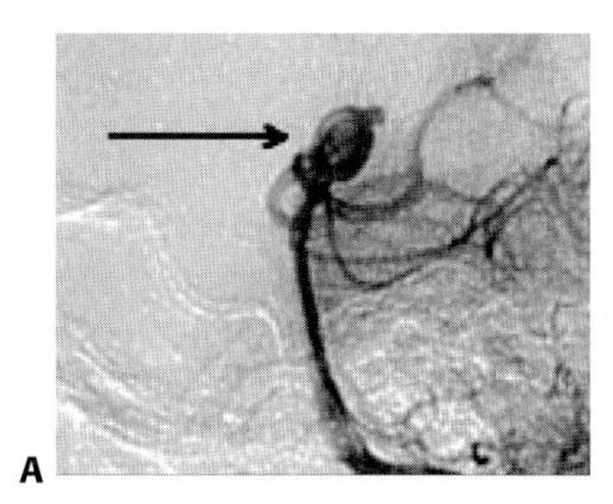

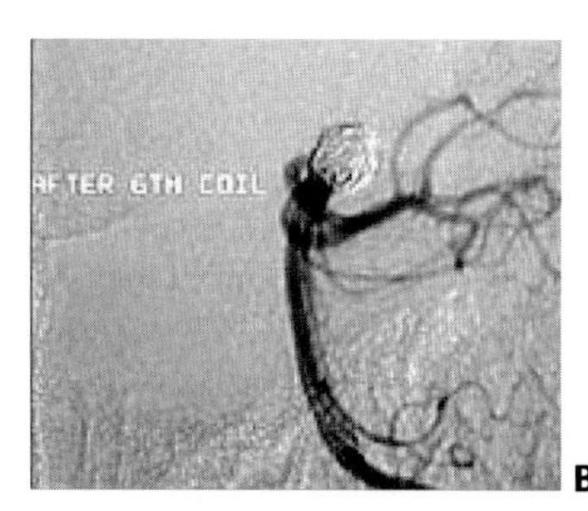

FIGURE 28.7. An aneurysm of the basilar artery, situated at the base of the brain **(A)** and technically difficult to operate was successfully treated by endovascular coils **(B)**.

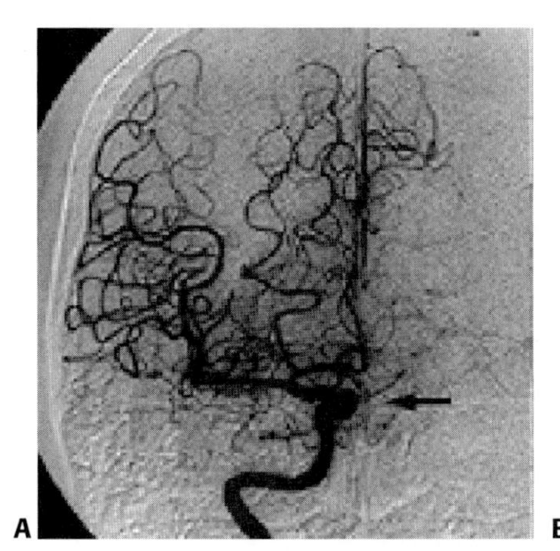

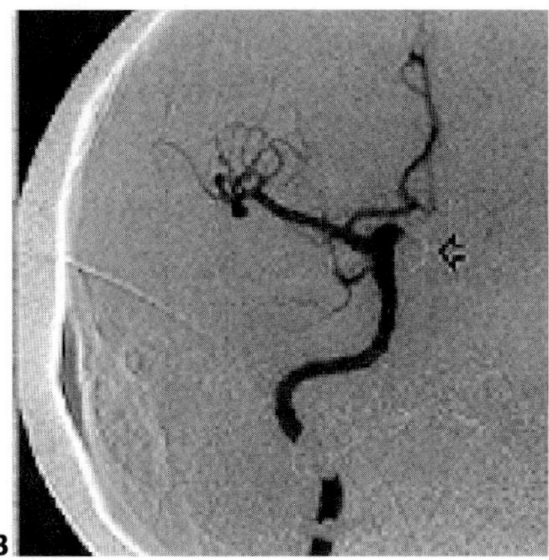

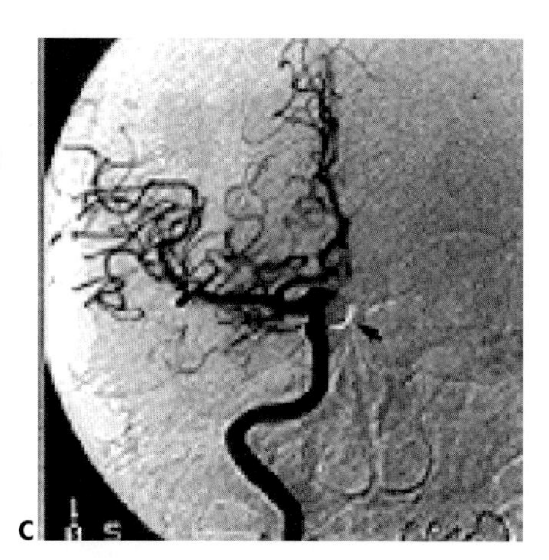

FIGURE 28.8. Angiographic study illustrating long-term complete GDC embolization. **A:** *Left:* Right internal carotid angiogram showing an unruptured superior hypophysial aneurysm (*arrow*). **B:** Immediate postembolization angiogram showing complete GDC occlusion of the aneurysm with preservation of the internal carotid artery lumen (*open arrow*). **C:** Follow-up angiogram at 20 months demonstrating persistent complete aneurysm obliteration with GDCs (*arrowhead*).

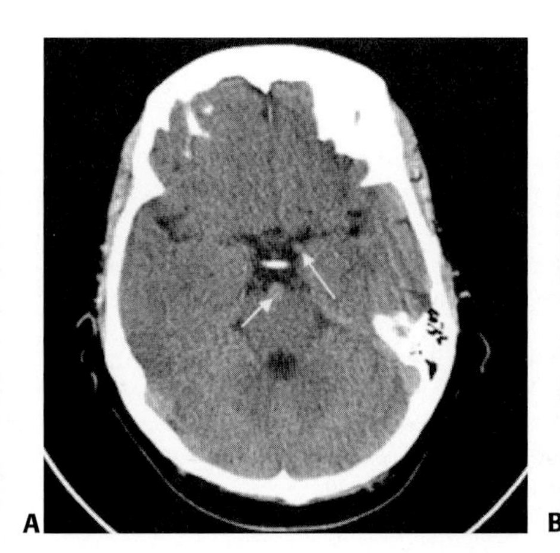

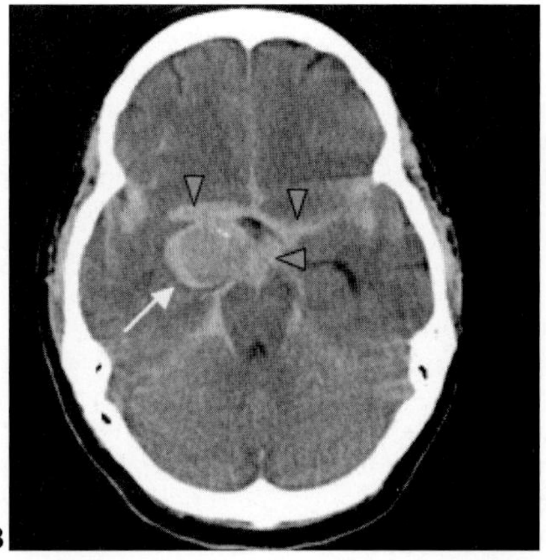

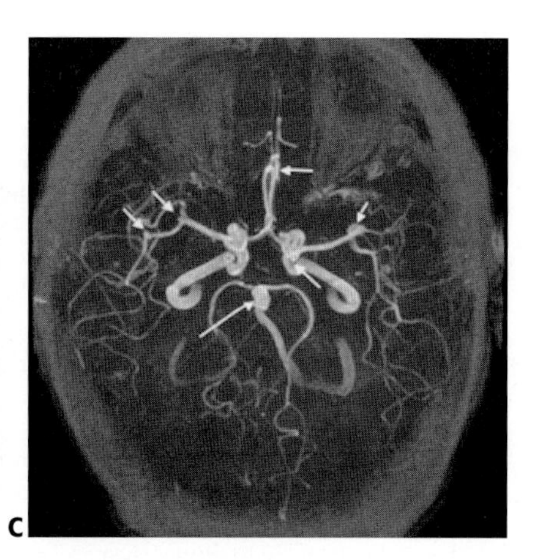

FIGURE 28.9 A: This is a brain computed tomography (CT) scan image. The *arrows* point to two aneurysms. **B:** This is also a brain CT scan image. The *arrow* points to a ruptured giant brain aneurysm with some clot (thrombus) within the main aneurysmal sac. The *arrowheads* point to blood in the subarachnoid space. This image therefore shows aneurysmal subarachnoid hemorrhage (SAH). **C:** This is a brain magnetic resonance angiogram (MRA). The image is a scout image of the Circle of Willis at the base of the brain. The *arrows* point to six different brain aneurysms. *(continued)*

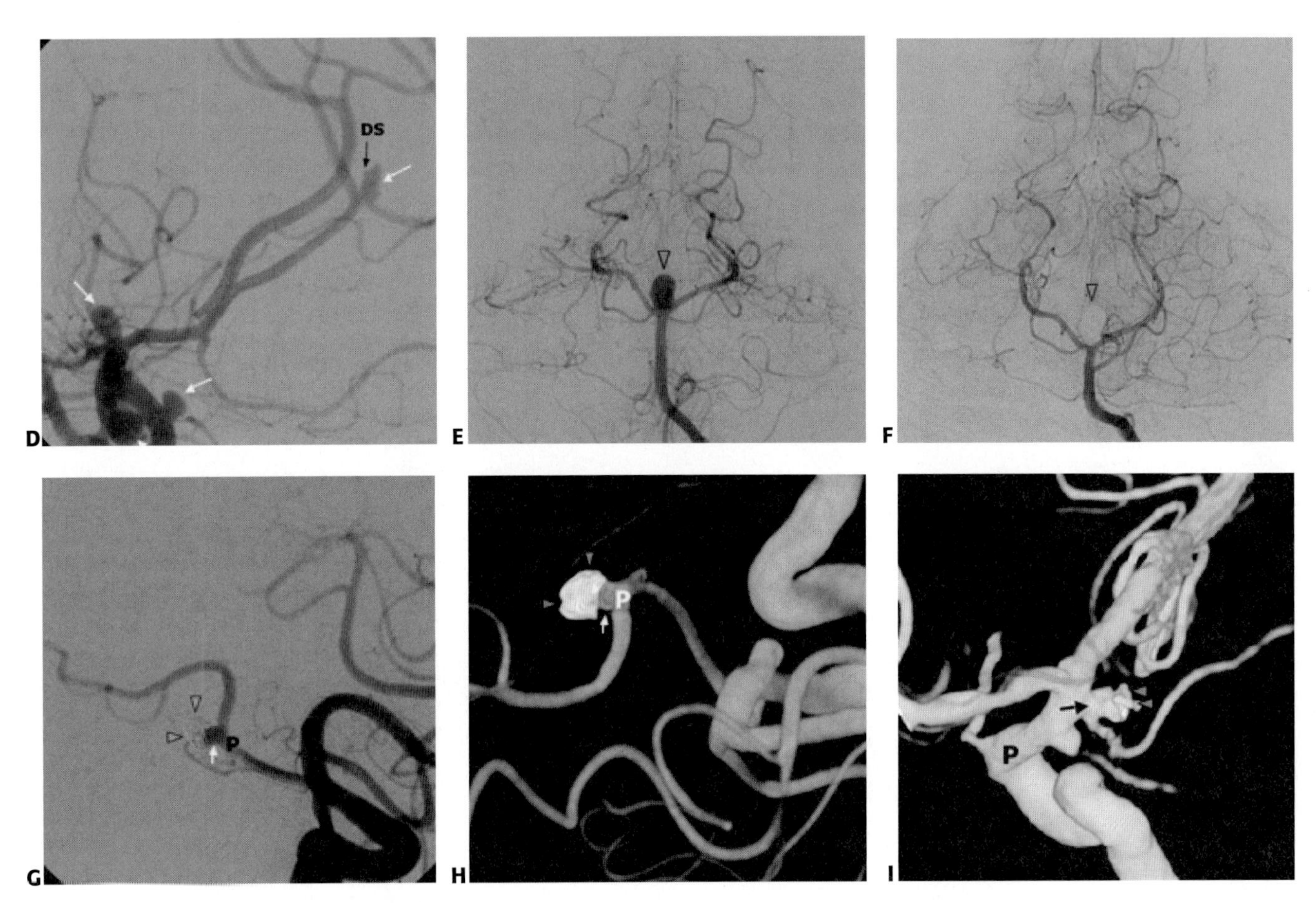

FIGURE 28.9 (continued) D: This is a formal cerebral angiogram image. This particular projection shows part of the roadmap of the brain arteries and happens to also show multiple brain aneurysms (*arrows*). One of the aneurysms has an irregular daughter sac (DS) coming off its dome. **E:** This a cerebral angiogram of the posterior circulation showing a basilar artery apex (or basilar caput) aneurysm (*arrowhead*). **F:** The same aneurysm shown in Figure 28.9E has now undergone endovascular coiling. The *arrowhead* points to the coiled aneurysm, packed with ultrafine aneurysm coils. This aneurysm has been completely obliterated by the coiling procedure. **G:** This is a cerebral angiogram image of an aneurysm that underwent apparently successful coiling (*arrowheads*), but on the follow-up study, the neck of the aneurysm (*arrow*) was found to have regrown. The parent artery *(P)* from which the aneurysm arose is also seen. **H:** This is an MRA image of the same aneurysm shown in Figure 28.9F. Again, the *arrowheads* show the coil mass in the aneurysm dome, while the *arrow* points to the regrown aneurysm neck. The parent artery *(P)* is also seen here. **I:** This MRA image shows an aneurysm that ruptured some time after coiling was carried out. The parent artery is shown *(P)*, as is the neck of the aneurysm (*black arrow*) and the coils (marked by the *arrowheads*) sticking out of the aneurysm's dome following rupture.

SELECTED REFERENCES

Allen GS, Ahn HS, Preziosi TJ, et al. Cerebral arterial spasm—a controlled trial of nimodipine in patients with subarachnoid hemorrhage. *N Engl J Med* 1983;308(11):619–624.

Baker CJ, Prestigiacomo CJ, Solomon RA. Short-term perioperative anticonvulsant prophylaxis for the surgical treatment of low-risk patients with intracranial aneurysms. *Neurosurgery* 1995;37(5):863–870.

Barker FG, II, Ogilvy CS. Efficacy of prophylactic nimodipine for delayed ischemic deficit after subarachnoid hemorrhage: a metaanalysis. *J Neurosurg* 1996;84(3):405–14.

Biller J, Godersky JC, Adams HP, Jr. Management of aneurysmal subarachnoid hemorrhage. *Stroke* 1988;19(10):1300–1305.

Biller J, Toffol GJ, Kassell NF, et al. Spontaneous subarachnoid hemorrhage in young adults. *Neurosurgery* 1987;21(5):664–667.

Bonita R. Cigarette smoking, hypertension and the risk of subarachnoid hemorrhage: a population-based case-control study. *Stroke* 1986;17(5):831–835.

Broderick JP, Brott T, Tomsick T, et al. Intracerebral hemorrhage more than twice as common as subarachnoid hemorrhage. *J Neurosurg* 1993;78(2):188–191.

Cioffi F, Pasqualin A, Cavazzani P, et al. Subarachnoid haemorrhage of unknown origin: clinical and tomographical aspects. *Acta Neurochir (Wien)* 1989;97(1–2):31-9.

Ciongoli AK, Poser CM. Pulmonary edema secondary to subarachnoid hemorrhage. *Neurology* 1972;22(8):867–870.

Consensus Conference. Magnetic resonance imaging. *JAMA* 1988;259:2132–2138.

Drake CG. Progress in cerebrovascular disease. Management of cerebral aneurysm. *Stroke* 1981;12(3):273–283.

Ferguson GG. Physical factors in the initiation, growth, and rupture of human intracranial saccular aneurysms. *J Neurosurg* 1972;37(6):666–677.

Findlay JM, Kassell NF, Weir BK, et al. A randomized trial of intraoperative, intracisternal tissue plasminogen activator for the prevention of vasospasm. *Neurosurgery* 1995;37(1):168–176; discussion 177–178.

Hunt WE, Kosnik EJ. Timing and perioperative care in intracranial aneurysm surgery. *Clin Neurosurg* 1974;21:79–89.

Kassell NF, Drake CG. Review of the management of saccular aneurysms. *Neurol Clin* 1983;1(1):73–86.

Kassell NF, Helm G, Simmons N, et al. Treatment of cerebral vasospasm with intra-arterial papaverine. *J Neurosurg* 1992;77(6):848–852.

Kassell NF, Sasaki T, Colohan AR, et al.Cerebral vasospasm following aneurysmal subarachnoid hemorrhage. *Stroke* 1985;16(4):562–572.

Kassell NF, Torner JC, Adams HP, Jr. Antifibrinolytic therapy in the acute period following aneurysmal subarachnoid hemorrhage. Preliminary observations from the Cooperative Aneurysm Study. *J Neurosurg* 1984; 61(2):225–230.

Kusske JA, Turner PT, Ojemann GA, et al. Ventriculostomy for the treatment of acute hydrocephalus following subarachnoid hemorrhage. *J Neurosurg* 1973;38(5):591–595.

Milhorat TH. Acute hydrocephalus after aneurysmal subarachnoid hemorrhage. *Neurosurgery* 1987;20(1):15–20.

Molyneux A, Kerr R, Stratton I, et al. International Subarachnoid Aneurysm Trial (ISAT) of neurosurgical clipping versus endovascular coiling in 2143 patients with ruptured intracranial aneurysms: a randomised trial. *Lancet* 2002;360(9342):1267–1274.

Nehls DG, Flom RA, Carter LP, et al. Multiple intracranial aneurysms: determining the site of rupture. *J Neurosurg* 1985;63(3):342–348.

Newell DW, Eskridge JM, Mayberg MR, et al. Angioplasty for the treatment of symptomatic vasospasm following subarachnoid hemorrhage. *J Neurosurg* 1989;71(5 Pt 1):654–660.

Okawara SH. Warning signs prior to rupture of an intracranial aneurysm. *J Neurosurg* 1973;38(5):575–580.

Rinkel GJ, Djibuti M, Algra A, et al. Prevalence and risk of rupture of intracranial aneurysms: a systematic review. *Stroke* 1998;29(1):251–256.

Ross JS, Masaryk TJ, Modic MT, et al. Intracranial aneurysms: evaluation by MR angiography. *Am J Roentgenol* 1990;155(1):159–165.

Seiler RW, Grolimund P, Aaslid R, et al. Cerebral vasospasm evaluated by transcranial ultrasound correlated with clinical grade and CT-visualized subarachnoid hemorrhage. *J Neurosurg* 1986;64(4):594–600.

Shimoda M, Oda S, Tsugane R, et al. Intracranial complications of hypervolemic therapy in patients with a delayed ischemic deficit attributed to vasospasm. *J Neurosurg* 1993;78(3):423–429.

Solomon RA, Fink ME, Lennihan L. Early aneurysm surgery and prophylactic hypervolemic hypertensive therapy for the treatment of aneurysmal subarachnoid hemorrhage. *Neurosurgery* 1988;23(6): 699–704.

Vermeulen LC, Jr, Ratko TA, Erstad BL, et al. A paradigm for consensus. The University Hospital Consortium guidelines for the use of albumin, nonprotein colloid, and crystalloid solutions. *Arch Intern Med* 1995; 155(4):373–379.

Wiebers DO, Whisnant JP, Sundt TM, Jr, et al. The significance of unruptured intracranial saccular aneurysms. *J Neurosurg* 1987;66(1):23–29.

Weir B, Grace M, Hansen J, et al. Time course of vasospasm in man. *J Neurosurg* 1978;48(2):173–178.

Wirth FP. Surgical treatment of incidental intracranial aneurysms. *Clin Neurosurg* 1986;33:125–135.

SECTION IV

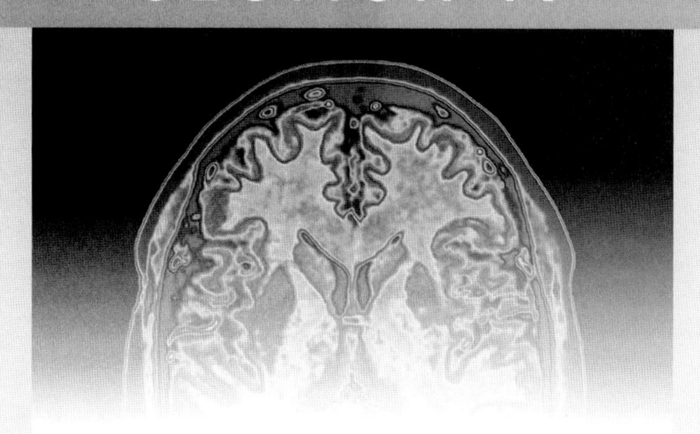

Inpatient Stroke Management

CHAPTER

29 Risk Stratification of Ischemic Stroke Patients

JAMES D. GEYER AND CAMILO R. GOMEZ

OBJECTIVES

- Why should a risk stratification be performed?
- What is included in the risk stratification of an ischemic stroke patient?
- What additional tests can be included in the risk stratification and when should these tests be added?

Cerebrovascular disorders continue to be one of the most common causes of death in the United States and the most important cause of disability for adults. The last decade has brought with it significant progress in the diagnosis and treatment of cerebrovascular disorders. Advances in imaging technology have played a key role in some of the progress made, facilitating the identification, classification, and documentation of the types of stroke and vascular abnormalities. Imaging, more specifically neuroimaging, is an integral part of the evaluation of stroke patients.

Stroke risk stratification is based on the concept of double jeopardy, or the possibility that more than one potential cause or complicating factor may exist in a given patient. For example, identifying a 70% stenosis in a carotid artery does not mean that the stenosis is the cause of the stroke. A more comprehensive evaluation of the patient is needed to reach a conclusion about the optimal course of therapy. Neuroimaging combined with the cardiac and laboratory evaluations provides the information necessary to select the most appropriate treatment paradigms (*See* Table 29.1). This chapter provides the framework for the risk stratification.

CLINICAL APPLICATIONS AND METHODOLOGY

The most practical approach to a discussion of the application of imaging techniques in cerebrovascular disorders is to first address the tasks, diagnostic or therapeutic, that require the use of imaging. Only this type of approach will allow the issuing of guidelines for choosing the appropriate technique for each clinical situation. From this perspective, the clinical scenarios in which imaging techniques are likely to be needed must be assessed along the following lines: (a) What information is being sought, and how quickly is it needed? (b) Which of the available imaging techniques is most likely to answer the question being asked? (c) How will the information obtained by imaging affect further diagnostic algorithms, the treatment, and the prognosis of the patient? Based on these considerations, the tasks that require the use of imaging during clinical care of cerebrovascular patients include imaging of the brain, brain vessels, and extracranial cerebral vasculature, and identifying potential sources of emboli (whether cardiac or arterial in origin). In addition to these factors, laboratory evaluation provides information about potential etiologies for the vascular abnormalities and risk factors for recurrent stroke.

Imaging of the Brain and Brain Vessels

Direct imaging of the brain is necessary in order to assess the status of the tissue, often documenting the damage caused by the stroke, and also to differentiate between ischemic and hemorrhagic strokes. The techniques available to complete this task include computed tomography (CT) and magnetic resonance imaging (MRI). Choosing between these involves considerations of speed, sensitivity, type of stroke, and temporal profile of the event.

Imaging of the brain blood vessels is part of the standard risk stratification algorithm that every stroke patient must undergo. As such, documentation of vascular abnormalities causally associated with the stroke not only allows determination of the level of risk for subsequent stroke but also helps plan preventive therapy. In general, the tests that are available for the completion of this task can be divided into two groups: (a) noninvasive, i.e., extracranial vascular ultrasound, transcranial Doppler (TCD) ultrasound, computed tomographic angiography (CTA), and magnetic resonance angiography (MRA), and (b) invasive, i.e., catheter angiography. In addition to its diagnostic capabilities, the latter also allows the application of endovascular therapeutic techniques.

Documentation of the Ischemic Process

The selection of the initial imaging modality is based largely on the availability and the timetable for potential thrombolytic therapy. CT is an excellent tool for rapid screening for hemorrhage and evaluating prior ischemic lesions. MRI provides much more detail about the new ischemic event as well as information on prior infarctions and ischemia. Magnetic resonance–based techniques [diffusion-weighted MRI (DW-MRI) and perfusion-weighted MRI] assist in the identification of ischemic tissue that may be salvageable, possibly having a role in the selection of patients for specific therapies.

TABLE 29.1 Stroke Etiologies and Their Findings on Risk Stratification

A. Atherothromboembolic
  1. Clinical criteria
    a. Sudden, gradual, stepwise, or fluctuating
    b. Absence of a cardioembolic source
    c. Prior TIA in the same vascular distribution
    d. Concurrent coronary or peripheral artery disease
  2. Imaging
    a. CT: Bland or hemorrhagic infarct
      (1) Possible hyperdense artery
    b. MRI: Bland or hemorrhagic infarct
      (1) Possible absent flow void
      (2) Acute infarction results in hyperintensity on DWIs and hypointensity on the ADC map
    c. Carotid U/S: Stenosis >50% or ulcer >2 mm
    d. Arteriography: Stenosis >50% or ulcer >2 mm
    e. TCD: Normal, collateralization, or absent flow

B. Cardioembolic
  1. Clinical criteria
    a. Sudden onset but may be stepwise/progressive
    b. High Risk—atrial fibrillation, prosthetic valve, left ventricular thrombus, left atrial thrombus, dilated cardial myopathy, sick sinus syndrome, MI in the prior 4 wk
    c. Moderate risk—CHF, atrial flutter, mitral valve prolapse, atrial septal defect, PFO, bioprosthetic valve, ventricular hypokinesis, MI between 4 and 6 wk
    d. Recent TIA/stroke in other vascular territories
    e. Evidence of systemic embolization
  2. Imaging
    a. CT: Bland or hemorrhagic infarct
      (1) Possible hyperdense artery
      (2) May have infarctions in multiple vascular distributions
    b. MRI: Bland or hemorrhagic infarct
      (1) Possible absent flow void
      (2) May have infarctions in multiple vascular distributions
    c. Carotid U/S: Various; stenosis typically <50%
    d. Arteriography: May show occlusion of a vessel
    e. TEE: May show thrombotic etiology
    f. TCD: Normal, absent flow or distal occlusion

C. Lacunar
  1. Clinical criteria
    a. Abrupt or gradual onset
    b. H/O hypertension or diabetes mellitus
    c. No cortical findings
    d. Compatible with a lacunar syndrome
    e. No evidence of embolic sources
  2. Imaging
    a. CT: Infarct <1.5 cm
    b. MRI: Infarct <1.5 cm
    c. TCD: Normal or unrevealing

TIA, transient ischemic attack; CT, computed tomography; MRI, magnetic resonance imaging; DWIs, diffusion-weighted images; ADC, apparent diffusion coefficient; U/S, ultrasound; TEE, transesophageal echocardiography ; TCD, transcranial Doppler, CHF, congestive heart failure; PFO, patent foramina ovale; MI, myocardial infarction.

Documentation of Cardiac Sources of Embolism

Although it is technically not part of the process of imaging of the brain, it is important to include documentation of cardiac sources of embolism during the care of the patients. Cardiogenic embolism is more frequent than it was once suspected. Transthoracic echocardiography (TTE) and magnetic resonance cardiac imaging provide noninvasive information about the heart and potential sources of emboli. The introduction and development of transesophageal echocardiography (TEE) represented a major advance in the identification of cardiac sources of cerebral embolism, and changed how stroke patients can be evaluated.

Imaging Scenarios

The tasks noted in the preceding section must also be placed in the practical context of two distinct clinical scenarios: (a) the emergency evaluation of the stroke patient and (b) the nonemergent risk stratification of patients with cerebrovascular disease. Depending on the scenario, the choice of imaging technique is then guided by the question being asked, the diagnostic characteristics inherent to each imaging modality, and the expectations of results based on the natural history of the process being investigated.

Emergency Imaging of Stroke Victims

Most patients with acute stroke are initially evaluated in emergency departments by physicians whose priorities include answering specific questions with direct relevance to the management of the patient, both immediately and during the days that follow. The first set of clinical questions confronted by stroke specialists is as follows:

- Does the patient have a stroke?
- Is it an ischemic or a hemorrhagic stroke?
- What vascular territory or territories have been compromised?
- What is the risk of death or significant neurological disability?
- What is the likelihood of neurological deterioration?

Once the presumptive diagnosis of stroke is made, imaging of the brain becomes an imminent necessity. It is important to know whether (a) the event is ischemic or hemorrhagic, (b) the brain has already undergone damage, and (c) there is any alternative diagnostic possibility. In the past, it was thought that astute clinicians could easily make the differentiation between hemorrhagic and ischemic stroke at the bedside. The introduction of CT in the 1970s, however, clearly revealed this as a fallacy. In fact, at present, emergency CT scanning is of paramount importance in the early evaluation of patients with acute stroke, as well as a pivotal point in any emergency stroke treatment algorithm.

Nonemergent Risk Stratification

The diagnostic perspective of patients with cerebrovascular disorders revolves around defining the stroke subtype (i.e., identifying the cause and mechanism of the stroke). This information allows for a more educated prediction of the risk of subsequent strokes and enables the physician to implement secondary prevention strategies tailored to the individual patient. In this context, the importance of imaging techniques cannot be overemphasized. Three categories of disorders are capable of leading to the production of stroke: cardiac abnormalities, cerebrovascular abnormalities per se, and hematological disorders.

Computed Tomography

The introduction of CT in the 1970s changed the way all neurological diseases are diagnosed and treated. Furthermore, CT allowed a rapid differentiation between the two main types of stroke (cerebral infarction and cerebral hemorrhage) and has ultimately made possible the application of aggressive treatment strategies, such as thrombolysis.

The usefulness of CT in the evaluation of cerebrovascular disorders is primarily related to the emergency assessment of patients with acute stroke. In this context the technique allows the determination of hemorrhagic changes, and the identification of early signs of ischemic tissue damage, and most recently, it has become a determining factor for the selection of patients for specific types of treatment (e.g., thrombolysis). The CT findings in patients with acute stroke can be divided into six categories:

1. *Normal brain tissue*: Many patients presenting early with acute or hyperacute ischemic brain processes have normal CT scans. This results from the low sensitivity of the test for the detection of ischemic tissue within the first few hours of evolution. A normal CT scan in the context of a patient with an acute focal neurological deficit by no means excludes the diagnosis of ischemic stroke, and, in fact, should be considered a good sign. The fact that the tissue is not shown as being irreparably damaged should open numerous possibilities for therapeutic intervention. Clearly, for patients suspected of having hemorrhagic stroke, a normal CT scan almost completely excludes the diagnosis.
2. *Abnormal, demonstrating the acute stroke:* The appearance of infarction on CT during the first few hours largely depends on the size and location of the affected tissue. Large territories supplied by the carotid artery system [e.g., middle cerebral artery (MCA) and anterior cerebral artery] have a tendency to be displayed earlier than smaller territories supplied by the vertebrobasilar system (e.g., penetrating pontine arteries). The early signs of infarction include changes in gray matter density with loss of gray–white matter differentiation, evolving very subtle to more noticeable hypodensity and early signs of edema over the subsequent 12 to 24 hours. Hemorrhagic strokes are displayed as hyperdense areas corresponding to the extravasated blood, for which CT is highly sensitive. It is not uncommon to see areas of petechial hemorrhage in areas of infarction.
3. *Abnormal, with findings related to the acute stroke:* Frequently, CT scans show abnormalities that bear a relationship with the ischemic stroke. For example, in patients with occlusion of the MCA, the hyperdense MCA sign has been described. A vessel acutely occluded by a blood clot may appear as a hyperdense structure within the Sylvian fissure. In addition, calcification of the brain arteries (e.g., carotid or vertebral) is a more common finding and implies the presence of atherosclerotic plaques that are capable of causing narrowing of these vessels. For patients with hemorrhagic strokes, it is possible sometimes to identify an aneurysm by calcification, thrombosis, or location.
4. *Abnormal, displaying previous strokes*: Often, patients who present with acute stroke are found to have abnormal CT scans that demonstrate preexisting strokes. These represent the evidence of cerebrovascular abnormalities, either intrinsic or secondary to other processes, and they can help in the diagnostic process. For example, evidence of infarctions in multiple bilateral territories suggests the possibility of cardiogenic or aortogenic emboli. On the other hand, previous infarctions clustered within one hemisphere may represent the effect of unilateral severe carotid or intracranial vascular stenosis.
5. *Abnormal, displaying an alternative diagnostic process:* Not every patient who presents with a clinical syndrome suggestive of stroke has one. CT is helpful in uncovering other conditions that mimic stroke and require alternative treatment (e.g., subdural hematoma and tumor).
6. *Abnormal, showing a combination of the various above:* The routine use of contrast during CT examination of the emergency stroke patient is, in our opinion, unwarranted. The potential enhancement of any of the tissue in patients with acute ischemia serves no clinical purpose since it does not help guide treatment. Furthermore, there is at least some suggestion in the literature that contrast media may be somewhat neurotoxic to ischemic tissue. For the patient with hemorrhagic stroke, it adds even less unless used as a part of CTA. Furthermore, in certain clinical scenarios, such a practice is dangerous. The intense nausea that can be produced by intravenous contrast administration, in fact, can jeopardize the fate of patients with ruptured aneurysms.

Over time, the appearance of the two major forms of stroke on CT scanning changes. Infarcted tissue develops swelling and its margins become progressively better demarcated. Its density decreases progressively as the damaged tissue shrinks, producing ex vacuo enlargement of adjacent structures (i.e., ventricles) and possibly cystic-appearing regions following resorption of the infracted tissue.

Another practical aspect of CT in the management of patients with cerebrovascular disorders is the ease with which it allows follow-up imaging in patients who evolve, either positively or negatively. An example of the former is the resolution of hydrocephalus in a patient who requires ventriculostomy following an intraventricular hemorrhage. On the other hand, the latter is best exemplified by the follow-up of a patient with malignant brain edema secondary to a large hemispheric infarction.

Computed Tomography Angiography

CTA is a noninvasive imaging technique that couples CT scanning with contrast enhancement to obtain vascular images. A series of axial images are reconstructed into three-dimensional angiographic images. Several studies have compared CTA with conventional angiography, finding agreement of 80% to 95% between the two techniques, when studying extracranial carotid atherosclerotic stenotic plaques. As with any other technique, CTA has advantages and disadvantages. It is not susceptible to flow perturbations and complex flow patterns like MRI. On the other hand, it uses ionizing radiation and contrast administration, which limit its use in patients with renal insufficiency or contrast allergy.

Magnetic Resonance Imaging

The increased sensitivity of MRI, as compared with CT, for the detection of abnormalities in brain structure makes it the imaging modality of choice in the demonstration of infarction of the brain parenchyma. MRI allows the documentation of ischemic brain lesions earlier and more precisely, particularly in regions that had remained relatively unavailable to previous imaging modalities, such as the brainstem. Various MRI sequences can be used in the imaging of the brain vessels, and in the study of the degree of ischemia and viability of the tissue.

The detection of abnormalities in patients with acute stroke, using MRI, depends on both the alteration of flow within the vessels and the changes produced by the disease process on the parenchyma. Normally, high velocity flow is displayed as a flow-void on conventional MRI sequences. This is easily seen both on T2-and T1-weighted images, and its absence implies slowed or stagnant flow within the vessel. In fact, arterial enhancement has been described among the MRI findings of patients with acute ischemic stroke as a sign of vascular occlusion or a low flow state.

Parenchymal abnormalities in patients with ischemic stroke respond to the accumulation of water within ischemic cells, first producing cytotoxic edema secondary to cellular membrane incompetence and later due to blood brain barrier (BBB) breakdown. Increased tissue signal on T2-weighted, proton-density, and fast low-angled inversion recovery (FLAIR) images is associated with infarction and neuroangiopathic change. In many cases there are no significant changes on T1-weighted images but in some patients there is a less pronounced drop in signal with this pathophysiological process. As opposed to the flow-related findings noted earlier, the parenchymal changes evolve over a period of hours to days. As time goes by, the changes observed on MRI give way to a picture most representative of encephalomalacia, necrosis, and gliosis. Thus, in the chronic stages, infarcted tissue appears as an area of high intensity on T2-weighted images, low intensity on T1-weighted images, and moderate intensity on proton density imaging.

The MRI appearance of hemorrhagic stroke is one of the most complex subjects to discuss, for it largely depends on the natural evolution of hemoglobin degradation within the tissue and the strength of the magnetic field. Typically, the sequence of conversion from oxyhemoglobin to deoxyhemoglobin (first intracellular and then extracellular, as the erythrocytes disappear), and then from deoxyhemoglobin to methemoglobin, and, finally to hemosiderin occurs as part of a continuum over weeks to months. Acute hemorrhage is isointense or slightly hypointense on T1-weighted images, while it is either isointense (low field strength) or markedly hypointense on T2-weighted images. This finding represents the presence of intracellular deoxyhemoglobin. As erythrocytes undergo lysis, extracellular deoxyhemoglobin is converted to aqueous methemoglobin, and a peripheral ring of hyperintensity develops first in T1-weighted imaging and later in T2-weighted imaging. Subsequently, the center of the lesion becomes progressively hyperintense because of subsequent oxidation. Finally, the rim becomes extremely hypointense on T2-weighted images because of the deposit of hemosiderin. The use of gradient-echo images makes the identification of hemorrhage much easier, and according to some studies superior to that achieved by CT scans.

Diffusion-weighted MRI. Ischemia of brain tissue results in disruption of oxidative phosphorylation due to impaired oxygen delivery to tissue. The brain cells resort to anaerobic glycolysis, a more inefficient form of energy production. These changes lead to impaired function of the Na-K pump function of the cell membrane, with consequent accumulation of intracellular sodium. Other high-energy phosphates are depleted, with accumulation of inorganic phosphate and lactic acid within the tissue. The osmotic gradient created by the accumulation of intracellular sodium facilitates the influx of water into the cells with the production of cytotoxic edema.

Signal intensity on DW-MRI is related to the random microscopic motion of water protons (Brownian motion), while conventional MRI sequences depend on the accumulation of water within the tissue. It is thus possible to detect slower proton motion within the ischemic tissue, with lower diffusion coefficients, as early as minutes following the onset of ischemia. Regardless of the exact cause of these findings, it is apparent that DW-MRI findings represent the earliest sign of ischemic injury, perhaps at stages in which the tissue can still be recovered. Increased signal intensity on DW-MRI can be related to T2 shine-through and can lead the neuroimager and clinician to the erroneous conclusion that the increased signal is the result of acute infarction. Regions of ischemia have a decreased apparent diffusion coefficient (ADC) and high signal intensity on DW-MRI, reflecting restricted diffusion of protons relative to normal brain. Using the combination of ADC and DW-MRI, the risk of such a false positive is drastically reduced.

Perfusion-weighted MRI. The ability to induce enhancement of MRI with magnetic susceptibility agents that facilitate T2* relaxation provides a method for assessing cerebral blood volume and tissue perfusion. These agents, dysprosium or gadolinium DTPA-BMA (DyDTPA-BMA and GdDTPA-BMA, respectively) are confined to the intravascular space by the intact BBB. A field gradient is created at the capillary level, resulting in significant signal loss in regions with normal blood flow. In contrast, nonperfused areas appear relatively hyperintense. This technique has been shown to significantly advance the time of detection of focal brain ischemia and reveal small infarctions not shown by conventional MRI sequences. In addition, ultrafast MRI techniques (i.e., echo-planar and turbo FLASH) allow resolution of the passage of contrast through the vascular bed, with kinetic modeling of regional blood flow and volume. The most important use for perfusion MRI is in combination with DW-MRI to assess the vascular penumbra.

Magnetic Resonance Spectroscopy

Ischemia causes a detectable decrease in intracellular pH concurrently with an increase in lactic acid concentration. These findings are accompanied by depletion of adenosine triphosphate (ATP) and phosphocreatine, and by increase of inorganic phosphate. With the development of better techniques for spectral editing and localization, it is possible to separate the tissue in question. This technique may be most useful in the assessment of the reversibility of ischemic brain damage. MR spectroscopy is not available on many clinical scanners, and interpretation may be hampered by the limited number of neuroimagers to read this type of study.

Magnetic Resonance Angiography

The discussion of MRI in the preceding sections only applies to spin-echo pulse sequences. These produce images in which there is negative visualization of the cerebral blood vessels owing to their characteristic signal void. Fast-scanning MRI pulse sequencing, particularly gradient-echo and bipolar flow-encoding gradient, has allowed direct vascular imaging, resulting in the development of MRA.

Visualization of the cerebral vasculature by MRA implies the use of either of two different techniques: time-of-flight (TOF) and phase-contrast (PC) angiography. The technique of TOF angiography is based on the phenomenon of flow-related enhancement, and it can be performed with either two- or three-dimensional volume acquisitions. It uses flip angles of <60 degrees and no refocusing 180 pulse (the echo is refocused by reversing the readout gradient). This technique, also known as *gradient refocused echo* (GRE), can be carried out using one of several methods, including fast low-angle shot (FLASH), free-induction steady-state precession (FISP), and gradient-recalled acquisition study state (GRASS). On the other hand, PC angiography is based on the detection of velocity-induced phase shifts to distinguish flowing blood from the surrounding stationary tissue. By using bipolar flow-sensitized gradients it is possible to subtract the two acquisitions of opposite polarity and no net phase (stationary tissue) from one another. The data that remain reflect the phase shift induced by flowing blood. The use of cardiac gating helps overcome the sensitivity of PC angiography to pulsatile and nonuniform flow. From this point of view, PC is somewhat impractical for three-dimensional imaging.

Neurovascular Ultrasonography

Ultrasound provides noninvasive methods by which it is possible to obtain diagnostic anatomical and physiological information. All of these methods are based on the interaction of ultrasound waves transmitted into the tissues and the echoes generated and returning from the tissues. The domain of vascular ultrasonography includes all the ultrasonic methods that are primarily used for the study of blood vessels and blood flow. It is possible to apply the principles of vascular ultrasonography to the evaluation of patients with disorders of the cerebral circulation.

Extracranial Ultrasound. The association between ischemic cerebrovascular events and atherosclerosis of the extracranial portion of the carotid arteries has been the main factor behind the development of neurovascular ultrasonography. In theory, carotid atheromatous plaques can be assessed to determine (a) the degree of stenosis they cause, (b) their surface characteristics, and (c) their histomorphology. Using duplex ultrasound, plaques can be fully studied by direct visualization, both sagitally and transversely. It is also possible to assess the hemodynamic derangements caused by atheromatous plaques, and it helps in the risk stratification of the patient.

The degree of stenosis caused by atheromatous plaques can be readily evaluated by duplex ultrasound, as follows: The B-mode image displays the spatial relationship between the plaque and the vessels, while the pulsed wave (PW) Doppler shows the turbulence and flow acceleration caused by it. This acceleration, accompanied by disruption of normal laminar flow, increases progressively as the lumen narrows and allows estimation of the degree of stenosis and the hemodynamic impact of the plaque. The evaluation of plaque surface characteristics is geared toward the determination of whether the plaque is ulcerated, a factor that has been believed to contribute to the increased risk for stroke. Unfortunately, ulceration implies a disruption in the endothelium continuity, a characteristic not easily discernible by any of the available diagnostic techniques. From this perspective, ulcers would have to be differentiated from plaque surface irregularities (craters) that are probably more frequent and that are associated with an intact endothelium. The ability of B-mode ultrasound to identify ulcers is not considered optimal, although it is similar to that of angiography. Craters are, however, much more easily visualized. In regard to the assessment of plaque morphology, the literature suggests that soft plaques, as well as unstable plaques, represent a greater risk for the development of stroke. Plaque morphology can be assessed as follows: The B-mode images show whether the plaque is soft (fibrofatty), fibrous, or calcific depending on its echogenic characteristics (i.e., fibrofatty plaques are echolucent, while calcific plaques and echodense). Other characteristics, such as intraplaque hemorrhage, another finding believed to be a risk factor for stroke, can also be identified by B-mode ultrasound.

The main role of duplex ultrasound is in the early assessment (screening) of patients at risk of ischemic stroke, and their follow-up. The recent results of multicenter studies designed to assess the effectiveness of carotid endarterectomy have placed significant pressure on clinicians because of the need for quick identification of patients with ischemic brain events resulting from atheromatous plaques that meet the criteria for surgical treatment. In spite of suggestions that these results (which are based on strict and often peculiar angiographic criteria) demand the absolute need for angiographic evaluation, clinical practice dictates that duplex ultrasound is a reliable tool that allows clinicians to plan further evaluation and care. Finally, the discussion so far has been centered on the ultrasonic evaluation of the carotid artery system. It must be noted, however, that the flow direction and velocity of the vertebral arteries within the vertebral canal of the cervical spine can also be assessed with duplex ultrasound.

Color Doppler Imaging. Color Doppler imaging (CDI) presents two-dimensional cross-sectional Doppler shift information superimposed on gray-scale anatomical images. It uses the pulse-echo imaging principle by which a pulse of ultrasound is emitted into the tissues and its echoes are then received and analyzed. Echoes returning from stationary tissues are detected and presented in gray scale in appropriate locations within the scan line. When a returning echo has a frequency different from when it was emitted, it implies the occurrence of a Doppler shift. Such Doppler shifts can be detected along the scan line and their sign (positive or negative), magnitude, and variance recorded. These variables are used by the instrument to determine the hue, saturation, and luminance of the color pixel at its location on the display. Each pixel is then updated multiple times per second, creating dynamic images of the flowing blood.

The main advantages of CDI over duplex are as follows:

1. It allows easier identification of vascular structures, leading to faster scan time.
2. It helps in differentiating plaque stenoses from other problems, such as kinks.
3. It allows appreciation of flow disturbances, even in the absence of stenosis.
4. It helps identify very small amounts of flow (e.g., critical stenosis or string sign).
5. It rapidly identifies echolucent plaques based on the absence of flow.
6. It allows better delineation of surface features.

In general, the application of CDI is quite similar to that of conventional duplex ultrasound. However, the sophisticated nature of the images produced has resulted in its application in the evaluation of conditions other than carotid atherosclerosis, including carotid body tumors, intimal fibroplasia, and dissection. Finally,

CDI has expanded the ability to evaluate the vertebral arteries as they course through the vertebral canal of the cervical spine extracranially.

A major limitation of extracranial ultrasound is that it is limited to an analysis of the extracranial vessels from the clavicle to the angle of the mandible. Visualization of the vertebral arteries is further limited by the surrounding bony elements.

Transcranial Doppler. TCD ultrasound is a diagnostic technique based on the use of a range-gated pulse-Doppler ultrasonic beam of 2 MHz frequency to assess the hemodynamic characteristics of the major cerebral arteries. The ultrasonic beam crosses the intact adult skull at points known as the *windows*, bounces off the erythrocytes flowing within the larger basal brain arteries, and allows the determination of blood flow velocity, direction of flow, collateral patterns, and state of cerebral vasoreactivity. By sampling of multiple cerebral blood vessels using TCD, it is possible to identify patterns pointing to lesions localized intra- or extracranially, followup their natural history over time, and even monitor the effects of therapeutic strategies. Although certainly having its own inherent limitations, TCD provides physiological information about the brain circulation that cannot be obtained by any other means. In addition to the uniqueness of the information gathered by TCD, the other attractive characteristics are that it is noninvasive (i.e., safe), reproducible, versatile, and dynamic.

The most important established (Class II and III evidence) clinical applications of TCD are evaluation of ischemic cerebrovascular disorders and cerebral vasospasm.

Evaluation of Ischemic Cerebrovascular Disorders: Atherosclerosis of the cerebral vasculature is by no means restricted to the common carotid bifurcation. In fact, the second most common location of atherosclerotic plaques in the carotid circulation is the cavernous portion of the internal carotid artery. Intracranial atherosclerotic stenosis is relatively common and can certainly alter the prognosis and management of patients in whom it is discovered. TCD provides a noninvasive way of screening and following up these patients. Characteristically, TCD shows that the intracranial stenotic vessel displays increased blood flow velocities to levels greater than two standard deviations of normal. In addition to local stenosis causing increased velocities in the affected vessel, other patterns of collateralization may be identified. In addition to intracranial lesions, those causing significant hemodynamic narrowing of the extracranial portions of the cerebral blood vessels lead to decreased TCD velocities. The degree of the decrement depends on the existence of collateral flow through the communicating arteries. Such a pattern, in turn, will be characterized by increased blood flow velocities in the vessel acting as the collateral supplier. In these patients, it is also possible to show reduced vasoreactivity in the hemisphere ipsilateral to the stenosis.

TCD is also capable of detecting embolic particles as they traverse the cerebral blood vessels. Due to the differences in impedance between the embolic material, TCD has a greater ultrasonographic impedance than do the red blood cells resulting in ultrasound reflection with greater intensity by the emboli. This produces the characteristic signature of emboli within the Doppler waveform. These signals are known as high-intensity transients (HITs) and they vary in intensity, duration, and appearance within the cardiac cycle. It has been possible to detect HITs not only during surgical procedures that place patients at risk for cerebral embolism (e.g., carotid endarterectomy and cardiopulmonary bypass) but also at the bedside. This has allowed for the detection of spontaneous asymptomatic emboli in patients with atrial fibrillation and mechanical heart valves. Such a finding has carried with itthe implication that cerebral embolism may occur continuously under certain circumstances and that the factors that motivate the development of symptoms are yet to be determined. In addition, the technique can be combined with the intravenous injection of agitated saline solution, allowing clinicians to diagnose patent foramina ovale (PFO) and right-to-left shunts.

Evaluation of Cerebral Vasospasm: The diagnosis of vasospasm by TCD depends on the finding of velocities greater than two standard deviations of normal, in the appropriate clinical context. Vasospasm is a very dynamic process requiring serial evaluations for its documentation and follow-up. It is because of these characteristics that TCD is so useful in the assessment of patients with vasospasm. The test should be performed as soon as a condition known to be associated with vasospasm is diagnosed (e.g., subarachnoid hemorrhage). This is followed by repeat TCD studies with a frequency that depends on the condition of the patient being studied. In patients with aneurysmal subarachnoid hemorrhage or closed head injury, daily TCD studies are performed to identify trends that will alert the clinicians that vasospasm is developing and that therapeutic measures should be instituted. Along these lines, TCD can also be used to follow up the response to treatment, particularly the institution of interventional procedures.

Catheter Angiography

Cerebral angiography carries with it a certain amount of risk and potential complications. In the first place, just as any other type of angiography, allergic reactions to iodinated contrast may occur. Another negative aspect of the use of contrast agents involves their potential nephrotoxic effect. The variables that have an effect on this type of complication include (a) state of hydration, (b) amount of contrast used, and (c) pre-existing renal dysfunction (particularly diabetic nephropathy). Finally, the most dreaded complication of angiography is stroke. This relates to either clot formation in the catheterization instruments with embolism or dislodging of plaque material during catheter and wire manipulation. It is our opinion that emboli are very common during angiography, yet only occasionally do they become symptomatic. One factor that seems to make the patient prone to develop neurological symptoms during angiography is the state of hydration. The fact that a dehydrated patient is more likely to have symptoms of ischemia is important, when one considers that patients are kept without oral intake for hours before angiography. Therefore, the use of isotonic crystalloid intravenously should be consistent to avoid complications. The current incidence of permanent neurological complications following diagnostic angiography is $<1\%$.

Cerebral angiography allows clear visualization of the lumen of the cerebral blood vessels, arteries, arterioles, capillaries, veins, and venous sinuses. From this point of view, the technique can be considered vascular lumenography. Angiography does not provide information about the vascular wall. For this purpose, ultrasound is a much better tool.

Cardiac Evaluation

The cardiac evaluation begins at the time of the initial presentation. The heart should be evaluated by auscultation and palpation. A 12-lead electrocardiogram (ECG) is a component of the initial code stroke evaluation. The patient should then be maintained on cardiac telemetry monitoring.

After the initial screening assessments, detailed imaging of the heart, valves, and proximal vessels provides information on the risk for a proximal source of emboli as a potential cause for stroke. Several options are available for cardiac imaging, including TTE, TEE, and cardiac MRI. The choice of the individual imaging modality depends on the availability and expertise at each center and on the individual patient characteristics.

Every patient should be evaluated with at least a TTE. The images may be adequate for screening evaluation of wall motion, valvular function, ejection fraction, and thrombus. In obese patients or in other situations, the imaging window may be small and the images may be insufficient for adequate diagnosis.

TEE allows for better imaging of the heart and proximal great vessels because the probe is in the esophagus, and therefore, the ribcage does not obscure the heart. While these images are typically superior in terms of the image quality and the screening sensitivity, the procedural risk is higher (given the invasive nature of the study) and the procedure may not be available at all centers.

Cardiac MRI is an emerging imaging modality that can provide excellent structural detail of the heart but again is new and therefore even more subject to interpretative error. This imaging modality is, at present, unavailable at most community based centers. In the future, this type of imaging may surpass even TEE for image quality and sensitivity for important cardiac abnormalities.

Laboratory Evaluation

Abnormalities of the blood itself represent one of the three primary causes of stroke. Even if they are not the primary cause for the stroke, certain abnormalities can direct treatment pathways (e.g., hyperlipidemia). The laboratory evaluation is divided into three separate compartments. The initial phase is the acute presentation. This is followed by the subacute evaluation, primarily collection of lipid studies. Finally, the third phase is needed only in a small number of cases: the analysis of a potential hypercoagulable state or possible vasculitic condition.

These initial laboratory studies include a comprehensive metabolic profile (basic chemistry studies and hepatic profile), complete blood count, cardiac enzymes, coagulation panel [prothrombin time (PT), partial thromboplastin time (PTT), international normalized ratio (INR)], and pregnancy test if applicable. The cardiac enzymes are an important part of the evaluation as is the ECG since concomitant myocardial infarction is common in the acute stroke setting. These studies should be performed on every patient presenting with acute ischemic stroke. Additional studies such as C-reactive protein and alcohol level may be of some benefit. Furthermore, urine drug screening can provide important information about stroke etiology as well as risk for withdrawal during the hospitalization.

Lipid studies are an important component of the evaluation and subsequent future selection of secondary stroke preventatives. Typically in the morning following admission, a lipid profile is obtained. A lipid profile consisting of total cholesterol, high-density lipoprotein (HDL), low-density lipoprotein (LDL), very low density lipoprotein (VLDL), and triglycerides is sufficient in most situations. On rare occasions, further evaluation with genetic studies and subclassification of the lipid constituents may be of benefit.

TABLE 29.2 Causes of Secondary Hypercoagulable States

Hypercoaguable state (secondary)
a. Malignancy
b. Pregnancy
c. Oral contraceptives
d. Disseminated intravascular coagulation
e. Nephrotic syndrome
f. Dehydration
Rheology
a. Homocystinuria (cystathione synthase deficiency)
b. Polycythemia vera
c. Sickle cell disease
d. Thrombotic thrombocytopenia purpura

In a young adult, additional studies for hypercoagulable states should be drawn. If the patient is going to be given recombinant tissue plasminogen activator (rt-PA) or heparin, these studies should be obtained before beginning their administration because these medications can alter the results of some laboratory tests. Some hypercoagulable states are secondary (e.g., dehydration, malignancy, and pregnancy), as described in Table 29.2. Others states are primary [e.g., antithrombin III (ATIII) deficiency, factor V Leiden, and protein C or S deficiency] and require detailed and often costly laboratory evaluation. Given the cost of these studies, they should not be ordered as part of a standing protocol for every patient, or even every young patient with a stroke. The potential causes of a primary hypercoagulable state are reviewed in Table 29.3 with the appropriate laboratory studies are reviewed in Table 29.4.

The vasculitides also represent an uncommon cause of stroke that requires specialized laboratory testing. A number of different vasculitic processes may contribute to the risk of stroke (e.g., infectious vasculitis, systemic lupus erythematosis). These vasculitides are shown in Table 29.5 with laboratory studies shown in Table 29.4.

TABLE 29.3 Causes of Primary Hypercoagulable States

ATIII deficiency
Protein C deficiency
Protein S deficiency
Dysfibrinogenemia
Factor XII deficiency
Antiphospholipid antibodies
Fibrinolytic abnormalities
Activated protein C resistance, factor V Leiden mutation (gene on 1q23)
Hyperhomocysteinemia (gene on 1q36)
CADASIL (gene on 19p13): Recurrent subcortical infarcts with spared U fibers
MTHFR polymorphism

CADASIL, cerebral autosomal dominant arteriopathy with subcortical infarcts and leukoencephalopathy; MTHFR, methylenetetrahydrofolate reductase.

TABLE 29.4 Stroke Risk Stratification Testing

Evaluation
A. Imaging
 1. CT head without contrast
 2. MRI/MRA
  DWIs may identify ischemic lesions within minutes of symptom onset.
  Diffusion perfusion imaging may identify a mismatch (potentially salvageable tissue).
 3. Carotid ultrasound
 4. TCD
 5. TEE or TTE or cardiac MRI
 6. Cerebral angiography
B. ECG
C. Chest x-ray
D. Initial laboratory testing
 1. CBC, chem 20, PT, PTT, cholesterol, triglycerides, β-HCG (if applicable)
 2. Cardiac enzymes, urine drug screen
E. Further laboratory testing
 1. Vasculitis: RA, ANA, C-reactive protein, ESR, complement (C3, C4, CH50), P-ANCA, C-ANCA, Scl-70, anticentromere antibody, ACE level, immunoglobulins, cryoglobulins, Coomb's test, CSF
 2. Hypercoagulable: Serum viscosity, fibrinogen, ATIII, protein C, protein S, bleeding time, SPEP, HIV, factor V Leiden mutation, factor VII, VIII, IX, X, XI, XII, XIII, thrombin time, fibrin degradation products, sickle prep, antiphospholipid antibodies

CT, computed tomography; MRI, magnetic resonance imaging; MRA, magnetic resonance angiography; DWI, diffusion-weighted image; ECG, electrocardiogram; CBC, complete blood cell; PT, prothrombin time; PTT, partial thromboplastin time; RA, rheumatoid arthritis; ANA, antinuclear antibodies; ESR, erythrocyte sedimentation rate; ANCA, anti-neutrophilic cytoplasmic antibody; ACE, angiotensin-converting enzyme; CSF, cerebrospinal fluid; SPEP, serum protein electrophoresis.

PRACTICAL RECOMMENDATIONS

The use of imaging techniques for the evaluation of patients with cerebrovascular disorders must be guided by the specific needs of the clinical situation. Newer tests being introduced will not necessarily replace the old ones but rather will provide additional dimensions to our ability to diagnose and treat different conditions capable of causing stroke. It is important to keep in mind that every one of these diagnostic techniques is operator dependent, to different degrees. As such, another aspect of choosing the appropriate diagnostic technique requires the recognition of the quality of the resources available.

All patients should be assessed with the described initial screening evaluation that occurs on admission, as a part of the code stroke protocol.

Imaging with MRI, including gradient echo images for hemorrhage, should be obtained on all patients unless there is a contraindication to MRI (e.g., pacemaker). If the patient is unable to undergo MRI and MRA, additional evaluation with repeat CT on day 2 with CTA (when possible) can provide some of the information from the MRI.

TABLE 29.5 Causes of Vasculitides

Vasculitis
 Infectious
 Necrotizing
  PAN
  Wegener's syndrome
  Churg-Strauss syndrome lymphomatosis
 Collagen vascular disease
  SLE
  RA
  Sjögren's disease scleroderma
 Systemic disease
  Behçet's disease
  Sarcoid
  Ulcerative colitis
 Giant cell arteritis
  Takayasu's syndrome
  Temporal arteritis
 Hypersensitivity (drug, chemical)
Neoplastic
 Primary CNS vasculitis

PAN, polyarteritis nodosa; SLE, systemic lupus erythematosus; RA, rheumatoid arthritis; CNS, central nervous system.

All patients should also have at least TTE. In certain cases TEE may also be of benefit. Cardiac MRI is an excellent system but at this point of time is reserved for a relatively small number of centers.

SELECTED REFERENCES

Atkinson DS, Jr. Computed tomography of pediatric stroke. *Semin Ultrasound CT MR* 2006;27(3):207–218.

Brobeck BR, Forero NP, Romero JM. Practical noninvasive neurovascular imaging of the neck arteries in patients with stroke, transient ischemic attack, and suspected arterial disease that may lead to ischemia, infarction, or flow abnormalities. *Semin Ultrasound CT MR* 2006;27(3):177–193.

DeMarco JK, Huston J, III, Nash AK. Extracranial carotid MR imaging at 3T. *Magn Reson Imaging Clin N Am* 2006;14(1):109–121.

Ferro JM. Update on intracerebral haemorrhage. *J Neurol* 2006;253(8):985–999.

Forsting M. CTA of the ICA bifurcation and intracranial vessels. *Eur Radiol* 2005;15(suppl 4):D25–D27.

Graves MJ, U-King-Im J, Howarth S, et al. Ultrafast magnetic resonance imaging protocols in stroke. *Expert Rev Neurother* 2006;6(6):921–930.

Heiss WD, Sorensen AG. Advances in imaging 2006. *Stroke* 2007;38(2):238–240; epub January 4, 2007.

Hillis AE. Rehabilitation of unilateral spatial neglect: new insights from magnetic resonance perfusion imaging. *Arch Phys Med Rehabil* 2006;87(12 Suppl 2):S43–S49.

Janjua N. Cerebral angiography and venography for evaluation of cerebral venous thrombosis. *J Pak Med Assoc* 2006;56(11):527–530.

Kane I, Sandercock P, Wardlaw J. Magnetic resonance perfusion diffusion mismatch and thrombolysis in acute ischaemic stroke: a systematic review of the evidence to date. *J Neurol Neurosurg Psychiatr* 2007;78(5):485–491.

Kavlak ES, Kucukoglu H, Yigit Z, et al. Clinical and echocardiographic risk factors for embolization in the presence of left atrial thrombus. *Echocardiography* 2007;24(5):515–521.

Korsten HH, Mischi M, Grouls RJ, et al. Quantification in echocardiography. *Semin Cardiothorac Vasc Anesth* 2006;10(1):57–62.

Lauzon ML, Sevick RJ, Demchuk AM, et al. Stroke imaging at 3.0 T. *Neuroimaging Clin N Am* 2006;16(2):343–366, xii.

Meltzer SM, Rigby MJ, Meltzer RS. Transthoracic echocardiographic diagnosis of mobile aortic arch atherothrombosis associated with stroke. *Echocardiography* 2007;24(3):267–268.

Molina CA. Monitoring and imaging the clot during systemic thrombolysis in stroke patients. *Expert Rev Cardiovasc Ther* 2007;5(1):91–98.

Moustafa RR, Baron JC. Imaging the penumbra in acute stroke. *Curr Atheroscler Rep* 2006;8(4):281–289.

Muir KW, Buchan A, von Kummer R, et al. Imaging of acute stroke. *Lancet Neurol* 2006;5(9):755–768.

Nedeltchev K, Mattle HP. Contrast-enhanced transcranial Doppler ultrasound for diagnosis of patent foramen ovale. *Front Neurol Neurosci* 2006;21:206–215.

Ovbiagele B, Saver JL, Sanossian N, et al. Predictors of cerebral microbleeds in acute ischemic stroke and TIA patients. *Cerebrovasc Dis* 2006;22(5–6):378–383.

Platt OS. *Prevention and Management of Stroke in Sickle Cell Anemia.* Washington DC: American Society of Hematology, 2006:54–57.

Rustemli A, Bhatti TK, Wolff SD. Evaluating cardiac sources of embolic stroke with MRI. *Echocardiography* 2007;24(3):301–308; discussion 308.

Sankaranarayanan R, Msairi A, Davis GK. Stroke complicating cardiac catheterization—a preventable and treatable complication. *J Invasive Cardiol* 2007;19(1):40–45.

Srinivasan A, Goyal M, Al Azri F, et al. State-of-the-art imaging of acute stroke. *Radiographics* 2006;26(Suppl 1):S75–S95.

Warburton L, Gillard J. Functional imaging of carotid atheromatous plaques. *J Neuroimaging* 2006;16(4):293–301.

Weiller C, May A, Sach M, et al. Role of functional imaging in neurological disorders. *J Magn Reson Imaging* 2006;23(6):840–850.

Wolf RC, Spiess J, Vasic N, et al. Valvular strands and ischemic stroke. *Eur Neurol* 2007;57(4):227–231.

CHAPTER 30

Complications of Acute Stroke

JAMES D. GEYER, CAMILO R. GOMEZ, A. ROBERT SHEPPARD, AND NADEEM AKHTAR

OBJECTIVES

- What are the common complications of stroke?
- What methods should be used to monitor for these complications?
- What are the methods of treatment and prevention for these potential complications?

It is rare for a stroke patient who is admitted, treated, and discharged to have no neurological, medical, or psychiatric complications. Therefore, it should be expected that something will arise to complicate the hospitalization. The most important factors in the management of the acute stroke patient are to be aware of the potential complications and be ready to treat them in an expeditious and aggressive manner.

Virtually every organ system is at risk for dysfunction during the acute phase of a stroke. Infections are commonplace. Neurological problems range from seizures to herniation syndromes. These complications are reviewed briefly in the following sections.

CLINICAL APPLICATIONS AND METHODOLOGY

Infection

Aspiration Pneumonia

While the risk of aspiration pneumonia is well known as a complication of stroke, even rudimentary procedures for limiting its occurrence are often not initiated. Patients requiring nasogastric tube feedings appear to be at the highest risk for aspiration. A number of factors predispose the stroke patient to aspiration including dysphagia, large hemispheric stroke, brainstem stroke, impaired consciousness, seizures, and mechanical ventilation.

Every patient should be screened for evidence of dysphagia with a bedside swallowing evaluation by nursing. Patients with evidence of dysphagia or with any significant dysarthria should have more detailed evaluation by speech therapy. A formal swallowing study may be necessary at that point. A more detailed discussion of this complex issue is covered in Chapter 35.

A slight elevation of the head of the bed, accounting for the need to maintain optimal cerebral hemodynamics, may be of some benefit. The family should be instructed to clear any food or beverage with the nursing staff.

Pneumonia (Hospital Acquired)

The debilitated, bedridden patient is at risk for developing a hospital-acquired pneumonia. The organisms causing pneumonia are frequently resistant to standard antibiotics and can be extremely difficult to treat.

Prophylactic antibiotic therapy has not shown benefit, but an aggressive course of management should be instituted at the earliest signs of infection. Chest X-ray, blood cultures, sputum culture, and complete blood cell (CBC) should be obtained. The patient should be started on regimented pulmonary toilet with percussion and drainage.

Urinary Tract Infection

Urinary tract infections are common in the stroke population, occurring in approximately 15% of patients. Diabetic patients are at an even higher risk. The presence of a catheter is the most important predisposing factor. Sepsis with associated hypotension can ensue, worsening the stroke and in some cases resulting in death.

Hydration is of some benefit in preventing urinary tract infection. The addition of cranberry juice or vitamin C can also decrease the risk of infection. When possible the use of an indwelling catheter should be avoided.

Sinusitis

Sinusitis is not often thought of as a complication of stroke but may occur more frequently than suspected. Nasogastric tubes and nasal intubation increase the risk of sinus infection. If fever occurs, sinus X-rays should be obtained. The sinuses should be inspected each time a neuroimaging study is obtained.

Sepsis

Sepsis can occur secondary to any of the infectious complications of stroke described earlier. Infections must be treated aggressively to avoid sepsis and its cascade of effects. In the worst case, sepsis is life threatening. The complications of sepsis can be devastating even when not directly life threatening. Hypotension decreases cerebral perfusion pressure and can cause an enlargement of the stroke. Severe shift in blood sugar can occur as well.

Neurological Complications

Seizures

Seizures are relatively uncommon in patients with ischemic stroke. The risk is considerably higher in patients with hemorrhage, especially subarachnoid hemorrhage. Seizures usually occur at the onset of symptoms but may occur as a late or remote complication. The seizures occurring in the remote phase of a large cortical infarction are more likely to be recurrent than those occurring in the acute phase.

Patients with intracranial hemorrhage are typically treated with prophylactic anticonvulsants. Patients with ischemic stroke, given their lower risk of seizure activity, are not treated prophylactically. Once a seizure occurs, an antiepileptic medication must be selected. The selection must take into account several factors. Medications that might result in hypotension should be avoided. Drug–drug interactions must also be taken into account. Finally, medications with multiple routes of administration (PO/NG/IV) are preferable. For discussions on hemorrhagic transformation and cerebral edema see Chapters 27 and 32, respectively.

Altered Mental Status/Encephalopathy

Confusion is a common problem in the acute phase of stroke, occurring in at least 25% of patients. Many patients are elderly and are at risk for cognitive dysfunction. The extreme psychophysiologic stress related to the stroke itself, hospitalization, and loss neurological function increase the risk of an acute encephalopathy. While this is often transient, the confusion increases the risk of injury and increases the demands on nursing and family alike. Other patients may have a dementia, recognized or not, which may worsen dramatically during hospitalization. Hallucinations, paranoia, and delusions are common.

Maintaining a reasonable environment for rest is important as described in Chapter 38. If necessary, medications such as haloperidol, risperdal, and quietapine may be used acutely to manage hallucinations and delusions. Physicians, nurses, and family should understand that the impairment in cognitive function related to the hospitalization itself rarely resolves during the hospitalization.

Strokes, both ischemic and hemorrhagic can result in declining cognitive function. Even a single stroke can result in cognitive decline. This is most apparent in the demented patient but may be seen to a lesser degree in the cognitively healthy patient. Conversely, multiple strokes in the otherwise normal patient can cause a significant vascular dementia.

Hemiballismus

Movement disorders are relatively uncommon in the stroke patient. A stroke or hemorrhage in the subthalamic nucleus results in hemiballismus. The movements are usually violent and can result in injury to the patients, and even the caregiver. In many cases the extremity must be restrained for a short time. In severe cases, treatment with phenothiazines or haloperidol may be of benefit. Fortunately, this complication typically improves over time.

Parkinsonism

Infarction of the globus pallidus may, in rare cases, cause contralateral parkinsonism. Multiple infarctions can also create a parkinsonian-like syndrome. These complications are difficult to treat.

Falls

Stroke patients are at high risk for falls. Ataxia, hemiparesis, sensory loss, and confusion all may contribute to the risk. Even bed-bound patients can fall from bed. As patients are mobilized, the risk increases. The patients should be evaluated by physical therapy for appropriate therapy and assist devices.

Contractures

Spasticity followed by contractures can occur quickly after a stroke. These should be assessed by physical therapy and treated with range-of-motion exercises, splinting, and in some severe cases injection with botulinum toxin. Left unchecked, the spasticity can become painful and significantly limit function.

Stroke-related Pain

Poststroke pain syndrome typically follows thalamic or medullary infarctions. The so-called thalamic pain syndrome can be associated with infarction or hemorrhage involving the contralateral ventroposterolateral (VPL) nucleus of the thalamus or the dorsolateral medulla. The pain is usually a boring-type pain occurring with minimal stimulation. These syndromes can be disabling and adversely affect the patient's quality of life. Treatment with agents such as pregabalin, gabapentin, tricyclic antidepressants, and other chronic pain management medications may be of some benefit.

Shoulder pain

Several factors contribute to shoulder pain. Weakness of the shoulder girdle muscles increases the risk of subluxation and associated pain. The patient should not be pulled up in bed or pulled up to a sitting or standing position using the arms. The nursing staff should be aware of these issues and should educate the family about this risk during their orientation to the unit.

Adhesive capsulitis may result from paralysis. Although the use of slings or other immobilizing devices may make the patient feel transiently better, they actually worsen the problem. The best prevention is an aggressive course of physical therapy with range-of-motion exercises.

Hiccups

Hiccups usually occur following lower brainstem infarction but occasionally occur following large cortical stroke. The hiccups may last for days or in some cases for weeks but usually improve. In rare cases, the hiccups can last much longer. For severe cases, especially when the hiccups interfere with nutrition or rest, there are several treatment options. Haloperidol, risperdal, quietapine, chlorpromazine, cabamazepine, and baclofen may help control the symptoms.

Compression Neuropathy

Prolonged bedrest increases the risk of compression neuropathy, especially involving the ulnar and peroneal nerves. The patient should be turned on a regular schedule. The patient should not be left in positions felt to be high risk for compression.

Sleep-related Complications

For discussions on obstructive sleep apnea syndrome, insomnia, and restless legs syndrome see Chapter 38.

Parasomnias, including sleep walking and rapid eye movement (REM) sleep behavior disorder, are relatively uncommon but can result in serious injury. The staff should be aware of these types of disorders and report any potential episodes to the physician.

Cardiac Complications

Myocardial Infarction

Heart disease including myocardial infarction is one of the most common causes of death in a stroke patient. The patient should be monitored, at least for the initial few days of the hospitalization, for evidence of myocardial ischemia. As described elsewhere, electrocardiogram (ECG) and cardiac enzymes are obtained on admission. The patient is then placed on cardiac telemetry monitoring. Many of the treatments used for acute stroke are also beneficial in the treatment of myocardial ischemia. Blood pressure management may need adjustment in the presence of concomitant myocardial ischemia.

Cardiac Arrhythmia

Arrhythmias are seen in the poststroke phase for several different reasons. The arrhythmia may predate the stroke and may have even contributed to it. The arrhythmia could be a result of the physiological stress of the stroke and some of its treatments. Finally, myocardial ischemia, as described earlier, can contribute to the occurrence of cardiac arrhythmias.

Heart Failure

Heart failure is not typically a result of a stroke. The treatments of acute stroke, most important the use of intravenous crystalloids, increase the risk of heart failure decompensation and pulmonary edema. The patient must be monitored for signs of heart failure and treated accordingly.

Deep Vein Thrombosis

Though uncommon, deep vein thrombosis (DVT) is an important and usually avoidable complication. All patients should be placed on DVT prophylaxis. At our center, sequential compression hose following screening lower extremity ultrasound and subcutaneous heparinoids are used in most patients.

Hypertension, Hypotension and Endocrine Complications

For discussions on hypertension and hypotension see Chapter 36. Endocrine complications are covered in Chapter 5.

Psychiatric Complications

Depression associated with stroke is covered in detail in Chapter 40.

Anxiety is common in the general population. The stresses associated with a stroke and the tests that the patients are required to endure only serves to wosen this problem. Some patients require treatment only for claustrophobia-enhancing procedures such as magnetic resonance imaging (MRI), while others require daily treatment with benzodiazepines or anxiolytic antidepressants such as selective serotonin reuptake inhibitors (SSRIs).

Other Complications

Other complications include urinary incontinence as well as fecal incontinence, which may be related to diarrhea or may be situational and related to the inability to notify staff of the need to defecate. This problem causes skin irritation, increases the risk of urinary tract infection, and is psychologically distressing to the patient and family alike. Constipation is a far more common problem. A bowel program initiated on admission and followed throughout the hospitalization can limit the severity of the constipation.

Gastrointestinal Hemorrhage

Severe, life-threatening hemorrhages are uncommon. So-called stress ulceration, related to the profound physiological stress of the stroke, may occur. Furthermore, the use of aspirin and other antiplatelet medications increases the risk of gastrointestinal bleeding. Prophylactic histamine blockers may be of benefit but should be administered with care since they can cause drowsiness and confusion.

Pressure Ulcerations

Decubitus ulcers are relatively common, occurring in 10% to 15% of stroke patients. Elderly, thin, or malnourished patients are at higher risk. Severe weakness and being bed bound compound the problem. The patient should be turned frequently. Skin care for even the earliest signs of skin breakdown can help prevent a much worse problem.

End-of-Life Care

In some cases, the question is not "what can we do?" but "what should we do?" The patient's family should be advised of the severity of the neurological deficit and the potential for meaningful neurological recovery. Resuscitation options should be discussed with every patient/family. A more directed frank discussion of end-of-life options is necessary for the patient with a poor prognosis for meaningful recovery. Palliative care, including pain management for the patient and psychological support for the family, is an important component of any stroke care program.

SELECTED REFERENCES

Bayer T. Key advances in care for the elderly. *Practitioner* 2005; 249(1670):311–314, 316.

Boz C, Velioglu S, Bulbul I, et al. Baclofen is effective in intractable hiccups induced by brainstem lesions. *Neurol Sci* 2001;22(5):409.

Bravata DM, Ho SY, Meehan TP, et al. Readmission and death after hospitalization for acute ischemic stroke: 5-year follow-up in the medicare population. *Stroke* 2007;38(6):1899–1904.

Bruno A, Williams LS, Kent TA. How important is hyperglycemia during acute brain infarction? *Neurologist* 2004;10(4):195–200.

Carey TS, Hanson L, Garrett JM, et al. Expectations and outcomes of gastric feeding tubes. *Am J Med* 2006;119(6):527.e11–527.e16.

Daly JJ. Response of gait deficits to neuromuscular electrical stimulation for stroke survivors. *Expert Rev Neurother* 2006;6(10):1511–1522.

Grau AJ, Buggle F, Schnitzler P, et al. Fever and infection early after ischemic stroke. *J Neurol Sci* 1999;171(2):115–120.

Jones SA, Shinton RA. Improving outcome in stroke patients with visual problems. *Age Ageing* 2006;35(6):560–565.

Kappelle LJ, Van Der Worp HB. Treatment or prevention of complications of acute ischemic stroke. *Curr Neurol Neurosci Rep* 2004;4(1):36–41.

Katzan IL, Dawson NV, Thomas CL, et al. The cost of pneumonia after acute stroke. *Neurology* 2007;68(22):1938–1943.

Kong KH, Young S. Incidence and outcome of poststroke urinary retention: a prospective study. *Arch Phys Med Rehabil* 2000;81(11):1464–1467.

Kumar A, Dromerick AW. Intractable hiccups during stroke rehabilitation. *Arch Phys Med Rehabil* 1998;79(6):697–699.

Mancia G. Prevention and treatment of stroke in patients with hypertension. *Clin Ther* 2004;26(5):631–648.

Moretti R, Torre P, Antonello RM, et al. Gabapentin as a drug therapy of intractable hiccup because of vascular lesion: a three-year follow up. *Neurologist* 2004;10(2):102–106.

Pertoldi S, Di Benedetto P. Shoulder-hand syndrome after stroke. A complex regional pain syndrome. *Eura Medicophys* 2005;41(4): 283–292.

Roth EJ, Lovell L, Harvey RL, et al. Delay in transfer to inpatient stroke rehabilitation: the role of acute hospital medical complications and stroke characteristics. *Top Stroke Rehabil* 2007;14(1):57–64.

Shigemitsu H, Afshar K. Aspiration pneumonias: under-diagnosed and under-treated. *Curr Opin Pulm Med* 2007;13(3):192–198.

Singh S, Hamdy S. Dysphagia in stroke patients. *Postgrad Med J* 2006;82(968):383–391.

Witt BJ, Ballman KV, Brown RD, Jr, et al. The incidence of stroke after myocardial infarction: a meta-analysis. *Am J Med* 2006;119(4): 354.e1–354.e9.

Wu J, Baguley IJ. Urinary retention in a general rehabilitation unit: prevalence, clinical outcome, and the role of screening. *Arch Phys Med Rehabil* 2005;86(9):1772–1777.

CHAPTER 31

Cerebral Angiography in the Evaluation of Stroke Patients

CAMILO R. GOMEZ

OBJECTIVES

- What are the indications for diagnostic cerebral angiography in patients with stroke?
- How is the benefit:risk ratio assessed for diagnostic angiography in patients with stroke?
- What measures can be taken to improve the chances of a successful outcome during diagnostic angiography?
- What are the limitations of angiography as a diagnostic tool?

Diagnostic cerebral angiography has been considered the gold standard for the assessment of cerebral vascular pathology. As such, it has been used as a point of comparison for every other diagnostic technique applied to this patient population. However, the invasive nature of angiography is what has motivated the sequential and progressive introduction of less invasive diagnostic techniques. This has resulted in an unintended consequence. There are fewer angiograms performed every day and the skills of the angiographers have suffered, perhaps increasing the risk of complications. Nevertheless, despite the advances in noninvasive vascular imaging, the role that cerebral angiography plays in the management of stroke patients is unique and irreplaceable. The following are the most important concepts on the use of diagnostic cerebral angiography in the management of stroke patients.

CLINICAL APPLICATIONS AND METHODOLOGY

Technique

Catheter cerebral angiography, as it is presently being performed, most commonly involves access to the intravascular space via the femoral artery. From this point of entry, catheters measuring approximately 100 cm in length are used to engage the cerebral vessels and inject iodinated contrast that can then be imaged fluoroscopically and by digital subtraction. Traditionally, the procedure involved the injection of the aortic root via a pigtail catheter connected to a power injector. The latter is necessary because of the high volume required to opacify the aortic arch and the great vessels. This technique (i.e., arch aortography) has advantages and disadvantages. It allows the operator to clearly map out the position and size of the great vessels, thereby facilitating their direct catheterization. In addition, pathology of the great vessels (e.g., subclavian artery stenosis) often occurs at their ostium, and this is a relatively easy way to diagnose these lesions. However, this technique involves the use of a relatively large volume of contrast (typically 40 to 50 mL), which adds to the risk of contrast-induced nephropathy and limits the amount of additional contrast to be used during the rest of the procedure. The latter problem becomes magnified when diagnostic angiography is immediately followed by an intervention. In general, the routine performance of arch aortograms has been abandoned because they have been found to be unnecessary in most patients.

From the author's point of view, the first step of cerebral angiography involves catheterization of the main cerebral arteries. The favored approach, which derives from more than a decade of experience in performing cerebral angiography (>3,000 angiograms undertaken), involves one principle: catheterizing the target vessel (i.e., the vessel in question) last. Such an approach has several advantages, the most important of which is evident when the diagnostic procedure has to be converted to an intervention. Under such a circumstance, the diagnostic catheter is perfectly located, and there is no need to recatheterize the target vessel after injecting the remaining vessels. Furthermore, since the decision to proceed with an intervention requires knowledge of the condition of all cerebral vessels, catheterizing the target vessel last affords the operator the ability to make decisions immediately, having already reviewed the remaining arterial information. From this perspective, and considering that there are four major vascular target regions (two carotid and two vertebral systems), the course to follow is quite predictable. In turn, predictability is important because it facilitates the day-to-day performance of angiograms in patients by decreasing variability while facilitating the tasks required by the catheterization laboratory personnel.

In general, every angiogram must include catheterization of both common carotid arteries, both subclavian arteries, and at least one vertebral artery (the one that is dominant). This approach provides the necessary diagnostic information in >90% of cases and does not require catheterization or injection of every cerebral vessel. However, there are instances in which additional information is required and the operator must catheterize both vertebral arteries and, sometimes, the internal carotid arteries. Arterial catheterization sequence is planned ahead of time (see Critical Pathway: Catheterization Sequence) to expedite the procedure and minimize risk for the patient. The left subclavian artery is typically the first vessel to be catheterized because it is the most accessible, and the information derived from its images has significant effect on the procedure (see Fig. 31.1A). Typically, the innominate artery is then injected (see Fig. 31.1B), providing the opportunity to plan the rest of the procedure, which depends on the target vessel in question (see Critical Pathway: Angiography in Practice2). The remaining injections must include orthogonal views (typically anteroposterior and lateral) of the extracranial (see Fig 31.2) and intracranial segments (i.e., cerebrovascular bed; see Figs. 31.3 and 31.4) of the each catheterized vessel. Care must be taken when imaging the intracranial vessels to include all phases of the angiogram—arterial, arteriolar, capillary, and venous (including the sinuses). Additional angiographic views may require different angulations and/or magnification to better define specific vascular structures. A particular circumstance arises when one of the vertebral arteries, typically the left, arises directly from the aortic arch (see Fig. 31.5). This is usually suspected because the vessel is not found during the subclavian injection, but it is briefly seen during the contralateral vertebral artery injection. Selective catheterization of the vertebral artery, as it arises from the aortic arch, then becomes necessary. Moreover, visualization of the vessel is important because of the incidence of ostial stenosis in this location.

Traditionally, all injections of the major cerebral arteries were carried out manually. More recently, however, small power injectors designed to infuse low volumes of contrast at programmable pressures have been made available. The force required to opacify the cerebral vessels can easily be generated with these devices, the risk of trapping air in the line is diminished, and the speed of the procedure is enhanced. The latter point is important because there is a direct correlation between the amount of time the patient spends on the table during catheterization and the incidence of thromboembolic complications.

In the emergency use of angiography for the treatment of stroke, it could be argued that the strategy of injecting the target vessel last may not be the most reasonable one. On the contrary, the author has found that decisions about the injection of thrombolytic drugs or coiling of ruptured aneurysms can be more easily made when the operator has information about the status of the entire cerebral vasculature. In any case, the delay incurred by following the described approach is in the magnitude of 10 to 15 minutes, a small price to pay for diminishing the speculative position of not having all the angiographic information necessary at the time of treatment.

A final practical point to consider involves the management of the arteriotomy site. In the past, removal of the angiographic sheath (typically 5 or 6 Fr) following the procedure was the only method for handling this situation. Sheath removal was usually followed by the use of pressure dressings, sandbags, or compression devices (e.g., FemStop RADI Medical Systems), and the necessity for the patient to remain supine for many hours following the procedure (typically 1 hour for every 1 Fr of the sheath's size). As time elapsed, it became increasingly difficult to handle patients who were concurrently treated with antithrombotic or thrombolytic agents. This resulted in the development of a variety of closure devices the sole purpose of which was to secure the arteriotomy site

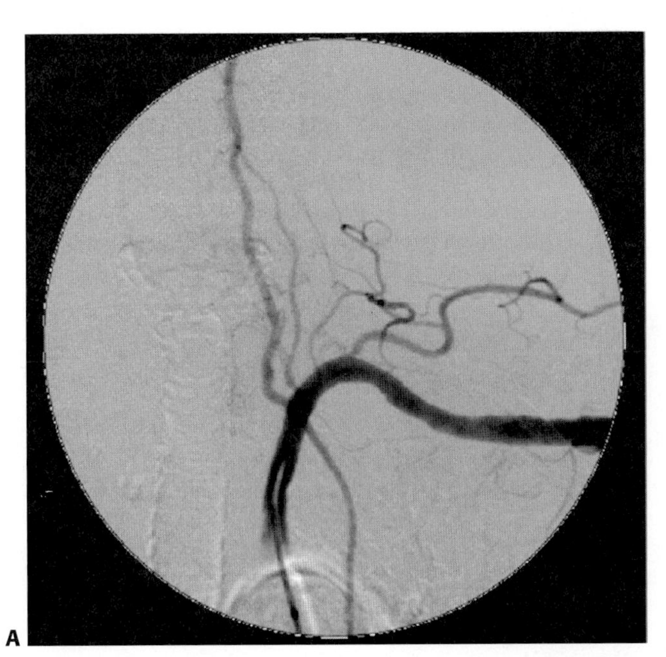
A

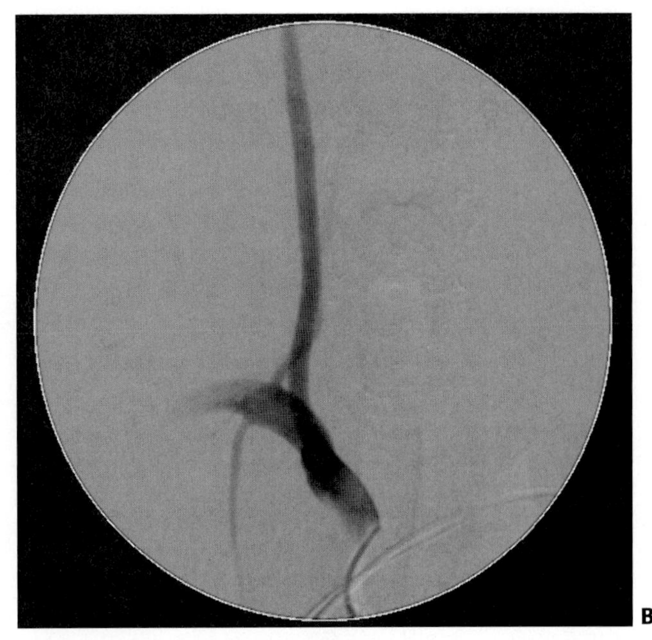
B

FIGURE 31.1. A: Injection of the left subclavian artery, typically the first one performed in most angiograms, allows demonstration of the origin and most proximal portion of the left vertebral artery. In this case, it demonstrates widespread atherosclerotic changes, with brisk and antegrade flow in the left vertebral artery, which is of reasonably large size. **B:** Injection of the innominate artery demonstrates the right common carotid and subclavian arteries, while also allowing visualization of the proximal right vertebral artery. Injecting this vessel immediately after the left subclavian artery provides sufficient information to plan the rest of the procedure, based on the target vessel.

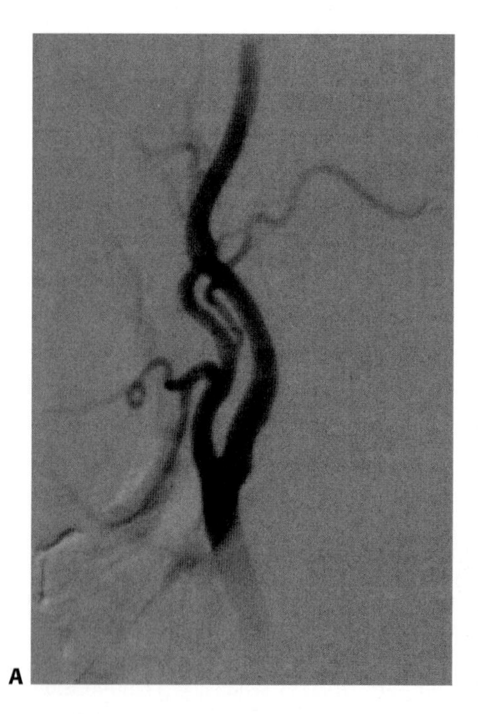

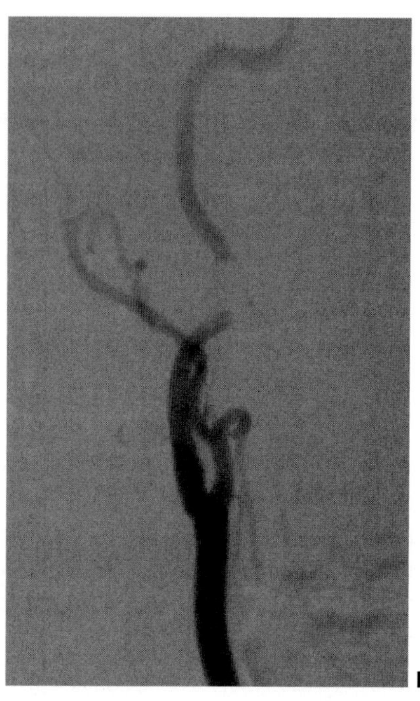

FIGURE 31.2. Typical orthogonal angiographic views (lateral on the left and anteroposterior on the right) of the extracranial segments of the carotid system. Notice that the images not only center on the common carotid bifurcation but also extend to the entrance of the internal carotid artery into the skull.

at the end of the procedure, decreasing the risk of hemorrhagic complications, and at least theoretically, the development of pseudoaneurysms. These devices varied in their design, but their premise was to facilitate clotting of the needle track with a collagen plug (e.g., VasoSeal, Datascope Corp.), suturing the arteriotomy (e.g., Perclose, Abbott Vascular, Inc.), or a combination (e.g., Angio-Seal, St. Jude Medical). The author has had the opportunity to use nearly all of these devices over the last decade. At present, the author favors the StarClose (Abbott Vascular, Inc.), which consists of a device that allows deployment of a very small nickel–titanium star-shaped clip that closes the arteriotomy. Patients are then taken from the catheterization laboratory to their room and are allowed to ambulate within 60 to 120 minutes. The clip can be later visualized fluoroscopically and is small enough that it does not interfere with subsequent attempts at vascular access. All arteriotomy sites are closed, since this is the best overall approach to endovascular procedures, providing comfort to the patients and reduction of hemorrhagic complication.

Indications for Angiography

The most important indication for cerebral angiography is the need to define cerebral vascular pathology before therapeutic intervention. This is true whether the intervention is surgical, endovascular, or medical, and requires a keen understanding of the types of intervention possible for every pathological process. From this point of view, angiography has been traditionally indicated before treatment of aneurysms, vascular malformations, or carotid artery pathology. At present, because of the growth of endovascular therapeutic options, it is important to consider cerebral angiography in

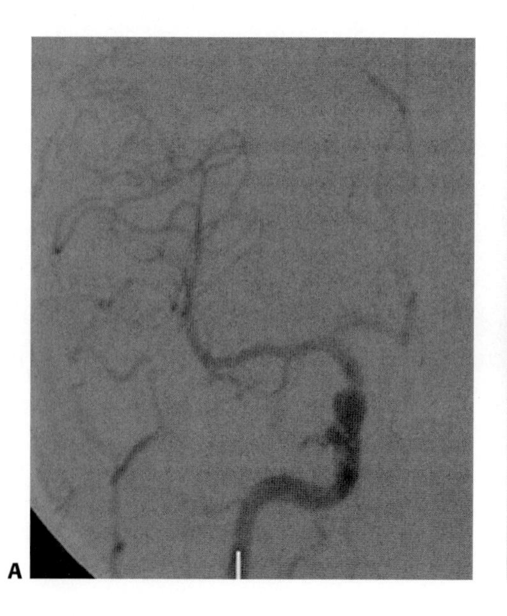

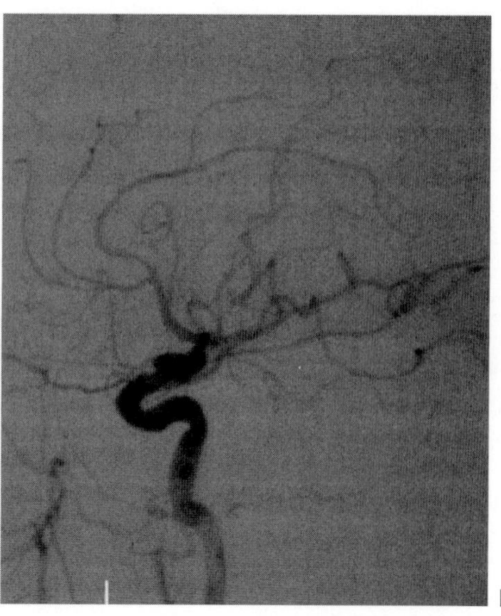

FIGURE 31.3. Orthogonal views, anteroposterior **(A)** and lateral **(B)** of the intracranial segments (early arterial phase) following injection of the common carotid artery. The anteroposterior view is most commonly obtained with a 10 to 15 degree cranial angulation above the orbitomeatal line (i.e., Caldwell's view).

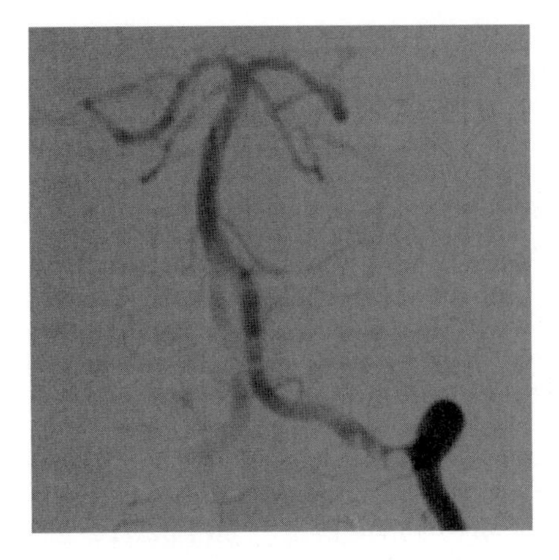
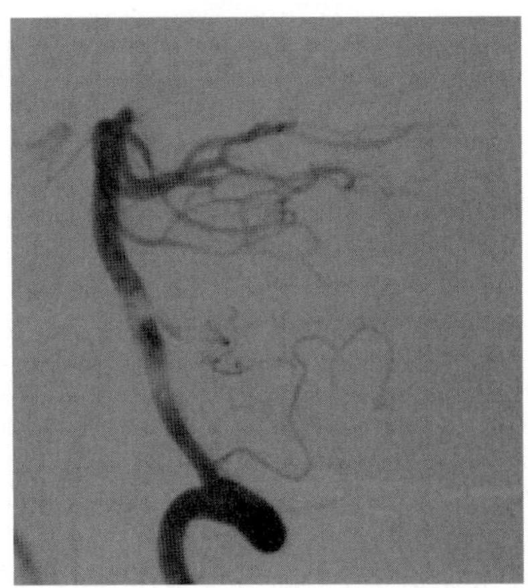

FIGURE 31.4. Typical orthogonal views of the intracranial vertebrobasilar system (early arterial phase) following injection of the left vertebral artery. The anteroposterior view is generally gained (*left*) without any angulation. However, at times it is necessary to angulate the image intensifier about 20 to 25 degrees cranially (i.e., Towne's view) to visualize the top of the basilar artery further. (*right*)

cases where other less traditionally accepted interventions may be of benefit to the patient.

It is also imperative to have a clear idea about the questions that the angiogram must answer before placing the patient on the table. Otherwise, the angiogram becomes a "fishing expedition," increasing the chances of complications and changing the benefit:risk ratio of the procedure. Another aspect that must also be discussed is the fact that angiography is a highly operator-dependent imaging modality. Thus, a poorly performed and uninformative angiogram is worse than no angiogram at all since it exposes the patient to risk and does not contribute to his or her care. Cerebral angiography should not being carried out unless the findings are likely to guide the therapeutic strategy. The most simplistic interpretation of this statement relates to therapeutic intervention, either surgical or endovascular. However, there are occasions when the results of the angiogram may help define the best medical course to follow. For example, choosing the most reasonable antithrombotic regimen in some instances requires a definition of the underlying pathology that only angiography can provide.

Contraindications of Cerebral Angiography

The most important contraindication of cerebral angiography is the inability to articulate what difference the results will make in the treatment or the outcome of the patient. It has been the author's experience that complications more likely take place under circumstances where the angiogram lacks clear indications, which leads to the following rule of thumb: *The less clear the indication, the more likely the complication!*

The next relative contraindication for cerebral angiography is the presence of renal insufficiency or one of its predisposing conditions (e.g., diabetes). Thus, the risk of contrast-induced nephropathy, with worsening of renal function and possibly the need for dialysis, must be always considered in the benefit:risk analysis. One of the simplest strategies to reduce the risk of contrast-induced nephropathy is to limit the volume of contrast used during the procedure. In general, a cerebral angiogram can be performed, as described in the preceding text, with 50 to 60 mL of contrast, largely by diluting it in half with saline. In instances when an angiogram is absolutely necessary, the procedure can be made

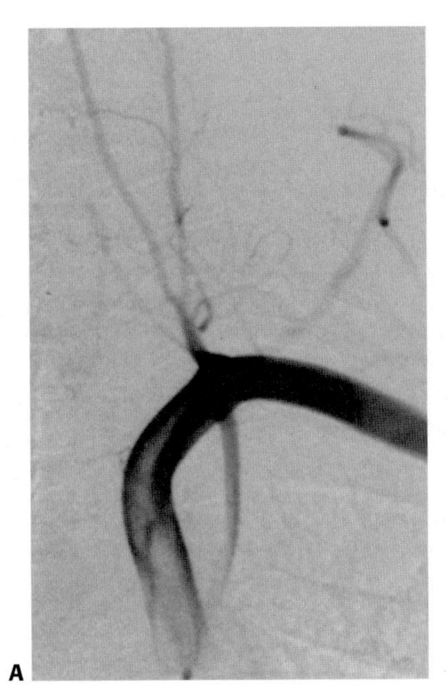

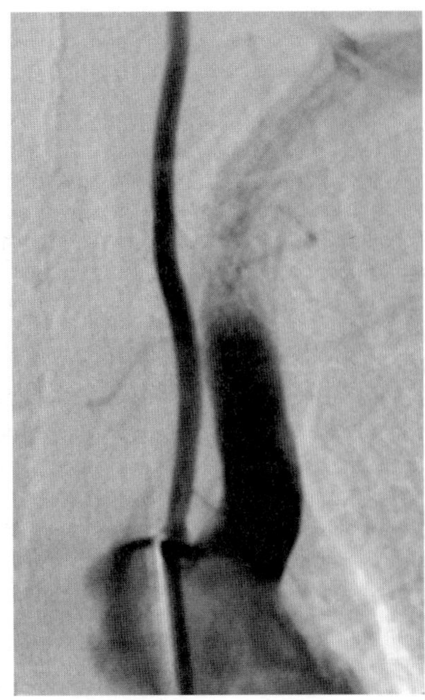

FIGURE 31.5. Injection of the left subclavian artery **(A)** at times fails to show the left vertebral artery. In these circumstances, a search for a left vertebral artery originating directly from the aortic arch usually leads to its identification and injection **(B)**. Most commonly the vessel can be found immediately proximal to the origin of the left subclavian artery.

safer if precautions are taken, including aggressive preoperative hydration, preprocedural treatment with certain medications (i.e., acetylcysteine), significantly limitation of the amount of iodinated contrast, or the use of non-nephrotoxic contrast agents (e.g., gadolinium). The latter are incapable of opacifying the vessels to the same degree that iodinated contrast agents do, but they can be mixed with regular contrast to minimize the danger to renal function.

Another relative contraindication for cerebral angiography is allergy to iodinated contrast agents. However, this can also be overcome relatively easily by premedication of the patient with steroids and histamine receptor blockers. Finally, a less common concern is that of patients with dysplastic vessels (e.g., Marfan syndrome). The fact that their vessels do not have normal arterial walls suggests an increased risk for catheter- or wire-induced injury. In this particular type of patient, the indications and contraindications of cerebral angiography need to be carefully weighed to decide the importance of carrying out the procedure.

Limitations of Angiography

As noted earlier, cerebral angiography has been traditionally considered the gold standard by which other diagnostic vascular techniques are measured. Although a discussion of all imaging techniques is beyond the scope of this chapter, it is important to understand that angiography provides primarily a lumenographic image of the vessel and that any information about vascular structure must be inferred. However, experienced angiographers will also admit that there is a certain dynamic aspect to angiography, which is typically not displayed in the static images but that relates to the flow of contrast as it is visualized during the catheterization procedure.

One particular aspect of angiography relates to the need in certain populations to discriminate the percentage of stenosis in a pathological vessel as part of assessing the need for intervention. In fact, the results of the North American Symptomatic Carotid Endarterectomy (NASCET) study were based on angiographic calculations of the percentage of carotid stenosis. The author has taken a rather skeptical approach to this whole subject because the introduction of digital subtraction technology to produce angiographic images carries with it the feasibility of changing images during postprocessing. As such, it is possible to manipulate the brightness and contrast of an image and change the measured percentage of stenosis of the vessel by as much as 10% to 15%. Furthermore, it is imperative to note that the percentage of stenosis measured may also vary depending on the catheters used and magnification of the image being studied. From this point of view, vessels that are being considered for intervention consistently have a higher degree of stenosis when measured in the diagnostic images (following injection through a small-bore diagnostic catheter) than during the intervention. The latter includes images obtained by injecting through a large -bore interventional guide catheter, allowing for a larger volume of contrast, and using larger magnification.

In general, and on the basis of what has been explained, the author has largely abandoned the use of percentage of stenosis in daily practice, reverting to a more qualitative nomenclature (see Fig. 31.6). The critics may see this as a retrograde move from the more popular, and "scientifically sound," quantitative methodology. However, inaccurate quantification is not any better than reasonable qualification. The typical internal carotid artery measures approximately 5 mm in diameter. Thus, a 10% error in quantification corresponds to 0.5 mm, a magnitude that cannot be reliably resolved by the human eye. The problem becomes compounded in smaller vessels, particularly when postprocedural brightness and contrast manipulations are used to better visualize the arteries. In addition, we have found that the lack of a unified method for measuring vascular stenoses by practitioners leads to significant confusion among patients, particularly when numbers are quoted across diagnostic platforms (e.g., angiography versus ultrasound).

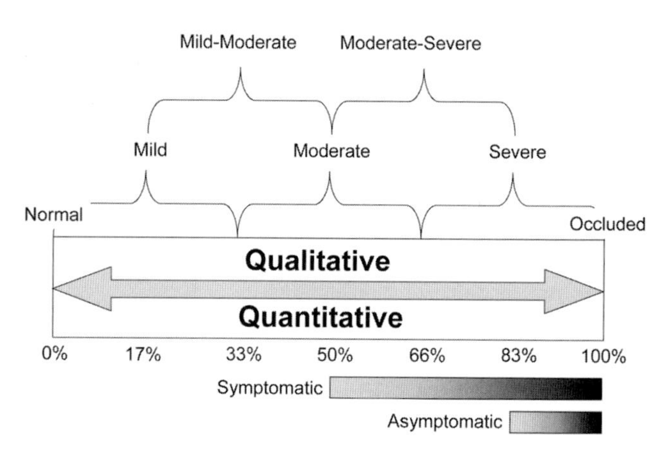

FIGURE 31.6. Schematic comparison of both qualitative and quantitative methods for describing arterial stenoses.

Clinical Applications of Cerebral Angiography

The consideration to undertake diagnostic cerebral angiography in a stroke patient typically arises after noninvasive testing has suggested the presence of an underlying pathology that may require one or another form of intervention. Even for cerebral aneurysms, at the present time, computed tomographic angiography (CTA) has largely replaced cerebral angiography as the initial test of choice. From this point of view, several scenarios must be considered when thinking about CTA as the next diagnostic step (see Table 31.1):

Scenario 1

A lesion is not clearly defined and therefore it is difficult to choose the optimal treatment. This represents one of the most common situations encountered in daily practice. Here, the angiogram must address two separate issues: lesion definition and optimal therapy. Patients in this scenario are likely to have been evaluated by one or more noninvasive imaging techniques, and the results are conflictive or incongruent. Angiography becomes the procedure to clearly

TABLE 33.1 Scenarios that Indicate Cerebral Angiography

	Lesion Definition	Optimal Treatment	Treatment Approach
Scenario 1	?	?	?
Scenario 2	✓	?	?
Scenario 3	✓	✓	?

See text for definitions of each scenario.

define the lesion and decide what form of therapy to implement. An interesting example of this type of scenario is found in patient with lateral medullary ischemia ipsilateral to a nondominant vertebral artery. Typically, ultrasound shows antegrade flow with decreased velocities in the vertebral artery, while magnetic resonance angiography (MRA) shows decreased vertebral signal but cannot resolve whether the vessel is occluded or highly stenotic. At this time one could argue in favor of the use of CTA. However, it would be difficult to decide which segment of the vertebral artery to image, and if the entire vessel is to be imaged, the amount of contrast may be prohibitive. Furthermore, CTA would provide little or no information about interventional feasibility. Finally, if it is determined that intervention is indicated, yet another procedure would be needed: angiography! And so it is concluded that angiography was probably the best way to proceed to begin with, answering all issues relevant to such clinical situation.

A variant of this scenario is the application of cerebral angiography during the emergent treatment of acute stroke. These patients, usually very ill, cannot be evaluated extensively using noninvasive imaging techniques. Thus, their suspected lesion is not as well defined as one would prefer, but in the interest of time, angiography must be carried out under somewhat hasty conditions so treatment can be expedited. Typically, the operator does not really know what the best treatment will be until the angiogram is completed and a better definition of the lesion exists.

Scenario 2

A lesion is well defined but its optimal treatment is uncertain. This situation arises when a lesion that has been reasonably well defined by noninvasive testing requires further investigation to decide about an optimal management strategy. For example, given a symptomatic patient in whom both ultrasound and MRA suggest the presence of a carotid plaque that moderately narrows the lumen, the decision to revascularize rests on the demonstration of at least a 50% diameter stenosis using the NASCET method. Such information can only be acquired using angiography. In this case, should the degree of stenosis be <50%, the patient's treatment would be eminently medical. In addition to supporting the choice of therapeutic strategy, angiography would also provide critical information that can be used for surveillance during the follow-up period, especially if a change in treatment strategy is eventually considered.

Scenario 3

A lesion is well defined, its optimal treatment is certain, but the approach to this treatment is uncertain. This scenario is slightly different, as it involves a lesion that is well defined and whose optimal treatment is known, but for which angiography can provide necessary tactical information about the best therapeutic approach. This is true for most lesions to be treated endovascularly, since issues of access to the target vessel, collateral patterns under specific circumstances, and choices of interventional equipment rest on angiographic knowledge of the vascular environment of the patient. This is another reason for performing diagnostic angiograms rather than of relying on those performed by others. An example of this situation relates to planning endovascular treatment for an arteriovenous malformation (AVM). In these cases, angiography allows a better definition of the vascular compartments of the AVM, its feeding pedicle, and the flow–pressure relationship within the anomaly.

PRACTICAL RECOMMENDATIONS

Once the stroke patient has been studied using noninvasive testing (see Chapter 22) and one of the scenarios described in this chapter has been identified, a decision to proceed with diagnostic angiography must be made. The next step for practitioners involves an honest and dispassionate assessment of the resources and assets available in their institution. Just as surgeons and interventionists must document a competitively low complication rate, so do angiographers. At present, the author's practice performs approximately 400 angiograms per year, a number that allows for skills maintenance and optimization of outcomes. The angiographic equipment must be state-of-the-art, and the catheterization laboratory personnel conversant with the management of neurology patients. If an interventional procedure is contemplated, angiography should not be carried out unless the intervention can also be completed in the same institution. In fact, unless all of these issues are well covered, the patient should be referred to an institution that meets all of these criteria.

Once the results of the noninvasive tests are examined and a decision to proceed with angiography is made, the patient needs to be hydrated aggressively to avoid any complications from the procedure. In particular, this is important when patients are kept without oral intake for many hours prior to the procedure as is commonly done. We recommend the use of isotonic crystalloid (0.9% sodium chloride) at rates of 60 to 100 mL per hour depending on the patient's underlying cardiovascular reserve. Unless there is a contraindication, it is recommended that these patients be pretreated with both aspirin and clopidogrel (Plavix), particularly if there is a possibility that the procedure will be converted into an intervention. Typically, when time permits, patients are started on 75 mg per day of clopidogrel for at least 4 days prior to the procedure. When the procedure is to be carried out immediately, or within a few hours, a loading dose of 375 mg of clopidogrel will suffice. Patients with renal dysfunction at baseline should receive, in addition to the hydration protocol noted here, 600 mg of acetylcysteine (Mucomyst) twice a day for 2 days, starting the day before the procedure. Finally, patients with history of iodinated contrast allergy should receive 60 mg of prednisone daily for at least 2 days before the procedure if possible. Regardless, these patients are routinely treated with 125 mg of methylprednisolone (Solu-Medrol) PLUS 20 mg of famotidine (Pepcid) PLUS 12.5 mg of diphenhydramine (Benadryl) intravenous immediately before the procedure.

Although the specifics of the procedure are within the purview of the operator, it is imperative that the technique maintain focus on the questions that need clinical answers and that every aspect of it is subordinate to those clinical questions. This cannot be overemphasized, as it will allow the operator to construct a procedural blueprint that is based on necessity and not curiosity. Furthermore, the use of predetermined catheterization sequences as outlined in this chapter is strongly recommended, particularly since they have led to significantly good outcomes in the past.

Once the procedure is completed, the care of the patient requires additional hydration and extra attention to the possibility of delayed complications. Several of these warrant further discussion. The first is the development of pseudoaneurysms at the arteriotomy site, a complication that has become less common in the era of closure devices. Pseudoaneurysms are suspected when the patient complains of unusually severe pain at the arteriotomy site and can often be diagnosed at the bedside by the auscultation of a femoral bruit that had not previously been present. At the first sign of the possibility of a postprocedural femoral pseudoaneurysm, color Doppler ultrasound should be used to identify and measure it. In most cases, direct pressure of the pseudoaneurysm under ultrasound guidance results in its obliteration. Such a maneuver can be painful to the patient, and parenteral analgesics may need to be administered to be able to carry it out. If the pseudoaneurysm does not respond to external compression, an alternative approach is to inject it with thrombin under ultrasound guidance. This results in obliteration of nearly all aneurysms. It is uncommon to have to refer a patient to surgical repair of a femoral pseudoaneurysm.

Another complication of the arteriotomy site is acute closure with limb ischemia. This is most common in patients with preexisting aortofemoral grafts, whose sheath removal is followed by extended manual compression. The patient typically complains of pain in the affected limb, which feels cold and pulseless. This situation represents a vascular emergency and requires prompt surgical intervention. In less dramatic cases, distal embolization to feet and toes are also observed infrequently. These patients generally require medical treatment, reserving surgical intervention for those who require toe amputation if the process does not improve. It has been found to be useful, on occasion, to apply nitroglycerin ointment to the skin surrounding the area of embolism, in an attempt to improve collateral flow to the toe. Its effect is somewhat unpredictable.

Finally, the most dreaded delayed complication of angiography is retroperitoneal hematoma. This occurs when the femoral artery is inadvertedly accessed higher than the inguinal ligament, leading to arterial bleeding into the retroperitoneal space following sheath removal. These patients can become critically ill within a short period and require aggressive diagnosis and treatment. The first sign may be an ill-defined discomfort or pain in the ipsilateral flank. However, we have seen patients whose first manifestation of a retroperitoneal hematoma is the development of frank hypovolemic shock. The diagnosis and management of these patients depends on their hemodynamic stability, and it is imperative that we take this into account when deciding how to proceed. The patient who is suspected of having a retroperitoneal hematoma on the basis of pain or drop in hematocrit, but whose vital signs are stable, can be sent for abdominal CT, which provides the diagnosis in all instances. Care must be exercised about not sending a hemodynamically unstable patient to CT, at least until measures of hemodynamic support have been instituted. The first aid of the unstable patient involves (a) starting isotonic crystalloid resuscitation (i.e., patients with hemorrhagic shock invariably have a crystalloid deficit), (b) measuring hematocrit plus type and crossing the patient for at least four units of blood, and (c) using plasma expanders if necessary (e.g., 5% to 25% albumin). Vasopressors should be used only after volume replacement has begun, and the decision to hold any ongoing parenteral antithrombotic or thrombolytic agents must be carefully considered on the basis of appropriate benefit:risk assessment. Vascular surgery consultation must not be delayed, particularly in the hemodynamically unstable patient who is likely to require surgical intervention.

SELECTED REFERENCES

Brook AL, Mirsky DM, Bello JA. Stroke prevention: carotid intervention based on catheter angiography versus noninvasive vascular imaging. *Tech Vasc Interv Radiol* 2004;7(4):196–201.

Bull JW, Marshall J, Shaw DA. Cerebral angiography in the diagnosis of the acute stroke. *Lancet* 1960;1:562–565.

Bunt TJ, Cropper L. The role of complete cerebral angiography in the evaluation of patients with prior stroke. *Am Surg* 1987;53(2):77–79.

Burger IM, Murphy KJ, Jordan LC, et al. Safety of cerebral digital subtraction angiography in children: complication rate analysis in 241 consecutive diagnostic angiograms. *Stroke* 2006;37(10):2535–2539.

Caplan LR, Wolpert SM. Angiography in patients with occlusive cerebrovascular disease: views of a stroke neurologist and neuroradiologist. *Am J Neuroradiol* 1991;12(4):593–601.

Ganesan V, Savvy L, Chong WK, et al. Conventional cerebral angiography in children with ischemic stroke. *Pediatr Neurol* 1999;20(1):38–42.

Gerraty RP, Bowser DN, Infeld B, et al. Microemboli during carotid angiography. Association with stroke risk factors or subsequent magnetic resonance imaging changes? *Stroke* 1996;27(9):1543–1547.

Johnson AC. Stroke with special reference to cerebral angiography. *Rocky Mt Med J* 1958;55(5):57 passim.

Kassem-Moussa H, Graffagnino C. Nonocclusion and spontaneous recanalization rates in acute ischemic stroke: a review of cerebral angiography studies. *Arch Neurol* 2002;59(12):1870–1873.

Kuhn RA. Importance of accurate diagnosis by cerebral angiography in cases of stroke. *J Am Med Assoc* 1959;169(16):1867–1875.

Kuhn RA. The revolution produced by cerebral angiography in management of the patient with stroke. *J Med Soc N J* 1959;56(2):68–75.

Leffers AM, Wagner A. Neurologic complications of cerebral angiography. A retrospective study of complication rate and patient risk factors. *Acta Radiol* 2000;41(3):204–210.

Malik GK, Chhabra DK, Shukla R, et al., The pediatric stroke: a prospective study of cerebral angiography. *Indian J Pediatr* 1981;48(391):169–174.

Ohaegbulam SC. The value of angiography in the management of stroke. *Afr J Med Med Sci* 1981;10(1–2):29–32.

Soderman M, Bystam J. Cerebral air emboli from angiography in a patient with stroke. A case report. *Acta Radiol* 2001;42(2):140–143.

Vigman MP, Byrne RJ. Cerebral complications of angiography for transient ischemia and stroke. *Neurology* 1980;30(9):1018–1019.

CRITICAL PATHWAY
Catheterization Sequence

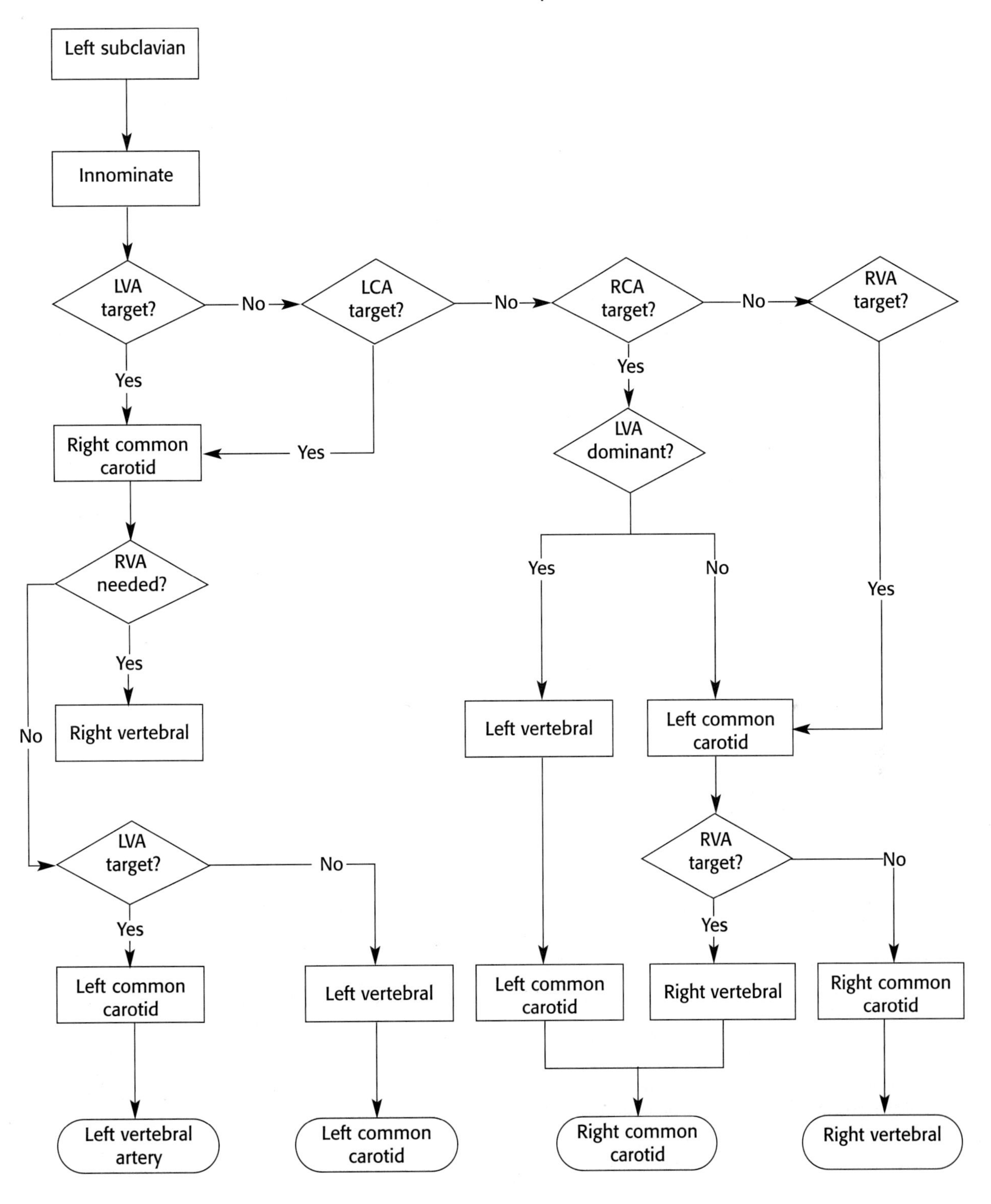

LVA, left vertebral artery; LCA, left carotid artery; RCA, right carotid artery; RVA, right vertebral artery.

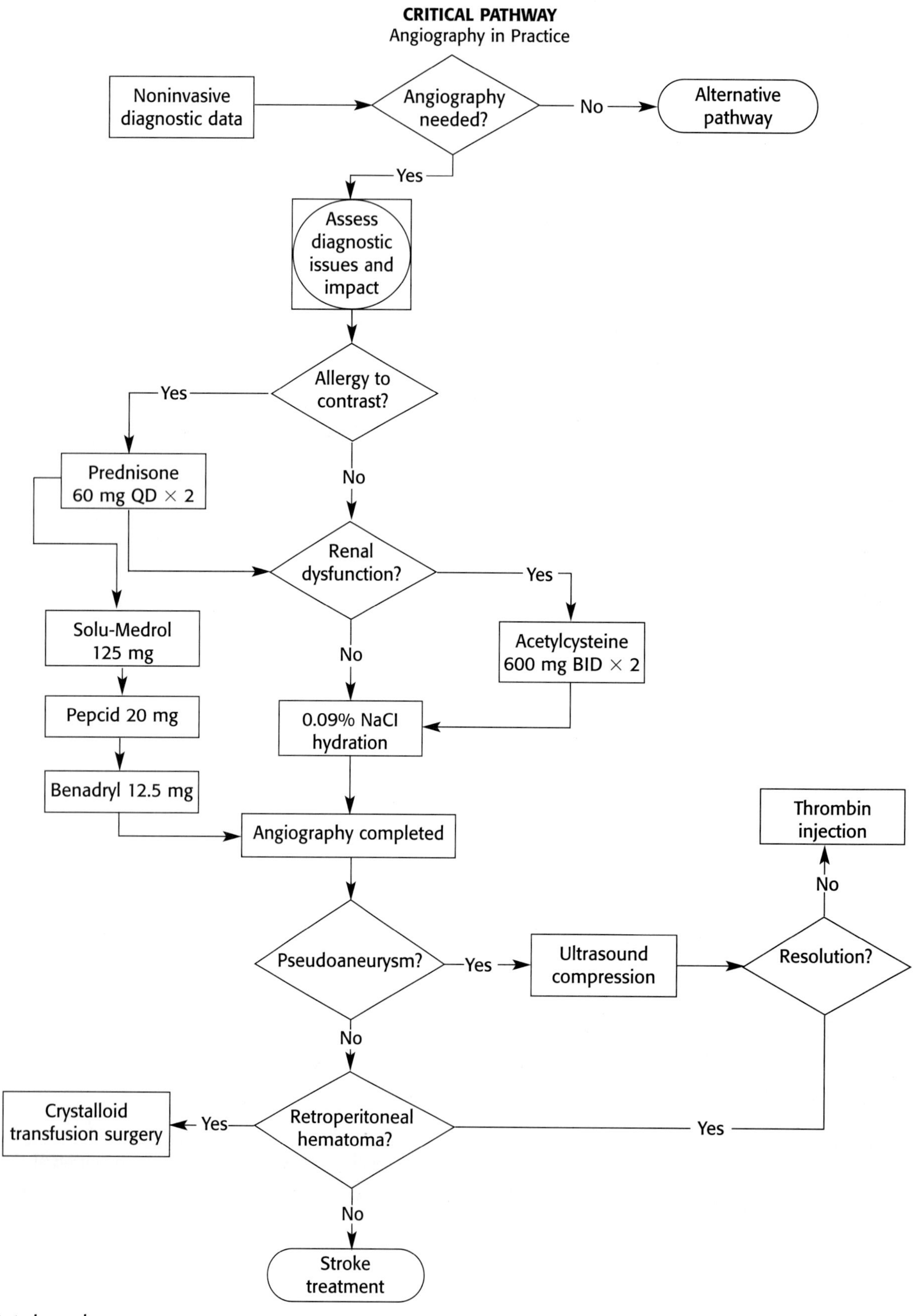

BID, twice a day.

CHAPTER

32 Management of Cerebral Edema after Stroke

CHAD M. MILLER AND MARC MALKOFF

OBJECTIVES

- What role does edema play in secondary injury after stroke?
- What are the predictors for malignant edema?
- What medical therapies are available for the treatment of stroke-related edema?
- What is the role for hemicraniectomy and duraplasty in the treatment of malignant edema?

Treatments of acute stoke traditionally fall into two categories: efforts directed toward the goals of revascularization and subsequent management designed to avoid secondary injury. Secondary injury results in further deterioration after the acute event and is attributable to additional ischemia, cerebral-free radical production, medical complications, fever, systemic metabolic disturbances, edema, mass effect, and other causes. This chapter outlines the contribution of cerebral edema to secondary injury and reviews the rationale and methodology associated with common treatments aimed at limiting this process.

BACKGROUND AND RATIONALE

The healthy brain maintains proper homeostasis among the intracellular, interstitial, and intravascular fluid compartments. During ischemia, cellular ion channels are no longer able to maintain this balance and cellular swelling and death ensues. This early rise in intracellular fluid volume is termed *cytotoxic edema*. Restriction of interstitial flow among the swollen cells accounts for the abnormalities observed on diffusion-weighted magnetic resonance images (DW-MRIs). Cytotoxic edema is quite common in cerebral ischemia and is the principal disturbance in brain volume state. However, eventual breakdown of the blood–brain barrier with subsequent increase in intracellular fluid volume does occur in the later stages of injury. This second type of edema is aptly named *vasogenic edema*, and edematous complications after stroke are likely a result of both of these forms of edema.

The time course of edema in stroke is variable but typically begins within the first 24 hours, peaking around 72 hours after the ictus. Preservation or infarction of the penumbral region likely affects the rate and extent of edema progression. While most brain edema resolves within the first week, massive and secondary infarction can prolong the typical course of resolution. The consequences of edema after stroke are variable. Most swelling is asymptomatic or produces only a transient headache, while in other patients vascular compression, hydrocephalus, and herniation syndromes may result. The initial size and location of the infarct, as well as the amount of preceding brain atrophy, determine the effect of the edema.

A particular type of swelling, termed *malignant edema*, deserves special consideration. Malignant edema complicates 10% of large hemispheric infarcts and is associated with disproportionate morbidity and mortality. Malignant edema commonly occurs after embolic infarcts, carotid dissections, and acute large vessel occlusions, presumably when insufficient time exists for the development of collateral perfusion. The mortality rate for this stroke subset is 78% to 80%, underscoring the importance of predicting the onset of this complication and pursuit of aggressive treatment. While young full brains would appear to be most intolerant of significant edema, age of <45 years is associated with improved survival.All severities of edema warrant consideration in poststroke care; however, identification of patients who are at risk for a malignant course merits special consideration. Patients with a history of hypertension or heart failure, an elevated white blood cell count at admission, higher presenting National Institute of Health Stroke Scale (NIHSS) scores, younger age, or nausea and vomiting within the first 24 hours of onset are particularly at risk for malignant edema. Multiple radiographic markers may also be predictive for extensive swelling. These include an acute DWI (6 hour) lesion >145 cm^3, attenuated corticomedullary contrast on the initial head computed tomography (CT) scan, and severe perfusion deficits involving greater than half of the middle cerebral artery (MCA) distribution on multiphasic helical CT scans. In addition, larger apparent diffusion coefficient (ADC) volumes with time-to-peak (TTP) $>+4$ seconds, smaller TTP/ADC ratios, and evidence of infarct in multiple vascular territories are associated with progression to malignant edema. In one cohort of 37 patients with proximal vessel occlusion and acute MCA infarction, 11 patients developed malignant edema. Kucinski et al. have reported that identification of a carotid T-occlusion is a better predictor of outcome than a large cortical hypodensity, supporting the belief that mechanism of stroke is closely tied to clinical course (see Table 32.1).

TABLE 32.1 Predictors of Malignant Brain Edema

Predictors of Malignant Brain Edema
Age <45 y
Nausea and vomiting present within first 24 h
Early hypodensity seen on initial CT scan
Attenuated corticomedullary contrast
Acute DWI lesion >145 cm^3
Proximal vessel occlusion
History of heart failure or hypertension
Elevated white blood cell count on admission
CT hypodensity >50% of MCA distribution
Strokes in multiple vascular territories

CT, computed tomography; DWI, diffusion-weighted MRI images; MCA, middle cerebral artery.

Because the course of edema after stroke can be predicted, monitoring of the stroke patient should allow for appropriate identification of those at risk for additional injury. The foundation of monitoring in the stroke care unit is physical assessment. Identification of a new deficit, worsening of a prior deficit, or deterioration in level of alertness should prompt radiographic evaluation with a CT scan. Unfortunately, changes in the physical examination are often a late sign of impending injury. The premise of neuromonitoring is that brain at risk can be identified earlier and appropriate interventions can be made. Positron emission tomography (PET) scans and cerebral microdialysis (MD) have been used to predict the onset of malignant edema. Reductions in penumbral size and cerebral blood flow within the ischemic core have been identified in those patients progressing to malignant edema. Similarly, a multitude of neurochemical disturbances correlate with progressive edema, though the timing of these changes makes them more correlative than predictive. Transcranial ultrasound has been used to follow midline shift, a parameter strongly correlated with risk of uncal herniation. The role of other devices, such as brain tissue oxygen monitors, is currently being defined. Intracranial pressure (ICP) monitoring after massive stroke has become a common practice in many units. However, elevation of ICP is often a late event or rather herniation occurs related to compartmental pressure discrepancies as opposed to frank ICP elevations. Further research is needed to clarify the utility of each monitor for use in observing progressive edema. Regardless of these uncertainties, changes in the patient's condition necessitate prompt re-evaluation and a noncontrast head CT. In addition to brain edema, hemorrhagic transformation, hydrocephalus, and other changes may require specific and unanticipated interventions (see Fig. 32.1).

CLINICAL APPLICATIONS AND METHODOLOGY

Many therapies exist for the treatment of cerebral edema after stroke. This would imply that the management of edema is a well-defined and evidence-based process. In truth, few of the strategies for combating the untoward effects of brain edema have undergone stringent clinical investigation in humans. Therefore, each of the following treatments will be discussed with an emphasis on that data that exists, as well as commonly accepted treatment protocols. The following approach will also make the assumption that edema that is sufficient to require management exists, recognizing that some of these therapies have variable effects on the goal of optimizing cerebral perfusion.

The first step in treatment of cerebral edema should be moderate elevation of the head of the patient's bed. A maneuver as simple as raising a patient's head to 30 degrees has significant and competing effects on venous drainage, ICP, and cerebral perfusion.

A

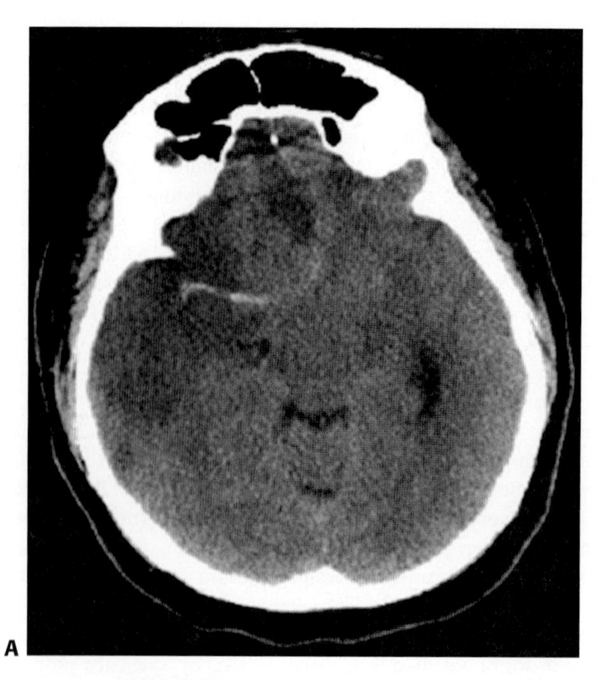

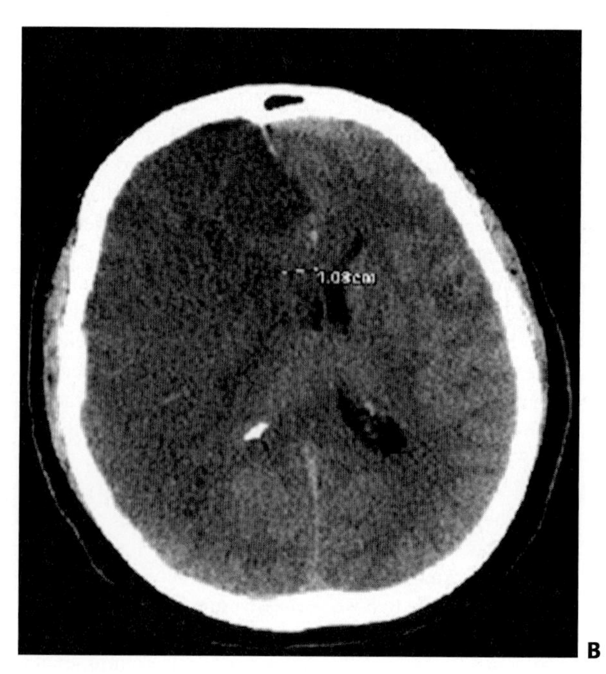

B

FIGURE 32.1. Noncontrasted head computed tomographic (CT) demonstrating massive right hemispheric infarct, hyperdense middle cerebral artery (MCA) sign, and midline shift 24 hours after right carotid occlusion.

The net effect, in a patient with substantial edema, favors elevation with close attention paid to the maintenance of cerebral perfusion pressures.

Hyperventilation is often used to treat critical and acute elevations in ICP. Increases in respiratory rate or tidal volume induce hyperventilation and lowering of serum CO_2 levels. Hypocarbia causes cerebral vasoconstriction with resultant reduction in intracranial blood volume and lowered ICP. Though this maneuver can occur at the expense of cerebral perfusion, most stroke and critical care experts believe that limiting hyperventilation to a CO_2 of 30 mm Hg avoids concerns for deleterious vasoconstriction. While hyperventilation has profound effects on reducing ICP in stroke, the ultimate effect on patient outcome has not been studied. The lasting effects of this therapy are variable but ultimately limited. Hyperventilation is a maneuver designed to buy time for more definitive treatments.

Hyperosmolar therapy attempts to reduce edema by creating an osmolar gradient between the intravascular and intracellular spaces. Water then equilibrates between these compartments to deplete the total brain water volume. The effectiveness of this physiological strategy is contingent on the maintenance of an intact blood brain barrier. Hypertonic saline, mannitol, and glycerol are the most commonly used hyperosmolar agents.

The interest in hypertonic NaCl in stroke was derived from its efficacy in small-volume resuscitation of hypovolemic shock. Improvements in cardiac output, intravascular volume, systemic blood pressure, and microvascular perfusion are all seen after the administration of hypertonic saline. The concentration of saline used and the rate of delivery vary among physicians. Some of the most convincing data for the use of hypertonic saline in stroke comes from the studies of Schwarz et al., who administered a 75 mL 10% saline bolus to stroke patients with elevated ICPs refractory to mannitol treatment. Effective reduction of ICP occurred in all patients, was maximal at the end of the infusion, and lasted for up to 4 hours. Other physicians prefer constant infusions of more dilute NaCl solutions to minimize excessive serum sodium elevations. The optimal dose and infusion rate of hypertonic saline to minimize edema after stroke will require additional research.

Mannitol is an attractive agent to treat stroke-related edema due to its multiple potential mechanisms of action. Mannitol is thought to reduce brain water volume, improve red blood cell rheology, act as a cellular neuroprotectant and free radical scavenger, and reduce production of cerebrospinal fluid. Mannitol has been shown to effectively reduce high ICP after stroke; however, its effect on outcome and the duration of effect are not well established. Treatment may be complicated by hypovolemia and electrolyte disturbance if each of these parameters is not monitored carefully. There is concern of nephrotoxicity with prolonged use and widespread belief that dosing should be stopped when serum osmolarity exceeds 320 mOsm per kg. This caveat is not supported by the literature. Critics of mannitol's use believe that it preferentially shrinks the healthy brain and may actually potentiate midline shift in patients at risk. While Diringer et al. have shown that the reduction in brain volume is probably greatest in the hemisphere with a preserved blood–brain barrier, worsening of midline shift or neurological deterioration does not appear to occur.

The combination of intravenous albumin followed by furosemide is also a treatment option for cerebral edema. Double-blind, placebo-controlled trials are again lacking but there is considerable clinical evidence that this combination may improve cerebral edema. The albumin and lasix combination is typically initiated when significant cerebral edema is identified by neuroimaging and continued until the edema has at least stabilized. The albumin is then slowly tapered off over several days.

Glycerol is a hyperosmolar agent less commonly used in the United States. It may be given enterally or intravenously and may be associated with volume overload, hemolysis, lactic acidosis, and electrolyte disturbance. Hemolysis can usually be minimized by concomitant infusion of solutions containing fructose. Sakamaki et al have published their success in infusing a 300 mL solution of 10% glycerol and 5% fructose over 2 hours (see Table 32.2).

Hypothermia is an attractive treatment for malignant edema given its success as a neuroprotectant for patients having cardiac arrest. Hypothermia is known to preserve the blood brain barrier, decrease the generation of free radicals and release of excitatory amino acids, reduce cerebral metabolism, and blunt the injurious inflammatory cascade. The adverse effect of hyperthermia on infarct volume has led to a series of animal and human studies evaluating variable degrees of induced hypothermia. The success demonstrated in animal studies has not always translated to human research, particularly because of the intolerability of the treatment and complicating side effects. Impressive reductions in ICP can be achieved safely with moderate surface cooling. Complications of pneumonia and hypokalemia as well as concern for rebound edema during rewarming are among the greatest obstacles for this therapy. Numerous mechanisms for rapid cooling now exist and include cool air blankets, intravascular catheters, topical alcohol rubs, ice water nasogastric lavages, room temperature intravenous boluses, and ice packs. Shivering severely limits the effectiveness of cooling and may require treatment with meperidine or neuromuscular blockers in extreme cases.

Corticosteroids would appear to benefit patients with malignant edema, particularly in the latter stages when a significant component of swelling may be vasogenic in origin. Despite this hope, level 1 evidence states that corticosteroids do not reduce cerebral edema after stroke or improve stroke outcome. Use of corticosteroids is fraught with complications such as hyperglycemia and immunosuppression, which may mask beneficial effects of this therapy. Future studies that account for these side effects may return corticosteroids to the list of therapeutic options for late-onset edema.

The potential for edema to cause secondary injury is related to its propensity to cause mass effect. For this reason, surgical therapies aimed at relieving pressure and allowing outward herniation of brain tissue have attracted interest. Steiner et al. have reported their experience with hemicraniectomy and duraplasty for the treatment of malignant edema after stroke. Mortality was decreased from

TABLE 32.2 Treatment Options for Brain Edema After Stroke

Treatment Options
Adjustment of head position
Hyperventilation
Hyperosmolar therapy
Hypertonic saline
Mannitol
Glycerol
Induced hypothermia
Hemicraniectomy and duraplasty
Sedation

76% in patients treated medically to 32% in those treated surgically. The surgery was performed when patients demonstrated evidence of neurological worsening. Half of their subjects had Barthel indices >75 and most subjects were retrospectively pleased with their decision to have undergone surgery. The Heidelberg group later published data showing that a reduction of mean operative time, from 39 to 21 hours after stroke, further reduced mortality to 16%. Of the 11 patients enrolled with dominant hemisphere strokes, none were left with global aphasia. Mori et al. published similar data retrospectively comparing three groups of patients with malignant edema. Subjects treated conservatively were compared with those who underwent surgery after clinical worsening and an additional cohort deemed to be at risk but who underwent an early operation. The 1- and 6-month mortalities for the early surgery group were superior and this subset enjoyed improved scores on the Barthel index and Glasgow Outcome Scale, compared to the conservatively managed cohort. Success in all of these studies was greatly influenced by adequate hemicraniectomy size and an early decision to undergo surgery. The available data stimulate hope that hemicraniectomy with duraplasty may improve outcome and survival, though data on the value of this treatment awaits completion of a randomized study. Many neurosurgeons believe that temporal lobectomy and removal of infracted tissue may add benefit to hemicraniectomy and duraplasty. (see Fig. 32.2).

Another treatment used to control elevated ICP related to ischemic edema is sedation. Sedation is thought to lower ICP by decreasing cerebral metabolic demand and subsequent blood flow. There is a paucity of data describing the success of sedative medications for this purpose. Schwab et al reported that only 5 of their 60 patients treated with thiopental for malignant edema survived. One quarter of the patients suffered significant side effects related to the treatment. Treatment with sedatives is often one of the last therapies attempted for refractory edema. This fact may account for its poor efficacy.

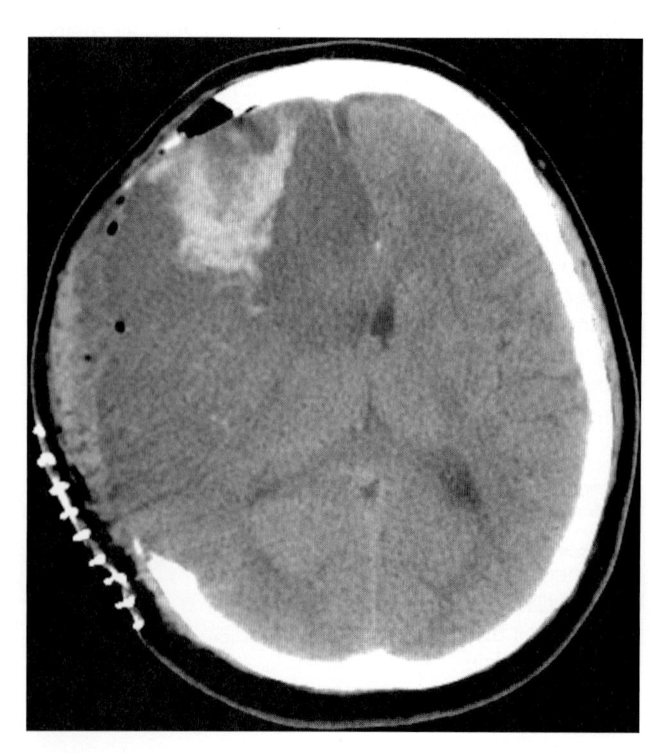

FIGURE 32.2. Noncontrast head computed tomography (CT) demonstrating hemicraniectomy and duraplasty complicated by reperfusion hemorrhage of a right hemispheric infarct.

Control of pain and agitation is crucial in the patient with malignant stroke edema. Likewise, monitoring for complications known to exacerbate edema, such as nonconvulsive status epilepticus, should occur.

PRACTICAL RECOMMENDATIONS

The lack of randomized data on the treatment of stroke-related edema has forced physicians to provide care based on current knowledge gathered largely from personal experience, expert opinion, and retrospective data. Among the initial challenges facing physicians is determination of those patients likely to progress to malignant edema. The absence or presence of the previously discussed predictors should guide either a watchful or aggressive course of care (Table 32.1). If marked edema and risk factors for development of edema are absent, a conservative course of observation should ensue. Avoidance of hyponatremia to minimize cerebral edema is not supported by the literature, but makes practical sense and probably carries minimal risks. Rapid deterioration of the patient is often marked by impaired alertness, new focal signs, and finally, pupillary asymmetry. This progression heralds impending herniation and constitutes a neurological emergency. The patient's head of bed should be raised to 30 degrees to lessen ICP. The patient should be intubated to secure an oral airway and to allow for hyperventilation to a CO_2 goal of approximately 30 mm Hg. A 1 g per kg mannitol bolus should be given immediately and a 3% NaCl infusion should be started at 25 mL per hour. Because, most of these measures are temporizing, neurosurgical consultation should be sought for consideration of prompt hemicraniectomy and duraplasty.

Care of the currently stable patient at risk for deterioration proves to be more uncertain. The authors' practice is to elevate the head of bed to 30 degrees and begin a hypertonic saline infusion with a goal sodium in excess of 140 mmol per L. Saline is chosen as the preferred hyperosmolar agent because of its safety profile and reduced risk of systemic dehydration. Moderate hypothermia is then achieved through the use of surface cooling measures or intravascular cooling devices. This patient requires attentive hourly neurological assessments. This is best achieved in a dedicated neurointensive care unit. Daily head CTs are obtained and additional scans are indicated for any change in examination. Central venous pressure monitoring is appropriate to ensure maintenance of adequate volume state. The neurosurgical consultant should be made aware that the patient is at risk for requiring emergent surgical decompression. The benefits of additional monitoring with brain tissue oxygen probes or cerebral MD await further study. A patient demonstrating massive progressive edema on serial scans despite clinical stability is likely to eventually deteriorate. Considering the available data on the timing of hemicraniectomy, a patient destined to deteriorate would derive greater benefit from an early surgery. Future decision making on these difficult issues will be facilitated by the results of Hemicraniectomy and Durotomy on Deterioration from Infarction Related Swelling Trial (HeADDFIRST). While it is hoped that hemicraniectomy and duraplasty may demonstrate survival and outcome benefit, family and patient counseling should stress that the outcomes for this procedure are still uncertain (see Critical Pathway).

The recognition and prompt treatment of cerebral edema after stroke is crucial to minimize clinical deterioration related to secondary injury. Multiple promising treatments exist, though all balance uncertain effectiveness with varying levels of therapeutic risk. Current research of these therapies has laid the groundwork for larger randomized prospective trials to be completed. Until the results of these trials are known, the clinical significance of cerebral edema demands that physicians manage aggressively on the basis of the best available data.

SELECTED REFERENCES

Abou-Chebl A, DeGeorgia MA, Andrefsky JC, et al. Technical refinements and drawbacks of a surface cooling technique for the treatment of severe acute ischemic stroke. *Neurocrit Care* 2004;1(2):131–143.

Bauer RB, Tellez H. Dexamethasone as treatment in cerebrovascular disease, 2: a controlled study in acute cerebral infarction. *Stroke* 1973;4: 547–555.

Broderick JP, Hacke W. Treatment of acute ischemic stroke: Part II: neuroprotection and medical management. *Circulation* 2002;106(13): 1736–1740.

Diringer MN, Zazulia AR. Osmotic therapy: fact and fiction. *Neurocrit Care* 2004;1(2):219–233.

Dohmen C, Bosche B, Graf R, et al. Prediction of malignant course in MCA infarction by PET and microdialysis. *Stroke* 2003;34:2152–2158.

Frank JI.Large hemispheric infarction, deterioration, and intracranial pressure. *Neurology* 1995;45(7):1286–1290.

Gerriets T, Stolz E, Konig S, et al. Sonographic monitoring of midline shift in space-occupying stroke: an early outcome predictor. *Stroke* 2001; 32(2):442–447.

Haring HP, Dilitz E, Pallua A, et al. Attenuated corticomedullary contrast: an early cerebral computed tomography sign indicating malignant middle cerebral artery infarction. A case-control study. *Stroke* 1999;30(5): 1076–1082.

Heinsius T, Bogousslavsky J, Van Melle G. Large infarcts in the middle cerebral artery territory: etiology and outcome patterns. *Neurology* 1998;50: 341–350.

Kasner SE, Demchuk AM, Berrouschot J, et al. Predictors of fatal brain edema in massive hemispheric ischemic stroke. *Stroke* 2001;32(9):2117–2123.

Kramer GC, Perron PR, Lindsay DC, et al. Small-volume resuscitation with hypertonic saline dextran solution. *Surgery* 1986;100:239–247.

Kucinski T, Koch C, Grzyska U et al. Kromer l-volume resuscitation with hypertronic saline dextran solution. *Surgery* 1986;100:239–2247.

Kucinski T, Koch C, Grzyska U, et al. The predictive value of early CT and angiography for fatal hemispheric swelling in acute stroke. *American Journal of Neuroradiology* 1998;19(5):839–846.

Mori K, Nakao Y, Yamamoto T, et al. Early external decompressive craniectomy with duraplasty improves functional recovery in patients with massive hemispheric embolic infarction: timing and indication of decompressive surgery for malignant cerebral infarction. *Surg Neurol* 2004;62(5):420–429.

Norris JW. Steroids may have a role in stroke therapy. *Stroke* 2004; 35(1):228–229.

Oppenheim C, Samson Y, Manai R, et al. Prediction of malignant middle cerebral artery infarction by diffusion-weighted imaging. *Stroke* 2000; 31:2175–2181.

Plum F. Brain swelling and cerebral edema in cerebral vascular disease. *Res Publ Assoc Res Nerv Ment Dis* 1961;41:318–348.

Sakamaki M, Igarashi H, Nishiyama Y, et al. Effect of glycerol on ischemic cerebral edema assessed by magnetic resonance imaging. *J Neurol Sci* 2003;209(1–2):69-74.

Schwab S, Spranger M, Schwarz S, et al. Barbiturate coma in severe hemispheric stroke: useful or obsolete? *Neurology* 1997;48(6): 1608–1613.

Schwab S, Steiner T, Aschoff A, et al. Early hemicraniectomy in patients with complete middle cerebral artery infarction. *Stroke* 1998;29(9): 1888–1893.

Schwarz S, Georgiadis D, Aschoff A, et al. Effects of hypertonic (10%) saline in patients with raised intracranial pressure after stroke. *Stroke* 2002;33(1):136–140.

Schwartz S, Schwab S, Bertram M, et al. Effects of hypertonic saline hydroxyethyl starch solution and mannitol in patients with increased intracranial pressure after stroke. *Stroke* 1998;29(8):1550–1555.

Steiner T, Ringleb P, Hacke W. Treatment options for large hemispheric stroke. *Neurology* 2001;57(suppl 2):S61–S68.

Thomalla GJ, Kucinski T, Schoder V, et al. Prediction of malignant middle cerebral artery infarction by early perfusion- and diffusion-weighted magnetic resonance imaging. *Stroke* 2003;34:1892–1900.

Vassar MJ, Fischer RP, O'Brien PE, et al. A multicenter trial for resuscitation of injured patients with 7.5% sodium chloride: the effects of added dextran 70. *Arch Surg* 1993;128:1003–1013.

Videen TO, Zazulia AR, Manno EM, et al. Mannitol bolus preferentially shrinks non-infarcted brain in patients with ischemic stroke. *Neurology* 2001;57(11):2120–2122.

Wijdicks EF, Diringer MN. Middle cerebral artery territory infarction and early brain swelling: progression and effect of age on outcome. *Mayo Clin Proc* 1998;73(9):829–836.

CRITICAL PATHWAY
Approach to the Treatment of Stroke-Related Cerebral Edema

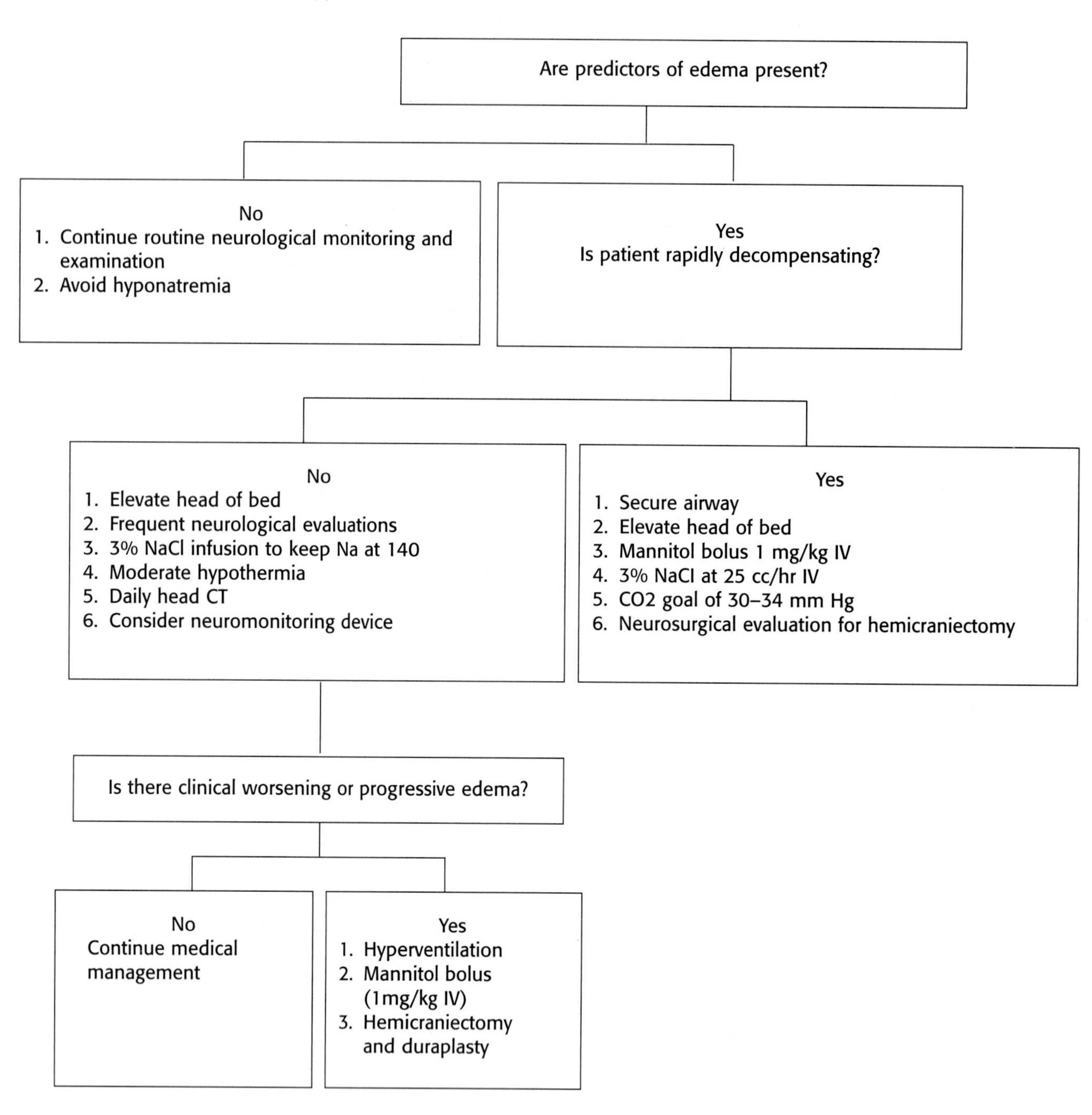

CT, computerized tomography.

CHAPTER

33 Ventilator Management for Critically Ill Stroke Patients

CAMILO R. GOMEZ

OBJECTIVES

- What are the indications for mechanical ventilation in patients with stroke?
- What modes of ventilation are most appropriate for patients with stroke?
- What are the goals and parameters that guide ventilation of stroke patients?
- When and how is hyperventilation a therapeutic tool for patients with stroke?
- When and how is it safe to discontinue mechanical ventilation in patients with stroke?

The typical patient with stroke is unlikely to need mechanical ventilation. Only those individuals with stroke of significant severity to compromise their airway are liable to require mechanical ventilation as part of their overall critical illness support. In fact, patients whose level of consciousness is depressed to the point of rendering them unable to protect their airways are almost invariably in need of intubation and mechanical ventilation. Over the course of years, it has become apparent that strokes of such severity generally lead to worse outcomes, and therefore, it is imperative that the decision to ventilate a patient is made in the context of the overall prognosis and plan of care. Otherwise, treating a patient by means of mechanical ventilation will interfere at times with end-of-life decisions and patients' preferences for long-term life support. The concepts and methodology outlined in this chapter are drawn from more than 25 years of experience with managing critically ill patients, many of whom have had one or another form of stroke as a primary diagnosis. The author's approach takes into consideration not only the primary neurological event but also concurrent medical problems that may influence decisions about the timing, style, and intensity of mechanical ventilation.

BACKGROUND AND RATIONALE

There are two types of clinical problems that influence decisions about instituting mechanical ventilation. First, the neurological event itself may be of such severity that it interferes with airway protection and renders the patient sufficiently unconscious to require mechanical ventilatory support. Furthermore, many of these severe types of stroke are accompanied by evolutional changes (e.g., edema) that lead to increased intracranial pressure (ICP), which can also benefit from mechanical ventilation as a therapeutic tool. The second reason to ventilate stroke patients relates to the presence of comorbid conditions that lead to either hypoxemia or hypercarbia, and result in a threat both to the patient's life and to the outcome of the stroke care. For example, it is not unusual for stroke patients to have congestive heart failure or chronic obstructive pulmonary disease (COPD), which can lead to either pulmonary edema or ventilatory failure, respectively. Still, it is imperative for the practitioner to realize that a decision to ventilate a stroke patient must take into consideration not only the potential benefit in terms of improved oxygenation but also the impact that intubating and ventilating a patient will have on the care of the stroke itself. Along these lines, one must not lose focus of the fact that the reason the patient is in the hospital in the first place may be the stroke, and therefore, one must not compromise the treatment of this by instituting therapeutic maneuvers that are counterproductive.

CLINICAL APPLICATIONS AND METHODOLOGY

Institution of Mechanical Ventilation

The first decision relative to the institution of mechanical ventilation in a critically ill stroke patient (i.e., how much ventilatory support to provide) depends on the objective of the intubation and ventilation. There is a substantial difference between ventilating a patient whose only need is for airway protection and the support of an individual who has concurrent pulmonary problems (e.g., aspiration pneumonia) that induce hypoxemia. The patient who requires ventilation for airway protection is better off when managed by minimal ventilatory support, being allowed to breathe independently as much as possible. Conversely, the patient with a concurrent pulmonary disorder may require more support, and if the severity is sufficiently high, it may be necessary for the providers to completely take over ventilatory function. This is not only a philosophical but also a practical decision, one that influences the modes of ventilation and settings to be used for each patient. The characteristics of the most important modes of ventilation we will discuss are summarized in Table 33.1.

TABLE 33.1 Most Important Modes of Ventilation Available for Use in Stroke Patients

Mode of Ventilation	Primary Setting	Spontaneous Breathing
AC	Provider sets VT to be delivered at a set rate	Every patient's effort triggers the delivery of a breath equal to VT
SIMV	Provider sets VT to be delivered at a set rate	Patient is able to breathe between the set ventilator breaths
PSV	Provider sets the amount of pressure to be delivered with every patient's effort	Patient's effort determines the rate since there is no baseline mandatory rate

AC, Assist-control; VT, tidal volume; SIMV, synchronized intermittent mandatory ventilation; PSV, pressure support ventilation.

At present, general guidelines for mechanical ventilation require for patients to be treated using relatively low tidal volumes (VT), with as low a fraction of inspired oxygen (FIO_2) as possible, and using modes of ventilation that are comfortable without completely overcoming the effort to breathe inherent to every patient. Along these lines, the use of synchronized intermittent mandatory ventilation (SIMV) combined with pressure support ventilation (PSV) is favored as the most useful approach to ventilating stroke patients. The reason for this is simple—these patients do not need more than minimal ventilatory support— and, therefore, it is possible to take advantage of their relatively intact neuropulmonary functional unit. Furthermore, having the patient's spontaneous ventilatory function available for assessment provides another dimension that allows for the bedside evaluation of the nervous system status. As noted earlier, low VT has been the rule across the critical care community for more than a decade. This preference obeys the need to prevent barotrauma (and volutrauma) such as it was previously seen in patients treated with exceedingly large VT . Eight to 10 mL per kg of ideal body weight is recommended at the start, with the respiratory rate set so that the minute ventilation (Ve) equals 100 mL/kg/minute. For example, the ventilator settings of a 70 kg individual can be set to a VT = 560 mL and SIMV = 12, for a Ve = 6,720 mL (i.e., 96 mL/kg/minute). The addition of PSV provides some degree of comfort to the patient, as it facilitates breathing against the resistance of the ventilator circuit tubing.

The patient who also has a concurrent pulmonary disorder that causes hypoxemia or hypercarbia may need to have ventilation instituted differently. These patients have significantly increased work of breathing (WOB), requiring ventilator settings that promote comfort and rest. As such, assist-control (AC) ventilation can be used to provide ventilatory support with the least amount of energy expenditure by the patient. The only limitation of AC as a mode of ventilation relates to patients for whom indiscriminate hyperventilation may be dangerous since this type of ventilation may result in greatly exaggerated Ve when patients trigger the ventilator beyond the set rate, leading to unwanted results.

Maintenance of Mechanical Ventilation

Once the patient is on ventilation, the goal of therapy in most circumstances will be to maintain normocapnia. It is critical to understand that one of the most common myths of the management of neurological patients is that they need to be hyperventilated regardless of the circumstances. This not only represents a deviation from the standard of care and the needs of the patient but also in many cases may become counterproductive. For example, patients with acute cerebral ischemia (an infarction) are likely to have an ischemic penumbra that is kept viable by collateral circulation provided by microarterioles. These patients are at significant risk of being harmed by hyperventilation because of the resulting vasoconstriction of the arterioles with subsequent worsening of the ischemic process, and further ischemic damage. In addition, even patients who have increased ICP, for whom hyperventilation is often a lifesaving maneuver, may be harmed if hyperventilation is used indiscriminately.

Maintenance of normocapnia is the direct result of balancing the ventilator settings to achieve an optimal Ve (i.e., the product of VT and the respiratory rate). As such, most individuals who breathe 100 mL/km/minute will maintain a partial pressure of carbon dioxide (pCO_2) of approximately 40. As the Ve increases, the resulting pCO_2 decreases, and the relationship between these two parameters allows the provider to set the ventilator such that the results are congruent with the objective of treatment. Another important consideration is that a certain amount of Ve is required to provide adequate oxygenation. In patients with intact lungs, this relationship does not represent a problem. However, in individuals who also have lung parenchymal abnormalities or reactive airway pathology, higher Ve than is commonly used may be required to maintain oxygenation. When this presents a problem because of the effect on pCO_2 and hence on cerebral microarteriolar caliber, additional ventilatory settings such as positive end-expiratory pressure (PEEP) maybe used to improve oxygenation without compromising pCO_2 and pH. Once the practitioner is satisfied with the initial ventilator settings, maintenance becomes subordinate to the evolution of the process that led to the need for mechanical ventilation. As such, patients intubated for airway protection will remain ventilated until the cause of their inability to protect their airway is corrected, either naturally or therapeutically. Others, with underlying respiratory problems, will require correction of these before withdrawal of ventilatory support.

An important aspect of ventilatory support maintenance relates to the use of ancillary measures to guide therapy. Arterial blood gases (ABGs) have been the traditional test that allows practitioners to decide how to steer ventilatory changes. However, when one considers the predictability of ABGs relative to the ventilatory settings, we highly recommend the use of pulse oximetry to guide oxygenation and actual Ve (measured by the ventilator) to guide gas exchange in most circumstances. Using this method limits the number of ABGs obtained, which ends up in saving time and money. Clearly, there will be circumstances and occasions when the ABGs will be irreplaceable as a guide for ventilatory therapy but these are a minority.

Sedation

One of the most important aspects of mechanical ventilation is to maintain patients in a state in which they do not fight the ventilator settings, while they are capable of being examined at the bedside. Stroke patients who are to be intubated for periods longer than a few hours require sedation, and in these circumstances, the ideal agent for sedation is one that (a) has rapid onset of action, (b) does not accumulate rapidly, and (c) has a short half-life. The latter characteristic allows the rapid discontinuation of the agent, with the consequent ability to examine the patient as necessary. The author favors the use of propofol as the agent of choice for sedation of all neurological patients requiring ventilation, and more specifically for stroke patients. Following its introduction >20 years ago, this medication has come to occupy a niche that has made it irreplaceable because of its effectiveness and its ease of titration. The existing literature supports this recommendation, favoring it over the use of opiates and benzodiazepines in terms of the overall effectiveness and lack of undesirable side effects (e.g., prolonged ventilation withdrawal times). In general, it is recommend for the patient to be sedated to the point that displayed behavior is consistent with a Ramsay Scale Score = 3 (see Table 33.2). An exception to this rule involves patients with increased ICP and labile neurological function. In these patients, a deeper state of sedation (Ramsay Scale Score = 5 to 6) is warranted because of the ill effects of stimuli on intracranial hemodynamics.

An important issue directly related to sedation is the ability to examine patients. Traditionally, neurologyl patients are followed up by means of the neurological examination. Stroke patients being managed on ventilators are no exception. However, this is an aspect of their care that can be guided by the expertise of the practitioner. Indeed, knowledge of the natural history of the underlying type of stroke allows the treatment team to predict the clinical evolution of the patient, allowing for tactically scheduled short periods of sedation pauses that permit examination of the patient. In this context, propofol is also the ideal agent because it can be stopped and restarted at will owing to its short half-life. Finally, the nutritional effect of propofol must be highlighted. Because it is a lipid-based compound, propofol delivers approximately 1 kcal per mL, a fact that must be taken into account when calculating nutritional support of the patients.

TABLE 33.2 Ramsay Sedation Scale

Score	Description
1	Patient is anxious and agitated or restless, or both
2	Patient is cooperative, oriented and tranquil
3	Patient responds to commands only
4	Patient exhibits brisk response to loud auditory stimulus
5	Patient exhibits sluggish response to loud auditory stimulus
6	Patient exhibits no response

Management of Increased Intracranial Pressure

The management of increased ICP in patients with severe forms of stroke requires a keen understanding of the volume–pressure relationship of the intracranial contents. This relationship is guided by the Monro-Kellie doctrine, which specifies that the contents of the skull belong in three compartments: brain parenchyma, cerebrospinal fluid (CSF), and cerebral blood volume (CBV), and that the overall intracranial volume must remain constant, as follows:

$$Vk = V_{\text{Parenchyma}} + V_{\text{CSF}} + V_{\text{CBV}}$$

As such, in the intact skull, any attempt to augment the volume of any of the compartments will lead to a compensatory displacement of the other two—the volume–pressure relationship is illustrated in Figure 33.1. On the other hand, it is possible to use this same principle for therapeutic purposes. Thus, stroke patients with increased ICP secondary to brain tissue edema or hydrocephalus may benefit from active tactical reduction of CBV. In the mechanically ventilated patient, this can be accomplished by therapeutic hyperventilation. Increasing the Ve results in a reduction in pCO_2 and an increase in pH, leading to overall arteriolar vasoconstriction with reduction of CBV and ICP. Unfortunately, this effect is not permanent, and as time elapses, the cerebral arterioles adapt to the new pH and regain their baseline diameter (see Fig. 33.2). This results in a practical problem, as it reduces the margin of efficacy of the technique, while limiting the ability to normalize the pH and pCO_2. Since the effectiveness of hyperventilation to reduce ICP depends on the response of the cerebral microarterioles to changes in pH, it is relatively simple to apply some of the principles discussed here to the use of this technique as shown in Table 33.3.

Thus, a 70 kg individual (ideal body weight) will require Ve = 7 L per minute to maintain normocapnia and will be extremely hyperventilated when Ve = 14 L per minute, all other variables considered equal. The technique involves using hyperventilation only for as long as it is absolutely necessary, with protocols that

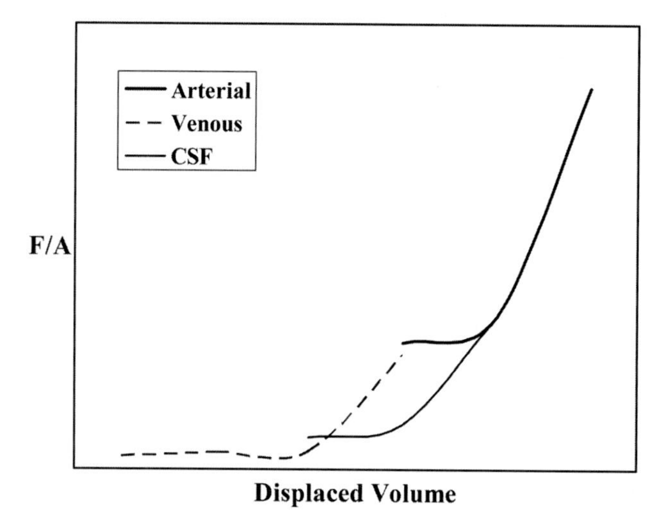

FIGURE 33.1. Relationship between the volume displaced from each of the three intracranial compartments and the intracranial pressure (F/A = force applied). Note that, as the force increases, the first compartment to be affected is the venous capacitance vessels. This is followed by the CSF, and finally by arterial vessels.

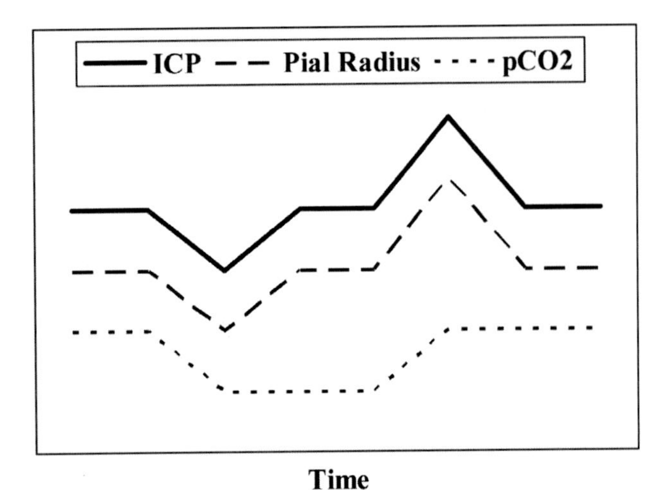

FIGURE 33.2. Relationship between pCO_2 changes and their effect over time on pial artery diameters [i.e., cerebral blood volume (CBV) and intracranial pressure (ICP)]. Rapid reduction of the pCO_2 results in generalized reduction of pial arterial diameters and ICP. However, the longer the pCO_2 is maintained at the new level, the greater the chance that the other two parameters will return to their baseline status. Therefore, subsequent correction of the pCO_2 will be accompanied by exaggerated diameter of the arterioles and consequent increase in ICP.

resume normocapnia and avoid undesirable ill effects of widespread cerebral arteriolar vasoconstriction.

Discontinuation of Mechanical Ventilation

Traditionally, one of the most popular topics of discussion related to mechanical ventilation is *weaning*. The medical literature is filled with data related to the various strategies, championed through the years, for discontinuation of ventilatory support. In reality, none of these strategies has been shown to be better than the others, underscoring the erroneous conceptual approach to this subject. Indeed, the word *weaning* refers to the act of detaching someone from something to which he or she is strongly habituated, an inaccuracy in relation to the practice of mechanical ventilation. Patients do not become habituated to ventilators, since the use of a ventilator does inherently suppress respiratory drive. From this point of view, it is easy to see why it does not really matter what strategy is used to discontinue ventilatory support, so long as one unequivocal criterion is met: *The reason for the patient needing ventilation in the first place must be corrected!*

Looking at this subject from this point of view is a departure from the traditional teachings, but it provides a more realistic and pragmatic method for managing ventilated patients. Following the original decisions made about institution of ventilation, the process of discontinuation begins with a realization of how much ventilatory support was being exercised on behalf of the patient. Patients for whom complete ventilatory support is being used (e.g., for increased ICP) require a different set of indicators than those only being provided partial support (e.g., for airway protection). The latter, as was noted earlier, can be ventilated with minimal support and are typically allowed to do most of the work. Thus, once their airway is protected, it is relatively easy to discontinue ventilation by simply extubating them if they demonstrate the capacity to breathe competently via T-piece (see following text).

On the other hand, the patient that requires major ventilatory support fits one of two scenarios: severe stroke with increased ICP or concurrent pulmonary pathology. The former cannot have ventilatory support discontinued until the ICP problem has resolved. Then, the situation becomes similar to the patient who requires partial support and can be quickly switched to such an approach. The patient with pulmonary pathology needs to have this corrected (e.g., aspiration pneumonia) or taken into consideration (e.g., emphysema) for withdrawal of support.

Once the decision to withdraw ventilatory support is made, the use of PSV with concurrent PEEP is preferred as the main mode of ventilation. Then, as soon as the patient is able to breathe through the ventilator circuit using PSV $\leq$8 cm H_2O, a 2-hour T-piece trial largely allows the patient to be successfully extubated. This entire exercise can be accomplished rapidly and without hesitation. If the patient is not able to tolerate any of these simple steps, the cause for failure must be identified and corrected before a subsequent attempt at the same steps. For example, a common problem arises in patients who have been in the intensive care unit for several weeks, whose nutritional status is less than optimal, or who have neuropathy of critical illness. Rapid withdrawal of ventilatory support may be tolerated for short periods, but as soon as they become fatigued, they are unable to maintain small alveoli inflated, and they develop atelectasis, and hypoxemia, and end up being reintubated. This type of scenario must be avoided at all costs, since reintubation may result in complications and disappointments. The best method for avoiding such an occurrence is to have clear goals and indicators of when to discontinue ventilatory support.

A special situation occurs when a patient remains intubated for >14 to 21 days. As time elapses, the risk of permanent airway injury by the cuff of the endotracheal tube increases. Thus, there is a general consensus that patients who require ventilatory support for >14 days ought to be considered for tracheostomy. Although we adhere to this principle, we must note that knowledge of the natural history of the underlying stroke type and close attention to the clinical evolution facilitate decisions regarding tracheostomy and its application. For example, patients with large intracerebral hemorrhages, who typically spend several weeks in intensive care, whose depressed levels of consciousness and inadequate ability to protect their airways that remain abnormal for a protracted period, may be considered for early tracheostomy. On the other hand, switching a patient from SIMV to PSV = 8 on day 14 of intubation should be followed by at least another 24 to 48 hours of an attempt to extubate if the original reason for ventilation is corrected.

TABLE 33.3 Relationship between Predicted pCO2, Predicted pH, and Ve

Measured Ve (mL/kg/min)	Predicted pCO_2	Predicted pH
100	~40	~7.40
150	~30–35	~7.45–7.48
200	~20–25	~7.48–7.52

PRACTICAL RECOMMENDATIONS

It is recommended that decisions on assisted ventilation in stroke patients should not be delayed unnecessarily. Thus, in the event of any doubt, the airways should be secured and ventilatory support provided. However, these decisions must be made in the context of the overall status and prognosis of the patient. The following initial ventilator settings should prove adequate for most patients:

Mode: SIMV
Rate: 10 per minute
VT: 10 mL per kg (IBW)
PSV: 12 cm H_2O
PEEP: 5 cm H_2O
FIO_2: 1.0

Once the patient is being ventilated, keep in mind the overall goal of ventilatory support for each patient and do not deviate from the path to fulfill this goal. The FiO_2 can be slowly decreased down to 0.3 to 0.4 based on continuous oximetric monitoring. Sedation with propofol should follow the institution of ventilatory support and titrated for a Ramsay Scale of 3. Finally, once the reason for providing ventilatory support is corrected, particularly if minimal support is provided, a trial of T-piece for a few hours is likely to demonstrate whether the patient's ventilatory support can be discontinued.

SELECTED REFERENCES

Bardutzky J, Georgiadis D, Kollmar R, et al. Energy demand in patients with stroke who are sedated and receiving mechanical ventilation. *J Neurosurg* 2004;100(2):266–271.

Berrouschot J, Rossler A, Köster J, et al. Mechanical ventilation in patients with hemispheric ischemic stroke. *Crit Care Med* 2000;28(8): 2956–2961.

Bestue M, Ara JR, Martín J, et al. Mechanical ventilation for ischemic stroke and intracerebral hemorrhage. *Neurology* 1999;52(9):1922–1923.

Burtin P, Bollaert PE, Feldmann L, et al. Prognosis of stroke patients undergoing mechanical ventilation. *Intensive Care Med* 1994;20(1):32–36.

Davies LC, Francis DP, Crisafulli A, et al. Oscillations in stroke volume and cardiac output arising from oscillatory ventilation in humans. *Exp Physiol* 2000;85(6):857–862.

el-Ad B, Bornstein NM, Fuchs P, et al. Mechanical ventilation in stroke patients—is it worthwhile? *Neurology* 1996;47(3):657–659.

Foerch C, Kessler KR, Steckel D, et al. Survival and quality of life outcome after mechanical ventilation in elderly stroke patients. *J Neurol Neurosurg Psychiatr* 2004;75(7):988–993.

Gujjar AR, Deibert E, Manno EM, et al. Mechanical ventilation for ischemic stroke and intracerebral hemorrhage: indications, timing, and outcome. *Neurology* 1998;51(2):447–451.

Leker RR, Ben-Hur T. Re: cost and outcome of mechanical ventilation for life-threatening stroke. *Stroke* 2001;32(6):1443–1448.

Lessire H, Denis B, Vankeerberghen L, et al. Prognosis of stroke patients undergoing mechanical ventilation. *Intensive Care Med* 1996;22(2): 174–175.

Magi E, Recine C, Patrussi L, et al. [Prognosis of stroke patients undergoing intubation and mechanical ventilation]. *Minerva Med* 2000;91 (5–6):99–104.

Mayer SA, Copeland D, Bernardini GL, et al. Cost and outcome of mechanical ventilation for life-threatening stroke. *Stroke* 2000;31(10): 2346–2353.

Santoli F, De Jonghe B, Hayon J, et al. Mechanical ventilation in patients with acute ischemic stroke: survival and outcome at one year. *Intensive Care Med* 2001;27(7):1141–1146.

Schielke E, Busch MA, Hildenhagen T, et al. Functional, cognitive and emotional long-term outcome of patients with ischemic stroke requiring mechanical ventilation. *J Neurol* 2005;252(6):648–654.

Steiner T, Mendoza G, De Geaorgia M, et al. Prognosis of stroke patients requiring mechanical ventilation in a neurological critical care unit. *Stroke* 1997;28(4):711–715.

Wijdicks EF, Scott JP. Causes and outcome of mechanical ventilation in patients with hemispheric ischemic stroke. *Mayo Clin Proc* 1997;72(3): 210–213.

CRITICAL PATHWAY
Ventilator Management for Critically Ill Stroke Patients

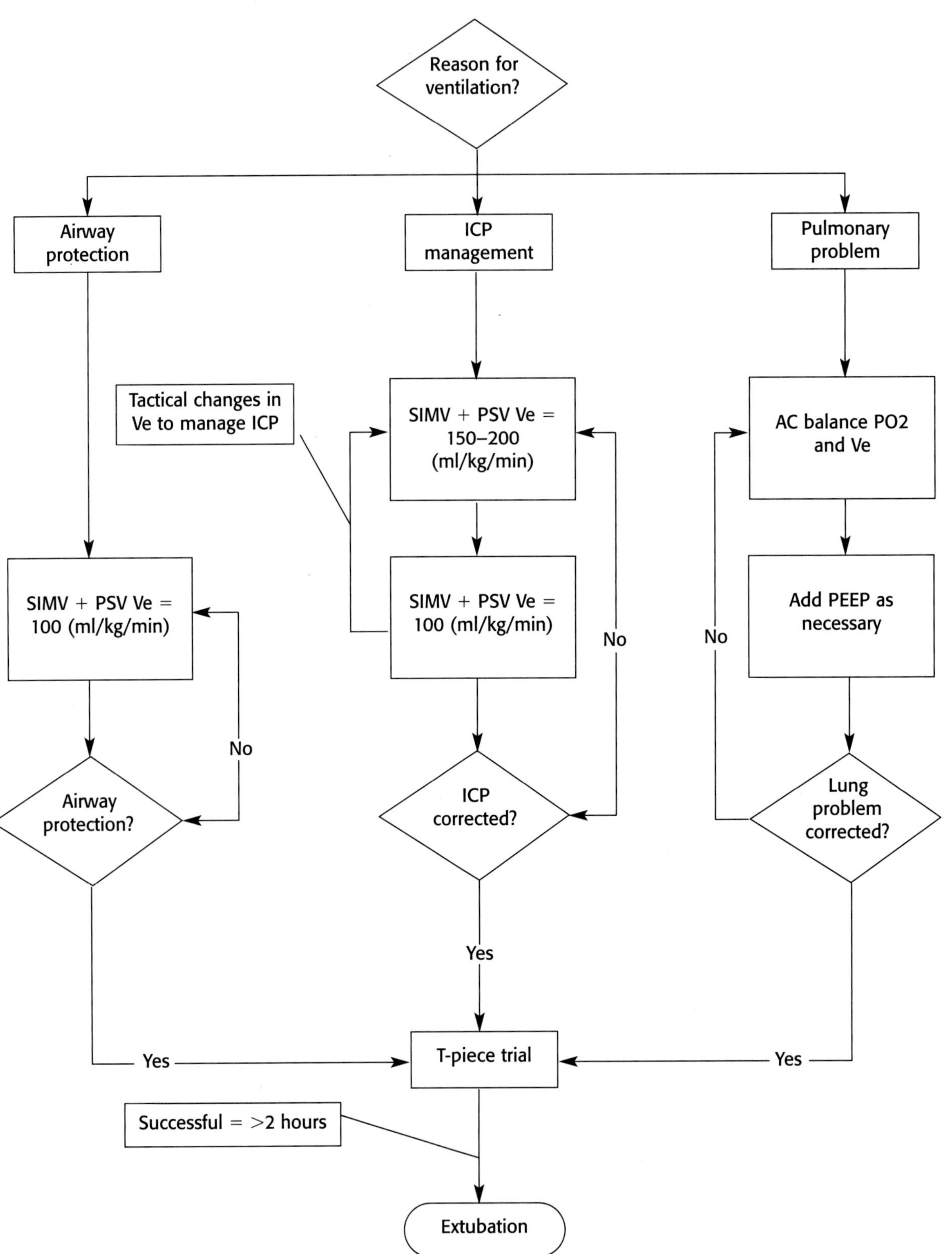

ICP, intracranial pressure; Ve, ventilation; SIMV, synchronized intermittent mandatory ventilation; PSV, pressure support ventilation; AC, assist control; PEEP, positive end-expiratory pressure.

CHAPTER

34 Fluid Management in Acute Ischemic Stroke

RONALD G. RIECHERS II AND GEOFFREY S.F. LING

OBJECTIVES

- What is the ischemic penumbra and how does dehydration impact it?
- What are the pathophysiological effects of dehydration in acute stroke?
- What are the clinical and laboratory parameters that indicate dehydration in stroke patients?
- What is the appropriate intravenous fluid to use for rehydration in stroke patients?
- Is there a role for hypertonic solutions in the management of acute ischemic stroke?

Optimizing cerebral perfusion is critical to improving outcome following acute stroke. Accomplishing this requires adequate circulating intravascular volume. This is most often achieved through intravenous fluid resuscitation. A basic medical intervention, it is generally not given adequate deliberation by the treating clinician. A number of considerations must be made. Specifically, one must rationally decide which resuscitative fluid to use [e.g., normal saline (NS), lactated Ringer's (LR) solution]. Is blood transfusion warranted? How much fluid is needed and how fast should it be administered? This basic medical intervention can greatly contribute to improved neurological and functional outcome.

BACKGROUND AND RATIONALE

Over the last decade, the approach to intravenous fluid therapy has changed dramatically. In the past, fluid restriction was considered the standard approach to ischemic stroke. This was based on the concern that hydration would worsen cerebral edema. This perspective changed with improved understanding of the pathophysiological events related to cerebral infarct and subsequent brain injury. In 1997, Yamaguchi et al noted that dehydration plays a significant role in early stroke recurrence and worsening outcome. The 1998 Trial of ORG 10172 in Acute Stroke Treatment (TOAST) study also provided evidence that dehydration is deleterious. TOAST was a randomized placebo-controlled study of danaparoid in acute stroke that was unsuccessful. On further analysis, an unexpectedly high incidence (29%) of patients presenting with ischemic stroke were dehydrated and this population had a trend ($p = 0.06$) toward worsened National Institute of Health (NIH) stroke scale at presentation. Furthermore, Bhalla et al. demonstrated that plasma osmolarity >296 mOsm per L on presentation in acute ischemic stroke patients was associated with increased mortality independent of stroke type.

This dehydration is likely caused by several factors, including inadequate fluid intake from dysphagia or decreased level of arousal, impaired thirst, and/or concurrent infection/fever. Furthermore, older patients, the population at highest risk for stroke, have diminished thirst perception, and when osmolarity is at high levels, thirst perception is further impaired.

Dehydration is deleterious during acute cerebral ischemia because the ischemic penumbra, which is inadequately perfused, is particularly sensitive to inadequate circulating volume. Normally, the brain has very high metabolic requirements. To meet this demand, cerebral blood flow (CBF) is maintained at a constant 50 to 55 mL/100 g/minute over a wide range of systemic blood pressures via cerebrovascular autoregulation. This level of perfusion is necessary to supply adequate oxygen and glucose. During cerebral ischemia, CBF in the affected region decreases because of mechanical obstruction of the supplying blood vessel and loss of cerebrovascular autoregulation. In the injured region, CBF becomes pressure passive, that is, directly proportional to systemic arterial pressure. Thus, neuronal function becomes proportional to arterial blood pressure. When blood pressure decreases to the level at which CBF falls to 25 mL/100 g/minute, electrical activity in neurons ceases as normal metabolic processes fail and lactic acid accumulates. If CBF further drops to <10 mL/100 g/minute, irreversible neuronal injury occurs. However, if CBF can hold at ≥25 mL/100 g/minute, neurons can remain viable for several hours. This viability accounts for the ischemic penumbra, a region of potentially salvageable tissue following an ischemic infarct.

When a stroke patient is dehydrated, several factors affect CBF. First, dehydration alters the rheologic properties of blood. Increased hematocrit results in increased blood viscosity, which in turn impairs CBF through the microcirculation. As dehydration worsens and intravascular volume decreases, hypotension will ensue. This decrease in blood pressure will further compromise CBF in the penumbra. Finally, dehydration may worsen preexisting hypercoagulable states and thus potentially increase the risk of recurrent stroke.

CLINICAL APPLICATIONS AND METHODOLOGY

Appropriate fluid management in patients with ischemic stroke is contingent on accurate assessment of each patient's current fluid status and identification of other pertinent medical conditions. It is better to tailor therapy to each patient's individual volume requirements than to use a standard rate and volume for every patient regardless of specific needs.

Dehydration can often be detected by physical examination. Clinical signs of dehydration include tachycardia, dry mucous membranes, poor skin turgor, orthostatic hypotension, and decreased urine output. These clinical bedside tests, however, are imperfect. Skin turgor is less predictive of volume status in elderly, patients who have loss of subcutaneous tissue, or obese patients, who have excessive subcutaneous tissue. Medications may cause dry mucous membranes or orthostasis. Disorders such as diabetes or Parkinson's disease can cause orthostatic blood pressure changes due to dysautonomia, which is not dehydration. While these individual tests have limitations, coexisting abnormalities detected by a combination of these tests are more predictive. For example, dry mucous membranes with normal blood pressure and heart rate suggest an approximate 5% total body water decrease, whereas positive orthostatic vital signs (>15 bpm increase, >10 mm Hg drop) along with decreased urinary output suggest a 15% decrease in total body water.

O'Neill et al., in a study of elderly patients, demonstrate that rehydration using individualized therapy based on laboratory measurements related to volume state, such as serum osmolarity or arginine vasopressin levels, is superior to using a standard rate and volume approach. Common useful laboratory measurements include serum sodium, blood urea nitrogen (BUN), hematocrit, uric acid, and urine specific gravity. In particular, serum sodium level can be used to determine free water deficit and serum osmolarity. This is important as the free water deficit can be used to guide how much fluid is required and the rate at which it needs to be administered to achieve euvolemia. The serum osmolarity provides clinical evidence of the patient's current state of hydration. This can be used to support the institution of volume therapy as well as provide a reference to determine how well resuscitation is succeeding in meeting clinical objectives.

Serum sodium values can be obtained almost immediately at bedside using point-of-care devices. Once serum sodium level is known, free water deficit can be calculated as follows:

$$H_2O \text{ deficit (mL)} = 10 \times (\%TBW) \times (wt) \times \frac{(\text{actual Na} - \text{desired Na})}{\text{desired Na}}$$

where TBW is total body water and can be estimated as 60% in men and 50% in women. Wt is body weight and is most practical if ideal body weight in kilograms is used. The actual Na is measured serum sodium and desired Na can be approximated to a value of 145 mEq per L. The calculated free water deficit represents the amount of volume that needs to be repleted.

From results of a standard chemistry panel, serum osmolarity can be calculated using the following equation:

$$\text{Serum Osm} = 2(\text{serum Na}) + \text{serum glucose}/18 + \text{BUN}/2.8 + \text{EtOH}/4.6$$

where serum Osm is the serum osmolarity in milliosmol per liter, serum Na is the measured serum sodium, BUN is blood urea nitrogen, and EtOH is measured alcohol level. Many clinicians find that a good ballpark value of serum osmolarity can be approximated by simply doubling the measured serum sodium.

For severely ill patients, placement of central venous access or a pulmonary artery catheter may be needed. Both allow accurate real time assessments of volume status and may also aid in determining the cause of hypotension if dehydration alone does not fit the clinical history. The treatment goal levels for euvoluemia using central venous pressure (CVP) or pulmonary capillary wedge pressure (PCWP) are 4 to 6 mm Hg or 12 to 14 mm Hg, respectively.

Fever can have an effect on stroke outcome through dehydration. Reith et al demonstrate that during acute stroke, there is an inverse relationship between neurological outcome and body temperature. They provide evidence that for every elevated degree Celsius there is further worsening of clinical outcome. Part of this may be due to worsening dehydration. For each degree increase in temperature, an additional 300 mL per day of insensible fluid is lost. This, in combination with baseline insensible volume losses of 500 mL per day, can contribute significantly to dehydration.

The rate of restoration depends on a patient's clinical state and how much fluid is needed. If the patient is neurologically and physiologically stable and the free water deficit is relatively low (e.g., 1 L or less), it can be administered via peripheral intravenous infusion over the subsequent 24 hours. In general, at least during the first 24 hours and continuing as long as the patient is not taking anything orally (NPO), patients will generally require 75 to 100 mL per hour. This is needed to replete insensible losses and ensure adequate urine output. However, if the patient is in shock or otherwise severely ill, then aggressive fluid resuscitation via central venous access may be needed. Typically, this will be as large volume fluid boluses with high rate infusion. Under these circumstances, patients should be in an intensive care setting. Hemodynamic monitoring including CVP, continuous cardiac and arterial pressure measurements, and echocardiography will be invaluable in helping guide such therapy.

Just as dehydration can exacerbate neurological injury following ischemic stroke, restoration of volume either too quickly or too much can lead to untoward effects. One must be careful not to resuscitate too quickly such that the rate will exceed a serum sodium correction of 0.5 mEq/L/hour as this may place the patient at risk of central pontine myelinolysis. Patients having cardiac or renal diseases are highly sensitive to fluid volume [e.g., those with congestive heart failure (CHF) or renal insufficiency]. Fluid overload can decrease oxygenation via pulmonary edema or decrease blood pressure through compromised myocardial contractility (i.e., poor Starling relationship).

Patients who are dehydrated will need to be reassessed frequently. Acute stroke victims are often prohibited from oral intake because of risk of aspiration. As such, they will be dependent on what volume is administered intravenously. So, frequent bedside examination of volume state and serum sodium levels should be part of the routine assessment.

After determining that a patient requires intravenous fluid therapy, an appropriate fluid needs to be selected. In general, most investigators recommend the use of an isotonic crystalloid solution. The selection of an isotonic solution is based on the premise that hypotonic solutions worsen cerebral edema. Increases in cerebral edema from hypotonic solutions occur in infarcted tissues because of low plasma oncotic pressure and subsequent diffusion of water

TABLE 34.1 Common Intravenous Fluids

Solution	Na	Cl	Other Components	Osmolality (mOsm/L)	Notes
D5W	0	0	Glucose 50 mg/L	252	High free water
D5 0.5NS	77	77	Glucose 50 mg/L	406	–
NS	154	154	–	308	Hyperchloremic acidosis
Saline 3%	462	462	–	924	Requires central access for infusion
LR	130	109	K, Ca, Lactate	273	Hyperkalemia
Albumin 5%	154	154	Carbonate, acetate	–	~$80 per 300/L

D5W, 5% dextrose water; NS, normal saline; LR, lactated Ringer's.

from the intravascular space into injured brain tissue. Several isotonic solutions are available in clinical practice. The most common solutions are NS and LR solution. Table 34.1 lists the components and compares the benefits and risks of each fluid type and several other common fluids in clinical practice.

Crystalloid solutions are preferred as they are well tolerated by patients, relatively inexpensive, and stable when stored at room temperature for long periods. Furthermore, they have good clinical efficacy for restoring intravascular volume in a number of different disease states in addition to stroke. However, crystalloids have some limitations when used to support blood pressure as they redistribute quickly. Because the components can move relatively freely from the intravascular space to the interstitial and intracellular spaces, the water moves out of the intravascular space based on the tonicity. In other words, the volume of fluid administered has a relatively short half-life within the intravascular space where it serves to maintain or increase blood pressure. Because of these factors, other types of solutions, for example, colloids, have been evaluated for expansion of intravascular volume.

For most patients, NS is the preferred isotonic crystalloid solution for use in patients with ischemic stroke. NS has a favorable osmolality, is inexpensive, and is commonly found in every medical treatment facility, including ambulances. However, NS can cause a hyperchloremic metabolic acidosis when given in large amounts.

LR solution is another option. It does not cause acidosis due to the presence of buffers but has a significantly lower osmolality than NS and thus is not typically employed in the setting of acute stroke. There is also evidence that LR may worsen the inflammatory state associated with injury. Rhee et al demonstrated that LR but not NS will cause activation of neutrophils when used to resuscitate hemorrhagic shock.

Another caveat in selecting intravenous fluids is avoidance of fluid solutions containing dextrose. The ischemic penumbra has inadequate oxygen. The presence of dextrose and lack of oxygen will drive glycolosis toward an anaerobic pathway. This will result in lactic acid production as opposed to pyruvate, which is the product of aerobic respiration when oxygen is readily available. By producing more lactic acid, the regional acidosis is worsened, local CBF is further compromised, and ischemia is exacerbated. Parsons et al provided evidence in patients having acute stroke that hyperglycemia reduced salvage of the penumbra and thus worsened functional outcome following acute stroke. Thus, both hyperglycemia and use of dextrose containing solutions should be avoided in acute stroke.

Colloid solutions have been evaluated for stroke. These are solutions containing large molecules, such as albumin. Such fluids do not readily redistribute into extravascular spaces, and thus, colloid solutions persist in the intravascular spaces longer than crystalloids. There are disadvantages in using colloids. They are more expensive than crystalloids and have an infection risk attributable to the human-derived albumin. Importantly, there is presently no evidence that shows benefit in outcome when using colloids instead of crystalloids.

Hypertonic and hyperosmotic solutions have also been studied in acute stroke treatment. Hypertonic solutions are typically concentrated crystalloids. The most commonly used hypertonic solutions for neurological disorders are those that use sodium as the osmotic agent. A high sodium concentration (e.g. 2% to 7.5%) establishes the favorable osmolarity gradient. The most commonly used hyperosmotic solution for neurological emergencies is mannitol.

Hypertonic sodium solutions and hyperosmotic mannitol have revolutionized the therapy for elevated intracranial pressure (ICP). Because of the significant benefit in conditions associated with elevated ICP, such as traumatic brain injury, consideration has been given and studies performed to assess their benefit in ischemic stroke. Stroke-related elevated ICP is usually caused by cerebral edema. Edema, both cytotoxic and vasogenic, is a normal occurrence following ischemic stroke, with the peak edema occurring at 48 to 72 hours after ictus. The volume of edema, as one might expect, is proportional to the size of the infarct. In large infarcts such as that following complete middle cerebral artery occlusion, the development of edema can lead to malignant intracranial hypertension (i.e., very high ICP). The subsequent brain herniation is a leading cause of mortality in such large territory strokes.

Identifying the ideal osmotic agent is critical. Bhardwaj and Ulatowski offered useful criteria as listed in Table 34.2. In addition to these criteria, an important characteristic is the reflection coefficient, that is, the ability of an intact blood–brain barrier (BBB) to exclude the agent. The range of the potential coefficients is 0 to1, with 0 freely permeable and 1 entirely excluded. The more permeable an agent is to the BBB, the greater the risk of rebound edema. Rebound edema is interstitial edema that develops as the agent crosses the BBB and accumulates in the brain. This results in the passage of free water back into the brain, which paradoxically worsens ICP and the injury state. Sodium has a reflection coefficient of

TABLE 34.2 Criteria for Ideal Osmotic Agent

Criteria
Produces a favorable osmotic gradient by remaining in the intravascular compartment
Is inert
Is nontoxic
Has minimal systemic side effects

1 and mannitol has a reflection component of 0.9, whereas infrequently used agents glycerol and urea have reflection coefficients of 0.48 and 0.59, respectively. The reflection coefficient, however, may lose relevance in the setting of a damaged BBB. Without an intact BBB, there is no exclusion. However, at sites of injury, there is also poor perfusion, so the agent may not be distributed to the penumbra.

Mannitol has been in clinical use for >30 years, predominantly for treatment of ICP. Mannitol is an alcohol derivative of mannose, a simple sugar. Within the circulation, it acts as an osmotic diuretic, drawing fluid into the intravascular space. It is also proposed to act as a free radical scavenger and to alter the rheologic properties of blood. Interestingly, mannitol has been demonstrated to preferentially shrink uninjured rather than injured brain.

The preclinical evidence supporting mannitol efficacy is more compelling than clinical findings. Work in animal models of ischemic stroke shows decreases in cerebral edema, infarct size, and neurological deficits when mannitol is administered within 6 hours of onset of ischemia. Despite this encouraging animal data, human clinical evidence remains lacking. In spite of this, mannitol is used throughout the world for acute stroke. Because of this discrepancy, the Cochrane Database performed a review of mannitol use in ischemic stroke. Because of the lack of well-controlled studies, no clear recommendations could be made for mannitol in treating acute ischemic stroke. Subsequent to the publication of the Cochrane review, Bereczki et al. reported several clinical studies evaluating mannitol treatment of acute ischemic stroke. Conducted in Hungary where mannitol use for stroke is based on consensus recommendations, these studies revealed that mannitol is not effective for treating this disease. The initial retrospective study of 1,000 patients demonstrates a higher case fatality rate among mannitol-treated patients independent of age or level of consciousness on admission. The subsequent prospective study reveals higher case fatality rates among mannitol-treated stroke patients. The authors of this study acknowledge that the prospective observational nature of their study has limitations but assert that "it raises concerns and emphasizes the need for properly designed, randomized, clinical trials to decide whether the practice of routine mannitol use in patients with acute stroke is justified, should be restricted to subgroups, or should be stopped altogether."

Mannitol also has serious side effects. The primary effect is related to mannitol's diuretic effect. As an osmotic diuretic, mannitol can induce significant fluid losses. As detailed in the preceding text, stroke patients should be euvolemic to mildly hypervolemic. Thus, fluid losses associated with mannitol if not corrected can exacerbate cerebral hypoperfusion. Other common complications include fluid/electrolyte imbalances (hyponatremia, hyperosmolarity), cardiopulmonary edema, hypersensitivity reactions, and renal failure. As mannitol shrinks normal brain, there is concern that mannitol will increase the likelihood of herniation as edematous injured brain will shift accordingly. However, this does not appear to be clinically relevant as studies have not shown midline tissue shifts following mannitol therapy.

The effects of hypertonic saline on brain volume were first described in 1919 by Weed and McKibben, but this description was largely forgotten until the early 1980s when hypertonic saline was rediscovered as a treatment for hemorrhagic shock. Experimental studies of hemorrhagic shock demonstrate decreased ICP and increased CBF following treatment in animal models. When hypertonic saline therapy is applied to laboratory models of ischemic stroke, effects have been mixed. Toung et al demonstrated decreased global brain water with 7.5% saline infusion started 24 hours following induced cerebral ischemia. This reduction in edema is equivalent to that seen with scheduled dosing of mannitol. However, Bhardwaj et al showed that infusion of hypertonic saline (7.5%) during reperfusion following 2 hours of middle cerebral artery occlusion increases infarct volume. These mixed results are not fully understood. It may be due to hypertonic saline's differential effects on healthy- versus glutamate-injured neurons. These discrepancies perhaps indicate that there is a critical time factor in initiation of hypertonic therapy.

Similarly, clinical studies evaluating the use of hypertonic saline in ischemic infarct have been inconclusive. An early prospective study comparing hypertonic saline–hydroxyethyl starch solution with mannitol demonstrates a more robust decrease in ICP with hypertonic saline. A subsequent study by the same investigators evaluates hypertonic saline (10%) in patients with elevated ICP who have failed mannitol. In this nonrandomized study, infusion of hypertonic saline (10%) decreases ICP and increases cerebral perfusion pressure (CPP). In light of this second study, Ziai et al raised concerns about conclusions based on the relatively uncontrolled data and urged caution on the use of hypertonic saline for the treatment of acute ischemic stroke. Aside from the effects on ischemic tissue, hypertonic saline has systemic effects and complications. These include hemolysis, fluid/electrolyte abnormalities (hypernatremia, hypokalemia), cardiopulmonary edema, hyperchloremic acidosis, and coagulopathy. The hyperchloremic acidosis can be minimized if the sodium used in the hypertonic solution is made as 50% sodium chloride:50% sodium acetate mix. Finally, treatment with hypertonic saline solutions requires central venous access because of possible phlebitis associated with 2% or greater sodium solutions.

Investigators have also attempted to assess the clinical utility of hydroxyethyl starch and colloids such as albumin for ischemic stroke. The use of hydroxyethyl starch solutions is primarily in the setting of hemodilution. Unfortunately, these studies demonstrate no benefit for this agent for ischemic stroke. A recent retrospective review of patients treated with high-dose serum albumin for ischemic stroke demonstrated the rate of cardiopulmonary complications in patients treated with albumin twice as high as that of controls. This study was primarily a safety study, so neurological outcome was not assessed. Thus, the currently available data either do not support the use of these therapies or are insufficient for further conclusions as they pertain to acute stroke management.

Using blood as a routine means of restoring euvolemic state or acute stroke treatment is not recommended. This therapy should be reserved for patients who require blood transfusion due to severe anemia or other medical conditions. Blood is a scarce resource that has significant attendant complications, including infection, fever, and transfusion reaction. Furthermore, the optimal hematocrit for acute stroke management is unknown. As early as 1972, Sunder-Plassmann et al provided animal evidence that a lower hematocrit is better than a normal value. They suggested a hematocrit of 33%. Others have suggested a hematocrit as low as 30%. These low levels are felt to provide optimal rheology and maximal oxygen delivery. However, this has not been rigorously evaluated in acute stroke patients. Berrouschot et al reported a randomized placebo-controlled study in acute stroke patients where extracorporeal rheopheresis is used to reduce blood viscosity and erythrocyte aggregation to optimize regional CBF, particularly in the microcirculation. Reduction of blood viscosity is considered an important benefit of low hematocrit. There is no improvement with rheopheresis treatment but there is no adverse effect either. A study conducted by Hebert et al. in critically ill patients compared a liberal transfusion approach against a restrictive one. The liberal approach allows transfusion for hemoglobin values of 10 g/dL. The restrictive approach does not allow transfusion until hemoglobin values are <7 g per dL. The study reports improved survival and fewer complications in the restrictive group. However, this study did not include acute stroke patients. So, although there are theoretical and limited clinical reasons for tolerating a lower than normal hematocrit, (e.g., 30% to 33%) or hemoglobin (e.g., 10 to 11 g/dL) (or lower), there is no compelling evidence to support transfusion for acute stroke treatment.

PRACTICAL RECOMMENDATIONS

Despite the controversies detailed in the preceding sections, the fluid management of patients with ischemic stroke can be fairly straightforward (see flowchart). Begin with an assessment of hydration state and establish venous access. This can all be part of the initial clinical assessment. In general, unless the patient is in extremis, peripheral IV catheter is sufficient. While taking the medical history, the review of systems should include obtaining important information that may impact the rate of resuscitation. It is important to identify medical conditions that are common in the stroke population, such as CHF, renal failure, orthopnea, and peripheral edema. From the typical acute stroke workup laboratory studies, free water deficit and serum osmolarity should be calculated and/or measured. Subsequently, the resuscitative fluid should be decided. The most common fluid of choice is NS, generally without dextrose unless the patient is hypoglycemic on presentation or persistently thereafter. If a patient is normotensive to mildly hypertensive on presentation and does not have a significant free water deficit, one can begin with a rate of 75 to 100 mL per hour. This can be lowered to 25 to 50 mL per hour in cases of CHF or renal failure with fluid retention. If the patient is mildly hypotensive or has a significant free water deficit on presentation, intravenous boluses should be considered, again using NS and then starting a continuous infusion, which will correct the deficit within 12 to 24 hours and at a rate not to exceed a serum Na correction of 0.5 mEq/L/hour. When severely hypotensive or when the stroke has occurred in the setting of severe CHF or renal failure, monitoring of cardiac function becomes more critical. In these cases, central access with invasive hemodynamic monitoring may be needed. Clearly, such patients should be managed in an intensive care unit. In general, a euvolemic to slightly positive fluid balance is desirable during the first 24 hours following ischemic stroke. As such, strict I/Os should be monitored.

Implementing hypertonic/osmotic therapies in acute ischemic stroke should be reserved for severe situations such as intracranial hypertension and herniation. In cases of elevated ICP with herniation syndromes, mannitol or hypertonic saline can be instituted. Care, however, must be taken with these therapies as diuresis may follow, and aggressive fluid replacement is the rule to avoid cerebral hypoperfusion. Continuous infusion or scheduled dosing of these therapies in cases where ICP is not elevated is clearly not beneficial. Until clear benefit is demonstrated in randomized clinical trials for mannitol, hypertonic saline, or other colloid or osmotic therapies, their use should generally be limited.

In conclusion, patients who have acute stroke can benefit from restoration of euvolemic state. Conversely, allowing a dehydrated state to persist can contribute to worsening neurological outcome. A rational clinical approach to patient assessment and institution of volume resuscitation is required. Selection of the appropriate fluid and rate of administration are important considerations. Although not difficult, this often overlooked aspect of clinical stroke management is an important component of a comprehensive acute stroke management plan.

Disclaimer

The opinions expressed herein belong only to the authors. They do not nor should they be interpreted as belonging to, endorsed by, or otherwise representative of the Uniformed Services University of the Health Sciences, Walter Reed Army Medical Center, U.S. Army, Dept of Defense or U.S. government.

SELECTED REFERENCES

Adams HP, Adams RJ, Brott T, et al. Guidelines for the early management of patients with ischemic stroke. *Stroke* 2003;34:1056–1083.

Bereczki D, Liu M, do Prado GF, et al. Cochrane Report: a systematic review of mannitol therapy for acute ischemic stroke and cerebral parenchymal hemorrhage. *Stroke* 2000;31:2719–2722.

Bereczki D, Mihalka L, Szatmari S, et al. Mannitol use and outcome in acute stroke: results from the Mures-Uzhgorod-Debrecen stuffy. *Eur J Neurol* 2002;9:293–296.

Bereczki D, Mihalka L, Szatmari S, et al. Mannitol use in acute stroke: case fatality at 30 days and 1 year. *Stroke* 2003;34:1730–1735.

Berrouschot J, Barthel H, Köster J, et al. Extracorporeal rheopheresis in the treatment of acute ischemic stroke. *Stroke* 1999;30:787–792.

Bhalla A, Sankaralingam S, Dundas R, et al. Influence of raised plasma osmolality on clinical outcome after acute stroke. *Stroke* 2000;31: 2043–2048.

Bhalla A, Tilling K, Kolominsky-Rabas P, et al. Variation in the management of acute physiological parameters after ischemic stroke: a European perspective. *Eur J Neurol* 2003;10:25–33.

Bhalla A, Wolfe CDA, Rudd AG. Management of acute physiological parameters after stroke. *Q J Med* 2001;94:167–172.

Bhardwaj A, Harukuni I, Murphy SJ, et al. Hypertonic saline worsens infarct volume after transient focal ischemia in rats. *Stroke* 2000;31: 1694–1701.

Bhardwaj A, Ulatowski JA. Hypertonic saline solutions in brain injury. *Curr Opin Crit Care* 2004;10:126–131.

Fulgham JR, Ingall TJ, Stead LG, et al. Management of acute ischemic stroke. *Mayo Clin Proc* 2004;79:1459–1469.

Hakim AM. The cerebral ischemic penumbra. *Can J Neurol Sci* 1987;14:557–559.

Hebert PC, Wells G, Blajchman MA, et al. A multicenter, randomized, controlled clinical trial of transfusion requirements in critical care. Transfusion Requirements in Critical Care Investigators, Canadian Critical Care Trials Group. *N Engl J Med* 1999;340:409–417.

Heiss WD, Graf R. The ischemic penumbra. *Curr Opin Neurol* 1994;7: 11–19.

Hemodilution in Stroke Study Group. Multicenter trial of hemodilution in acute ischemic stroke, I: results in the total patient population. *Stroke* 1987;18:691–699.

Himmelseher S, Pfenninger E, Morin P, et al. Hypertonic-hyperoncotic saline differentially affects healthy and glutamate injured primary rat hippocampal neurons and cerebral astrocytes. *J Neurosurg Anesthesiol* 2002;13:120–130.

Italian Acute Stroke Study Group. Hemodilution in acute stroke: results of the Italian hemodilution trial. *Lancet* 1988;1:318–320.

Kagansky N, Levy S, Knobler H. The role of hyperglycemia in acute stroke. *Arch Neurol* 2001;58:1209–1212.

Karibe H, Zarow GJ, Weinstein PR. Use of mild intraischemic hypothermia versus mannitol to reduce infarct size after temporary middle cerebral artery occlusion in rats. *J Neurosurg* 1995;83:93–98.

Koch S, Concha M, Wazzan T, et al. High dose human serum albumin for the treatment of acute ischemic stroke: a safety study. *Neurocrit Care* 2004;1:335–341.

Kraus JJ, Metzler MD, Coplin WM. Critical care issues in stroke and subarachnoid hemorrhage. *Neurol Res* 2002;24:547–557.

Laureno R, Karp BI. Myelinolysis after correction of hyponatremia. *Ann Intern Med* 1997;126:57–62.

Malkoff MD, Gomez C, Tulyapronchote R, et al. Incidence and significance of dehydration in patients with ischemic stroke. *Stroke* 1994;25:246.

Manno EM, Adams RE, Derdeyn CP, et al. The effects of mannitol on cerebral edema after large hemispheric cerebral infarct. *Neurology* 1999;52:583–587.

Meinke L, Lighthall GK. Fluid management in hospitalized patients. *Comp Ther* 2005;31:209–223.

Miller CM, Vespa P. Intensive care of the acute stroke patient. *Tech Vasc Interventional Rad* 2005;8:92–102.

O'Neill PA, Davies I, Fullerton KJ, et al. Fluid balance in elderly patients following acute stroke. *Age Ageing* 1992;21:280–285.

Paczynski RP, He YY, Diringer MN, et al. Multiple dose mannitol reduces brain water content in a rat model of cortical infarction. *Stroke* 1997; 28:1437–1443.

Parsons MW, Barber PA, Desmond PM, et al. Acute hyperglycemia adversely affects stroke outcome: a magnetic resonance imaging and spectroscopy study. *Ann Neurol* 2002;52:20–28.

Pulsinelli W. Pathophysiology of acute ischemic stroke. *Lancet* 1992;339: 533–536.

Qureshi AI, Suarez JI. The use of hypertonic saline solutions in treatment of cerebral edema and intracranial hypertension. *Crit Care Med* 2000;28: 3301–3313

Reith J, Jorgensen HS, Pedersen PM, et al. Body temperature in acute stroke: relation to stroke severity, infarct size, mortality, and outcome. *Lancet* 1996;347:1415–1416.

Rhee P, Sun L, Austin B, et al. Lactated ringers resuscitation causes immediate cytokine release. *J Trauma* 1998;44:313–319.

Rosner M, Coley I. Cerebral perfusion pressure: a hemodynamically mechanism of mannitol and the pre-mannitol hemogram. *Neurosurgery* 1987;21:147–156.

Schwarz S, Georgiadis D, Aschoff A, et al. Effects of hypertonic saline in patients with raised intracranial pressure after stroke. *Stroke* 2002;33: 136–140.

Schwarz S, Schwab S, Bertram M, et al. Effects of hypertonic saline hydroxyethyl starch solution and mannitol in patients with increased intracranial pressure after stroke. *Stroke* 1998;29:1550–1555.

Sunder-Plassmann L, Klovekorn WP, Messmer K. Hemodynamic and rheologic changes induced by hemodilution with colloids. In: *Hemodilution: theoretical basis and clinical applications*. Messmer K, Schmid-Schonbein H (eds.). Basal: Karger. pp. 184–202; 1972.

Suzuki J, Tanaka S, Yoshimoto T. Recirculation in the acute period of cerebral infarction: brain swelling and its suppression using mannitol. *Surg Neurol* 1980;14:467–472.

Thomas, DJ. Hemodilution in acute stroke. *Stroke* 1985;16:763–764.

Toung TJK, Hurn PD, Traytsman RJ, et al. Global brain water increases after experimental focal cerebral ischemia: effect of hypertonic saline. *Crit Care Med* 2002;30:644–649.

Videen TO, Zazulia AR, Manno EM, et al. Mannitol bolus preferentially shrinks non-infarcted brain in patients with ischemic stroke. *Neurology* 2001;57:2120–2122.

Yamaguchi T, Minematsu K, Hasegawa Y. General care in acute stroke. *Cerebrovasc Dis* 1997;7(suppl 3):12–17.

Ziai WC, Mirski MA, Bhardwaj A. Use of hypertonic saline in ischemic stroke. *Stroke* 2002;33:1166–1167.

CRITICAL PATHWAY
Fluid Flows

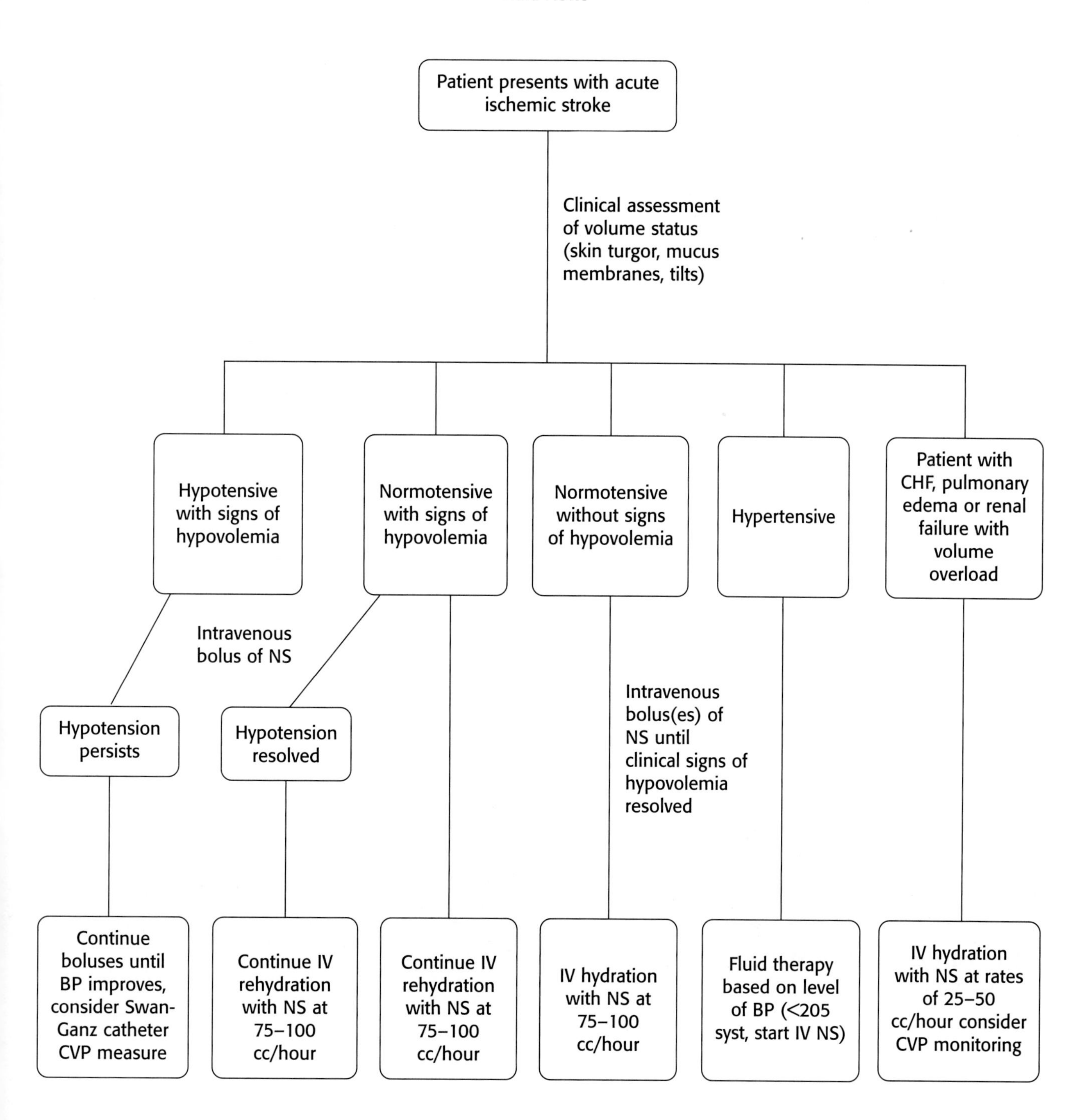

NS, normal saline; CHF, congestive heart failure; BP, blood pressure; CVP, central venous pressure.

CHAPTER

35 Enteral Feeding after Stroke

DAVID J. TEEPLE, CHAD M. MILLER, AND MARC MALKOFF

OBJECTIVES

- What steps should be taken to monitor nutritional status?
- How should patients be fed?
- Which stroke patients require enteral feeding?

Evidence of undernourishment is commonly found in stroke patients. In this setting of inadequate nutrition, metabolic needs are often increased in those with stroke and acute brain injury, and the rigors of rehabilitation require an adequate diet. Of the >90% of persons who will survive an acute stroke, as many as 50% will suffer from at least a transient dysphagia, and even more will have impairment in maintaining sufficient nutrition. There are several factors that lead to problems in maintaining nutrition including deficits in motor function, communication, level of alertness, or cognitive function. On admission, 16% to 31% of patients with stroke and as many as 50% of stroke patients admitted to rehabilitation units show evidence of undernourishment. These patients are unable to initiate or maintain a sufficient diet. Malnourished patients have increased rates of immune compromise, development of pressure sores, prolonged hospital stay, and a higher morbidity and mortality. To prevent these sequelae of malnutrition, it is critical to determine the answers to questions on which stroke patients need to be fed, when to feed them, and how to deliver the feedings to ensure every chance for good recovery.

CLINICAL APPLICATIONS AND METHODOLOGY

First, malnourished patients need to be identified. This can be accomplished by evaluating nutrition status in all hospitalized patients. The initial screening can be done by any health care individual with simple questions to assess nutritional risk, for example: Is the patient dysphagic? Has the patient had significant weight loss? Are there pressure ulcers? Once high risk patients have been identified, a comprehensive nutritional assessment should be performed. A nutrition assessment is defined by the American Dietetic Association as a comprehensive approach completed by a registered dietitian for defining nutrition status using medical, social, nutritional, and medication histories; physical examination; anthropometric measures; and laboratory data.

Nitrogen balance is used as an index of protein status and can be used to assess the adequacy of nutrition (see Table 35.1). A negative nitrogen balance indicates that there is net nitrogen loss, which may be secondary to inadequate protein intake, inadequate caloric intake, or accelerated protein catabolism. The goal of nutrition therapy is a positive balance of 4 g of nitrogen per day. Often, in the critically ill patient this is not possible, and a more realistic goal is to minimize nitrogen loss. Nitrogen balance is a valuable means to evaluate whether an anabolic state has been reached with the current nutritional therapy. It is important to remember that calculations for the nitrogen balance are underestimated in patients with burns, significant gastrointestinal (GI) losses, and hemorrhage, and it is invalid in patients with renal disease. It is well known that malnutrition negatively affects protein synthesis. Visceral proteins are made up of circulating serum proteins and proteins found in organs. They are albumin, transferrin, and prealbumin. Measurements of these proteins are useful as an index of protein energy malnutrition (see Table 35.2). Albumin is a valuable indicator

TABLE 35.1 Common Nutritional Formulas

Nitrogen Balance

Nitrogen balance = (Protein intake in 24 h/6.25) − (Urinary urea + 2 g + 0.02 g/kg body weight)

Harris–Benedict Equation

BEE (men) (kcal/d) = 66.47 + (13.75 × W) + (5.0 × H) − (6.76 × A)

BEE (women) (kcal/d) = 655.1 + (9.6 × W) + (1.8 × H) − (4.7 × A)

Where W is weight in kilograms, H is height in centimeters, and A is age in years

Stress factors to be multiplied with BEE for increased caloric requirement

Infection: 1–1.8 depending on severity

Fever: 1.13 per 1 degree >37 °C

Activity: 1.2 for patients confined to bed

1.3 for patients out of bed

BEE, basal energy expenditure.

TABLE 35.2 Visceral Proteins

Albumin
Normal: 3.5–4 g/dL
Mild depletion: 2.8–3.4 g/dL
Moderate depletion: 2.1–2.7 g/dL
Severe depletion: <2.1 g/dL
Transferrin
Normal: 200–400 mg/dL
Mild depletion: 150–200 mg/dL
Moderate depletion: 100–150 mg/dL
Severe depletion: <100 mg/dL
Prealbumin
Normal: 19–38 mg/dL
Mild depletion: 10–15 mg/dL
Moderate depletion: 5–10 mg/dL
Severe depletion: <5 mg/dL

of protein synthesis, with levels <2.1 g per dL indicating severe depletion. Nutrition is probably the single most important factor regulating albumin synthesis. However, serum albumin level is also affected by the hypercatabolic stress response to acute stroke, and not just undernourished states. Despite this, Gariballa has demonstrated that low serum albumin concentrations at admission and during hospital stay is a strong independent predictor of death at 3 months after an acute stroke and predicts poor functional status and increased morbidity. Transferrin is a slightly more sensitive indicator of visceral protein status because of its shorter half-life with levels <100 ng per dL consistent with severe depletion. Finally, prealbumin is a much more sensitive indicator of protein status with a serum half-life of only 2 to 3 days. It is one of the first metabolic variables to register increased demands for protein synthesis during stress.

Enteral nutrition is preferred over parenteral administration whenever possible. This route has several advantages over parental nutrition including lowering the risk of infection by providing fuel to the intestine to keep the local defense barrier intact and prevent translocation of bacteria, using the normal physiological functions of digestion, and it is less expensive. In the rat model, the intestinal villi have been demonstrated to become severely atrophic and develop increased permeability when not used for relatively short periods. By using normal digestive functions, enteral nutrition has traditionally been thought to prevent villous atrophy and prevent bacterial overgrowth, limiting the ability of these pathogens to migrate from the intestinal lumen to the systemic circulation, thus reducing the incidence of sepsis. Intestinal function and motility must be closely monitored and supported by a stimulant when necessary. Feeding can be initiated either by mouth or via a feeding tube placed in the stomach or duodenum. The proposed advantage of duodenal placement is a reduced risk of reflux of the feeding solution into the esophagus and subsequent pulmonary aspiration. However, the rate of reflux in gastric feedings is the same as that in duodenal feedings. Elevating the head of the bed to 45 degrees can reduce, although not eliminate, the risk of reflux. Contraindications for using enteral nutrition support include complete bowel obstruction, ileus or severe intestinal hypomotility, a high-output enterocutaneous fistula, severe GI hemorrhage, intestinal ischemia, and severe acute pancreatitis. In these cases, it may be necessary to consider total parenteral nutrition.

As mentioned earlier, there are many hospitalized patients with stroke who have dysphagia. In these patients, the risk of aspiration precludes intake of food by mouth. There is no established timeline for the placement of a feeding tube. The FOOD trial was a large randomized, controlled, multicenter trial to evaluate whether there was any advantage to enterally feeding dysphagic stroke patients within the first 7 days of admission versus no feedings during that time. This study found that there was a nonsignificant absolute risk reduction of 1.2% of death or poor outcome in patients who were given enteral nutrition within the first 7 days. This study, however, did not stratify the most malnourished patients on admission to determine whether these patients received more benefit from early nutrition compared with patients without evidence of undernourishment. At this time, we attempt to establish a route for feedings as soon as possible in patients with hemispheric or bulbar strokes.

There has been debate on whether early placement of a percutaneous endoscopic gastrostomy (PEG) tubes offers decreased risk of mortality. Several studies have suggested that PEG tubes do not offer protection from aspiration. A randomized prospective study at a single center demonstrated a lower case fatality rate in patients fed via early PEG tube placement (13%) rather than nasogastric tubes (57%). The FOOD trial also assessed the utility of early PEG placement, as opposed to a nasogastric feeding tube, in dysphagic patients who received enteral feedings. There was no survival benefit discovered for early PEG tube placement. In fact, there was a nonsignificant increased absolute risk of death or poor outcome of 7.8%. The FOOD trial also demonstrated no increased risk for aspiration pneumonia in patients who received early tube feedings via either PEG or nasogastric tube compared with matched controls. However, early tube feeding was associated with a two- to threefold increased risk of GI bleeding.

Most patients with significant bulbar dysfunction secondary to brainstem or substantial hemispheric strokes will necessitate long-term enteral nutritional support. These patients, once the critical period has elapsed, should be given a PEG tube that is better tolerated and causes fewer local complications than nasally placed tubes. PEG tube complications include aspiration pneumonia, infection at the PEG site, and obstruction of the PEG. PEG tubes will be removed from 20% to 30% of patients when their ability to safely swallow returns. The median duration for PEG tube placement is 4 months.

To determine the caloric needs of a patient one can use indirect calorimetry or the Harris Benedict (HB) Equation. The HB equation is often used to calculate the basal energy expenditure (BEE) (see Table 35.1). A person's weight, height, gender, and age factor in the calculation. The equation is often multiplied by a factor of 1.25 to 1.3, accounting for metabolic stress of being ill, to approximate the total energy expenditure of the patient. Variables that will increase a person's metabolic rate are fever, infection, and seizures. The use of glucocorticoids, hypothermia, and barbituate coma will decrease the metabolic rate. Standard enteral feeding preparations contain essential fatty acids, amino acids, and vitamins. However, protein requirements in the critically ill patients are higher (1.2 to 1.5 g per kg of body weight) than in nonstressed persons (0.8 g per kg). The FOOD trial did not show any improved outcome in stroke patients treated with oral supplementation high in protein in addition to the regular oral diet. Two possibilities for the lack of benefit are that few participants were malnourished on admission (8%) and that oral supplements may have contributed to hyperglycemia. Hyperglycemia is an independent risk factor for worse outcome in stroke patients. It is important to remember that propofol, a commonly used sedative in the intensive care unit (ICU), is 10% lipid, and because of this it has high caloric content, 1.1 kcal/mL. Therefore, nutritional requirements need to be adjusted accordingly.

Hyperglycemia should be rigorously controlled. As noted earlier, numerous studies have demonstrated that hyperglycemia is linked to increased mortality and morbidity in stroke patients. The possible etiologies for a hyperglycemic-mediated increase in cerebral infarct are glucose-mediated increase in oxidative stress, increased local edema, increased *N*-methyl-D-aspartic acid (NMDA) receptor–mediated calcium entry, changes in cerebral metabolism, and poor blood flow to the penumbra. Insulin may help protect the ischemic brain not only through its glucose-lowering properties but also through a direct anti-inflammatory effect. Evidence supporting benefits from aggressive intravenous insulin therapy to control blood glucose have been demonstrated in surgical intensive care units and for patients with myocardial infarctions. Attempts to aggressively control blood glucose in stroke patients seem rational, and studies are currently underway to evaluate this question.

Appropriate selection of an enteral feeding product is important. The enteral feeding products are generally classified by content, and each is suitable for different types of patients. Patients with normal GI function and minimal stress should receive supplements with intact protein. Patients with normal GI function requiring volume restriction or subjected to severe metabolic stress should receive supplements with intact protein and high caloric density. A semielemental or peptide formula is desirable for patients with moderately to severely altered GI function. These patients include those with acquired immunodeficiency syndrome (AIDS), malabsorption syndrome, irritable bowel syndrome, and short gut. A free amino acid or elemental formula is reserved for patients with more severely altered GI function and conditions of more severe metabolic stress. Supplements with intact protein, high caloric density, and low electrolyte content are indicated for dialysis patients whose fluid restriction and electrolyte administration need to be carefully followed. Finally, high-fat, low-carbohydrate feedings that are calorie dense are appropriate for patients with significant respiratory and pulmonary conditions where it is desirable to minimize CO_2 production. A careful selection of the appropriate formula is necessary in each patient.

Initiating a diet in severely malnourished patients can result in refeeding syndrome. This occurs when nutrition is introduced in a patient with severe malnutrition, and the body's metabolism abruptly changes from relying on fat stores to relying on carbohydrates as a source of energy. Insulin levels rise, causing intracellular shifts in electrolytes. The sequelae of refeeding syndrome adversely affect nearly every organ system, resulting in cardiac arrhythmias, heart failure, coma, paralysis, nephropathy, and liver dysfunction. Patients at risk for developing refeeding syndrome are those with anorexia nervosa, classic kwashiorkor or marasmus, chronic alcoholism, or any chronic fasting. To avoid this problem, it is best to start slowly, and carefully monitor electrolytes including potassium, magnesium, and phosphate bothbefore and after initiation of feedings.

PRACTICAL RECOMMENDATIONS

Many stroke patients are undernourished at presentation, and a variety of factors contribute to a worsening of this problem during hospitalization. These patients have undesirable clinical outcomes. Adequate nutrition needs to be addressed early. At our institution, we attempt to secure a route for feeding in dysphagic patients as early as possible (i.e., by the first hospital day). Attempts to place nasogastric or duodenal tubes can sometimes be difficult, delaying the final placement of these devices. An appropriate tube feeding regimen is started with tube placement. A nutrition assessment is done by a dietician, and adequacy of nutrition is monitored through the hospitalization. Strict control of blood glucose, usually with an insulin sliding scale, but in some instances an insulin drip, is required. If dysphagia is prolonged >1 week, if there is a significant brainstem stroke, or if there is a large hemispheric stroke, PEG placement is initiated.

SELECTED REFERENCES

Adams H, Adams R, Del Zoppo G, et al. Stroke Council of the American Heart Association. Guidelines for the early management of patients with ischemic stroke: 2005 guidelines update a scientific statement form the stroke council of the American Heart Association/American Stroke Association. *Stroke* 2005;36(4):916–923.

Becker K. Intensive care unit management of the stroke patient. *Neurol Clin* 2000;18(2):439–454.

Bruno A, Biller J, Adams HP, Jr, et al. Acute blood glucose level and outcome from ischemic stroke. Trial of ORG 10172 in Acute Stroke Treatment (TOAST) Investigators. *Neurology* 1999;52(2):280–284.

Capes SE, Hunt D, Malmberg K, et al. Stress hyperglycemia and prognosis of stroke in nondiabetic patients: a systematic overview. *Stroke* 2001;32:2426–2432.

Choi-Kwon S, Yang YH, Kim EK, et al. Nutritional status in acute stroke: undernutrition versus overnutrition in different stroke subtypes. *Acta Neurol Scand* 1998;98(3):187–192.

Davalos A, Ricart W, Gonzalez-Huix F, et al. Effect of malnutrition after acute stroke on clinical outcome. *Stroke* 1996;27(6):1028 1032.

Dandona P, Aljada A, Mohanty P, et al. Insulin inhibits intranuclear nuclear factor kappa B and stimulates I kappa B in mononuclear cells in obese subjects: evidence for an anti-inflammatory effect? *J Clin Endocrinol Metab* 2001;86:3257–3265.

Dennis MS, Lewis SC, Warlow C et al. Routine oral nutritional supplementation for stroke patients in hospital (FOOD): a multicentre randomised controlled trial. *Lancet* 2005;365(9461):755–763.

Dennis MS, Lewis SC, Warlow C et al. Effect of timing and method of enteral tube feeding for dysphagic stroke patients (FOOD): a multicentre randomised controlled trial. *Lancet* 2005;365(9461):764–772.

Dziewas R, Ritter M, Schilling M, et al. Pneumonia in acute stroke patients fed by nasogastric tube. *J Neurol Neurosurg Psychiatr* 2004;75(6): 852–856.

FOOD Trial Collaboration. Poor nutritional status on admission predicts poor outcomes after stroke: observational data from the FOOD trial. *Stroke* 2003;34(6):1450–1456; epub May 15, 2003.

Gariballa SE. Nutritional factors in stroke. *Br J Nutr* 2000;84(1):5–17 [Review].

Gariballa SE. Malnutrition in hospitalized elderly patients: when does it matter? *Clin Nutr* 2001;20(6):487–491.

Garg R, Chaudhuri A, Munschauer F, et al. Hyperglycemia, insulin, and acute ischemic stroke: a mechanistic justification for a trial of insulin infusion therapy. *Stroke* 2006;37(1):267–73; epub 2005.

Malmberg K, Ryden L, Efendic S, et al. Randomized trial of insulin-glucose infusion followed by subcutaneous insulin treatment in diabetic patients with acute myocardial infarction (digami study): effects on mortality at 1 year. *J Am Coll Cardiol* 1995;26:57–65.

Marino, P. *The ICU Book*. 2nd ed. Williams & Williams. pp. 737–753; 1998.

Nicholson FB, Korman MG, Richardson MA. Percutaneous endoscopic gastrostomy: A review of indications, complications, and outcome. *J Gastroenterol Hepatol* 2000;5:21–25.

Norton B, Homer-Ward H, Holmes GKT. A randomised prospective comparison of percutaneous endoscopic gastrostomy. *Br Med J* 1996;312: 13–16.

Perry L, McLaren S. Implementing evidence-based guidelines for nutrition support in acute stroke. *Evid Based Nurs* 2003;6(3):68–71.

Strong RM, Condon SC, Solinger MR, et al. Equal aspiration rates from post-pylorus and intragastric placed small bore nasoenteric feeding tubes: a randomized, prospective study. *J Parent Ent Nutr* 1992;16:59–63.

Suarez J, Nancy N. *Critical Care Neurology and Neurosurgery*. Totowa, NJ: Humana Press. pp. 267–285; 2004.

Unosson M, Ek AC, Bjurulf P, et al. Feeding dependence and nutritional status after acute stroke. *Stroke* 1994;25(2):366–371.

Van den Berghe G, Wouters P, Weekers F, et al. Intensive insulin therapy in the surgical intensive care unit. *N Engl J Med* 2001;345: 1359–1367.

Williams LS. Patients after stroke: who, when, and how. *Ann Intern Med* 2006;144(1):59–60.

Williams LS, Rotich J, Qi R, et al. Effects of admission hyperglycemia on mortality and costs in acute ishemic stroke. *Neurology* 2002; 59:67–71.

CHAPTER

36 Blood Pressure Management

LORENZO BLAS AND JENNIFER A. FRONTERA

OBJECTIVES

- What are the goals for blood pressure management in patients with acute ischemic stroke?
- What are the goals for blood pressure management in patients with the two major types of hemorrhagic strokes: intracerebral hemorrhage and subarachnoid hemorrhage?
- How is hypertensive encephalopathy managed?

According to the National Center for Health Statistics, in the United States approximately 30% of Americans ≥20 years of age develop hypertension. Approximately 30% of adults are unaware of their hypertension, >40% of individuals with hypertension do not receive treatment, and two thirds of hypertensive patients receiving treatment do not have adequate blood pressure (BP) control. Hypertension defined by the Joint National Committee 7 (JNC7) as a BP >140/90 mm Hg occurs in up to 75% of patients with acute ischemic stroke. Within the first 24 hours of the onset of stroke symptoms, elevations in BP [systolic blood pressure (SBP) >160 mm Hg and diastolic blood pressure (DBP) >90 mm Hg] have been detected in >60% of patients.

BACKGROUND AND RATIONALE

Ischemic Stroke

A U-shaped relationship exists between BP and rate of death after ischemic stroke such that both elevated and low BPs are associated with increased rates of death after ischemic stroke. Potential advantages to lowering BP acutely following ischemic stroke include lower risk of brain edema and hemorrhagic transformation and prevention of recurrent stroke. Acute elevations in BP following ischemic stroke have been found to be associated with worse outcome. The risk of neurological deterioration is increased by 40% and the risk of poor outcome by 23% for every 10 mm Hg rise in SBP >180 mm Hg. Analysis of the Glycine Antagonist in Neuroprotection (GAIN) study reveals that variables that describe the course of BP over the first 60 hours [higher weighted average mean arterial pressure (MAP) and a 30% increase from baseline MAP] have a marked and independent relationship with poor outcomes from ischemic stroke at 1 and 3 months.

The potential risk of lowering BP after ischemic stroke is perfusion failure in acutely injured brain with impaired cerebral autoregulation. Cerebral autoregulation is the mechanism by which cerebral blood flow (CBF) remains constant through a wide range of cerebral perfusion pressures (CPPs). CPP, which is the net pressure of blood flow to the brain, can be defined as CPP = MAP − ICP. CPP is normally between 70 and 90 mm Hg in an adult human. Under normal conditions, vasodilation and constriction of small arterioles help maintain CBF. However, autoregulation can be impaired after acute brain injury and CBF can become directly dependent on systemic BP. Under these circumstances, elevation of BP after an acute stroke may be beneficial in terms of increasing CBF to ischemic or penumbral areas.

The concept of an ischemic penumbra, as described in animal models, is that there is a critical threshold of CBF below which neurons cease to function but continue to survive for a time. These neurons can potentially return to a normal functional state with restoration of blood flow, and ischemia seems to be reversible within a window of several hours. Presuming impaired autoregulation, permissive hypertension may allow for penumbral perfusion and potential salvage.

In most ischemic stroke patients, acutely elevated BP is self-limited and begins to fall spontaneously in the following 10 to 14 days, without any specific medical treatment. The effect of BP-lowering drugs in the acute phase is not well understood. The Intravenous Nimodipine West European Stroke Trial (INWEST) found that acute lowering of BP with nimodipine conferred worse outcomes. Others have found that early administration of antihypertensive medications was associated with early deterioration, poor outcome, and death. The Acute Candesartan Cilexetil Therapy in Stroke Survivors (ACCESS) trial, a large, multicenter randomized placebo-controlled safety trial, tested the use of an angiotensin-converting enzyme inhibitor (ACEI) candesartan within 24 hours of ischemic stroke and targeted a 10% to 15% BP reduction within 24 hours. The trial was stopped early because of excessive deaths and recurrent strokes among the placebo-treated group, however, differences in outcome were seen only after a year. The authors concluded that administering an ACEI within 24 hours of ischemic stroke is safe and may have similar beneficial effects in acute cerebral ischemia as with myocardial ischemia.

The 2007 American Heart Association (AHA) guidelines on early management of adults with ischemic stroke recommend that markedly elevated BP may be lowered by approximately 15% during the first 24 hours of onset of stroke. The level of BP that should instigate treatment is an SBP >220 mm Hg or a DBP >120 mm Hg. Until more definitive data is available, a cautious approach should be taken to lowering BP acutely. Initiation of long-term antihypertensive treatment for secondary prevention after acute stroke may be initiated within approximately 1 day of ischemic stroke according to AHA recommendations, depending on the patient's neurological status and underlying stroke mechanism. Most patients can safely resume antihypertensive treatment within 1 week. Special care should be taken in patients with clinical perfusion failure.

There are two circumstances during which BP should be acutely lowered after ischemic stroke: if the patient is a candidate for thrombolysis or if the patient is has end-organ damage due to hypertension. Patients with end-organ injury (i.e., myocardial ischemia, hematuria, or hypertensive encephalopathy) should be managed as hypertensive crises. Since excessively elevated BP is a risk for hemorrhagic conversion after intravenous tissue plasminogen activator (IV-tPA), efforts to lower SBP <185 mm Hg and DBP <110 mm Hg must be undertaken before a patient can be considered a candidate for recombinant tPA (rt-PA). The AHA recommends that after rt-PA is administered, BP should be maintained <180/105 mm Hg for at least the first 24 hours. Patients with sustained BP greater than the 185/110 mm Hg threshold may not be treated with rt-PA because of safety concerns. Similarly, patients undergoing other acute interventions to recanalize occluded vessels should meet the same BP goals.

Intracerebral Hemorrhage

Approximately 37,000 to 52,400 people in the United States have intracerebral hemorrhages (ICH) every year. Worldwide, the incidence of ICH ranges from 10 to 20 cases per 100,000 population and increases with age. According to the Oxfordshire Community Stroke Project, spontaneous ICH accounts for 10% to 15% of all cases of stroke, is associated with the highest mortality rate, and can be classified further into primary or secondary. Primary ICH results from chronic hypertension and amyloid angiopathy, while secondary ICH is usually due to underlying vascular malformations, coagulation abnormalities, or intracranial tumors. ICH is more common in men than women, and, in certain populations, among blacks more than whites. It has been noted that in people aged <75 years, the risk of ICH among blacks is 2.3 times that of whites, whereas the risk among blacks aged ≥75 years was one quarter that of whites.

Elevated BP is common after ICH. As with ischemic stroke, hypertension is the most important risk factor for spontaneous primary ICH. In a large cross-sectional study involving 563,704 adult patients evaluated with stroke, SBP of ≥140 mm Hg was observed in 63%, DBP of ≥90 mm Hg in 28%, and MAP of ≥107 mm Hg in 38% of the patients.

Hypertensive hemorrhages tend to occur in the territory of penetrating arteries that branch off major intracerebral arteries. Degenerative changes in the wall of small blood vessels, induced by chronic hypertension, reduce the compliance and increase the likelihood of spontaneous rupture.

Patients with secondary ICH due to aneurysm or vascular malformation rupture are at the highest risk for hematoma expansion due to rerupture, and more aggressive BP control is warranted in these patients. Treatment of acute hypertension in patients with primary ICH remains controversial. Lowering BP may theoretically reduce hemorrhagic expansion at the risk of inducing cerebral ischemia in penumbral tissue.

A few studies have postulated that autoregulation may be disrupted in the perihematoma area; therefore, decreasing BP may impair CBF and provoke ischemia. PET studies in animals and humans have largely dispelled the notion of perihematomal ischemia and have shown reduced CBF, oxygen extraction fraction, and reduced metabolic rate in perihematomal tissue representing appropriate metabolic coupling. Recent publications have described three phases for CBF and metabolic changes in the perihematoma region based on laboratory and clinical studies. A hibernation phase is seen in the first 2 days after injury. During this time there is a decrease in metabolism in the perihematoma region with a concomitant decrease in CBF. In this particular phase, reducing BP would have no adverse consequences. From days 2 to 14 a reperfusion phase is seen. This consists of a heterogeneous pattern that includes areas of normal, hypocerebral, and hypercerebral perfusion. After 14 days, a normalization phase occurs where CBF and metabolism normalize. Kim-Han et al studied the perihematomal region in brain tissue samples from six patients with acute ICH. They were able to measure the oxygen consumption in isolated brain mitochondria within 2 hours of ICH and demonstrate that mitochondrial dysfunction is responsible for reduced oxygen metabolism ICH.

Initially, ICH was believed to be a monophasic event; however, studies have demonstrated that hematoma expansion occurs in 26% of patients within 1 hour and in another 12% of patients within 20 hours. It is unclear whether aggressive BP lowering within the first few hours of ICH onset decreases hematoma expansion. Baseline BP was not found to be related to ICH expansion in the Recombinant Activated Factor VII Intracerebral Hemorrhage Trial and isolated SBP ≤210 mm Hg was not related to hematoma expansion or neurological worsening in one study. Other studies have been unable to find an association between baseline and peak hemodynamic parameters or changes in hemodynamic parameters and ICH expansion. In one study, reducing BP <160/90 mm Hg within 6 hours of ICH onset showed a trend toward improved neurological outcomes. A target BP <160/90 mm Hg was associated with neurological deterioration in 7% (compared to 25% in untreated patients) and hemorrhagic expansion in 9% (compared to 13% in untreated patients).

The Antihypertensive Treatment of Acute Cerebral Hemorrhage (ATACH) and INTegrelin and Enoxaparin Randomized Assessment of acute Coronary Syndrome (INTERACT) trials are currently underway to determine whether acute BP lowering improves outcomes after ICH.

Subarachnoid Hemorrhage

Nontraumatic subarachnoid hemorrhage (SAH) occurs in >30,000 individuals per year in the United States and the 30-day mortality can be up to 50%. Acute hypertension after SAH occurs more frequently than with any other stroke subtype. The proportion of patients with SBP ≥140 mm Hg according to stroke subtypes was as follows: subarachnoid hemorrhage (100%), ICH (75%), and ischemic stroke (67%).

A major contributor to morbidity and mortality within the first few days of SAH is aneurysm rebleeding, which is most frequent in the first 24 hours of SAH and occurs in up to 30% of patients in the first month if untreated. The mortality in the population that rebleeds can reach 80%.

Elevated BP may be a determinant of acute rebleeding of unprotected aneurysms and some have found a significantly higher risk of rebleeding in patients with SBP >160 mm Hg, though others have been unable to demonstrate this effect. There are no well-controlled studies showing that BP control lowers the risk of rebleeding and elevated BP may, in fact, be secondary to the rebleed itself. Nonetheless, based on theoretical risk, it is reasonable to lower the BP acutely after SAH to keep an SBP <140 to 160 mm Hg.

A balance must be struck between avoiding the risk of aneurysmal rebleeding and maintaining adequate CPP. On the basis of extrapolations from traumatic brain injury literature, most clinicians attempt to maintain a CPP >60 mm Hg when intracranial pressure (ICP) monitoring is available. When ICP monitoring is unavailable, a minimum SBP of 90 mm Hg should be maintained to ensure adequate brain perfusion. Extremes of CPP can lead to elevated ICP. ICP is proportional to parenchymal volume, venous and arterial blood volume, cerebrospinal fluid volume, and any space-occupying lesion volume. According to the Monroe-Kellie doctrine, ICP is maintained relatively constant over a range of intracranial volumes up to a critical point at which compliance exponentially decreases and ICP increases. In the perfusion breakthrough zone of autoregulation, elevated BP overwhelms the arterioles capacity to autoregulate and leads to passive vascular dilation, elevated cerebral blood volume, and consequently elevated ICP. Conversely, in the vasodilatory zone of autoregulation, when CPP is low, cerebral arterioles are maximally vasodilated to maintain perfusion, cerebral blood volume increases, and ICP in turn increases causing plateau waves. Lowering BP in states of hyperperfusion can improve ICP, whereas induced hypertension in cases of vasodilatory cascade can attenuate arteriolar dilation and terminate ICP plateau waves.

Other complications of SAH may be related to hypertension. Elevated admission BP (MAP >130 mm Hg) has been associated with the development of symptomatic vasospasm, delayed cerebral ischemia, and worse outcome. Nimodipine, a calcium channel blocker, lowers BP and has been shown to reduce rates of delayed cerebral ischemia and improve outcomes when used for 21 days after SAH though there is mixed evidence of its effect on angiographic vasospasm. This agent may have neuroprotective effects apart from its antihypertensive effects.

Prophylactic volume expansion and hypertensive, hypervolemic therapy (HHT) in nonsymptomatic patients have not proven useful. Permissive and induced hypertension for patients experiencing symptoms related to vasospasm, however, can improve CBF to brain at risk, though strong evidence supporting the use of HHT is lacking. Typically, vasopressors may be used to increase BP by at least 20 mm Hg over baseline BP, and observation is made for a clinical improvement. Patients may be safely pressed up to 220/120 mm Hg, but surveillance is essential for any evidence of end-organ damage [i.e., daily electrocardiogram (ECG) and troponin levels while vasopressors are used]. Patients with coincident unruptured aneurysms can be safely pressed at least up to an SBP of 200 mm Hg without rupture of coexisting unruptured aneurysms.

Hypertensive Encephalopathy

Hypertensive crisis is an acute, life-threatening event, associated with marked increases in BP, generally >180/120 mm Hg. Hypertensive crisis is subdivided into hypertensive emergency or hypertensive urgency. Hypertensive emergency is characterized by acute end-organ damage (cardiovascular, cerebrovascular, or renal) and requires a prompt reduction in BP within minutes to hours. End-organ damage can consist of hypertensive encephalopathy, hematuria, cardiac ischemia, aortic dissection, pulmonary edema, microangiopathic hemolytic anemia, and obstetric complications. Although hypertensive emergencies have become less common, it is estimated that about 1% of hypertensive patients will develop a hypertensive crisis. Hypertensive urgency is not associated with end-organ damage and a reduction in BP can be attained within 24 to 48 hours.

Oppenheimer and Fishberg introduced the term *hypertensive encephalopathy*, describing the encephalopathic findings associated with the malignant phase of hypertension. Hypertensive encephalopathy refers to the transient migratory neurological symptoms associated with the malignant hypertensive state in hypertensive emergency. Typical symptoms include nausea, vomiting, confusion, seizures, and coma. Papilledema may be seen on clinical examination. The symptoms are due to the presence of signs of cerebral edema caused by the breakthrough hyperperfusion from the sudden elevation in BP. The increased cerebral perfusion from the loss of blood brain barrier integrity, resulting in exudation of fluid into the brain, accounts for the pathophysiology behind the illness. The clinical symptoms are usually reversible with prompt initiation of therapy. Classic magnetic resonance imaging (MRI) findings include posterior white matter hyperintensities on fast low-angled inversion recovery (FLAIR) consistent with edema in the parietal and occipital lobes that are reversible on repeat imaging and are often termed *reversible posterior leukoencephalopathy syndrome* (RPLS). Efforts should be made to rule out cerebral sinus thrombosis and CNS infection.

CLINICAL APPLICATIONS AND METHODOLOGY

General Considerations

The cerebral circulation and CBF have features that differ from those of other vascular beds in the body. The brain's blood vessels have a limited amount of vessel-wall connective tissue at the arteriolar and capillary level. This makes the brain vasculature more susceptible to volume and pressure overload in states of extreme hypertension. Under these conditions, the precapillary arteriolar system can become overwhelmed, leading to hyperperfusion states that can induce cerebral edema and elevated ICP. The cerebral vasculature is not primarily susceptible to effects of α-, β-, or calcium channel blockade since vascular tone is largely mitigated by nitric oxide, pH, and CO_2 levels. However, under conditions of extreme hypertension and perfusion breakthrough, lowering systemic BP will have a beneficial effect on the brain.

BP is the product of systemic vascular resistance and cardiac output. Medications targeting β-receptors present both in the myocardium and peripheral vasculature can reduce cardiac output by reducing heart rate and stroke volume and can also act as peripheral vasodilators. Drugs with combined α- and β-blockade can provide additional afterload reduction via the effect of α-blockade on peripheral vasculature. Calcium channel blockers provide an alternative means of afterload reduction and are particularly useful in patients who cannot tolerate β-blockade.

In general, the agent used during the first 48 hours of acute brain injury should be fast acting and administered as a continuous infusion rather than recurrent bolus dosing. This allows for safer and easier titration to reach target BP. Similarly, the half-life of infusion agents is typically shorter allowing for better control than can be afforded by PO agents. Ideal agents should have a reliable dose–response relationship and not have a significant effect on cerebral vasculature since vasodilation could increase ICP. The preferred continuous infusion agents are nicardipine, labetalol, esmolol, and enalaprilat.

Ischemic Stroke

Medications such as β-blockers, calcium channel blockers, and ACEIs effectively reduce BP during the acute phase of ischemic stroke according to a Cochrane Database Systematic Review. Because of the precipitous drops in BP associated with sublingual nifedipine, this medication is not recommended by the AHA consensus panel. In addition, because of the potential for elevated ICP, cyanide toxicity, and profound BP drops associated with nitroprusside, this medication should be reserved for patients refractory to other medications.

There is insufficient data to recommend any given antihypertensive over another during the acute ischemic stroke period, and medications should be chosen on an individualized basis, taking into account individual patient contraindications (i.e., β-blockers should be avoided in those with asthma or bradycardia). The ACCESS trial demonstrated that ACEIs are probably safe within the first 24 hours of ischemic stroke and may convey outcome benefit.

Long-term secondary stroke prevention was addressed in the PROGRESS trial, which randomized patients with a history of stroke or transient ischemic attack (TIA) within the last 5 years to placebo or the ACEI perindopril ± the diuretic indapamide. The combination of ACEI plus diuretic lowered BP more than either agent alone, and the combination conveyed a 28% risk reduction for stroke, with benefit across all stroke subtypes for hypertensive and normotensive patients. Based in part on this data, the AHA recommends antihypertensive treatment for prevention of both recurrent stroke and other vascular events in persons who have had an ischemic stroke or TIA (Class I, Level A evidence). Furthermore, because of benefit to persons with or without a history of hypertension, this recommendation is extended to all ischemic stroke patients. Benefit has been demonstrated with average BP reductions of 10/5 mm Hg, and normal BP levels have been defined as <120/80 mm Hg.

Primary stroke prevention has also been extensively studied. The Antihypertensive and Lipid-Lowering Treatment to Prevent Heart Attack Trial (ALLHAT) trial found that in patients >55 years with at least one coronary heart disease risk factor, the thiazide chlorthalidone was superior to amlodipine, lisinopril, and doxazosin for preventing cardiovascular disease. Thiazides are considered first-line antihypertensive therapy by the JNC7. The Heart Outcomes Prevention Evaluation (HOPE) trial showed that ramipril, an ACEI, significantly reduced the rates of death, myocardial infarction, and stroke in high-risk patients without a history of prior stroke. The Losartan Intervention for Endpoint Reduction (LIFE) study provided an additional basis for the use of angiotensin-receptor blockers (ARB)–based therapy as primary stroke prevention in the treatment of hypertension. A 25% reduction in stroke rates was found with losartan compared to the atenolol group, demonstrating a medication class benefit apart from BP-lowering effect. The combination of diuretics and ACEIs seems to convey the most potent risk reduction for stroke and other vascular events. The Comparison of AMlodipine to Enalapril to Limit Occurrences of Thrombosis (CAMELOT) trial compared the usage of two classes of antihypertensive agents—amlodipine, a calcium channel blocker, and enalapril, an ACEI. The trial was designed to see if either agent could reduce adverse cardiovascular events in normotensive patients with coronary artery disease (CAD). The investigators concluded that in patients with CAD who were treated with high-dose statins and aspirin, the usage of amlodipine for 24 months yielded a 31% relative reduction and 5.6% absolute reduction in adverse cardiovascular events. The effects observed in the enalapril group, although directionally similar, were smaller and nonsignificant.

Intracerebral Hemorrhage

Recommended guidelines for the acute management of elevated BP after ICH have been issued by the American Heart Association/American Stroke Association (AHA/ASA) (see Fig. 36.1.) In general, in patients with an MAP >130 mm Hg or an SBP >180 mm Hg, BP should be lowered modestly, with suggested goals of MAP ≤110 mm Hg or a BP of 160/90 mm Hg. In patients with elevated ICP and ICP monitoring, a goal CPP of at least 60 to 80 mm Hg should be targeted. The AHA suggests either intermittent bolusing or continuous infusion of antihypertensive medications in these cases. When BP is extremely elevated (SBP >200 mm Hg or MAP >150 mm Hg) a continuous infusion is suggested. Patients should be monitored frequently, at least every 5 to 15 minutes, while BP is being lowered.

After the first 24 to 48 hours and once the patient is stabilized, oral antihypertensive medications can be initiated and titrated to enable weaning from intravenous antihypertensives. A reasonable initial BP goal is <160/100 mm Hg. After approximately 1 week, dose escalation can be initiated to reach a BP goal <140/90 and <130/90 mm Hg in diabetic patients. Frequently, patients with hypertensive ICH require several oral agents. Agent selection should be made on the basis of patient-specific comorbidities and contraindications. Possible choices include β-blockers, mixed α- and β-blockers, ACEIs, ARBs, calcium channel blockers, diuretics, α-blockers, α_2-agonists (such as clonidine), direct vasodilators (such as hydralazine), and nitrates.

Subarachnoid Hemorrhage

BP management strategies in SAH vary during a patient's hospital course. Duringpre-aneurysm treatment, SBP can be maintained <140 to 160 mm Hg using either nicardipine or labetalol infusion. Labetalol should be avoided in patients with bradycardia but may be useful in patients with concomitant

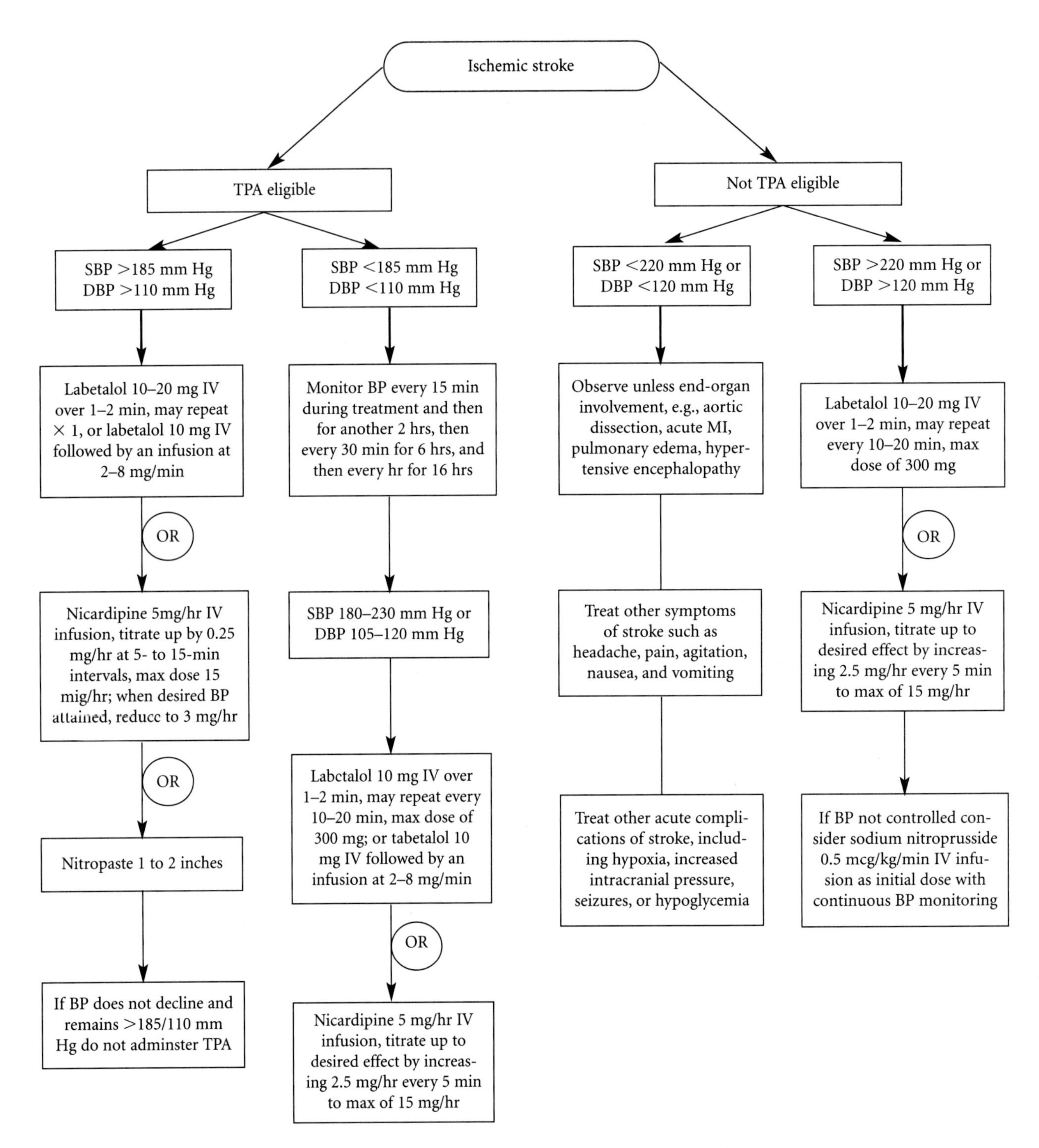

FIGURE 36.1. Approach to arterial hypertension in acute ischemic stroke TPA, tissue plasminogen activator; DBP, diastolic blood pressure, SBP, systolic blood pressure; MI, myocardial infarction. (Adapted from Adams H, del Zoppo G, Alberts MJ, et al. Guidelines for the early management of adults with ischemic stroke. *Stroke* 2007;38: 1655–1711, with permission.)

tachycardia. Infusions are preferred to IV boluses as they minimize BP fluctuations and allow for a more even control. Esmolol and enalaprilat infusions are also options, but are less commonly used. Nitroprusside, a powerful venodilator and indiscriminate nitric oxide donor, should be avoided because of its ability to elevate ICP.

Once a ruptured aneurysm has been secured, many clinicians will liberalize BP parameters as patients enter the vasospasm risk period and allow patients to autopress to a BP of up to 220/120 mm Hg. If patients develop evidence of end-organ damage related to hypertension, BP should be lowered and the patient treated as a hypertensive emergency.

In patients who develop symptomatic vasospasm, hypertensive, hypervolemic therapy (HHT) is typically used along with intra-arterial vasodilators and angioplasty. Typical vasopressors used for HHT include phenylephrine and norepinephrine. Dopamine gives a variable BP and CBF response when compared to norephineprine because of its dose-dependent effect on dopamine, α-blockers, and β-receptors, and it should be considered a second-line agent. A β-agonist, such as dobutamine, or a phosphodiesterase inhibitor, such as milrinone, can be used to support cardiac output and improve BP. Such agents are typically used in conjunction with a pulmonary artery catheter or noninvasive cardiac output monitor. Both dobutamine and phenylephrine increase SBP and CBF (as measured by Xenon flow study) in patients with vasospasm. In patients experiencing neurogenic stunned myocardium, hypotension is commonly refractory to β-agonist pressors because of catecholamine surge–related damage to β-receptors. In these circumstances, phosphodiesterase inhibitors, such as milrinone, are more effective vasopressors.

Hypertensive Encephalopathy

When managing hypertensive emergency, short-acting continuous infusion titratable medications are indicated to rapidly lower BP by 10% within the first hour and then by another 15% gradually over the next 2 to 6 hours. In hypertensive encephalopathy the main goal should be to decrease the MAP by 20% or DBP to 100 to 110 mm Hg within the first hour. The maximum initial fall in BP should not exceed 25% of the presenting value. Parenteral medications that can be used to treat hypertensive emergency are listed in Table 36.1. Once the BP is controlled the patient should be switched to an oral agent if possible and JNC7 BP targets of <140/90 and 130/90 mm Hg in diabetic patients.

PRACTICAL RECOMMENDATIONS

Ischemic Stroke

Patients who are candidates for thrombolysis after acute ischemic stroke should undergo BP lowering to a target BP of 185/110 mm Hg before treatment and should then be maintained with a BP <180/105 mm Hg for the next 24 hours (Fig. 36.1). Patients who are undergoing intra-arterial thrombolysis or mechanical clot retraction should be treated similarly. Possible medications include intravenous nicardipine or labetalol, preferably administered as a continuous infusion. Patients who are not candidates for thrombolysis should receive antihypertensives if their BP exceeds 220/120 mm Hg or if they have concomitant end-organ damage. Within the first 24 hours to 1 week following ischemic stroke, patients should be started on long-term BP medications for secondary stroke and vascular event prevention. BP targets should be compliant with JNC7 recommendations of BP <140/90 or <130/90 mm Hg for diabetic patients. There is evidence to suggest that normotensive patients also benefit from antihypertensive medications for secondary stroke and vascular event prevention. The strongest evidence for secondary stroke prevention exists for the combination of a diuretic and ACEI, but medication selection should be based on an individual patient's comorbidities and contraindications to medications.

Intracerebral Hemorrhage

It is generally considered safe to lower BP acutely following ICH to a target MAP <110 to 120 mm Hg or SBP <160 mm Hg (see Fig. 36.2). If ICP monitoring is available, a goal CPP of 60 to 80 mm Hg should be targeted. Intravenous infusions of labetalol or nicardipine are commonly used. Patients should begin oral antihypertensives within 24 to 48 hours to allow for weaning off intravenous medications.

Subarachnoid Hemorrhage

In pre-aneurysm treatment, SBP should be maintained <140 to 160 mm Hg to minimize the risk of aneurysm rebleed. This can be accomplished with intravenous continuous infusion labetalol or nicardipine in addition to PO nimodipine. Once the culprit aneurysm is secured, BP parameters should be reset to allow patients to autopress to SBP 200 to 220 mm Hg. Prophylactic HHT is not indicated for patients without symptoms of vasospasm. Once a patient develops symptoms of spasm, hypertensive therapy can be initiated, usually with either phenylephrine or norepinephrine, though other agents such as milrinone or dobutamine coul be used to maximize cardiac output. Dopamine has a less consistent effect on CBF and should not be a first line agent. Side effects from HHT include arrhythmia, pulmonary edema, myocardial infarction, elevated ICP, and ICH. If HHT is initiated, daily screening of ECG and cardiac enzymes is required to monitor for cardiac side effects.

Hypertensive Encephalopathy

Hypertensive encephalopathy is a type of hypertensive emergency requiring immediate lowering of BP by 10% to 15% within the first few hours of management. Reversible clinical findings such as headache, seizure, confusion, and coma are typical as are reversible posterior white matter changes on MRI.

TABLE 36.1 Intravenous Medications That May Be Considered for Control of Elevated Blood Pressure

Antihypertensive	Standard Dosage	Contraindications	Drug Interactions	Main Side Effects	Special Points
Labetalol	5–100 mg/h by intermittent IV bolus doses of 10–40 mg or continuous drip (2–8 mg/min)	Hypersensitive to labetalol or any component of its formulation; cardiogenic shock; heart block; bradycardia; bronchial asthma; pregnancy (second and third trimester)	Use with α-blockers may cause orthostasis; CYP2D6 inhibitors may increase labetalol effects; avoid use with diltiazem or verapamil; caution with digoxin; enhances hypoglycemic effect of sulfonylureas	Hypotension, bradycardia	Caution if impaired hepatic function; lower response rate and higher toxicity may occur in elderly patients; caution in compensated heart failure
Nicardipine	5 mg/h increased by 2.5 mg/h every 15 min to maximum of 15 mg/h intravenously	Hypersensitivity to nicardipine or any components of its formulation	Digoxin, cimetidine, fentanyl	Hypotension, orthostasis, tachycardia	N/A
Esmolol	250–500 μg/kg loading dose, then 50–200 μg/kg/min maintenance IV infusion	Hypersensitivity to esmolol or any components of its formulation; cardiogenic shock; heart block; sinus bradycardia; bronchial asthma; pregnancy (second and third trimester)	α-Blockers may worsen orthostasis; BBs and CCBs may worsen hypotension. Enhances hypoglycemic effect of sulfonylureas	Hypotension, bradycardia, and thrombophlebitis	May mask hypoglycemic symptoms and signs of thyrotoxicosis
Enalapril	1.25–5 mg intravenously every 6 h	Hypersensitivity to enalapril or any components of its formulation; history of angioedema	May cause excessive reduction in BP in conjunction with diuretics; hyperkalemia with potassium-sparing diuretics	Hypotension, rash, angioedema, cough	Caution in patients with renal insufficiency, bilateral renal artery stenosis, or elevated potassium
Enalaprilat	0.625–1.25 mg intravenously every 6 h. Max: 5 mg IV every 6 h	Hypersensitivity to enalaprilat or any components of its formulation; history of angioedema	Significant hyperkalemia when combined with potassium-sparing diuretics	Hypotension, angioedema, rash, cough	Caution in patients with renal insufficiency, bilateral renal artery stenosis, or elevated potassium
Hydralazine	5 to 20 mg intravenously every 30 min, then 1.5 to 5 μg/kg/min maintenance IV infusion	Hypersensitivity to hydralazine or any components of its formulation; history of lupus erythematosus	Careful if using in combination with BBs or with diazoxide. Careful with MAO inhibitors	Can have an unpredictable and precipitous drop in BP; reflex sympathetic stimulation; lupus-like syndrome	It is indicated for pre-eclampsia and eclampsia; can increase ICP
Nitroprusside	0.5 to 10 μg/kg/min intravenously. Maximum dose: 1.5 μg/kg/min	Hypersensitivity to nitroprusside or any component of its formulation; signs of increased ICP	None	Increased ICP and decreased CBF; hypotension	Hepatic or renal dysfunction increases risk of cyanide toxicity; rapid or profound drop in blood pressure

IV, intravenous; BBs, β-blockers; CCBs, calcium channel blockers; ICP, intracranial pressure; CBF, cerebral blood flow; MAO, monoamine oxidase.

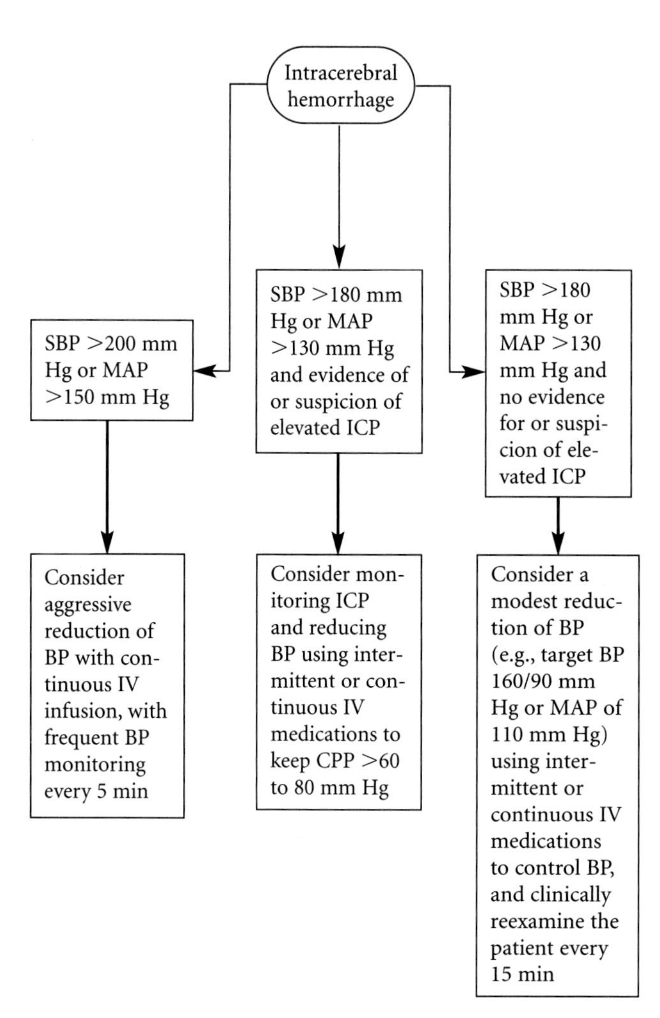

FIGURE 36.2. Recommended guidelines for treatment of elevated blood pressure in spontaneous intracerebral hemorrhage. SBP, systolic blood pressure; MAP, mean arterial pressure; BP, blood pressure; ICP, intracrainal pressure. (Adapted from Broderick et al. Guidelines for the management of spontaneous intracerebral hemorrhage in adults. *Stroke* 2007;38:2001–2023, with permission.)

SELECTED REFERENCES

Acute Hypertension in Intracerebral and Subarachnoid Hemorrhage: Strategies in Emergent Care 1-6 Mayer

Adams H, del Zoppo G, Alberts MJ, et al. Guidelines for the Early Management of Adults with Ischemic Stroke: a Guideline from the American Heart Association/American Stroke Association Stroke Council, Clinical Cardiology Council, Cardiovascular Radiology and Intervention Council, and the Atherosclerotic Peripheral Vascular Disease and Quality of Care Outcomes in Research Interdisciplinary Working Groups: the American Academy of Neurology affirms the value of this guideline as an educational tool for neurologists. *Stroke* 2007;38:1655–1711.

Ahmed N and Wahlgren NG. Effects of blood pressure lowering in the acute phase of total anterior circulation infarcts and other stroke subtypes. *Cerebrovasc Dis* 2003;15(4):235–243.

Allen GS, Ahn HS, Preziosi TJ, et al. Cerebral arterial spasm—a controlled trial of nimodipine in patients with subarachnoid hemorrhage. *N Eng J Med* 1983;308:619–624.

ALLHAT Officers and Coordinators for the ALLHAT Collaborative Research Group. Major outcomes in high-risk hypertensive patients randomized to angiotensin-converting enzyme inhibitor or calcium channel blocker vs diuretic: the antihypertensive and lipid-lowering treatment to prevent heart attack trial (ALLHAT). *JAMA* 2002;288: 2981–2997.

Aslanyan S, Fazekas F, Weir CJ, et al. Effect of blood pressure during the acute period of ischemic stroke on stroke outcome. *Stroke* 2003;34: 2420–2425.

Astrup J, Siesjö BK, Symon L, et al. Thresholds in cerebral ischemia—the ischemic penumbra. *Stroke* 1981;12:723–725.

Blood Pressure in Acute Stroke Collaboration (BASC). Vasoactive drugs for acute stroke. Cochrane Database of Systematic Reviews 2000, (4). Art. No.: CD002839. DOI: 10.1002/14651858.CD002839.

Brain Trauma Foundation. Guidelines for The Management of Severe Traumatic Brain Injury. 3rd edn *J Neurotraum* 2007;24(Suppl 1).

Broderick J, Connolly S, Feldmann E, et al. Guidelines for the Management of Spontaneous Intracerebral Hemorrhage in Adults: 2007 Update: A Guideline From the American Heart Association/American Stroke Association Stroke Council, High Blood Pressure Research Council, and the Quality of Care and Outcomes in Research. *Stroke* 2007;38: 2001–2023.

Broderick JP, Diringer MN, Hill MD, et al. Determinants of intracerebral hemorrhage growth: an exploratory analysis. *Stroke* 2007;38(3): 1072–1075.

Broderick JP, Brott T, Tomsick T, et al. The risk of subarachnoid and intracerebral hemorrhages in blacks as compared with whites. *N Eng J Med* 1992;326:733–736.

Brott T, Broderick J, Kothari R, et al. Early hemorrhage growth in patients with intracerebral hemorrhage. *Stroke* 1997;28:1–5.

Castillo J, Leira R, Garcia MM, et al. Blood pressure decrease during the acute phase of ischemic stroke is associated with brain injury and poor stroke outcome. *Stroke* 2004;35:520–527.

Chobanian AV, Bakris GL, Black HR, et al. Seventh Report of the Joint National Committee on prevention, detection, evaluation, and treatment of high blood pressure. *Hypertension* 2003;42:1206–1252.

Claassen J, Vu A, Kreiter KT, et al. Effect of acute physiologic derangements on outcome after subarachnoid hemorrhage. *Crit Care Med* 2004;32(3): 832–838.

Dennis MS, Burn JP, Sandercock PA, et al. Long-term survival after first-ever stroke: the Oxfordshire Community Stroke Project. *Stroke* 1993; 24(6):796–800.

Haas AR, Marik PE. Current diagnosis and management of hypertensive emergency. *Semin Dial* 2006;19(6):502–512.

Heart Outcomes Prevention Evaluation (HOPE) Study Investigators. Effects of an angiotensin-converting-enzyme inhibitor, ramipril, on cardiovascular events in high-risk patients. *N Engl J Med* 2000;342:145–153.

Hoh BL, Carter BS, Ogilvy CS. Risk of hemorrhage from unsecured, unruptured aneurysms during and after hypertensive hypervolemic therapy. *Neurosurgery* 2002;50(6):1207–1211.

Jauch EC, Lindsell CJ, Adeoye O, et al. Lack of evidence for an association between hemodynamic variables and hematoma growth in spontaneous intracerebral hemorrhage. *Stroke* 2006;37(8):2061–2065.

Jones TH, Morawetz RB, Crowell RM, et al. Thresholds of focal cerebral ischemia in awake monkeys. *J Neurosurg* 1981;54(6):773–782.

Joseph M, Ziadi S, Nates J, et al. Increases in cardiac output can reverse flow deficits from vasospasm independent of blood pressure: a study using xenon computed tomographic measurement of cerebral blood flow. *Neurosurgery* 2003;53(5):1044–1051.

Kazui S, Minematsu K, Yamamoto H, et al. Predisposing factors to enlargement of spontaneous intracerebral hematoma. *Stroke* 1997;28(12): 2370–2375.

Kim-Han JS, Kopp SJ, Dugan LL, et al. Perihematomal mitochondrial dysfunction after intracerebral hemorrhage. *Stroke* 2006;37(10):2457–2462.

Lennihan L, Mayer SA, Fink ME, et al. Effect of hypervolemic therapy on cerebral blood flow after subarachnoid hemorrhage: a randomized controlled trial. *Stroke* 2000;31:383–391.

Naidech A, Janjua N, Kreiter KT, et al. Predictors and impact of aneurysm rebleeding after subarachnoid hemorrhage. *Arch Neurol* 2005;62:410–416

Nissen SE, Tuzcu EM, Libby P, et al. Effect of antihypertensive agents on cardiovascular events in patients with coronary disease and normal blood pressure: the CAMELOT study: a randomized controlled trial. *JAMA* 2004;292:2217–2225.

Ohkuma H, Tsurutani H, Suzuki S. Incidence and significance of early aneurysmal rebleeding before neurosurgical or neurological management. *Stroke* 2001;32:1176–1180.

Patel SC and Mody A. Cerebral hemorrhagic complications of thrombolytic therapy. *Prog Cardiovasc Dis* 1999;42:217–233.

Powers WJ, Zazulia AR, Videen TO, et al. Autoregulation of cerebral blood flow surrounding acute (6 to 22 hours) intracerebral hemorrhage. *Neurology* 2001;57(1):18–24.

PROGRESS Collaborative Group. Randomised trial of a perindopril-based blood-pressure-lowering regimen among 6105 individuals with previous stroke or transient ischaemic attack. *Lancet*, 2001;358 (9287):1033–1041.

Qureshi A, Tuhrim S, Broderick JP, et al. Spontaneous intracerebral hemorrhage. *N Engl J Med* 2001;344:1450–1460.

Qureshi A, Ezzeddine M, Nasar A, et al. Prevalence of elevated blood pressure in 563 704 adult patients with stroke presenting to the ED in the United States. *Am J Emerg Med* 2007;25(1):32–38.

Qureshi AI, Mohammad YM, Yahia AM, et al. A prospective multicenter study to evaluate the feasibility and safety of aggressive antihypertensive treatment in patients with acute intracerebral hemorrhage. *J Intensive Care Med* 2005;20(1):34–42.

Qureshi AI, Wilson DA, Hanley DF, et al. Pharmacologic reduction of mean arterial pressure does not adversely affect regional cerebral blood flow and intracranial pressure in experimental intracerebral hemorrhage. *Crit Care Med* 1999;27(5):965–971.

Rashid P, Leonardi-Bee J, Bath P. Blood pressure reduction and secondary prevention of stroke and other vascular events: a systematic review. *Stroke* 2003;34:2741–2748.

Robinson T, Waddington A, Ward-Close S, et al. The predictive role of 24-hour compared to causal blood pressure levels on outcome following acute stroke. *Cerebrovasc Dis* 1997; 7:264–272.

Sacco R, Adams R, Albers G, et al. Guidelines for Prevention of Stroke in Patients with Ischemic Stroke or Transient Ischemic Attack: a Statement for Healthcare Professionals from the American Heart Association/American Stroke Association Council on Stroke: Co-sponsored by the Council on Cardiovascular Radiology and Intervention: the American Academy of Neurology affirms the value of this guideline. *Circulation* 2006;113: e409–e449.

Schrader J, Lüders S, Kulschewski A, et al. The ACCESS Study: evaluation of acute candesartan cilexetil Therapy in stroke survivors. *Stroke* 2003;34: 1699–1703.

Shah QA, Ezzeddine MA, Qureshi AI. Acute hypertension in intracerebral hemorrhage: pathophysiology and treatment. *J Neurol Sci* 2007;261 (1–2):74–79.

Sica DA , Weber Michael. The Losartan Intervention for Endpoint Reduction (LIFE) Trial—have angiotensin-receptor blockers come of age? *J Clin Hypertens* 2002;4(4):301–305.

Steiner LA, Johnston AJ, Czosnyka M, et al. Direct comparison of cerebrovascular effects of norepinephrine and dopamine in head-injured patients. *Crit Care Med* 2004;32(4):1049–1054.

Zazulia AR, Diringer MN, Videen TO, et al. Hypoperfusion without ischemia surrounding acute intracerebral hemorrhage. *J Cereb Blood Flow Metab* 2001;21(7):804–810.

CHAPTER 37

Temperature Management in Acute Stroke

MAXIM D. HAMMER AND TUDOR G. JOVIN

OBJECTIVES

- What are the effects of elevated temperature on the stroke patient?
- What is the effect of avoiding hyperthermia?
- What treatment options are available for the treatment of hyperthermia?

There are two potential goals for temperature management in acute stroke: treating hyperthermia and inducing hypothermia. The rationale for each of these goals is discussed in this chapter. In addition, methods of monitoring and controlling temperature are reviewed. For the purpose of this chapter, the definitions presented in Table 37.1 are used with respect to core temperature.

It should be noted that the term *hyperthermia* is used generically to refer to any temperature elevation, regardless of cause. In other words, the distinction between fever (elevation of the temperature set point) and hyperthermia (heat production resulting in temperature above the set point) will not be made here. Finally, the effects of temperature on cerebral metabolism and the molecular mechanisms of neuroprotection by hypothermia are beyond the scope of this chapter. For more information on these subjects, the reader is referred to the most recently published expert review.

CLINICAL APPLICATIONS AND METHODOLOGY

Treating and Preventing Hyperthermia

Animal studies have shown that hyperthermia worsens neuronal damage in focal and global ischemia models. Fever also worsens clinical outcomes in humans. Recent prospective clinical data reveal that body temperature is directly related to stroke severity, infarct volume, and mortality. This presents a target for therapeutic intervention because fever is common among stroke victims. Fever occurs in approximately 27% to 40% of ischemic stroke patients and is usually caused by infection (nosocomial pneumonia being the most common), although up to one third of febrile stroke patients have no identifiable source. Hyperthermia is deleterious to stroke patients regardless of the cause.

TABLE 37.1 Definitions

Term	Temperature
Hyperthermia	≥38°C
Normothermia	36–38°C
Hypothermia	
Mild	34–36°C
Moderate	28–34°C
Severe	20–28°C
Deep	15°C
Profound	10°C

A logical conclusion may be that maintaining normothermia in acute stroke patients can improve neurological outcomes, although this remains to be clinically proven. It also remains to be seen whether the treatment of hyperthermia is sufficient, or whether prevention of hyperthermia may be beneficial.

Treatment of hyperthermia requires the identification of the underlying cause, if any. It is understood that identification and treatment of the cause of fever is the standard of care. This includes the use of appropriate antibiotics for infection, and antithrombotics for deep venous thrombosis (DVT) or pulmonary embolism (PE), if applicable. In addition, antipyretic medications are often used. Nonsteroidal anti-inflammatory drugs (NSAIDs) have been tested in febrile patients with concomitant acute neurological illness. In this patient population, up to one third will remain febrile despite the treatment, and the overall temperature reduction may be <1°C. Continuously infused diclofenac may be effective in achieving temperature control more uniformly than intermittently bolused NSAIDs, but this has not been tested as yet in ischemic stroke patients, let alone for clinical efficacy. Finally, active body cooling can achieve temperature reduction in hyperthermic patients and can be achieved by external or internal cooling methods.

External cooling can be achieved by various means. For example, ice water lavage is used, with conflicting data on the efficacy of fever reduction. The use of water-circulating cooling blankets is still common clinical practice, but the efficacy of fever reduction is questionable. Newer external cooling devices have also been tested. One such device has proven efficacy over more conventional cooling blankets in a prospective clinical trial: Patients treated using the newer device attained normothermia faster, and maintained normothermia longer, than patients treated with a more conventional cooling blanket. Internal cooling devices, which work by intravenous heat exchange, have also recently been developed. These have demonstrated efficacy in controlling hyperthermia in neurointensive care unit (NICU) patients. Both the external and internal cooling devices are described in more detail in the section Methodology.

In contrast to hyperthermia treatment (i.e., fever control), the *prevention* of hyperthermia has been less well explored. Acetaminophen has been tested in the prophylaxis of fever. The effect of acetaminophen on temperature reduction is at best modest, and the ability of even high doses to prevent fever is not clear. Active cooling, such as with either external or internal cooling devices, has not been well explored for the *prophylaxis* of fever.

Inducing Hypothermia for Treatment of Acute Ischemic Stroke

Preclinical Data

Tisherman's initial studies in dogs demonstrated that deep hypothermia (15°C) confers significant neuroprotection in the setting of global cerebral ischemia. This set the stage for even more dramatic resuscitations of clinically dead dogs that were protected with profound hypothermia (10°C). Such extreme degrees of hypothermia render a state of suspended animation to the canine brain. Deep and profound levels of hypothermia cannot be safely produced clinically. However, a wealth of less dramatic animal data suggests that milder degrees of hypothermia are also neuroprotective.

There have been numerous animal models of global ischemia that have demonstrated neuroprotection by mild hypothermia. Animal experiments performed between 1987 and 1990 demonstrated that inducing mild hypothermia (34°C to 35°C) during global cerebral ischemia confers significant protection from histologically measured cell damage in the most sensitive areas of the brain (CA1 region of the hippocampus). In 1991, Sterz et al. showed that inducing hypothermia (33°C to 34°C) either during or immediately following cardiac arrest, significantly improved neurobehavioral outcome in dogs. Immediate postischemic hypothermia (30°C to 32°C) was also shown to be effective in preventing CA1 hippocampal ischemic neuronal injury in the setting of global ischemia, as measured histologically. The animal evidence suggests that the sooner the hypothermia is initiated after onset of ischemia, the more the cerebral tissue is preserved.

Animal models of focal ischemia (i.e., stroke) have also demonstrated neuroprotection by hypothermia. Rosomoff reported in 1956 that dogs that were cooled to 22°C to 24°C and then had permanent interruption of one middle cerebral artery (MCA) had significantly better neurobehavioral outcome than normothermic controls. Xue et al. more recently reported a study of rats that were cooled to 32°C and then received either permanent or transient focal ischemia. The hypothermic rats that received permanent focal ischemia had a 60% reduction in infarct size compared with normothermic controls; the rats that received transient focal ischemia had a 92% reduction in infarct size compared with normothermic controls. This same study also demonstrated that rats with delayed initiation of hypothermia, up to 90 minutes after onset of occlusion, had significantly smaller infarct volumes than normothermic controls. The benefit was greater with prolonged periods of postischemic hypothermia (49% to 73% reduction). Baker et al. showed similar results in rats using cooling to 24°C up to 1 hour postischemia. Others have shown that even minute changes in brain temperature by only 1°C to 2°C confer protection.

Clinical Data

Extreme levels of hypothermia (severe to profound) have long been employed as a means of providing neuroprotection for patients undergoing cardiothoracic surgeries, such as aortic arch reconstructions, and neurosurgeries, such as giant aneurysm repair, during which cerebral blood flow is electively interrupted.

In the past few years, several preliminary studies in humans have also shown that mild postischemic hypothermia is effective in improving neurological outcome after cardiac arrest. These have culminated in two randomized, controlled trials, published back-to-back in the *New England Journal of Medicine* in early 2002. The first study, by the European Hypothermia After Cardiac Arrest Study Group, randomly assigned patients after successful resuscitation for ventricular fibrillation (Vfib) cardiac arrest to either a hypothermia (n = 137) or a normothermia group (n = 138). The groups were treated identically except that the patients in the hypothermia group were cooled to a target of 32°C to 34°C (mild–moderate hypothermia). The median time to initiation of cooling was 105 minutes, and the time from initiation to arrival at the target temperature was 8 hours. Outcomes of survival and neurological status were measured at 6 months. There was a striking increase in survival (59% versus 45%) and favorable neurological outcome (55% versus 39%) in favor of hypothermia. The second study, by the Australian group lead by Bernard, evaluated the effect of moderate hypothermia on patients who remained comatose after resuscitation from out-of-hospital Vfib cardiac arrest. Eighty-six patients were enrolled and randomly assigned to the hypothermia or normothermia group. The hypothermia group reached their target temperature of 33°C approximately 120 minutes after return of spontaneous circulation. A total of 49% of the cooled patients survived and had good neurological outcome (discharged home or to a rehabilitation facility), as compared with 26% of the normothermia group. These two trials show that delayed, mild-to-moderate hypothermia improves mortality and neurological outcome in patients after Vfib arrest.

There have been two clinical feasibility trials of moderate hypothermia for massive ischemic stroke. The first, published in 1998 by Schwab et al., was a report of 25 patients with severe MCA infarction. The mean time from onset of symptoms to initiation of hypothermia was 14 hours, after which patients required 3.5 to 6.2 hours to achieve a target of 32°C to 33°C using surface cooling methods. Fifty-six percent of patients survived; herniation related to cerebral edema during rewarming was a prominent complication, being responsible for all of the mortalities. Among the survivors, the median Scandinavian Stroke Scale was 29 after 4 weeks and 38 after 4 months; the median Barthel index was 70 and the mean Rankin scale was 2.6.

The second feasibility trial of surface cooling for stroke was published by Krieger et al. in 2001. Hypothermia, by surface cooling, was induced in ten patients who suffered massive infarction. Surface cooling was initiated at a mean of 6.2 ± 1.3 hours after stroke onset, and patients arrived at the target 32°C at a mean of 3.5 ± 1.5 hours after initiation of cooling. Although not randomized, this study used concomitant patients with severe strokes who underwent thrombolysis but not hypothermia as a control group. Three-month neurological outcomes using the modified Rankin scale were better in the hypothermia group, although these numbers did not reach statistical significance.

A feasibility trial of endovascular cooling for acute stroke was recently published by DeGeorgia et al. Forty patients with acute ischemic stroke within 12 hours of onset (with or without thrombolysis) were randomized to receive either endovascular hypothermia ($n = 18$), or normothermia ($n = 22$). Endovascular cooling was generally rapid and well tolerated. Although this feasibility trial was not powered to detect clinical efficacy, there was a trend toward decreased stroke volumes in the hypothermia group, particularly among those patients who cooled rapidly.

Ongoing Trials of Hypothermia in Stroke

The Nordic Cooling Stroke Study (NOCSS) is an effort to enroll 1,000 patients with ischemic stroke (<6 hours) and randomize them to surface hypothermia (to 35°C) or normothermia and compare 90-day clinical outcomes. Similarly, the Controlled Hypothermia in Large Infarction (CHILI) trial is a phase II study of surface hypothermia (35°C) but with a much larger time window (72 hours from stroke onset). The Intravascular Cooling in the Treatment of Stroke-Longer tPA Window (ICTuS-L) is a phase I safety study that aims to test the combination of intravenous tissue plasminogen activator (IV-tPA) and hypothermia (33°C). Finally, the combination of hypothermia (34.5°C), caffeine, and alcohol is also currently being tested.

Methodology

Methods of Temperature Control

The three main categories of temperature control are surface, internal, and selective (see Table 37.2).

Surface cooling can be achieved by immersion in ice water or by rubbing the patient with alcohol and applying ice packs strategically over the groin, neck, and axillae. This triggers peripheral vasoconstriction and shivering, which generally impede decreasing core temperature <34°C without general anesthesia.

Surface cooling can also be achieved using a traditional cooling blanket that is available in many hospitals. These work by circulating a cold liquid (water or alcohol) from a refrigerated reservoir through channels within the blanket material. The efficiency of cooling depends in part on the extent of the body surface that is in contact with the blanket. Wrapping a patient (front and back) is ideal, if possible.

A more recent type of external cooling device has been found to be effective. Perhaps the archetype is the Arctic Sun Temperature Management System (Medivance). This system consists of an external reservoir of cold water that communicates with channels located inside special adhesive pads. The pads adhere to the skin by a biodegradable hydrogel that has a high thermal conductivity. This feature increases the cooling efficiency. The Arctic Sun device was compared with a traditional cooling blanket in a prospective trial that conclusively demonstrated the superiority of the specialized device: Patients treated using the newer device attained normothermia faster, and maintained normothermia longer, than patients treated with the more conventional cooling blanket.

The major disadvantage of surface cooling is the lack of precise control of the patient's temperature, which can result in overshooting to a lower level of hypothermia than desired (with possible medical complications) and in difficulty in controlling the rewarming process (which can lead to rapid cerebral edema and herniation).

Internal cooling is achieved using endovascular cooling catheters. A catheter is connected to an external reservoir of refrigerated water. The coolant is circulated between the reservoir and the catheter in a closed system. Feedback from a core temperature sensor is fed to a microprocessor that controls the temperature of the cooling catheter. The catheter is introduced into a vein, such as the femoral, jugular, or subclavian vein, but then is placed and remains in the inferior vena cava. The coolant circulates in the opposite direction of blood flow, and the central blood is cooled by convection. Once the catheter is in place, target temperatures of 33°C can be achieved rapidly (77 ± 44 minutes). Another advantage is that overshoot and uncontrolled rewarming are totally avoided by having an automated cooling process by which temperatures can be maintained within a tenth of a degree Celsius. A final advantage of endovascular cooling is that it is possible to cool patients to 33°C without general anesthesia, using only mild sedation and warming blankets. The disadvantages of internal cooling by endovascular catheters are primarily high cost and invasiveness. There are potential complications (e.g., infection, hematoma, DVT) that may offset the potential advantages of this technique.

Both external and internal cooling methods create systemic hypothermia, which presumably cools the brain. It is not clear to what extent brain temperature correlates with core temperature, nor whether the ischemic brain, as well as brain with normal blood delivery, is cooled. These problems are the basis for the development of selective brain cooling systems. The current prototypes are external in that they are applied externally, but selectively, to the head and neck. Selective brain cooling has been demonstrated in small pilot studies.

Hypothermia Technical Parameters

Fundamental questions about the target temperature and duration of hypothermia remain unanswered. However, answers may be forthcoming. The completion of the NOCSS trial, which should be powered to detect clinical efficacy, will help determine whether a target temperature of 35°C within 6 hours of stroke onset will improve clinical outcome. If this trial should be negative, then hopefully the ICTuS-L trial will proceed to phases II and III and help us determine the clinical efficacy of the more moderate target of 33°C.

Potential Complications

Hypothermia may cause a variety of cardiac, pulmonary, renal, electrolyte, infectious, and other complications. These complications tend to occur with more profound levels of hypothermia, and the mild to moderate hypothermia used in acute ischemic stroke is generally safe and well tolerated.

Various arrythmias have been documented in the setting of hypothermia. Ventricular ectopy is occasionally seen, but is more common with deeper levels of hypothermia. Vfib is not common with mild–moderate hypothermia, except in patients with prior history of arrhythmias, such as underlying atrial fibrillation (AF)—hypothermia should thus be avoided in this group. AF may also occur, again more commonly in patients with history of intermittent AF.

Hypothermia can cause decreases in systemic blood pressure, especially during the cooling phase. This tends to stabilize during the maintenance phase, and most patients do not require blood pressure support.

Pulmonary complications, especially aspiration pneumonia, are prevalent in stroke patients undergoing hypothermia. Pneumonia, urinary tract infections, and bacteremia may occur in hypothermic patients, but it is not entirely clear whether they relate

TABLE 37.2 Current Methods Used to Achieve Hypothermia

Modality	Method	Advantages	Disadvantages
Surface	Ice water or alcohol rubs	Inexpensive, omnipresent, noninvasive	Cannot get <34°C without general anesthesia, induction is slow, labor intensive
	Traditional cooling blanket	Inexpensive, omnipresent, easy to use, noninvasive	Cannot get below 34°C without general anesthesia, induction is slow
	Specialized external cooling systems	Easy to use, noninvasive, induction is the fastest of external methods	Expensive, induction is still not as fast as internal cooling
Internal	Endovascular cooling catheters	Rapid induction, precise control, automation	Expensive, invasive
Selective	Head coolers	Possible selective head cooling, avoidance of complications of systemic hypothermia, noninvasive	New technology

to hypothermia or to the procedures applied to the patients to prevent shivering and thermal discomfort. In addition, aspiration pneumonia is a frequent in dysphagic stroke patients.

Hypothermia causes mild hypokalemia, hyperglycemia, and metabolic acidosis due to intracellular shifts caused by lowering the temperature. These electrolyte changes are usually of little clinical consequence and revert on rewarming. Electrolyte shifts can cause rebound hyperkalemia on rewarming; therefore, replenishment of potassium or glucose in hypothermia should be avoided. Patients experience a mild diuresis during the cooling phase.

Pancreatitis, thrombocytopenia, and coagulopathy have been previously reported but may in fact be inherent to invasive measures to induce hypothermia, rather than caused by hypothermia itself.

TABLE 37.3 Summary of Temperature Management Strategies

Strategy	Treatment	Effectiveness
Treatment of hyperthermia[a] (i.e., fever control)	NSAIDs	Modest effect on temperature reduction. Future direction might be continuous infusion of Diclofenac **If specialized external cooling devices are unavailable, then NSAIDs in combination with traditional cooling blankets are recommended to treat fever in stroke patients[a]**
	Traditional cooling blanket	Modest effect on temperature reduction **If specialized external cooling devices are unavailable, then NSAIDs in combination with traditional cooling blankets are recommended to treat fever in stroke patients[a]**
	Specialized external cooling devices	Effective in normalizing temperature and maintaining normothermia **Recommended as first-line treatment, if available, in the treatment of fever in stroke patients[a]**
Prevention of hyperthermia	NSAIDs	Very small effect on temperature. Not recommended
Induction of hypothermia	Specialized external cooling devices	Slow cooling, mild hypothermia can be achieved Undergoing efficacy trials: NOCSS, CHILI **Cannot yet be recommended as a therapeutic strategy**
	Core cooling	Rapid cooling, moderate hypothermia can be achieved; undergoing efficacy trials: ICTuS-L **Cannot yet be recommended as a therapeutic strategy**
	Head cooling	Undergoing feasibility trials **Cannot yet be recommended as a therapeutic strategy**

NSAIDS, nonsteroidal anti-inflammatory drugs; NOCSS, Nordic Cooling Stroke Study; CHILI, Controlled Hypothermia in Large Infarction.
[a]It is understood that identification and treatment of the cause of fever is the standard of care. This includes the use of appropriate antibiotics for infection and antithrombotics for deep venous thrombosis or pulmonary embolism if applicable.

In patients in whom cooling is targeted to ameliorate effects of severe ischemic cerebral edema secondary to the stroke, hypothermia can reduce the extent of the edema and the level of intracranial pressure (ICP). However, the rewarming process, if it occurs too quickly, can precipitate severe increases in ICP with resulting transtentorial herniation. Deliberately slow rewarming (0.1°C to 0.5°C per hour) may be necessary to avoid this effect.

PRACTICAL RECOMMENDATIONS

Conclusion

There is a sound rationale for treating hyperthermia (i.e., fever) in stroke patients. Traditional treatment with intermittent doses of NSAIDs seems only modestly effective, and more data on continuous infusions of NSAIDs is needed. By contrast, it seems clearer that specially designed devices effectively control fever.

There is a wealth of animal and clinical data supporting the neuroprotective properties of extreme levels of hypothermia. It remains to be determined through clinical studies whether mild to moderate levels of hypothermia also confer neuroprotection in acute stroke. Multiple clinical trials are under way, and even more will be needed to answer fundamental efficacy questions. The routine clinical application of hypothermia in the setting of acute stroke cannot yet be recommended on the basis of current clinical data (see Table 37.3).

SELECTED REFERENCES

Azzimondi G, Bassein L, Nonino F, et al. Fever in acute stroke worsens prognosis. A prospective study. *Stroke* 1995;26:2040–2043.

Badjatia N, O'Donnell J, Baker J, et al. Achieving normothermia in febrile subarachnoid hemorrhage patients: feasibility and safety of a novel intravascular cooling catheter. *Neurocrit Care* 2004;1:145–156.

Baena R, Busto R, Dietrich W, et al. Hyperthermia delayed by 24 hours aggravates neuronal damage in rat hippocampus following cerebral ischemia. *Neurology* 1997;48:768–773.

Baker CJ, Onesti ST, Solomon RA. Reduction by delayed hypothermia of cerebral infarction following middle cerebral artery occlusion in the rat: a time-course study. *J Neurosurg* 1992;77:438–444.

Baumgartner WA, Silverberg GD, Ream AK, et al. Reappraisal of cardiopulmonary bypass with deep hypothermia and circulatory arrest for complex neurosurgical operations. *Surgery* 1983;94:242–249.

Behringer W, Safar P, Wu X, et al. Survival without brain damage after clinical death of 60–120 mins in dogs using suspended animation by profound hypothermia. *Crit Care Med* 2003;31(5):1523–1531.

Bernard SA, Gray TW, Buist MD, et al. Treatment of comatose survivors of out-of-hospital cardiac arrest with induced hypothermia. *N Engl J Med* 2002;346:557–563.

Bernard SA, Jones BM, Horne MK. Clinical trial of induced hypothermia in comatose survivors of out-of-hospital cardiac arrest. *Ann Emerg Med* 1997;30:146–153.

Busto R, Dietrich WD, Globus MY-T, et al. Small differences in intraischaemic brain temperature critically determine the extent of ischaemic neuronal injury. *J Cereb Blood Flow Metab* 1987;7:729–738.

Busto R, Dietrich WD, Globus MY-T, et al. Postischemic moderate hypothermia inhibits CA1 hippocampal ischemic neuronal injury. *Neurosci Lett* 1989;101:299–304.

Carroll M, Beck O. Protection against hippocampal CA1 cell loss by postischemic hypothermia is dependent on delay of initiation and duration. *Metab Brain Dis* 1992;7:45–50.

Castillo J, Martines F, Leira R, et al. Mortality and morbidity of acute cerebral infarction related to temperature and basal analytic parameters. *Cerebrovasc Dis* 1994;4:66–71.

Chyatte D, Flefteriades J, Kim B. Profound hypothermia and circulatory arrest for aneurysm surgery. *J Neurosurg* 1989;70:489–491.

Clifton GL, Miller EM, Choi SC, et al. Lack of effect of induction of hypothermia after acute brain injury. *N Engl J Med* 2001;344:556–563.

Clinicaltrials.Gov identifier nct00283088.

Clinicaltrials.Gov identifier nct00299416.

Commichau C, Scarmeas N, Mayer S. Risk factors for fever in the neurologic intensive care unit. *Neurology* 2003;60(5):837–841.

Cormio M, Citerio G, Spear S, et al. Control of fever by continuous, low-dose diclofenac sodium infusion in acute cerebral damage patients. *Intens Care Med* 2000;26:552–557.

Cormio M, Citerio G. Continuous low dose diclofenac sodium infusion to control fever in neurosurgical critical care. *Neurocrit Care* 2007;6(2): 82–89.

De Georgia MA, Krieger DW, Abou-Chebl A, et al. Cooling for acute ischemic brain damage (COOL AID): a feasibility trial of endovascular cooling. *Neurology* 2004;63(2):312–317.

Dippel D, vanBreda E, vanGemert H, et al. Effect of paracetamol (acetaminophen) and ibuprofen on body temperature in acute ischemic stroke. PISA, a phase II double-blind randomized placebo-controlled trial. *BMC Cardiovac Disord* 2003;3:22 [abstract].

Dippel D, vanBreda E, vanGemert H, et al. Effect of paracetamol (acetaminophen) on body temperature in acute ischemic stroke: a double-blind, randomized phase II clinical trial. *Stroke* 2001;32:1607–1612.

Diringer M. Treatment of fever in the neurologic intensive care unit with a catheter-based heat exchange system. *Crit Care Med* 2004;32:559–564.

Geogilis K, Plomaritoglou A, Dafni U, et al. Aetiology of fever in patients with acute stroke. *J Inter Med* 1999;246:203–209.

Ginsberg MA, Pulsinelli W. The ischemic penumbra, injury thresholds and the therapeutic time window for acute stroke. *Ann Neurol* 1994;36: 553–554.

Ginsberg MD, Sternau LL, Globus YT, et al. Therapeutic modulation of brain temperature: relevance to ischemic brain injury. *Cereb Brain Metab Rev* 1992;4:189–225.

Hajat C, Hajat S, Sharma P. Effects of poststroke pyrexia on stroke outcome: a meta-analysis of studies in patients. *Stroke* 2000;31:410–441.

Hindfelt B. The prognostic significance of subjebrility and fever in ischaemic cerebral infarction. *Acta Neurol Scand* 1976;53:72–79.

http://www.Strokecenter.Org/trials/trialdetail.Aspx?Tid=573.

http://www.Strokeconference.Org/sc_includes/pdfs/ctp8.

Ikonomidou C, Mosinger JL, Olney JW. Hypothermia enhances protective effect of MK-801 against hypoxic-ischemic brain damage in infant rats. *Brain Res* 1989;487:184–187.

Kapidere M, Ahiska R, Guler I. A new microcontroller-based human brain hypothermia system. *J Med Syst* 2005;29(5):501–512.

Kasner S, Wein T, Piriyawat P, et al. Acetaminophen for altering body temperature in acute stroke: a randomized clinical trial. *Stroke* 2002;33: 130–135.

Kielblock AJ, Van Rensburg JP, Franz RM. Body cooling as a method for reducing hyperthermia. An evaluation of techniques. *S Afr Med J* 1986; 69(6):378–380.

Koennecke H, Leistner S. Prophylactic antipyretic treatment with acetaminophen in acute ischemic stroke: a pilot study. *Neurology* 2001;57: 2301–2303.

Krieger DW, DeGeorgia MA, Abou-Chebl A, et al. Cooling for acute ischemic brain damage (COOL AID): an open pilot study of induced hypothermia in acute ischemic stroke. *Stroke* 2001;32:1847–1854.

Leonov Y, Stetz F, Saraf P, et al. Mild cerebral hypothermia during and after cardiac arrest improves neurologic outcome in dogs. *J Cereb Blood Flow Metab* 1990;10:57–70.

Liu L, Yenari MA. Therapeutic hypothermia: neuroprotective mechanisms. *Front Biosci* 2007;12:816–825.

Maher J and Hachinski V. Hypothermia as a potential treatment for cerebral ischemia. *Cereb Brain Metab Rev* 1993;5:277–300.

Marion DW, Penrod LE, Kelsery SF, et al. Treatment of traumatic brain injury with moderate hypothermia. *N Engl J Med* 1997;336:540–546.

Mayer S, Commichau C, Scarmeas N, et al. Clinical trial of an air-circulating cooling blanket for fever control in critically ill neurologic patients. *Neurology* 2001;56:292–298.

Mayer S, Kowalski R, Presciutti M, et al. Clinical trial of a novel surface cooling system for fever control in neurocritical care patients. *Crit Care Med* 2004;32:2508–2515.

Minamisawa H, Smith M, Siesjo B. The effect of mild hyperthermia and hypothermia on brain damage following 5, 10, and 15 minutes of forebrain ischemia. *Ann Neurol* 1990;28:26–33.

Nozari A, Safar P, Wu X, et al. Suspended animation can allow survival without brain damage after traumatic exsanguination cardiac arrest of 60 minutes in dogs. *J Trauma* 2004;57(6):1266–1275.

O'Donnell J, Axelrod P, Fisher C, et al. Use and effectiveness of hypothermia blankets for febrile patients in the intensive care unit. *Clin Infect Dis* 1997;24:1208–1213.

Poblete B, Romand J, Pichard C, et al. Metabolic effects of i.v. propacetamol, metamizol, or external cooling in critically ill febrile sedated patients. *Br J Anaesth* 1997;78:123–127.

Reith J, Joergensen H, Pedersen P, et al. Body temperature in acute stroke: relation to stroke severity, infarct size, mortality, and outcome. *Lancet* 1996;347:422–425.

Rosomoff H. Hypothermia and cerebral vascular lesions: Experimental interruption of the middle cerebral artery during hypothermia. *J Neurosurg* 1956;13:244–255.

Saccani S, Beghi C, Fragnito C, et al. Carotid endarterectomy under hypothermic extracorporeal circulation: a method of brain protection for special patients. *J Cardiovasc Surg* 1992;33:311–314.

Safar P, Tisherman SA, Behringer W, et al. Suspended animation for delayed resuscitation from prolonged cardiac arrest that is unresuscitable by standard cardiopulmonary-cerebral resuscitation. *Crit Care Med* 2000;28(11 Suppl):N214–N218.

Schwab S, Schwarz S, Spranger M, et al. Moderate hypothermia in the treatment of patients with severe middle cerebral artery infarction. *Stroke* 1998;29:2461–2466.

Spetzler RF, Hadley MN, Rigamonti D, et al. Aneurysms of the basilar artery treated with circulatory arrest, hypothermia, and barbiturate cerebral protection. *J Neurosurg* 1988;68:868–879.

Steiner T, Friede T, Aschoff A, et al. Effect and feasibility of controlled rewarming after moderate hypothermia in stroke patients with malignant infarction of the middle cerebral artery. *Stroke* 2001;32: 2833–2835.

Sterz F, Safar P, Tisherman S, et al. Mild hypothermic cardiopulmonary resuscitation improves outcome after prolonged cardiac arrest in dogs. *Crit Care Med* 1991;19:379–389.

Stocchetti N, Rossi S, Zanier E, et al. Pyrexia in head-injured patients admitted to intensive care. *Intens Care Med* 2002;28:1555–1562.

The Hypothermia after Cardiac Arrest Study Group. Mild therapeutic hypothermia to improve the neurologic outcome after cardiac arrest. *N Engl J Med* 2002;346(8):549–556.

Tisherman SA, Safar P, Radovsky A, et al. Deep hypothermic circulatory arrest induced during hemorrhagic shock in dogs: preliminary systemic and cerebral metabolism studies. *Curr Surg* 1990;47(5): 327–330.

Tisherman SA, Safar P, Radovsky A, et al. Therapeutic deep hypothermic circulatory arrest in dogs: a resuscitation modality for hemorrhagic shock with "irreparable" injury. *J Traum* 1990;30(7):836–847.

Wang H, Olivero W, Lanzino G, et al. Rapid and selective cerebral hypothermia achieved using a cooling helmet. *J Neurosurg* 2004;100(2): 272–277.

Wang H, Wang D, Lanzino G, et al. Differential interhemispheric cooling and ICP compartmentalization in a patient with left ICA occlusion. *Acta Neurochir (Wien)* 2006;148(6):681–683; discussion 683.

Wu X, Drabek T, Kochanek PM, et al. Induction of profound hypothermia for emergency preservation and resuscitation allows intact survival after cardiac arrest resulting from prolonged lethal hemorrhage and trauma in dogs. *Circulation* 2006;113(16):1974–1982.

Wu X, Drabek T, Tisherman SA, et al. Emergency preservation and resuscitation with profound hypothermia, oxygen, and glucose allows reliable neurological recovery after 3 h of cardiac arrest from rapid exsanguination in dogs. *J Cereb Blood Flow Metab* 2008:28;302–311.

Xue D, Huang ZG, Smith KE, et al.. Immediate or delayed mild hypothermia prevents focal cerebral infarction. *Brain Res* 1992;587:66–72.

Yanagawa Y, Ishihara S, Norio H, et al. Preliminary clinical outcome study of mild resuscitative hypothermia after out-of-hospital cardiopulmonary arrest. *Resuscitation* 1998;39:61–66.

Zeiner A, Holzer M, Sterz F, et al. Mild resuscitative hypothermia to improve neurological outcome after cardiac arrest: a clinical feasibility trial. *Stroke* 2000;31:86–94.

CHAPTER

38 Sleep and Acute Stroke

JAMES D. GEYER, PAUL R. CARNEY, KENNETH LICHSTEIN,
STEPHENIE C. DILLARD, AND MONICA M. HENDERSON

OBJECTIVES

- What are the effects of acute stroke on sleep-related breathing disorders?
- What are the effects of sleep-related breathing disorders on acute stroke?
- What role does insomnia play in acute stroke?
- What is the interaction between acute stroke and restless legs?
- What is the inter-relationship between excessive daytime sleepiness and acute stroke?
- What is the effect of acute stroke on the circadian rhythm?

More than 750,000 strokes occur in the United States each year with approximately 150,000 fatalities. Numerous studies have demonstrated that 31% to 54% of strokes occur during sleep, and the most common time of onset during wakefulness is in the first several hours following awakening. The Sleep Heart Health Study identified an increase in the prevalence of stroke in patients with obstructive sleep apnea, and other studies have shown the frequency of coexisting sleep apnea and stroke in 62.5% to 80% of patients with stroke.

BACKGROUND AND RATIONALE

Sleep-related Breathing Disorders—Obstructive Sleep Apnea

Obstructive sleep apnea syndrome is a common disorder in the general population but becomes extremely common, approaching epidemic proportions, in the stroke subpopulation. Studies have shown that obstructive sleep apnea occurs in 70% to 80% of stroke patients. Since obstructive sleep apnea results in multiple physiological changes that might increase the risk of stroke, sleep apnea should be treated in an aggressive manner for secondary stroke prevention.

During wakefulness, upper airway muscle tone maintains upper airway patency. With sleep onset, there is a decrease in voluntary muscle tone with a concomitant increase in upper airway resistance to airflow. Normal rapid eye movement (REM) sleep is associated with relative voluntary muscle atonia that further worsens the airway constriction. The narrowing of the airway may become pathological in people with anatomically crowded or weakened airways. Causes for this upper airway crowding include enlarged tonsils, macroglossia, low soft palate, micrognathia (typically manifested as an overbite), large neck circumference, and a large uvula.

Upper airway narrowing or collapse during sleep results in obstructive sleep apnea. *Apnea* is defined as complete upper airway obstruction lasting at least 10 seconds in an adult. A partial airway obstruction with increased work of breathing and sleep disruption or oxygen desaturation is known as *hypopnea.* Since the physiologic effects are the same, patients with hypopneas may present with the same symptoms as those with complete apneas.

The *apnea–hypopnea index* (AHI) is defined as the number of apneas and hypopneas per hour of sleep and is one of the measures of the severity of obstructive sleep apnea. An AHI >5 is considered abnormal, and if occurring with complaints of sleepiness or related symptoms, it defines obstructive sleep apnea–hypopnea syndrome. Symptoms of obstructive sleep apnea may include excessive daytime sleepiness, unrefreshing sleep, cognitive dysfunction, morning headaches, nocturnal sweating, nocturia, loud snoring, and insomnia.

Most patients with obstructive sleep apnea do not have oxygen desaturations or hypoventilation during wakefulness. *Obesity hypoventilation syndrome*, previously known as the *pickwickian syndrome*, occurs in patients with hypoventilation but without primary lung disease. This is a heterogeneous disorder with components of upper airway obstruction, impaired respiratory compliance secondary to mechanical factors related to the obesity and abnormalities of ventilatory drive. Most of these patients with obesity hypoventilation have severe obstructive sleep apnea with marked oxygen desaturation, but some patients have prolonged nocturnal oxygen desaturation unrelated to apnea or hypopnea.

Cerebral autoregulation is the process by which the brain attempts to control intracranial blood pressure to maintain adequate cerebral blood flow. Obstructive sleep apnea interferes with this process. While the change has not been shown to cause stroke, the inability of the brain to alter pressures to ensure adequate circulation may result in decreased cerebral perfusion and cause enlargement of an acute stroke that originated from other causes. Treatment of obstructive sleep apnea with continuous positive airway pressure (CPAP) results in improvement of the cerebral autoregulation and overall cerebral blood flow measured by transcranial Doppler ultrasound.

Obstructive sleep apnea interacts with multiple stroke risk factors and appears to significantly increase the risk of cerebral infarction. Aggressive management of obstructive sleep apnea is an important component in stroke prevention.

An overnight screening study with oximetry, capnography, and nasal pressure monitoring can be helpful in borderline or questionable cases. Unfortunately, these monitoring devices are not in widespread use. Overnight pulse oximetry provides information about the degree of oxygen desaturation but can miss significant obstructive sleep apnea and evidence of upper airway resistance syndrome. A negative oximetry study does not eliminate obstructive sleep apnea syndrome from the differential diagnosis.

Overnight laboratory-based polysomnography is the gold standard for the evaluation of a possible sleep-related breathing disorder. A standard polysomnogram should include limited electroencephalography (EEG), electro-oculography (EOG), electrocardiograph (ECG), evaluation of limb movement, snore monitoring, respiratory effort, and measurement of airflow. Additional monitoring with capnography and nasal pressure monitoring provides further information about hypoventilation and respiratory event–related arousals (RERAs). Overnight polysomnography should be obtained on any patient with a suspected sleep-related breathing disorder. These comprehensive studies can be extremely challenging to perform in the acute stroke setting.

Positive airway pressure (PAP), including both CPAP and bilevel positive airway pressure (BPAP), delivered by either a nasal or face mask is the most efficient way of treating obstructive sleep apnea. Concerns have been raised as to whether stroke patients will tolerate PAP, and results from two studies have shown PAP compliance rates of 50% to 70% in highly selected stroke patients in the stable phase following their stroke. Levels of compliance were lowest in those with worse disability and lower consciousness levels, which suggests that compliance may be even lower in the acute phase. A more recent study that aimed to implement PAP in the acute phase has reported even lower levels of compliance (<50% when starting at day 4 after the stroke). Careful adjustment of PAP and a wide array of mask selections are necessary for good compliance and effective use of PAP in the acute setting.

Circadian Factors

The sleep–wake cycle is the most apparent circadian rhythm in humans. Light is the strongest synchronizing agent for the circadian clock, and its ability to advance or delay circadian rhythms is dependent on the time of exposure. The desire for sleep and the tendency to sleep longer and more deeply after sleep loss is referred to as *sleep homeostasis*. This homeostatic drive for sleep is a function of the amount of prior wakefulness. Physiological sleepiness and alertness not only varies with prior waking duration but also exhibits circadian variation. In humans, daily variation in physiological sleep tendency reveals a biphasic circadian rhythm of wake and sleep propensity, with a mid-day increase in sleep tendency occurring around 2 to 4 PM, followed by a robust decrease in sleep tendency and increase in alertness that lasts through the early- to mid-evening hours.

The causes of circadian rhythm disruption during hospitalization, but most notably in the critical care setting, are poorly understood. The need for constant monitoring and assessment of neurological status and frequent interruptions for diagnostic testing not only causes frequent arousals but also disrupts the normal light–dark cycle, which may alter the circadian rhythm. Often the clinician is unaware of these arousals. One study found that postcardiotomy patients had their sleep interrupted approximately 60 times per night.

Noise is the environmental factor most commonly cited as disrupting sleep. The US Environmental Protection Agency (EPA) recommends that hospital noise levels should not exceed 45 dB during the day and 35 dB at night. Several studies have shown that noise levels in the intensive care unit (ICU) are commonly substantially higher than the EPA recommendations.

Several polysomnographic studies have demonstrated sleep deprivation and sleep fragmentation in patients in ICUs. Sleep in ICU patients has been characterized by a predominance of Stages 1 and 2 sleep, decreased or absent Stage 3 and 4 and REM sleep, shortened periods of REM sleep, frequent arousals, and profound sleep fragmentation. Day sleeping accounts for 50% of the total sleep time in an ICU. This percentage appears to be even higher in the poststroke patient. Altered sleep patterns frequently do not improve over the course of the patient's ICU stay and may actually worsen. Following transfer to a non-ICU bed, sleep may take several days to improve. The sleep may remain substantially abnormal over the remainder of the hospitalization and continue to lesser degrees well after discharge.

In one study, environmental noise was responsible for 11.5% and 17% of the overall arousals and awakenings from sleep, respectively. Environmental noise is in part responsible for sleep–wake abnormalities, but it is not responsible for most of the sleep fragmentation and may therefore not be as disruptive to sleep as previous literature suggests. This does not imply that the environmental noise should be ignored. On the contrary, it must be addressed in the context of a broader circadian management program.

Vital signs and diagnostic testing are also frequently disruptive to sleep. No single environmental factor was perceived as significantly more disruptive than any other.

A number of environmental factors [noise, light, nursing interventions (e.g., bathing), diagnostic tests (i.e., imaging, ECG), recording of vital signs, phlebotomy, and the administration of medications] may affect the quantity and quality of sleep in the hospitalized patient.

Poor sleep quality and decreased quantity can have a significant adverse affect on multiple physiological parameters, including negative nitrogen balance, reduced host immunity, attenuated ventilatory responses to hypoxemia and hypercapnia, and increased oxygen consumption and carbon dioxide production. Sleep disruption could prolong hospital stay, increase medication requirements, and decrease perceived quality of life.

A comprehensive circadian management protocol may dramatically affect a patient's perceived quality of sleep, quality of life, medical condition, and utilization of resources.

Insomnia

Sleep is sensitive to disturbance from many internal influences, such as excessive worry, anxiety, and depressed mood. Likewise, many external influences such as transient stress, an important life event, excessive noise, high or low room temperature, an uncomfortable bed, drug withdrawal, and sleeping in unfamiliar surroundings may disturb sleep or the ability to fall asleep. There are also many daily activities that influence the quality of sleep (see Table 38.1) Most of these factors are present in the acute stroke setting.

TABLE 38.1 Daily Living Activities That Influence Good Quality Sleep

Frequent napping
Variable bedtimes or morning rise times
Frequently spending an excessive length of time in bed
Regular use of sleep-disruptive substances near bedtime (e.g., alcohol, tobacco, caffeine)
Exercise too near bedtime
Stimulating activities too close to bedtime
Use of the bed for non–sleep-related activities (such as watching television, reading, snacking)
Using an uncomfortable bed
Poor control of the bedroom environment (e.g., too much light, heat, cold, or noise)
Performing activities that demand strong concentration near bedtime
Allowing oneself to persist in sleep-preventing mental activities while in bed, such as thinking, planning, reminiscing, etc. (When these mental activities persist, it is best to get out of bed for a while and do something relaxing until sleepy.)

Categories of Insomnia Subtype and Causes of Insomnia

It is not accurate to view insomnia as one single entity that has only one treatment. The International Classification of Sleep Disorders 2 (ICSD-2) presents over 30 insomnia diagnoses. As an aid to diagnosis and treatment planning, the diagnoses are grouped here into nine categories. The categories are defined by the type of cause for the sleep disturbance: (1) transient or short-term factors, (2) psychophysiological and/or conditioning factors, (3) associated with psychiatric disorders, (4) related to medications, drugs or alcohol, (5) associated with circadian rhythm disorders, (6) secondary to sleep-related physiological disorders, (7) related to neurological disorders, (8) associated with other medical illness, and (9) secondary to environmental factors (see Table 38.2).

Epidemiology

The high prevalence of insomnia is well documented; population surveys estimate that one third of all adults have one or more episodes every year. In one of the best US surveys, 15% reported having a serious problem with insomnia during the preceding year. Insomnia increases with age. Clinically significant insomnia prevalence in older adults is estimated at 25% and higher. In one U.S. poll, 67% of the adults aged 55 and above reported having symptoms of sleep disorders at least a few nights a week, but only 8% had been diagnosed with a sleep disorder and fewer received treatment. The epidemiology of insomnia in the acute stroke setting has not been fully described.

Clinical insomnia not only causes nights of restless, broken sleep, and frustration but also causes daytime sequelae that include depressed mood, anxiety, daytime fatigue, irritability, reduced concentration, and memory complaints. Daytime functioning impair-

TABLE 38.2 Insomnia Diagnoses by Type of Etiological Factor

Etiological Factor	Diagnosis
1. Transient or short-term factors	Adjustment sleep disorder
2. Insomnia related to psychophysiological and/or conditioning factors	Psychophysiological insomnia
	Idiopathic insomnia
	Sleep state misperception
	Inadequate sleep hygiene
3. Sleep disorders associated with psychiatric disorders	Psychoses associated with sleep disturbance
	Mood disorders associated with sleep disturbance
	Anxiety disorders associated with sleep disturbance
	Panic disorder associated with sleep disturbance
	Alcoholism associated with sleep disturbance
4. Insomnia related to medications, drugs, and alcohol	Hypnotic-dependent sleep disorder
	Stimulant-dependent sleep disorder
	Alcohol-dependent sleep disorder
5. Insomnia associated with circadian rhythm disorders	Delayed sleep phase syndrome
	Advanced sleep phase syndrome
	Shift work sleep disorder
	Irregular sleep–wake pattern
6. Insomnia secondary to sleep-related physiological disorders	Periodic limb movement disorder
	Restless legs syndrome
	Central sleep apnea
	Obstructive sleep apnea
	Narcolepsy
7. Insomnia related to neurological illness	Cerebral degenerative disorders
	Dementia
	Parkinsonism
8. Insomnia associated with other medical illness	Fibrositis syndrome
	Sleep-related gastroesophageal reflux
	Chronic obstructive pulmonary disease
9. Insomnia associated with situational factors	Environmental sleep disorder

ment that patients attribute to insomnia can affect the physical, emotional, cognitive, occupational, and social areas of one's life.

Transient and Short-term Insomnia

Most insomnia episodes last for 1 month or less. These are highly prevalent and they are classified as transient insomnia or short-term insomnia. When an episode lasts for more than 4 weeks, it is termed *chronic* or *persistent.*

The more brief insomnias raise the questions of treatment need and timing—whether to treat an insomnia complaint and whether to treat it right away when the patient first presents versus a decision not to treat, or at least, to delay a treatment choice until the problem is shown to be more persistent.

A decision to give no medical treatment offers the patient only support and sleep hygiene advice. A decision not to treat short-term insomnia is reasonable, based on the statistic that without treatment most transient and short-term insomnias do not progress to chronic insomnia.

The decision to treat insomnia of recent onset is a clinical one, based on patient distress and professional judgment about the need for intervention. Prevention of chronic insomnia is an additional treatment goal in a few cases. There is no research to document long-term benefits from early treatment, nor are there data showing long-term negative consequences from early treatment. Research on insomnia and stroke management is very limited.

Restless Legs Syndrome

Restless legs syndrome (RLS) is characterized by four primary diagnostic criteria: (1) an urge to move the legs usually accompanied by uncomfortable leg sensations, (2) temporary relief from the discomfort with movement, (3) worsening of the symptoms with rest or inactivity, and (4) worsening of the symptoms at night. Other features supporting the diagnosis of RLS include sleep disturbance (insomnia), involuntary leg movements, a family history of restless legs, and response to therapy with dopaminergic medications.

Patients typically have difficulty finding words to adequately describe the uncomfortable sensations and typically use a variety of descriptors: ache, discomfort, tingling, restless (plus comments such as, "have to move"), uncomfortable, creeping, crawling, pulling, or itching. The discomfort is usually in the lower leg muscles, but can involve the feet and thighs, and less commonly, the arms. The symptoms are typically present only at rest just before the sleep period, but can occur at other times, especially when lying in bed for long periods.

RLS is a pattern of subjective symptoms. To diagnose RLS, it is not necessary to perform sleep laboratory testing. RLS can be associated with anemia, uremia, and heavy caffeine intake. Predisposing factors also include rheumatoid arthritis, osteoarthritis, and peripheral vascular disease. RLS can cause severe insomnia and can be severely distressing resulting in significant psychological disturbance. In severe cases, it may lead to depression. Symptoms of RLS have been identified in 5% to 15% of healthy adults. The most common time of onset is middle age. In a recent study, moderate to severe restless legs occurred more frequently in patients with acute stroke than in age-matched controls, with as many as 62% of the stroke patients reporting at least an element of restless legs. The restlessness was most prominent in the weakened extremity. Patients confined to bed because of the stroke and associated complications reported a significant increase in RLS symptoms compared to their prestroke baseline.

Periodic Limb Movement Disorder

Periodic limb movement (PLM) disorder is characterized by frequent, rhythmic limb twitches or movements during sleep. Leg movements are most typical, but some patients have arm movements or both arm and leg movements. A key distinguishing feature is the timing of movements, which usually occur 20 to 40 seconds apart. The patient is not directly aware of the movements because they are initiated during sleep; a bed-partner may notice them, but often they occur when both parties are asleep, and go unobserved.

It is not possible to confirm the presence of a clinically significant PLM disorder without polysomnography. Physiological monitoring in a sleep laboratory reliably records all leg movements (and/or arm movements) and the degree of sleep fragmentation and restlessness caused by them.

The periodic movements can cause frequent, brief arousals leading to frequent awakenings, and/or unrefreshing sleep and excessive daytime sleepiness. The clinical significance of PLMs must be assessed on an individual basis by how much the sleep is disrupted and by the degree of daytime sleepiness. PLMs may occur as an incidental finding.

The general prevalence of PLM disorder is unknown. It shows increased incidence with age. Studies of older adults reveal PLMs in up to 45% of individuals aged 60 and above. Because PLMs are commonly associated with RLS and RLS occurs frequently in the stroke population, PLMs are likely to occur frequently in this population as well.

CLINICAL APPLICATIONS AND METHODOLOGY

Evaluation

All patients with acute stroke or transient ischemic attack (TIA) should be screened for sleep disorders, including obstructive sleep apnea, RLS, and insomnia. A number of complaints may accompany obstructive sleep apnea syndrome including sleepiness, fatigue, tiredness, and perceived laziness. A history of loud snoring, snorts, nocturnal coughing and gasping, and witnessed apneas can commonly be obtained from patients' bed-partners. Although uncommon, some patients may not have snoring or may be unaware of the nocturnal symptoms.

If possible, the patient should be evaluated with screening tools during the hospitalization. An overnight screening study with oximetry, capnography, and nasal pressure monitoring can be helpful. Unfortunately, these monitoring devices are not in widespread use. Overnight pulse oximetry provides information about the degree of oxygen desaturation but can miss significant obstructive sleep apnea and evidence of upper airway resistance syndrome. A negative oximetry study does not eliminate obstructive sleep apnea syndrome from the differential diagnosis.

All patients admitted with acute stroke or TIA should be evaluated with polysomnography following the acute phase of the stroke.

Treatment

The threshold for initiating therapy in patients with stroke or other vascular disorders should be lower than that in the general population. In this group, even relatively mild sleep apnea may warrant treatment, even if there is little or no associated daytime sleepiness. Special attention should be given to the severity of the obstructive sleep apnea during REM sleep and in each sleep position. The detrimental aspects of obstructive sleep apnea are frequently worse during REM sleep. In most patients, the severity of the sleep-related breathing disorder is worst in the supine position. Following strokes with hemiparesis, one lateral position may be associated with severe apnea while the other may be associated with relatively normal sleep.

Nasal PAP is the treatment of choice for most patients with obstructive sleep apnea. PAP treatment maintains upper airway patency via a pneumatic splint, with the air pressure preventing airway collapse. CPAP maintains a constant pressure throughout the respiratory cycle. A system of CPAP with a brief decrease in the pressure at the beginning of exhalation can significantly improve comfort and compliance, but these systems are not typically used in the hospital setting. BPAP provides a higher pressure on inhalation than on exhalation, which may be more comfortable, especially in patients with weakness from stroke or neuromuscular disease.

Empiric selection of a pressure setting for these devices is fraught with danger. An inadequate setting will leave the patient undertreated and an excessive pressure may result in patient non-compliance or central apnea. Use of auto-PAP technology can be of some benefit in the patient before formal polysomnoraphy, but this technique has not been fully developed and can inadvertently lead to incorrect titrations because of central apneas.

If CPAP is attempted during the hospitalization, the patient should be counseled on the system and treated with desensitization and acclimatization. The usual outpatient selection of masks and interfaces should be available since these are typically much more comfortable than those used in the inpatient setting. This factor may be one of the important reasons behind poor patient compliance seen in some studies. Furthermore, heated humidification makes the systems much more easily tolerated if allowed by the hospital infection control team.

Positional therapy is an option for patients with abnormal breathing isolated to a single position. Avoiding that position will then allow normal nocturnal respiration. This positional response should be documented by formal polysomnography. A wedge pillow can also be added to CPAP therapy to decrease the pressure requirement.

Supplemental oxygen alone is typically ineffective in treating the respiratory events and may actually prolong the duration of individual events. The use of stimulant medications to treat the degree of daytime sleepiness has little effect on the degree of obstructive sleep apnea. Treating the symptoms without addressing the primary problem does not significantly improve the quality of life or lower the associated vascular morbidity.

Restless legs should be treated if in the moderate-to-severe range. The effect of therapies for RLS has not been fully studied in the acute stroke setting. Patients may however report significant improvement in the quality of life once the RLS has been treated. At present two medications are approved by the Food and Drug Administration for the treatment of moderate to severe RLS—ropinirole and pramipexole. In many cases, initiation of therapy approximately 1 hour before typical bedtime can provide substantial relief from the symptoms. Many patients require more frequent dosing for symptom control since stroke patients are typically in bed and are frequently less able to move to obtain relief.

TABLE 38.3 Medications Used in the Treatment of Insomnia

Class	Medication	Half-life	Onset	Dosing (mg)
Benzodiazepine	Alprazolam	Medium	Medium	0.25–2.0
	Chlordiazepoxide	Long	Medium	10–25
	Clonazepam	Long	Medium	0.25–2.0
	Clorazepate	Long	Rapid	7.5–15
	Diazepam	Long	Rapid	2–10
	Estazolam	Medium	Rapid	1–2
	Flurazepam	Long	Medium	15–30
	Midazolam	Short	Medium	7.5–15
	Lorazepam	Medium	Medium	0.5–2
	Oxazepam	Medium	Slow	15–30
	Temazepam	Medium	Medium	15–30
	Triazolam	Short	Rapid	0.125–0.25
NBBRA	Zaleplon	Short	Rapid	10–20
	Zolpidem	Short	Rapid	5–10
	Eszopiclone	Long	Medium	1–3
TCA	Amitriptyline	Long	Medium	10–100
	Doxepin	Short	Rapid	10–100
	Imipramine	Medium	Rapid	10–100
	Nortriptyline	Long	Medium	10–100
Triazolopyridine	Trazodone	Medium	Rapid	25–100
Antiepileptic	Gabapentin	Short-medium	Medium	100–600
	Tiagabine	Medium	Medium	4–32
Dopamine antagonist	Quetiapine	Long	Medium	25–100
Other antidepressants	Mirtazapine	Long	Medium	5–45
Others	Ramelteon	Short	Rapid	8
	Melatonin	Short	Rapid	0.3–3

NBBRA, nonbenzodiazepine benzodiazepine receptor agonist; TCA, tricyclic antidepressant.

Treatment options for insomnia are reviewed in Table 38.3. The decision to initiate treatment for insomnia should be based on the severity of the symptoms and the impact on both psychological and physical functioning. The stress, anxiety, and depression associated with stroke should be taken into consideration when selecting a medication. Achieving multiple goals with a single medication may be possible in some patients.

PRACTICAL RECOMMENDATIONS

Sleep-disordered breathing disorders, including obstructive sleep apnea, occur so frequently in patients with stroke and TIA that strong consideration should be given to formal sleep evaluation with polysomnography in all cerebrovascular patients. Screening questions take only seconds to ask and can dramatically improve patient outcome. Patients may have had a sleep-related breathing disorder before the stroke or may develop it as a consequence of the associated weakness, so screening should occur both during the acute phase of stroke treatment and during follow-up examinations.

In the authors' experience, even patients with severe hemiparesis and aphasia tolerate the PAP treatment well. The importance of patient and family education cannot be overemphasized since compliance with treatment is closely related to the degree of improvement in symptoms and stroke risk reduction.

SELECTED REFERENCES

Ancoli-Israel S, Kripke DF, Klauber MR, et al. Sleep-disordered breathing in community-dwelling elderly. *Sleep* 1991;14:486–495.

Asplund R. Sleep disorders in the elderly. *Drugs Aging* 1999;14(2):91–103.

Bassetti C, Aldrich MS. Sleep apnea in acute cerebrovascular diseases: final report on 128 patients. *Sleep* 1999;22:217–223.

Bassetti CL. Sleep and stroke. *Semin Neurol* 2005;25(1):19–32.

Belozeroff V, Berry RB, and Khoo MC. Model-based assessment of autonomic control in obstructive sleep apnea syndrome. *Sleep* 2003;26:65–73.

Chan PH. Reactive oxygen radicals in signaling and damage in the ischemic brain. *J Cereb Blood Flow Metab* 2001;21:2–14.

Cherkassky T, Oksenberg A, Froom P, et al. Sleep-related breathing disorders and rehabilitation outcome of stroke patients. A prospective study. *Am J Phys Med Rehabil* 2003;82:452–455.

Cheyne J. A case of apoplexy in which the fleshy part of the heart was converted into fat. *Dublin Hospital Reports* 1818;2:216–223.

Davies DP, Rodgers H, Walshaw D, et al. Snoring, daytime sleepiness and stroke: a case-control study of first-ever stroke. *J Sleep Res* 2003;12:313–318.

Dawson SL, Manktelow BN, Robinson TG, et al. Which parameters of beat-to-beat blood pressure and variability best predict early outcome after acute ischemic stroke? *Stroke* 2000;31:463–468.

del Zoppo G, Ginis I, Hallenbeck JM, et al. Inflammation and stroke: putative role for cytokines, adhesion molecules and iNOS in brain response to ischemia. *Brain Pathol* 2000;10:95–112.

Dyken ME, Somers VK, Yamada T, et al. Investigating the relationship between stroke and obstructive sleep apnea. *Stroke* 1996;27:401–407.

Dyugovskaya L, Lavie P, and Lavie L. Increased adhesion molecules expression and production of reactive oxygen species in leukocytes of sleep apnea patients. *Am J Respir Crit Care Med* 2002;165:934–939.

Elwood P, Hack M, Pickering J, et al. Sleep disturbance, stroke, and heart disease events: evidence from the Caerphilly cohort. *J Epidemiol Community Health* 2006;60(1):69–73.

Foley D, Ancoli-Israel S, Britz P, et al. Sleep disturbances and chronic disease in older adults: results of the 2003 National Sleep Foundation Sleep in America Survey. *J Psychosom Res* 2004;56(5):497–502.

Foley DJ, Monjan A, Simonsick EM, et al. Incidence and remission of insomnia among elderly adults: an epidemiologic study of 6,800 persons over three years. *Sleep* 1999;22(Suppl 2):S366–S372.

Franklin KA. Cerebral haemodynamics in obstructive sleep apnoea and Cheyne-Stokes respiration. *Sleep Med Rev* 2002;6:429–441.

Good DC, Henkle JQ, Gelber D, et al. Sleep-disordered breathing and poor functional outcome after stroke. *Stroke* 1996;27:252–259.

Harbison J, Ford GA, James OFW, et al. Sleep-disordered breathing following acute stroke. *Q J Med* 2002;95:741–747.

Harbison J, Gibson GJ, Birchall D, et al. White matter disease and sleep-disordered breathing after acute stroke. *Neurology* 2003;61:959–963.

Harbison JA andGibson GJ. Snoring, sleep apnoea and stroke: chicken or scrambled egg? *Q J Med* 2000;93:647–654.

Hermann DM and Bassetti CL. Sleep apnea and other sleep–wake disorders in stroke. *Curr Treat Options Neurol* 2003;5(3):241–249.

Hui DSC, Choy DKL, Wong LKS, et al. Prevalence of sleep-disordered breathing and continuous positive airway pressure compliance. Results in Chinese patients with first-ever ischemic stroke. *Chest* 2002;122:852–860.

Iranzo A, Santamaria J, Berenguer J, et al. Prevalence and clinical importance of sleep apnea in the first night after cerebral infarction. *Neurology* 2002;58:911–916.

Kaneko Y, Hajek VE, Zivanovic V, et al. Relationship of sleep apnea to functional capacity and length of hospitalization following stroke. *Sleep* 2003;26:293–297.

Kato M, Roberts-Thompson P, Phillips B, et al. Impairment of endothelium-dependent vasodilation of resistance vessels in patients with obstructive sleep apnea. *Circulation* 2000;102:2607–2610.

Katsunuma H, Shimizu T, Ogawa K, et al. Treatment of insomnia by concomitant therapy with Zopiclone and Aniracetam in patients with cerebral infarction, cerebroatrophy, Alzheimer's disease and Parkinson's disease. *Psychiatr Clin Neurosci* 1998;52(2):198–200 [Review].

Kim YS, Lee SH, Jung WS, et al. Intradermal acupuncture on shen-men and nei-kuan acupoints in patients with insomnia after stroke. *Am J Chin Med* 2004;32(5):771–778.

Koskenvuo M, Kaprio J, Telakivi T, et al. Snoring as a risk factor for ischaemic heart disease and stroke in men. *Br Med J* 1987;294:16–19.

Kripke DF, Garfinkel L, Wingard DL, et al. Mortality associated with sleep duration and insomnia. *Arch Gen Psychiatr* 2002;59(2):131–136.

Lawrence E, Dundas R, Higgens S, et al. The natural history and associations of sleep disordered breathing in first ever stroke. *Int J Clin Pract* 2001;55:584–588.

Leppavuori A, Pohjasvaara T, Vataja R, et al. Generalized anxiety disorders three to four months after ischemic stroke. *Cerebrovasc Dis* 2003;16(3):257–264.

Leppavuori A, Pohjasvaara T, Vataja R, et al. Insomnia in ischemic stroke patients. *Cerebrovasc Dis* 2002;14(2):90–97.

Li Pi Shan RS and Ashworth NL. Comparison of lorazepam and zopiclone for insomnia in patients with stroke and brain injury: a randomized, crossover, double-blinded trial. *Am J Phys Med Rehabil* 2004;83(6):421–427.

McArdle N, Devereux G, Heidarnejad H, et al. Long-term use of CPAP therapy for sleep apnea/hypopnea syndrome. *Am J Respir Crit Care Med* 1999;159:1108–1114.

McArdle N, Riha RL, Vennelle M, et al. Sleep-disordered breathing as a risk factor for cerebrovascular disease: a case-control study in patients with transient ischaemic attacks. *Stroke* 2003;34:2916–2921.

Mohsenin V. Sleep-related breathing disorders and risk of stroke. *Stroke* 2001;32:1271–1278.

Nasr-Wyler A, Bouillanne O, Lalhou A, et al. Syndrome d'apnees du sommeil et accident vasculaire cerebral dans une population agee. *Rev Neurol (Paris)* 1999;155:1057–1062.

Neau JP, Meurice JC, Paquereau J, et al. Habitual snoring as a risk factor for brain infarction. *Acta Neurol Scand* 1995;92:63–68.

Neau JP, Paquereau J, Meurice JC, et al. Stroke and sleep apnoea: cause or consequence? *Sleep Med Rev* 2002;6:457–469.

Nobili L, Schiavi G, Bozano E, et al. Morning increase of whole blood viscosity in obstructive sleep apnea syndrome. *Clin Hemorheol Microcirc* 2000;22:21–27.

Palomaki H, Berg A, Meririnne E, et al. Complaints of poststroke insomnia and its treatment with mianserin. *Cerebrovasc Dis* 2003;15 (1–2):56–62.

Palomaki H. Snoring and the risk of ischemic brain infarction. *Stroke* 1991;22:1021–1025.

Parra O, Arboix A, Bechich S, et al. Time course of sleep-related breathing disorders in first-ever stroke or transient ischemic attack. *Am J Respir Crit Care Med* 2000;161:375–380.

Partinen M abd Palomaki H. Snoring and cerebral infarction. *Lancet* 1985;ii:1325–1326.

Robinson TG, Dawson SL, Eames PJ, et al. Cardiac baroreceptor sensitivity predicts long-term outcome after acute ischemic stroke. *Stroke* 2003;34:705–712.

Sandberg O, Franklin KA, Bucht G, et al. Nasal continuous positive airway pressure in stroke patients with sleep apnoea: a randomised treatment study. *Eur Respir J* 2001;18:630–634.

Sanner BM, Konermann M, Tepel M, et al. Platelet function in patients with obstructive sleep apnoea syndrome. *Eur Respir J* 2000;16:648–652.

Schulz R, Mahmoudi S, Hattar K, et al. Enhanced release of superoxide from polymorphonuclear neutrophils in obstructive sleep apnea. *Am J Respir Crit Care Med* 2000;162:566–570.

Shamsuzzaman ASM, Winnicki M, Lanfranchi P, et al. Elevated C-reactive protein in patients with obstructive sleep apnea. *Circulation* 2002;105:2462–2464.

Shepard JW. Gas exchange and hemodynamics during sleep. *Med Clin North Am* 1985;69:1234–1264.

Smirne S, Palazzi S, Zucconi M, et al. Habitual snoring as a risk factor for acute vascular disease. *Eur Respir J* 1993;6:1357–1361.

Spalletta G, Ripa A, and Caltagirone C. Symptom profile of DSM-IV major and minor depressive disorders in first-ever stroke patients. *Am J Geriatr Psychiatr* 2005;13(2):108–115.

Spriggs DA, French JM, Murdy JM, et al. Historical risk factors for stroke: a case control study. *Age Ageing* 1990;19:280–287.

Spriggs DA, French JM, Murdy JM, et al. Snoring increases the risk of stroke and adversely affects prognosis. *Q J Med* 1992;83:555–562.

Turkington PM, Allgar V, Bamford J, et al. Effect of upper airway obstruction in acute stroke on functional outcome at 6 months. *Thorax* 2004; 59:367–371.

Turkington PM, Bamford J, Wanklyn P, et al. Prevalence and predictors of upper airway obstruction in the first 24 hours after acute stroke. *Stroke* 2002;33:2037–2042.

Wessendorf TE, Teschler H, Wang YM, et al. Sleep-disordered breathing among patients with first-ever stroke. *J Neurol* 2000;247:41–47.

Wessendorf TE, Thilmann AF, Wang YM, et al. Fibrinogen levels and obstructive sleep apnea in ischemic stroke. *Am J Respir Crit Care Med* 2000;162:2039–2042.

Wessendorf TE, Wang YM, Thilmann AF, et al. Treatment of obstructive sleep apnoea with nasal continuous positive airway pressure in stroke. *Eur Respir J* 2001;18:623–629.

Yaggi H and Mohsenin V. Sleep-disordered breathing and stroke. *Clin Chest Med* 2003;24:223–237.

Yaggi K, Kernan W, and Mohsenin V. The association between obstructive sleep apnea and stroke. *Am J Respir Crit Care Med* 2003;167:A173.

CHAPTER

Cerebral Sinus Thrombosis

W. ALVIN MCELVEEN

OBJECTIVES

- What is the anatomy of the cerebral venous system?
- What are the symptoms of cerebral sinus thrombosis?
- What is the best way to test for cerebral sinus thrombosis?
- What are the treatment options for cerebral sinus thrombosis?
- What are the potential complications of cerebral sinus thrombosis?

Cerebral vein thrombosis occurs much less frequently as a cause of infarction when compared to arterial disease and can have a variety of clinical features. Its incidence has been reported at a frequency of 7 per 100,000 hospital admissions, with a ratio of venous to arterial strokes of 1:62.5.

BACKGROUND AND RATIONALE

Anatomy

Knowledge of the venous drainage patterns is helpful in determining the symptoms of cerebral venous thrombosis (CVT). However, the drainage patterns are not as defined as the arterial supply to the brain. Figure 39.1 shows the anatomy of the venous sinuses by magnetic resonance imaging (MRI).

The territories drained by the cerebral venous system are not sharply demarcated. The superficial and deep cerebral veins empty into the dural sinuses. These sinuses also communicate with the extracranial venous system, providing a collateral drainage system in case of venous sinus thrombosis. However, this may also provide a channel for intracranial spread of infection from extracranial sites. The superficial cerebral veins drain the cortex and subcortical white matter and empty into the superior sagittal sinuses (SSS). The deep cerebral veins drain the choroid plexus, the periventricular regions, diencephalon, basal ganglia, and deep white matter. They empty into the internal cerebral and great cerebral veins and basal sinuses.

There are 10 to 15 superficial veins, with only three being named. They are the superficial middle cerebral vein (SMCV), the vein of Trolard, and the vein of Labbe. SMCV drains into the cavernous sinus and receives branches from Trolard connecting SMCV to the SSS.

The vein of Labbe drains the lateral temporal lobe and empties into the transverse sinus. Branches also connect the SMCV to the transverse sinus.

The deep venous system drains centrally, with several small medullary veins draining into the subependymal veins such as the septal veins, thalamostriate veins, internal cerebral veins (ICV), basal vein of Rosenthal (BVR), and the great vein of Galen. Septal veins and thalamostriate vein (TSV) empty into the paired ICV. The ICVs join the BVR to form the vein of Galen. The vein of Galen then joins the inferior sagittal sinus to form the straight sinus. This terminates at the confluence of sinuses where it joins the SSS, giving rise to the transverse sinuses.

There are three major venous systems in the posterior fossa. The superior group consists of the precentral cerebellar vein, the

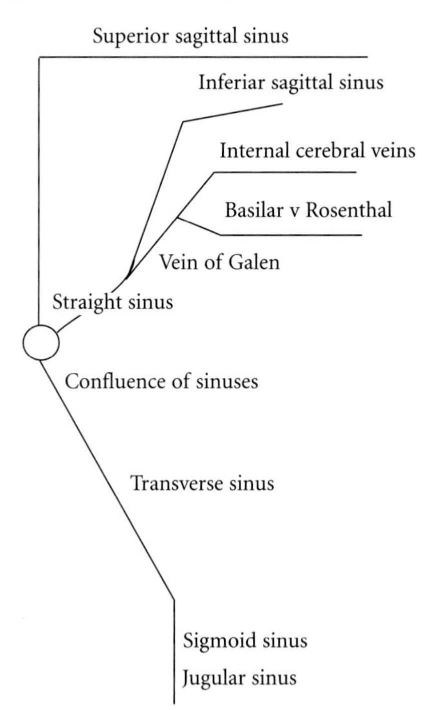

FIGURE 39.1. Schematic of major cerebral sinuses.

superior vermian vein, and the anterior pontomesencephalic veins. The PCV and SVV terminate in the vein of Galen. The anterior group consists of the petrosal vein, which receives tributaries from the cerebellum, pons, and medulla, with termination in the superior petrosal sinus. The most important veins of the posterior group are the inferior vermian veins, which terminate in the transverse, superior petrosal, and occipital sinuses.

Symptoms

Unlike arterial strokes, venous occlusion may present in a slower, progressive course. Patients with hormonal etiology usually present with a more sudden time course.

The presenting symptoms depend on the area of thrombosis. Many patients present with headaches. Although thunderclap headaches have often been considered to be the presenting symptoms for subarachnoid hemorrhage, this may also be seen in venous sinus thrombosis. Headaches are also seen with pseudotumor cerebri, which is often seen with lateral sinus thrombosis.

Sagittal sinus thrombosis may be associated with hemiparesis, lower extremity paresis, or bilateral lower extremity weakness. Seizures are often present with venous infarction. Decreased level of consciousness progressing to coma may occur and is more frequent in older patients.

Receptive aphasia may be seen with temporal lobe. Ataxia with cerebellar thrombosis is common. Nausea and vomiting are often associated symptoms. Many venous infarcts are hemorrhagic in nature.

Cranial nerve palsies including pulsatile tinnitus, vestibular neuronopathy, unilateral deafness, diplopia, facial weakness, and visual obscuration are seen. Findings on examination may include papilledema, hemianopsia, oculomotor nerve involvement, and abducens nerve deficit. If the jugular vein is involved at the jugular foramen, cranial nerves IX, X, and XI may be affected.

Cavernous sinus thrombosis is associated with ipsilateral periorbital edema, papilledema, and retinal hemorrhages. The first division of the trigeminal nerve as well as oculomotor paresis can be seen.

Cortical vein thrombosis in the absence of venous sinus thrombosis is unusual but does occur. Symptoms may include aphasia, hemiparesis, seizures, hemisensory loss, and hemianopsia.

Transient global amnesia is a condition associated with the loss of antegrade memory in the absence of other neurological symptoms, with recovery of function within 24 hours. The cause is unknown but the pathophysiology has been postulated to include migraine, transient ischemic attack (TIA), seizure, and paradoxical embolus through patent foramen ovale. One of the latest considerations is that of venous congestion with thrombosis of the deep cerebral venous system. This, however, may be difficult to see with newer imaging techniques.

Thrombosis of the deep veins classically involves the diencephalon resulting in coma and eye movement abnormalities. Prognosis is often poor. Partial symptoms may occur depending on collateral circulation, the territory of the involved venous structure, and the extent of thrombosis.

The presentation and prognosis in elderly patients may be somewhat different from that in younger patients. Isolated intracranial hypertension syndrome is seen less frequently in the elderly, while altered level of consciousness is more common.

Potential Etiologies

The occurrence of cerebral sinus thrombosis is more frequent in women, but there does not appear to be a racial predilection. There are higher number of cases of CVT in women between the ages of 20 and 35 compared to men. This may be related to pregnancy or the use of hormonal contraceptives. Many causative conditions are described in CVT. In addition to pregnancy and oral contraceptives, other hypercoagulable states may be causative. These include the antiphospholipid syndrome, factor V Leiden deficiency, protein S and C deficiency, antithrombin III deficiency, and the lupus anticoagulant syndrome. In addition, the use of oral contraceptives in women with the factor V Leiden mutation seems to be associated with a greater risk for venous thrombosis compared with nonusers of hormonal contraceptives with the mutation.

Another medical condition that seems to predispose to venous sinus thrombosis includes paranasal sinus infection. When the frontal sinus is involved, this may also be associated with direct extension of the infection with subdural empyema formation. Trauma may be associated with the occurrence of CVT.

Other medical conditions have been associated with venous sinus thrombosis. Inflammatory bowel disease such as Crohn disease and ulcerative colitis are described as risk factors. Corticosteroids are associated with increased risk of venous thrombosis. Hematological conditions including paroxysmal nocturnal hemoglobinuria, thrombotic thrombocytopenia purpura, sickle cell disease, and polycythemia are considered risk factors. Malignancies may be associated with hypercaoagulable states. Carcinoma as a cause of venous sinus thrombosis is more common in the elderly. Collagen vascular diseases such as systemic lupus erythematosis, Wegener's granulomatosis, and Behçet's syndrome have been reported to be associated with CVT. Nephrotic syndrome, dehydration, hepatic cirrhosis, and sarcoidosis have all been described as increasing the risk of CVT.

Several medications have been associated with development of CVT. Among these are oral contraceptives, corticosteroids, e-amino caproic acid, and L-asparaginase. Heparin therapy has been reported to produce thrombotic thrombocytopenia with associated venous sinus thrombosis.

Diagnosis

The development of MRI has improved the diagnostic capabilities in determining the presence of cerebral sinus thrombosis. MRI brain scan typically shows an infarct that does not follow an expected arterial distribution. The infarct is often hemorrhagic, and flow voids may be absent where flow was expected.

Magnetic resonance venography (MRV) visualizes the dural sinuses well. There may be normal variant anatomical narrowing of the left sinus, however. Computed tomogram (CT) angiography may be helpful in resolving questions related to flow voids or atypical venous drainage seen on MRV. CT venography with matched mask bone elimination technique may be a useful adjunct for the visualization of the intracranial venous circulation by removing bone from the image.

Carotid arteriography with delayed filming technique to visualize the venous system was the procedure of choice in the diagnosis of venous thrombosis before the advent of MRV. It is an invasive procedure and is therefore associated with a small risk. Direct venography can be performed by passing a catheter from the jugular vein into the transverse sinus with injection outlining the venous sinuses.

Clinical laboratory studies are useful for determining the possible cause of CVT. Diagnosis of the condition is made on the basis of clinical presentation and imaging studies. Complete blood count (CBC) is done to assess polycythemia as an etiologic factor. Decreased platelet count would support thrombotic thrombocytopenic purpura; leukocytosis might be seen in sepsis. In addition, if heparin is used for treatment, platelet counts should be monitored for thrombocytopenia. Antiphospholipid and anticardiolipin antibody levels should be obtained to evaluate for antiphospholipid syndrome. Other tests that may indicate hypercoagulable states include protein S, protein C, antithrombin III, lupus anticoagulant, and factor V Leiden mutation. These evaluations should not be made while the patient is on anticoagulant therapy.

Sickle cell preparation or hemoglobin electrophoresis should be obtained in individuals of African decent. Erythrocyte sedimentation rate and antinuclear antibody (ANA) should be performed to screen for systemic lupus erythematosus, Wegener granulomatosis, and temporal arteritis. If the values are elevated, further evaluation including complement levels, anti-deoxyribonucleic acid (DNA) antibodies, and neutrophil cytoplasmic antibodies (ANCA) could be considered. Urine protein levels should be checked, and if elevated, nephrotic syndrome should be considered. Liver function studies should be performed to rule out cirrhosis.

D-Dimer values may be beneficial in screening patients who present in the emergency department for headache evaluation. This test does not establish the diagnosis of CVT, and more definitive studies, such as MRV, are necessary. Likewise, if a high suspicion for CVT exists, the test does not definitely exclude the diagnosis, and imaging procedures should be done if clinical suspicion is high.

Treatment

The initial management of cerebral vein thrombosis involves stabilization similar to the management of arterial stroke patients. Patients with altered mental status or hemiplegia should be given nothing by mouth to prevent aspiration. Intravenous fluids should not be hypotonic solutions. Normal saline is recommended at a rate of approximately 1,000 mL in 24 hours. In the treatment of stroke patients, supplemental oxygen has not been shown to be beneficial unless the level of consciousness is decreased. Pulse oximetry may be used and supplemental oxygen used if pO_2 is $<95\%$.

The use of anticoagulation in CVT has been a subject of some debate among neurologists for many years. Concern has been expressed over the possibility of increasing hemorrhage in patients treated in this manner. Several studies, however, have indicated that anticoagulation could be used safely in this condition. The question of effectiveness of anticoagulation is not clear, but most articles tend to point toward improved outcome with its use. The prevention of propagation of the clot has been the goal of heparin therapy.

Thrombolytic therapy has been described in several case reports as being beneficial in cases of CVT. These patients were treated with an infusion of a thrombolytic agent into the dural venous sinus using the microcatheter technique. This treatment is at present limited to specialized centers but should be considered for patients with significant deficit. No data supporting the use of intravenous immunoglobulin (IVIG) have been described.

A recent report describes the use of a rheolytic catheter device in a patient who had not responded to microcatheter instillation of urokinase. The rheolytic catheter was designed for use in the coronary circulation and delivers six high-velocity saline jets through a halo device at the tip of the catheter. This leads to a Bernoulli effect that breaks up the thrombus. In addition, the particulate debris is directed into an effluent lumen for collection into a disposable bag. The catheter is advanced into the sagittal sinus, resulting in restoration of venous flow and reduction of intracranial pressure.

In cases of severe neurological deterioration, open thrombectomy and local thrombolytic therapy have been described as being beneficial. Patients selected for these procedures have progressed despite adequate anticoagulation and intensive medical care.

Outcome

Mortality in untreated cases of venous thrombosis has been reported to range from 13.8% to 48%; this high mortality rate may be a reflection of clinical severity at entrance into the study. Between 25% and 30% of patients will have full recovery.

The prognosis is less favorable in patients older than 65. Forty-nine percent of elderly patients make a complete recovery compared to 27% of younger patients. The death rate is 27% for the elderly group compared to 7% of the younger patients.

CLINICAL APPLICATIONS AND METHODOLOGY

Presenting symptoms such as thunderclap headaches, seizures, lower extremity or bilateral lower extremity weakness, and altered level of consciousness progressing to coma should lead to clinical suspicion and consideration of cerebral vein thrombosis as a diagnosis.

On occasion, findings on an MRI or CT scan may trigger suspicion of cerebral vein thrombosis. For example, a hemorrhagic posterior temporal lobe lesion is often seen in the condition and should trigger the appropriate imaging procedure. On routine MRI, one can often see a flow void in a thrombosed sinus. An infarct that does not correspond to an arterial distribution may suggest CVT.

MRV using phase contrast technique is presently the procedure of choice to diagnose CVT. CT venography may also add information in questionable cases. Direct angiography with venous phase filming or jugular venography were used before MR and CT techniques but are invasive procedures. However in select cases, these procedures can be considered.

Treatment consists of fluid and neurological stabilization similar to the care of arterial cerebral infarcts. However, the use of heparin is recommended in patients with CVT to prevent clot propagation. No increase in hemorrhagic complications has been seen in patients treated with heparin compared to those who were not. For patients who do not respond to these measures, direct injection of thrombolytic agents via microcatheter or rheolytic may be performed in those facilities that have expertise.

The clinical causes of CVT should be explored, including hypercoaguable states, oral contraceptive use or other hormonal conditions, medical conditions such as Crohn's disease, polycythemia, neoplasm, trauma, or infections.

PRACTICAL RECOMMENDATIONS

Brain MRI often gives a strong clue that CVT should be considered. The author finds that one can become suspicious, especially on a contrast scan, if a sinus is not visualized. The distribution of cerebral infarcts and hemorrhagic infarcts can be a significant indicator.

In evaluating patients with a diagnosis of stroke, if there is a risk factor for venous thrombosis, I will evaluate for CVT also. For example, a patient with Crohn's disease was found to have lateral sinus thrombosis after presenting with a temporal lobe hemorrhage.

Patients with pseudotumor cerebri may have lateral sinus thrombosis. The author obtains MRV in all such patients. In addition, patients should be checked for factors associated with CVT such as hypercoagulable laboratory evaluations, CBC, urine for protein, sedimentation rate and ANA.

Patients with thunderclap headaches are usually evaluated for subarachnoid hemorrhage. If that evaluation is negative, MRV should be considered.

Heparin, even in the presence of a hemorrhagic lesion, is recommended if the imaging procedure demonstrates cerebral vein thrombosis.

The author usually keeps the patient on warfarin for a period of 6 months, after which the imaging procedure is repeated to assess for recanalization of the vessel. If the patient is found to have hypercoagulation syndrome such as factor V Leiden, then that patient will likely be on anticoagulation indefinitely.

SELECTED REFERENCES

Adams WM, Laitt RD, Beards SC, et al. Use of single-slice thick slab phase-contrast angiography for the diagnosis of dural venous sinus thrombosis. *Eur Radiol* 1999;9(8):1614–1619.

Ameri A, Bousser MG. Cerebral venous thrombosis. *Neurol Clin* 1992;10(1):87–111.

Ayanzen RH, Bird CR, Keller PJ, et al. Cerebral MR venography: normal anatomy and potential diagnostic pitfalls. *Am J Neuroradiol* 2000;21(1): 74–78.

Benamer HT, Bone I. Cerebral venous thrombosis: anticoagulants or thrombolyic therapy? *J Neurol Neurosurg Psychiatr* 2000;69(4): 427–430.

Buccino G, Scoditti U, Patteri I, et al. Neurological and cognitive long-term outcome in patients with cerebral venous sinus thrombosis. *Acta Neurol Scand* 2003;107(5):330–335.

Cipri S, Gangemi A, Campolo C, et al. High-dose heparin plus warfarin administration in non-traumatic dural sinuses thrombosis. A clinical and neuroradiological study. *J Neurosurg Sci* 1998;42(1):23–23.

D'Alise MD, Fichtel F, Horowitz M. Sagittal sinus thrombosis following minor head injury treated with continuous urokinase infusion. *Surg Neurol* 1998;49(4):430–435.

Daif A, Awada A, al-Rajeh S, et al. Cerebral venous thrombosis in adults. A study of 40 cases from Saudi Arabia. *Stroke* 1995;26(7):1193–1195.

Dentali F, Crowther M, and Ageno, W. Thrombophillic abnormalities, oral contraceptives, and risk of cerebral vein thrombosis: a meta-analysis. *Blood* 2006;107(7):2766–2773.

Einhaupl KM, Villringer A, Meister W, et al. Heparin treatment in sinus venous thrombosis. *Lancet* 1991;338(8767):597–600.

Ekseth K, Bostrom S, Vegfors M. Reversibility of severe sagittal sinus thrombosis with open surgical thrombectomy combined with local infusion of tissue plasminogen activator: technical case report. *Neurosurgery* 1998;43(4):960–965.

Farb RI, Vanek I, Scott JN, et al. Idiopathic intracranial hypertension: the prevalence and morphology of sinovenous stenosis. *Neurology* 2003; 60(9):1418–1424.

Ferro JM, Lopes MG, Rosas MJ, et al. Long-term prognosis of cerebral vein and dural sinus thrombosis results of the venoport study. *Cerebrovasc Dis* 2002;13(4):272–278.

Ferro, JM, Lopes MG, Rosas MJ, et al. Cerebral vein and dural sinus thrombosis in elderly patients. *Stroke* 2005;36(9):1927–1932.

Gomez CR, Misra VK, Terry JB, et al. Emergency endovascular treatment of cerebral sinus thrombosis with a rheolytic catheter device. *J Neuroimaging* 2000;10(3):177–180.

Jacobs K, Moulin T, Bogousslavsky J, et al. The stroke syndrome of cortical vein thrombosis. *Neurology* 1996;47(2):376–382.

Meyer-Lindenberg A, Quenzel EM, Bierhoff E, et al. Fatal cerebral venous sinus thrombosis in heparin-induced thrombotic thrombocytopenia. *Eur Neurol* 1997;37(3):191–192.

Oppenheim C, Domigo V, Gauvrit JY, et al. Subarachnoid hemorrhage as the initial presentation of dural sinus thrombosis. *Am J Neuroradiol* 2005;26(3):614–617.

Solheim O, Skeidsvoll T. Transient global amnesia maybe caused by cerebral vein thrombosis. *Med Hypothes* 2005;65(6):1142–1149.

Smith AG, Cornblath WT, Deveikis JP. Local thrombolytic therapy in deep cerebral venous thrombosis. *Neurology* 1997;48(6):1613–1619.

Tardy B, Tardy-Poncet B, Viallon A, et al. D-Dimer levels in patients with suspected acute cerebral venous thrombosis. *Am J Med* 2002;113(3): 238–241.

Towbin A. The syndrome of latent cerebral venous thrombosis: its frequency and relation to age and congestive heart failure. *Stroke* 1973;4(3): 419–430.

van den Bergh WM, van der Schaaf I, van Gijn J. The spectrum of presentations of venous infarction caused by deep cerebral vein thrombosis. *Neurology* 2005;65:192–196.

Poststroke Depression

STEPHENIE C. DILLARD AND JAMES D. GEYER

OBJECTIVES

- What is the prevalence of poststroke depression?
- What is a simple, rapid, and reliable means for diagnosing patients with poststroke depression?
- What are the potential negative outcomes associated with poststroke depression and the benefits of treatment?
- What is the best approach to the management and follow-up of patients with poststroke depression?

Kudos to all physicians reading this chapter! Although depression is arguably the most common complication of stroke, it is the most underdiagnosed and untreated sequela of stroke. Since little is known about the etiology of poststroke depression (PSD), this chapter focuses on the clinical importance of the diagnosis and appropriate management of PSD. We have not addressed theories on its underlying pathophysiology, since, for the clinical physician, it is irrelevant whether the cause is biological and directly related to ischemic brain injury or whether it is primarily a psychological response to the disability, handicap, and sick role that may accompany stroke.

BACKGROUND AND RATIONALE

Although PSD is defined as depression that arises after stroke, surprisingly, the specific diagnostic criteria are not generally agreed on. Some researchers hold to the strict criteria of major depression as defined by the *Diagnostic and Statistical Manual of Mental Disorders*, Fourth Edition (*DSM-IV*), while others include minor depression in the diagnosis (Table 40.1). Still others have used abnormal results on a variety of neuropsychological tests that screen for depression, the most common of which include the Hamilton Depression Rating Scale, Montgomery and Asberg Depression Rating Scale, Beck Depression Inventory, and the Present Status Examination. Some of the prevalence studies have included cases using the physician's subjective impression of the presence of depressive symptoms. Given the variety of diagnostic criteria, the reported prevalence of PSD widely ranges from 16% to 62%, with the more reliable studies reporting 25% to 40% of stoke patients meeting the *DSM-IV* criteria of major or minor depression. Most cases develop soon after the stroke and persist from 6 to 12 months, with the frequency decreasing as time progresses, although a significant minority of patients may suffer from depression for 24 months or longer after the initial stroke. Since it appears that PSD occurs more frequently in patients with greater disability, its actual incidence may be much higher, since most studies have excluded aphasic patients and those with cognitive impairment. On the basis of a conservative estimate of 500,000 ischemic strokes in the United States per year, >150,000 stroke survivors meet the criteria for the diagnosis of PSD each year.

CLINICAL APPLICATIONS AND METHODOLOGY

As the average length of hospitalization decreases, the clinician may overlook the early symptoms of PSD as more urgent issues are addressed in the acute phase of stroke care. Further hindering diagnosis is the overlap that exists between depressive symptoms and somatic manifestations of stroke such as alterations in sleep patterns, fatigue, decreased appetite, and feelings of sluggishness or agitation. Language and cognitive impairment, emotional lability, and attentional disturbances further complicate the diagnostic picture. Often physicians recognize the early signs of PSD, but feel that such sadness is to be expected following a disabling stroke.

TABLE 40.1 Symptoms of Depression

Five (or more) of the following symptoms present during the same 2-wk period

1. Depressed mood most of the day
2. Markedly diminished interest or pleasure in activities
3. Significant weight change without purposeful diet change
4. Insomnia
5. Hypersomnia
6. Psychomotor agitation or retardation
7. Fatigue or loss of energy
8. Feelings of worthlessness or inappropriate guilt
9. Diminished ability to think or concentrate
10. Recurrent thoughts of death or recurrent suicidal ideation

Since the *DSM-IV* criteria require that the depressive symptoms persist for at least 2 weeks, the question arises as to who is responsible for making the diagnosis of PSD and managing treatment. By this time, many patients have returned to the care of their primary physician or are under the supervision of a rehabilitation facility.

Diagnosis

Unfortunately, there is no reproducible evidence that allows identification of patients at greatest risk of developing PSD. Numerous studies have demonstrated that there is no consistent association between stroke location, stroke volume, or the presence of preexisting lesions such as atrophy and an increased risk of developing PSD. PSD has been shown to arise more frequently in patients who have a history of prestroke depression, a lack of social support, and who have resulting severe disabilities including cognitive dysfunction, dysphasia/aphasia, or altered visual perception. Although hyperemotionalism can occur in nondepressed patients, one study concluded that those who display pathological crying, overt sadness, or catastrophic reactions immediately after stroke have an increased risk of having PSD at 3 and 12 months after the stroke. Apathetic patients did not show an increased risk of depression.

With 750,000 new ischemic strokes reported each year, physicians need a reliable and rapid means for diagnosing PSD since detailed psychiatric evaluation of all survivors is not practical. The single question, "Do you often feel sad or depressed?," has proved to have good correlation with the results of the Montgomery and Asberg Depression Rating Scale, showing 86% sensitivity, 78% specificity, 82% positive predictive value, and 82% negative predictive value. A single question can easily be used at the bedside or incorporated into a routine follow-up office visit, and it does not require the patient to read, write, or have normal speech to provide useful information.

Morbidity and Mortality Associated with Poststroke Depression

PSD has been shown to have a consistent, strong correlation with cognitive impairment, impaired functional recovery, poor perceived quality of life, and increased mortality. The relationship of PSD and poor outcome is akin to the question of the proverbial chicken-and-egg dilemma. In clinical practice, it does not matter what the inciting event is—the depression with accompanying decreased physical activity, impaired social relationships, and decreased compliance or the poor outcome. There is evidence that adequate treatment may not only improve the depressive symptoms but also improve the patient's quality of life, enhance the effective of rehabilitation, and possibly decrease the patient's long-term physical disabilities.

Cognitive impairment is common after stroke; reported in 14% to 35% of patients. Depression can result in pseudodementia or reversible dementia that improves on remission of the depression. In a double-blind, placebo-controlled study, stroke patients with major and minor depression showed improved cognition as measured by the Mini-Mental State Examination when their depression improved, regardless of whether the improvement came as a result of nortriptyline therapy or by spontaneous remission in the placebo group. A second study found that once cognitive function had improved following remission of PSD, it was likely to remain stable in the absence of recurrent stroke or other brain injury.

Both major and minor PSD have been shown to affect recovery of activities of daily living (ADL). When stroke patients were followed up in an acute rehabilitation facility, those reporting depressive symptoms made slower progress in regaining basic functional capacities such as mobility, dressing, and self-feeding. Interestingly, depressive symptoms but not cognitive impairment predicted how efficiently the patient could use rehabilitation services. Depression was not associated with longer stays in the rehabilitation facility but did correlate with poor functional outcome at home. (Owing to external pressures to maintain lower costs, the researchers reported the length of stay was routinely determined by functional status at the time of admission rather than response to therapy.) When patients diagnosed in-hospital with minor and major PSD were followed up for 3 or 6 months, the patients with remission of depression had significantly greater recovery of ADL functions than those whose mood did not improve. This finding occurred regardless of demographic variables, lesion characteristics, initial neurological deficits, cognitive impairment, or use of physical therapy and was comparable in patients with minor and major PSD.

Handicap is defined as the disadvantage resulting from ill health that limits fulfillment of societal roles, while disability is described as the inability to perform a given task. Handicap is common after stroke, even in nondisabled patients, and PSD may play an important role. Reduction of handicap by restoring function and teaching adaptive behaviors is the key aim of poststroke rehabilitation. When first-ever cases of stroke were evaluated 2 years after stroke for disability, physical impairment, depression, anxiety, and living arrangements, the independent determinants of handicap were disability, physical impairment, age, depression, and anxiety.

Quality of life encompasses both physical and mental components including socioemotional factors. The importance of addressing issues influencing quality of life has recently come to the forefront as patients have begun to expect greater satisfaction with health care. Stroke patients were assessed at 4 and 16 months following stroke using a questionnaire designed to assess the respondent's subjective view on different aspects of life, the Mini-Mental Status Examination and the Geriatric Depression Scale. Multivariate analysis showed that the most important determinants of perceived poor quality of life at 16 months were depression, poor functional status, older age, and female gender.

One could intuitively understand how depression could negatively affect poststroke recovery and perceived quality of life; however, the association of PSD and increased mortality following stroke is less obvious. A cohort of stroke patients was assessed for depression approximately 2 weeks after their initial stroke and their vital status was assessed at 10 years, by which time 53% of the patients had died. Patients who had been diagnosed with major or minor PSD were 3.4 times more likely to have died during the follow-up period. This finding was independent of other risk factors such as age, gender, social class, type of stroke, lesion location, and level of social function. The increased mortality was most notable in the first 5 years following the incident stroke, after which time the death rates of depressed and nondepressed patients were roughly the same. The study did not follow the depressive symptoms or report how many patients received treatment, so it is unclear whether remission of depression positively influenced mortality.

Treatment

Large double-blind, placebo-controlled studies of pharmacological agents for the prevention and treatment of PSD are lacking. Most studies are small and lack homogeneous clinical trial methodology. Meta-analysis of such trials is limited by the absence of consistent diagnostic criteria, lack of uniformity of the timeframe of treatment (both in time of initiation of treatment and duration of medication), variation in drug classes tested, and the end point sought (remission versus recovery versus documentable improvement in mood scores). Many studies limited the treatment window to 6 weeks or less, a very short period to assess the efficacy of an antidepressant. Meta-analysis of seven treatment and nine prevention placebo-controlled trials showed that although there was some evidence that medication can reduce depressive symptoms, given the heterogeneous results and wide confidence intervals, there was no clear reproducible evidence that therapy improved mood scores, cognitive function, or disability. Although a clear benefit of treatment was not detected, analysis failed to reveal any evidence of harm caused by pharmacological therapy.

The pharmacological treatment of PSD raises several questions. Although PSD is a common complication of stroke, many studies indicate that most patients will have spontaneous remission of depressive symptoms. Given the potential side effects of antidepressant medication, many clinicians feel that a wait-and-see approach is prudent; however, there is evidence that a relatively narrow therapeutic window exists for maximum benefit. Many of the placebo-controlled studies that showed no substantial recovery of ADLs in patients treated with antidepressants had initiated treatment months after the initial stroke. In a doubleblind, placebo-controlled randomized study, stroke patients, regardless of depressive symptoms, were randomized into one of six treatment groups: They were treated with fluoxetine, nortriptyline, or placebo, which was initiated within 1 month or after 1 month of stroke. Recovery of ADL of all patients was documented at 3, 6, 9, and 12 weeks and 12 and 24 months. Although both the early and late treatment groups improved gradually during the 3-month period, the early treatment group improved more rapidly, with ADL improvement exceeding the late treatment group at both 12 and 24 months. While the early treatment group remained stable during the second year, the late treatment group showed deterioration of ADL during the same period.

It is true that many cases of PSD will spontaneously remit, but treatment is associated with a higher rate of remission. A treatment study comparing the effects of nortriptyline versus placebo in improving ADL in a patient population with PSD demonstrated that there was a statistically significant functional improvement at 2 months in patients whose depression had remitted, regardless of whether the remission was spontaneous or following treatment; however, 70% of patients on nortriptyline had remission of depressive symptoms compared to 10% of the patients receiving placebo. Although short-term benefits of antidepressant therapy are questionable, the benefits of drug treatment may have long-term effects that continue even after the medication has been discontinued. In one study, patients diagnosed with moderate to severe PSD within 2 weeks of stoke were given fluoxetine or placebo for 3 months and then evaluated at 18 months. The depressive symptoms of both groups improved equally in the first 4 weeks of treatment, underscoring the high spontaneous remission rate of PSD; however, the patients who received fluoxetine were less likely to have clinical depression (18% versus 72%) at the 18-month follow-up.

As stated earlier, PSD is associated with poor quality of life. A randomized double-blind, placebo-controlled study treated patients diagnosed with major and minor PSD with either sertraline, a selective serotonin reuptake inhibitor, or placebo for 26 weeks. Although there was no statistical difference in the decrease in depression scores between the two groups at 6 and 26 weeks, and there was no substantial improvement in ADL or neurological deficit in either group, the patients receiving the antidepressant reported improved quality of life, which was significantly better than that of the non-treated group.

Finally, the effect of treatment of PSD on mortality rates was addressed in a double-blind, placebo-controlled study that treated depressed and nondepressed stroke patients within the first 6 months of stroke with a 12-week course of fluoxetine, nortriptyline, or placebo. They were followed up at 3, 9, 12, 18, and 24 months, and their vital status was determined 9 years poststroke. Of the patients who received the full 12-week course of antidepressant, 68% were alive at follow-up compared to 36% of those who received placebo. The increased probability of survival was seen in both the depressed and nondepressed groups. Of the depressed patients, 71% with chronic or relapsing depression were dead at follow-up compared to 27% of patients who responded to treatment and 36% of patients with no depressive disorder.

Prevention

Another point of study is whether the use of antidepressants in the acute phase of stroke can prevent PSD. In a randomized but not placebo-controlled study, patients with ischemic stroke were divided into a treatment group that was given the antidepressant mirtazapine and a nontreatment group that received no medication. Treatment was initiated on the first day of hospital admission, and the patients were examined on days 7, 44, 90, 180, 270, and 360. PSD developed in 40% of the untreated group compared to 6% of the patients receiving the antidepressant.

PRACTICAL RECOMMENDATIONS

It is estimated that less than one third of patients with PSD are treated. Although meta-analysis of combined trials failed to show statistically significant benefit of treatment, many studies have shown that treatment of PSD can influence functional recovery, improve quality of life, decrease mortality, and possibly reduce use of health care. There is speculation that some antidepressants used in the acute phase of stroke may enhance the plasticity of the brain and aid in maximum neurological recovery following ischemic injury. However, definitive evidence is lacking to support the use of antidepressants in all patients. In our experience, patients who exhibit pathological crying or excessive emotionalism in the acute phase benefit from antidepressant medications. We also recommend that each day during hospitalization and at each follow up visit within the first year, whether with the neurologist or primary care physician, the patient should be questioned about his/her emotional state, specifically including the question "Are you often sad or depressed?" Patients who answer "yes" should be offered a course of antidepressants. Patients expressing suicidal ideations should be referred to a psychiatrist for further evaluation.

The selection of an antidepressant should be based on its side effect profile. Nortriptyline, for example, is contraindicated in patients with cardiac conduction abnormalities, narrow angle glaucoma, and orthostatic hypotension. Medications that cause sedation such as mirtazapine should be used judiciously in patients with poststroke somnolence or in those with a tendency to fall, but this side effect may be beneficial in patients who have difficulty sleeping. Fluoxetine has been associated with weight loss, a benefit for some patients but a contraindication for others. No controlled studies of nonpharmacological treatments such as psychotherapy, cognitive behavioral therapy, family therapy, and electroconvulsive therapy have been performed.

In summary, a significant minority of stroke patients will develop PSD, an entity that has been associated with poor functional outcome and increased mortality. Remission of PSD appears to offer many long-term benefits, and physicians should routinely inquire about the psychological health of stroke patients, especially those with poor social support, and offer appropriate treatment to patients exhibiting depressive symptoms.

SELECTED REFERENCES

Aben I, Verhey F. Depression after a cerebrovascular accident. The importance of the integration of neurobiological and psychosocial pathogenic models. *Panminerva Med* 2006;48(1):49–57.

Amore M, Tagariello P, Laterza C, et al. Beyond nosography of depression in elderly. *Arch Gerontol Geriatr* 2007;44(Suppl 1):13–22.

Anderson CS, Hackett ML, House AO. Interventions for preventing depression after stroke. *Cochrane Database Syst Rev* 2004;(2):CD003689.

Annoni JM, Staub F, Bruggimann L, et al. Emotional disturbances after stroke. *Clin Exp Hypertens* 2006;28(3–4):243–249.

Bhogal SK, Teasell R, Foley N, et al. Lesion location and poststroke depression: systematic review of the methodological limitations in the literature. *Stroke* 2004;35(3):794–802.

Colle F, Bonan I, Gellez Leman MC, et al. Fatigue after stroke. *Ann Readapt Med Phys* 2006;49(6):272–276, 361–364.

Dieguez S, Staub F, Bruggimann L, et al. Is poststroke depression a vascular depression? *J Neurol Sci* 2004;226(1–2):53–58.

Farrell C. Poststroke depression in elderly patients. *Dimens Crit Care Nurs* 2004;23(6):264–269.

Hackett ML, Anderson CS, House AO. Interventions for treating depression after stroke. *Cochrane Database Syst Rev* 2004;(3):CD003437.

Hackett ML, Anderson CS, House AO. Management of depression after stroke: a systematic review of pharmacological therapies. *Stroke* 2005; 36(5):1098–1103.

Hackett ML, Anderson CS. Predictors of depression after stroke: a systematic review of observational studies. *Stroke* 2005;36(10):2296–2301.

Johnson JL, Minarik PA, Nystrom KV, et al. Poststroke depression incidence and risk factors: an integrative literature review. *J Neurosci Nurs* 2006;38(4 Suppl):316–327.

Kales HC, Maixner DF, Mellow AM. Cerebrovascular disease and late-life depression. *Am J Geriatr Psychiatr* 2005;13(2):88–98.

Kanner AM. Should neurologists be trained to recognize and treat comorbid depression of neurologic disorders? Yes. *Epilepsy Behav* 2005;6(3): 303–311.

Kappelle LJ, Van Der Worp HB. Treatment or prevention of complications of acute ischemic stroke. *Curr Neurol Neurosci Rep* 2004;4(1): 36–41.

Khan F. Poststroke depression. *Aust Fam Phys.* 2004;33(10):831–834.

Krishnan KR. Treatment of depression in the medically ill. *J Clin Psychopharmacol* 2005;25(4 Suppl 1):S14–S18.

Mast BT, Vedrody S. Poststroke depression: a biopsychosocial approach. *Curr Psychiatry Rep* 2006;8(1):25–33.

Mukherjee D, Levin RL, Heller W. The cognitive, emotional, and social sequelae of stroke: psychological and ethical concerns in post-stroke adaptation. *Top Stroke Rehabil* 2006;13(4):26–35.

Newberg AR, Davydow DS, Lee HB. Cerebrovascular disease basis of depression: post-stroke depression and vascular depression. *Int Rev Psychiatr* 2006;18(5):433–441.

Paranthaman R and Baldwin RC. Treatment of psychiatric syndromes due to cerebrovascular disease. *Int Rev Psychiatr* 2006;18(5):453–470.

Rampello L, Battaglia G, Raffaele R, et al. Is it safe to use antidepressants after a stroke? *Expert Opin Drug Saf* 2005;4(5):885–897.

Rickards H. Depression in neurological disorders: Parkinson's disease, multiple sclerosis, and stroke. *J Neurol Neurosurg Psychiatr* 2005; 76(Suppl 1):i48–i52.

Robinson RG. Poststroke depression: prevalence, diagnosis, treatment, and disease progression. *Biol Psychiatr* 2003;54(3):376–387.

Roman GC. Vascular depression: an archetypal neuropsychiatric disorder. *Biol Psychiatr* 2006;60(12):1306–1308.

Rosen HJ, Cummings J. A real reason for patients with pseudobulbar affect to smile. *Ann Neurol* 2007;61(2):92–96.

Sobel RM, Lotkowski S, Mandel S. Update on depression in neurologic illness: stroke, epilepsy, and multiple sclerosis. *Curr Psychiatr Rep* 2005; 7(5):396–403.

Spalletta G, Bossu P, Ciaramella A, et al. The etiology of poststroke depression: a review of the literature and a new hypothesis involving inflammatory cytokines. *Mol Psychiatr* 2006;11(11):984–991.

Whyte EM, Mulsant BH, Rovner BW, et al. Preventing depression after stroke. *Int Rev Psychiatr* 2006;18(5):471–481.

Williams LS. Depression and stroke: cause or consequence? *Semin Neurol* 2005;25(4):396–409.

CHAPTER

Stroke Rehabilitation

MURRAY E. BRANDSTATER

OBJECTIVES

- What useful rehabilitation interventions are important in the care of the acute stroke patient?
- What patient characteristics help in predicting survival and recovery of function?
- What are the overall functional outcomes in individuals who survive a stroke?
- What common physical complications can be avoided by early therapeutic intervention?
- How can therapy optimize motor recovery?

Rehabilitation is not a distinctly separate phase of care that begins after acute medical intervention. Rather, it is an integral part of medical management and continues longitudinally through acute care, postacute care, and community reintegration. Although diagnosis and medical treatment are the principal focus of early treatment, rehabilitation measures should be offered concurrently. Many of these can be considered preventive in nature. For example, patients who are paralyzed, lethargic, and have bladder incontinence are at high risk for developing pressure ulcers. Deliberate strategies should be followed to prevent skin breakdowns, including protection of skin from moisture such as urine, avoidance of undue pressure through use of heel-protecting pads, maintenance of proper position with frequent turning, and daily inspection and routine skin cleansing.

REHABILITATION DURING THE ACUTE PHASE

Many patients with acute stroke have dysphagia and are at risk for aspiration and pneumonia. Aspiration will usually result in coughing, but in up to 40% of patients with acute stroke, aspiration is silent, without coughing. Patients who are lethargic or have decreased arousal should not be fed orally. Even in alert patients, the ability to swallow should be assessed carefully before oral intake of fluids or food is begun. This is done with a bedside evaluation, and if any doubt exists about aspiration, a swallowing videofluoroscopy examination is performed. During the acute phase, nasogastric (NG) tube feeding is necessary. It should be noted that patients who are lying flat in bed are at significant risk for regurgitation and aspiration. Research has shown that patients who receive tube feedings have a better outcome because of improved intake of fluid and nutrition, and reduced risk of aspiration.

Impairment of bladder control frequently follows a stroke, which initially causes hypotonic bladder with overflow incontinence. If an indwelling catheter is used for drainage, it should be removed as soon as possible because reflex voiding returns quite quickly and retention is rarely a problem. The indwelling catheter may be useful in the first several days to monitor fluid balance, but it carries an increased risk of urinary tract infection. Regular intermittent catheterization is preferable to an indwelling catheter.

Hemiplegic patients are at high risk for the development of contractures. These are myogenic, induced by prolonged posturing with the muscles in a shortened position. When muscle fibers are unloaded there is rapid loss of sarcomeres and reduced fiber length, and some accumulation of connective tissue. The development of spasticity contributes to the development of contractures through sustained posturing of the limbs in certain positions. The harmful effects of immobility can be ameliorated by regular passive stretching and by moving the joints through a full range of motion, preferably twice daily.

There is a strong belief that early mobilization is beneficial to patient outcome by reducing the risks of deep vein thrombosis (DVT), gastroesophageal regurgitation and aspiration pneumonia, contracture formation, skin breakdown, and orthostatic intolerance. Early activation is assumed to have a strong positive psychological benefit for the patient. Mobilization involves a set of physical activities that may be started passively but that quickly progress to active participation by the patient. Specific tasks include turning from side to side in bed and changing position, sitting up in bed, transferring to a wheelchair, standing, and walking. Mobilization also includes self-care activities such as self-feeding, grooming, and dressing. The timing of patient participation and progression in these activities depends on the patient's condition. Progressive neurological signs, intracranial hemorrhage, coma, or cardiovascular instability would preclude these therapeutic activities. If the patient's condition is stable, however, active mobilization should begin as soon as possible, within 24 to 48 hours of admission.

EVALUATION FOR REHABILITATION PROGRAM

Within several days of admission, once the patient appears to be neurologically and medically stable, the patient should be evaluated for admission to a comprehensive rehabilitation program. The criteria for admission into a postacute rehabilitation program are listed in Table 41.1. A comprehensive rehabilitation program involving multiple professionals is justified when the patient has identified disability that affects multiple areas of function. A patient with an isolated disability such as a partial aphasia, visual loss, or monoparesis may need rehabilitation, but for these cases, rehabilitation can be provided by a therapist, perhaps one discipline only, usually in an outpatient setting. In the early postonset phase, it may not be possible to judge whether the patient has sufficient cognitive function or communicative ability to engage in the program or sufficient physical tolerance to participate fully. It may be necessary in such cases to offer a short trial of therapy to observe the patient's true capacity and potential before deciding on candidacy.

Evaluation of the acute stroke patient should include information about the patient's general medical status, including the presence of important comorbidities. Equally important, the patient's psychosocial status influences the way the patient copes with the disability, impacts motivation and physical outcome, and forms the basis of discharge planning. It is important to establish at the outset the nature of the patient's family support, living situation, and postdischarge environment. Knowledge of all of these factors will assist the team in counseling the patient and family and in planning for discharge.

Medical stability has traditionally been required for admission of a patient to a specialized rehabilitation unit. However, hospitals are increasingly transferring patients from acute wards to rehabilitation units at earlier stages, often when the patients still have unresolved medical problems. This practice has forced rehabilitation centers to expand their resources to care for these more complex cases and to provide closer medical and nursing monitoring. Local institutional referral patterns and practices will usually determine the timing of transfer, but if earlier transfer to rehabilitation can be accomplished safely, patient care may be enhanced by earlier active participation of the patient in the rehabilitation program.

The rehabilitation program may be offered in different settings, such as an acute inpatient rehabilitation unit, a subacute rehabilitation inpatient unit, home care, or an outpatient center. The acute rehabilitation inpatient setting is appropriate for those patients who meet the admission criteria and are able to tolerate 3 hours or more of active therapy per day. An acute rehabilitation setting is preferred if the patient requires close medical and nursing monitoring of the medical status. If the patient's medical status is stable, but the patient is unable to tolerate more than 1 hour of therapy a day, a subacute rehabilitation setting is more appropriate. Other patients who require only minor degrees of assistance in self-care and mobility would be suitable for outpatient therapy or a home-care program.

TABLE 41.1 Criteria for Admission to a Comprehensive Rehabilitation Program

Stable neurological status
Significant persistent neurological deficit
Identified difficulty affecting at least two of the following: mobility, self-care activity, communication, bowel or bladder control, or swallowing
Sufficient cognitive function to learn
Sufficient communication ability to engage with the therapist
Physical ability to tolerate the activities program
Achievable therapeutic goals

PRINCIPLES OF STROKE REHABILITATION

Although rehabilitation intervention is important during the acute phase of care, it is secondary to the activities involved in diagnosis and acute medical treatment. However, when a patient has a persisting major continuing impairment such as hemiplegia with disabilities, the rehabilitation components of care quickly become the main focus of management. The rehabilitation process for patients with complex problems requires a carefully planned and integrated program. Some general principles have evolved over time to form the basis of stroke rehabilitation. Some of these principles are based on conclusions from clinical trials, but many represent a general consensus based on clinical experience. They are as follows:

1. There is a clear need for a committed medical direction. The role of the physician includes provision of medical care. Many patients have ongoing associated medical problems that require appropriate monitoring and therapy. The physician must act as a medical counselor, offering reasonable prognostication to patient and family along with guidance in stroke risk factor reduction and ongoing medical care. The physician must also give leadership to the team and assist in developing treatment protocols and setting treatment expectations.
2. The multiple problems of a patient require the active participation of a team of professionals. The treatment activities of the team members must be coordinated so that detailed evaluations are shared, and goals and treatment interventions are agreed on.
3. Each of the professional therapists on the team should be knowledgeable about the appropriate interventions within his or her discipline for treating the disabilities of stroke patients.
4. The interventions should be directed at achieving specific therapeutic goals, which may be short term (e.g., week-to-week) or long term (e.g., goals to be achieved by discharge). Having achieved those goals, the patient moves on to the next phase of rehabilitation or is discharged home to continue treatment as an outpatient.
5. Rehabilitation should be started as early as possible. There is evidence from clinical trials that early initiation of therapy favorably influences the outcome. Any delay in starting therapy can lead to development of secondary avoidable complications such as contractures and deconditioning.
6. Therapy should be directed at specific training of skills and functional training. Therapy should be given with sufficient intensity to promote skill acquisition.
7. Planning for discharge from the inpatient rehabilitation program should begin on admission.

8. Psychosocial issues are obviously very important. Numerous studies have shown the influence of spouse, family, and the patient's own psychological adjustment and coping mechanisms on the ultimate outcome. Family involvement is essential throughout the treatment program and in discharge planning.
9. There should be an emphasis on patient and family education about stroke, risk factor reduction, and strategies to maximize functional independence.
10. Rehabilitation requires a functional approach. When impairments cannot be altered, every effort should be made to assist patients to compensate for deficits and to adapt with alternative methods to achieve optimal functional independence.
11. Discharge from the hospital is often thought of as the end of rehabilitation, with the assumption that a good program prepares the patient for reintegration into home and community. However, hospital discharge should instead be seen as the beginning of a new life, one in which the patient embarks on the challenge of adopting different roles and relationships and a search for new meaning in life. This will involve resuming as much as possible the former roles in the family and with friends and finding ways to live a meaningful life in the community.

RECOVERY FROM STROKE

Numerous studies have described the patterns of improvement in neurological deficits and in the recovery of function after stroke. There is marked variation among patients in the time course of recovery and in its degree. An important objective of many of these studies has been the identification of specific variables that would predict the course of recovery from neurological impairments.

Recovery from Impairments

Hemiparesis and motor recovery have been the most thoroughly studied aspects of all stroke impairments. As much as 88% of patients with an acute stroke have hemiparesis. In a classic report, Twitchell described in detail the pattern of motor recovery following stroke. At onset, the arm is more involved than the leg, and eventual motor recovery in the arm is less than that in the leg. The severity of arm weakness at onset and the timing of return of movement in the hand are both important predictors of eventual motor recovery in the arm. The prognosis for return of useful hand function is poor when there is complete arm paralysis at onset or no measurable grasp strength by 4 weeks. However, even among patients with severe arm weakness at onset, up to 11% may gain good recovery of hand function. Some other generalizations can be made. Among patients showing some motor recovery in the hand by 4 weeks postonset, as many as 70% will make a full or good recovery. Full recovery, when it occurs, is usually complete within 3 months of onset. Bard and Hirshberg claim that "if no initial motion is noticed during the first 3 weeks, or if motion in one segment is not followed within a week by the appearance of motion in a second segment, the prognosis for recovery of full motion is poor."

The patterns of motor recovery have been described in detail by the authors of the Copenhagen Stroke Study. Summary data are shown in Figure 41.1. Ninety-five percent of patients reached their

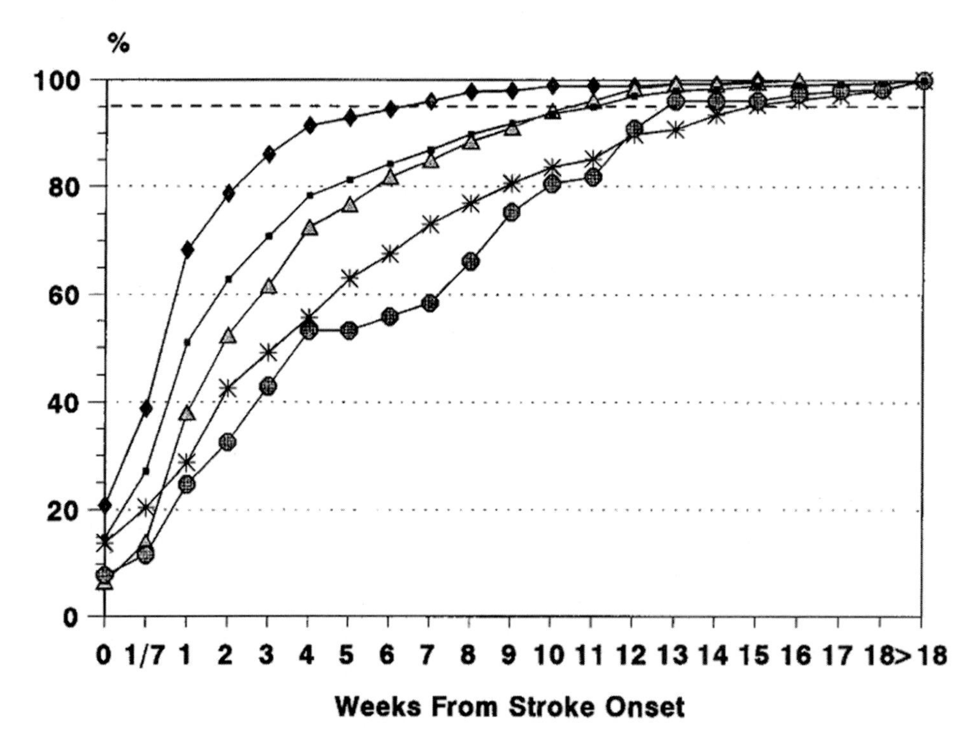

FIGURE 41.1. The time course of recovery in stroke survivors shown as the cumulative rate of patients having reached their best neurological outcome. The course of recovery is given for patients whose initial stroke severity was mild (◆), moderate (▲), severe (*), and very severe (•). All patients are represented by ■. From Jorgensen HS, Nakayama H, Raaschou HO, et al. Stroke rehabilitation: outcome and speed of recovery. Part II: speed of recovery. The Copenhagen Stroke Study. *Arch Phys Med Rehabil* 1995;76:406–412, with permission.

best neurological level within 11 weeks of onset. Patients with milder stroke recovered more quickly, and those with severe strokes reached their best neurological level within 15 weeks on average. The course of motor recovery reaches a plateau after an early phase of progressive improvement. Most recovery takes place in the first 3 months, and only minor additional measurable improvement occurs after 6 months postonset. However, in some patients who have significant partial return of voluntary movement, recovery may continue over a longer period.

About one third of patients with acute stroke have clinical features of aphasia. Language function in many of these patients improves, and at 6 months or more after stroke, only 12% to 18% have identifiable aphasia. Patients with aphasia continue to show some late improvement in language function, even beyond 1 year after onset. Patients who would be initially classified as having Broca aphasia have a variable outcome. In patients with large hemisphere lesions, Broca aphasia persists with little recovery, but patients with smaller lesions confined to the posterior frontal lobe often show early progressive improvement, the impairment evolving into a milder form of aphasia with anomia and word-finding difficulty. Patients with global aphasia tend to progress slowly, with comprehension often improving more than expressive ability. The communicative ability of patients who initially have global aphasia improves over a longer period, up to a year or more postonset. Patients with global aphasia associated with large lesions may show only minor recovery, but recovery may be quite good in those patients with smaller lesions. Language recovery in Wernicke's aphasia is variable.

About 20% of patients have a visual field defect. In general, the degree of visual improvement following stroke is not as impressive as recovery of motor and sensory function, and if the field defect persists beyond a few weeks, late recovery is less likely.

Mechanisms of Neurological Recovery

In the early phase poststroke, there is a prompt initial improvement in function as the pathological processes in the ischemic penumbra, metabolic injury, edema, hemorrhage, and pressure-resolve. The time frame for recovery of function in these reversibly injured neurons is relatively short, and this accounts for improvement in the first several weeks. The later, ongoing improvement in neurological function occurs by a different set of mechanisms that allow structural and functional reorganization within the brain. The processes involved in this reorganization represent neuroplasticity and may continue for many months. There is restitution of partially damaged pathways and expansion of representational brain maps, implying recruitment of neurons not ordinarily involved in an activity. A key aspect of neuroplasticity that has important implications for rehabilitation is that the modifications in neuronal networks are use dependent. Animal experimental studies and clinical trials in humans have shown that forced use and functional training contribute to improved function. On the other hand, techniques that promote nonuse may inhibit recovery. It used to be taught that benefits from rehabilitation are primarily achieved through training patients in new techniques to compensate for impairments (e.g., using the uninvolved hand to achieve self-care independence). This approach avoided intense therapy on the weak upper limb, its limited or nonuse forming a strategy, which is now known to lessen the potential for recovery. It is now recognized that repeated participation by patients in active physical therapeutic programs probably directly influences functional reorganization in the brain and enhances neurological recovery.

IMPAIRMENT EVALUATION

The focal neurological lesion that accompanies a stroke confers on the patient a set of neurological deficits that in rehabilitation medicine are referred to as *impairments*. Evaluation of these impairments constitutes an essential first step in the rehabilitation management of the patient. When the physician and the therapist understand the nature of a patient's impairments, they can provide specific targeted therapy to optimize the rehabilitation program. The relationship between medical diagnosis and rehabilitation diagnosis is described in Table 41.2. The initial clinical examination of a patient with an acute stroke includes a thorough, detailed neurological examination. The rehabilitation team uses the neurological findings for prognostication, development of specific details of the rehabilitation plan, and selection of the appropriate setting for rehabilitation. Reassessment of the patient during rehabilitation provides a means of monitoring progress and subsequently evaluating outcome. The initial rehabilitation assessment should begin immediately postonset, within 2 to 7 days, and then at repeated subsequent intervals.

The following sections summarize the important details of the neurological impairments encountered in postacute stroke patients.

Higher Mental Function

Focal brain lesions associated with a stroke frequently produce measurable impairments in higher mental function. Even small lesions may significantly impair cognition, particularly when they are multiple. However, interpretation of test information must be made in the context of the clinical situation because other nonstroke factors may contribute to impaired mental status. Many patients are elderly and may have had some premorbid decline in mental status. Furthermore, general medical disorders such as a fever, electrolyte disturbance, hypothyroidism, congestive heart failure, and reaction to medication may produce an encephalopathy. Such patients are often confused and may have a diminished level of consciousness; they have a generalized disturbance of mental status with abnormalities in most or all cognitive tests. The encephalopathy associated with these general medical problems is reversible following correction of the complicating disorder. Only when nonstroke factors have been excluded can changes in mental status be attributed to the focal lesion of the brain.

The cognitive impairments observed with focal lesions frequently show specific disturbances, for example, memory loss, neglect, or constructional apraxia. Disturbances such as these can usually be recognized at the bedside. Because cognitive impairments

TABLE 41.2 Medical Diagnosis versus Rehabilitation Diagnosis

Medical diagnosis
  Pathology (e.g., infarction) → Neurological deficits (e.g., hemiplegia)
Rehabilitation diagnosis
  Impairments (e.g., hemiplegia) → Disability (e.g., inability to walk)

TABLE 41.3 Mental Status Examination

Level of consciousness
  Alertness, response to stimulation
Attention
Memory
  Orientation, new learning, remote memory
Cognition
  Fund of knowledge, calculation, problem solving, abstract thinking, judgment
Perception, constructional ability, apraxia
Affect and behavior

can have a significant influence on the rehabilitation program and on outcome, the bedside mental status examination should be an essential part of the assessment of every stroke patient. The components of the examination are shown in Table 41.3. (For a more detailed description of this assessment see Strub and Black.) The Mini-Mental State Examination is a useful bedside tool that screens a variety of mental demands quickly and gives a well-validated measure of overall mental function. It requires less than 10 minutes to administer. Formal psychological tests may be used to establish global intellectual level and to reveal specific areas of diminished performance reflecting focal brain impairment. The Weschler Adult Intelligence Scale is commonly used in stroke patients.

Perceptual impairments are extremely important in stroke rehabilitation, and their recognition is an essential part of the higher mental function evaluation. A *perceptual deficit* is an impairment of the recognition and interpretation of sensory information when the sensory input system is intact. Impaired perception is caused by a lesion at the cortical level, almost always in the nondominant parietal lobe. The patient exhibits selective inattention, which can be detected by careful observation of behavior. A patient with hemisensory loss or homonymous hemianopia will also ignore the affected side. However, inattention is only referred to as true neglect when the sensory and visual pathways are intact. Unilateral neglect may be visual, tactile, spatial, or auditory. Visual neglect is demonstrated at the bedside when the patient, on request, attempts to draw numbers on a clock face, draw a stick figure, or bisect a horizontal line on a piece of paper. The patient is inattentive to the affected side. Other bedside tests of perceptual function are failure to recognize palm writing (graphesthesia), inability to identify objects in the hand (astereognosis), and extinction of simultaneous bilateral stimulation.

The term *apraxia* describes the inability of a patient to execute a willed movement when motor and sensory functions are apparently preserved. Apraxia may be detected when a patient is unable to carry out a task on command such as "comb your hair" or "wave goodbye" even though there is no paralysis. Patients with lesions of the nondominant parietal lobe may have apraxia of putting on their clothes and getting dressed.

Communication Disorders

Communication is a complex function involving reception, central processing, and sending of information. Communication occurs through the use of language and consists of a system of symbols that are combined to convey ideas (i.e., letters, words, or gestures). Impairment of language is called *aphasia*, and its presence reflects an abnormality in the dominant hemisphere. *Speech*, on the other hand, is a term that refers to the motor mechanism involved in the production of spoken words, that is, breathing, phonation, and articulation. Dysphonia and dysarthria are disorders of speech.

Although there are many classifications for aphasia, certain identifiable groups of patients are observed with clinically similar disorders of communication. In the simplest classification, aphasia is divided into two main categories: motor aphasia (sometimes called *expressive* or *anterior aphasia*), characterized by nonfluent speech, and sensory aphasia (sometimes called *receptive*, *posterior*, or *Wernicke aphasia*), characterized by fluent speech. A common system of classification of aphasia is listed in Table 41.4. By using simple bedside tests, the clinician can categorize the communication disorder according to this classification. During the evaluation of a patient, the clinician should avoid using nonverbal cues such as gestures. The questions addressed during the bedside assessment of aphasia are provided in Table 41.5.

Complete evaluations of patients can be performed using formal aphasia tests. Table 41.6 summarizes the more commonly used formal aphasia test instruments.

For assessment of dysarthria, clinicians subjectively rate the degree of impairment as a percentage intelligibility of speech.

Cranial Nerves

In patients with lesions involving the hemispheres, visual field defects may be present. Patients with hemianopia will often fail to detect objects on the affected side of the body, which confers significant disability. The precise nature of the defect can be characterized by confrontation testing. Extraocular palsies involving lesions of the midbrain or pons can produce characteristic dysfunction.

Dysphagia is a frequent impairment with unilateral hemisphere stroke, but it is much more pronounced in bilateral disease

TABLE 41.4 Classification of Aphasia

Classification	Fluency	Comprehension	Repetition	Naming
Global	Poor	Poor	Poor	Poor
Broca	Poor	Poor	Variable	Poor
Isolation	Poor	Poor	Good	Poor
Transcortical motor	Poor	Good	Good	Poor
Wernicke	Good	Poor	Poor	Poor
Transcortical sensory	Good	Poor	Good	Poor
Conduction	Good	Good	Poor	Poor
Anomic	Good	Good	Good	Poor

TABLE 41.5 Bedside Test of Language

Questions	Clinical Test
Can the patient understand?	Give verbal commands, ask patient to point to objects
Is the patient able to talk?	Ask the patient to name objects, describe them, count. Listen for spontaneous speech
Can the patient repeat?	Ask the patient to repeat words
Can the patient read?	Give commands in writing
Can the patient write?	Ask the patient to copy or to write dictated words

TABLE 41.6 Commonly Used Formal Aphasia Tests

- The Boston Diagnostic Aphasia Examination produces a classification of the aphasic features observed in a particular patient. Besides classifying the aphasia, it also provides a score of the severity of the aphasia, which can be compared with that of aphasic patients in general.
- The Western Aphasia Battery is somewhat similar to the Boston. It measures various parameters of spontaneous speech and examines comprehension, fluency, object naming, and repetition. It provides a total score called an aphasia quotient, which is a measure of severity of the aphasia.
- The Porch Index of Communication Ability is different from the other tests in that it evaluates verbal, gestural, and graphic responses. It is very structured in its format and must be given by a trained professional. It provides a useful statistical summary of the details of the language impairments and offers outcome prediction.
- The Functional Communication Profile provides an overall rating of functional communication. It is not a diagnostic test. The score indicates severity and can be a useful indicator of recovery.

and in brainstem lesions. Other cranial nerve lesions may be identified in lesions involving the brainstem.

Weakness and Paralysis

Paralysis is such a common feature among central nervous system impairments with stroke that the terms *hemiplegia* and *stroke* are often used interchangeably. Assessment of motor impairment includes an evaluation of tone, strength, coordination, and balance.

The most widely used scale to assess strength is the Medical Research Council (MRC) six-point scale 0 to 5, in which 0 represents complete paralysis, 3 is the ability to fully move the joint against gravity, and 5 indicates normal strength. The test is insensitive in its upper range, where the examiner must assess strength by offering manual resistance to maximum muscle activation. The MRC scale is designed to assess the strength of individual muscles, and it is therefore most useful in grading strength in patients with lower motor neuron lesions. There are drawbacks to the use of this scale in patients with upper motor neuron (UMN) lesions such as stroke. A patient recovering from hemiplegia may not be able to selectively activate a particular muscle in isolation and hence will be given a 0 grade on the MRC scale. However, the patient may be able to forcefully activate the muscle within a gross motor pattern in which groups of muscles contract together in synergy, for example, a flexor or extensor synergy pattern. Furthermore, as tone increases during recovery, the capacity of the patient to move a joint may be restricted by spasticity in the antagonists. Co-contraction of agonists and antagonists can diminish the force of muscle contraction recorded externally. Despite these shortcomings, the MRC scale may be quite useful in the early phases following a stroke, before significant spasticity develops.

Brunnstrom adopted a different approach for the assessment of motor function in hemiplegic patients. She developed a test in which movement patterns are evaluated and motor function is rated according to stages of motor recovery. The clinician assesses the presence of flexor and extensor synergies and the degree of selective muscle activation from the synergy pattern (see Table 41.7). The rating can be performed very quickly, and although the scale defines recovery only in broad categories, these categories do correlate with progressive functional recovery.

Rather than subjectively assess strength using the MRC scale, Bohannon advocated direct measurement of force with a dynamometer. Despite the limitations of assessing and interpreting muscle strength in patients with UMN lesions, strength does correlate with performance on functional tasks. Fugl-Meyer et al designed a more detailed and comprehensive motor scale in which 50 different movements and abilities were rated. The test evaluates strength, reflexes, and coordination, and a composite score is derived on a scale of 0 to 100. The Fugl-Meyer scale is reliable, and repeat scores reflect motor recovery over time. It is quite useful and informative but has not been widely adopted by clinicians because it is time consuming to complete each evaluation.

Muscle tone refers to the resistance felt when the examiner passively stretches a muscle by moving a joint. The rating is subjective and depends on the judgment of the examiner. Physiological conditions such as position of body segments and body posture strongly influence the level of muscle tone, and these must be controlled as much as possible. For example, tone will be increased if the patient is supine rather than prone, or standing rather than sitting. Tone in the leg muscles may be quite modest in a sitting hemiplegic patient

TABLE 41.7 Brunnstrom Stages of Motor Recovery

Stages	Characteristics
Stage 1	No activation of the limb
Stage 2	Spasticity appears, and weak basic flexor and extensor synergies are present
Stage 3	Spasticity is prominent; the patient voluntarily moves the limb, but muscle activation is all within the synergy patterns
Stage 4	The patient begins to activate muscles selectively outside the flexor and extensor synergies
Stage 5	Spasticity decreases; most muscle activation is selective and independent from the limb synergies
Stage 6	Isolated movements are performed in a smooth, phasic, well-coordinated manner

but may be very severe when the patient is standing. A high level of anxiety will also increase the degree of muscle tone. Quantitation of spasticity is difficult. The most widely used scale is the Ashworth scale.

Sensory Impairment

When sensory deficits exist as part of a clinical picture following a stroke, they frequently accompany motor impairment in the same anatomical distribution. Interpretation of sensory testing may be difficult in a confused or cognitively impaired patient. Clinical examination involves testing pain, temperature, touch, joint position, and vibration. Lesions of the thalamus may cause severe contralateral sensory loss. With lesions of the cortex, sensation, although preserved, is qualitatively and quantitatively reduced. Parietal lobe lesions cause perceptual deficits in which primary modalities of sensation may be intact. Typical tests to reveal the presence of perceptual impairment include simultaneous bilateral stimulation for inattention, two-point discrimination, object recognition for stereognosis, and recognition of digits drawn in the palm.

Balance, Coordination, and Posture

Impaired balance may be caused by deficits in motor and sensory function, cerebellar lesions, and vestibular dysfunctions. Clinical testing involves assessing coordination using finger-to-nose pointing and rapid alternating movements. The ability of the patient to sit unsupported or, if able, to stand and walk provides important information. Ataxia caused by sensory impairment can be differentiated from ataxia resulting from cerebellar loss because performance of a motor task with the eyes closed is much poorer in sensory ataxia, when the patient has no vision to compensate for sensory loss.

Evaluation of the neurological impairments should be made repeatedly during the course of the rehabilitation program. Ideally, evaluation should be made weekly in the early phases of rehabilitation, to allow monitoring of the recovery process and to guide the therapeutic intervention.

OUTCOME AND PROGNOSTICATION IN STROKE REHABILITATION

Prognostication about outcome for a stroke patient is often expressed in the simple question, "Is this patient a good candidate for rehabilitation?" The benefits of good prognostication are self-evident. Patients and family members need to know the prospects for survival, the degree of recovery that may be expected, and the extent of possible residual disability following rehabilitation. Professionals providing care need information with which to counsel patients and families. Knowledge of prognosis of individual patients can guide physicians and therapists in the selection of specific therapies and appropriate intensities of therapies. Finally, good prognostication can help reduce costs of care through reduction of misdirected therapy and optimal use of facilities and staff.

Accurate prognostication of the ultimate status of patients after recovery from stroke has proved to be elusive because of difficulties encountered in stroke outcome research. Some factors that have made conclusions about prognostication imprecise include the following: (a) the effects of cerebrovascular disease are heterogeneous, and pathologies are different; (b) some patients have only transient symptoms, whereas others have severe and lasting impairment; and (c) many studies are not comparable, for example, it is difficult to compare studies that aggregate all patients regardless of pathology, lesion site, time interval since onset, and degree of impairment with those studies of selected subgroups of patients. A major limitation in the interpretation of many early reports on prediction of stroke outcome has been the poor definition of prognostic variables and outcome variables. Methodological issues in stroke outcome research were reviewed in a symposium in 1989. Important recommendations were made to standardize methodologies in outcome studies in stroke research, and in 1989 the World Health Organization task force issued similar recommendations.

It is important to distinguish between prognostic and outcome variables. Prognostic variables influence the survival, recovery, and ultimate outcome of an individual who has sustained an acute stroke (see Table 41.8). These variables may be categorized into those that are patient related, those that are lesion related, those that are intervention and therapy related, and those that are psychosocial. Outcome variables, on the other hand, describe different aspects of the status of the patient at a particular end point. Typical outcome variables of interest are listed in Table 41.9.

TABLE 41.8 Classification of Prognostic Variables

Patient demographic variables
Age, race
General medical variables
Examples: hypertension, heart disease, diabetes
Lesion-related variables
Pathology
Lesion site and size
Impairment characteristics
Coma at onset
Bladder and bowel continence
Specific therapy interventions
Nature of therapy
Intensity of therapy
Psychosocial variables
Socioeconomic status
Premorbid personality
Patient family role

TABLE 41.9 Outcome Variables

Survival
Impairment; neurological deficit
Degree of paralysis
Aphasia
Visual field defect, neglect
Disability
Activities of daily living
Ambulation
Social variables
Discharge destination
Living arrangements
Social integration

Predicting Survival

Early death following a stroke is usually related to the underlying pathology and to the severity of the lesion. The 30-day survival for patients with cerebral infarction is 85%, but for patients with intracerebral hemorrhage, survival is reported to be only 20% to 52%. Better management of cardiac and respiratory disorders has decreased early mortality. Hypertension, heart disease, and diabetes, however, remain as risk factors for recurrence of stroke. Coma following a stroke onset indicates a poor prognosis, presumably because coma occurs frequently in cerebral hemorrhage, and when it occurs in relationship to cerebral infarction, it reflects a large lesion with cerebral edema.

Lacunar lesions are small and affect a very limited amount of tissue. The prognosis for recovery from lacunar lesions is usually excellent, although significant persisting deficits may occur when the lesion is strategically located. Because of their subcortical locations, lacunar lesions rarely, if ever, affect cortical functions. With large vessel infarctions, due to either thrombosis or embolism, prognosis is related to the volume of the lesion. Outcome is poorest when the lesion involves more than 10% of intracranial volume. Large intracerebral hemorrhages can be devastating, with a high mortality due to increased pressure and brain displacement. Small hemorrhages have a good prognosis because the pressure effects are minor.

Predicting Disability and Functional Status

The key outcomes from a rehabilitation perspective are those that describe the disability status of the patient. The central purpose of the rehabilitation program is to lessen ultimate disability; therefore, considerable attention has been directed at the identification of factors that will predict the late functional status of the patient, especially with respect to walking and activities of daily living (ADL).

Most patients admitted to an inpatient stroke rehabilitation program in the postacute phase have hemiparesis of sufficient severity that walking becomes impossible. Some recovery of leg function almost always occurs, and improvement in mobility follows. By 3 months postonset, 54% to 80% of patients become independent in walking. In a retrospective study of 248 patients with stroke treated at a rehabilitation center, Feigenson et al. reported that 85% of patients were ambulatory at discharge. The degree of recovery in walking ability depends on motor recovery. As measured on the Brunnstrom scale for stages of motor recovery, very few patients who remain in stage II (minimal voluntary movement) regain the ability to walk; however, most patients in stage III (active flexion and extension synergy through range of motion) do eventually walk. Data from the Framingham cohort reported by Gresham et al. indicate that long-term survivors of stroke show good recovery of functional mobility, with 80% being independent in mobility.

Most patients with significant neurological impairment who survive a stroke are dependent in basic ADL, that is, bathing, dressing, feeding, toileting, grooming, and transfers. The capacity of individuals to perform these activities is usually scored on disability rating scales such as the Functional Independent Measure. Almost all patients show improved function in ADL as recovery occurs. Most improvement is noted in the first 6 months, although as many as 5% of patients show continued measurable improvement up to 12 months postonset. Other patients may show some functionally worthwhile improvement beyond 6 months, which the disability scales usually fail to detect because of their limited sensitivity at the upper end of the functional range. The levels of functional independence eventually reached by stroke patients after recovery as reported by different authors are variable. This probably reflects differences between study populations and differences in methods of treatment, follow-up, and data reporting. In most reports, between 47% and 76% of survivors achieve partial or total independence in ADL.

Most authors who have attempted to determine which factors predict ultimate ADL functional outcome have used multivariate analysis. Of the many independent variables tested, those reported to have the most influence on outcome are listed in Table 41.10. Not all of these factors were shown in every study to statistically predict outcome status.

The effect of age on outcome may partly be related to more frequent co-impairments. If elderly patients are less functional prestroke, this alone could explain poorer outcomes following a stroke. Furthermore, elderly patients often do not receive as intensive therapy as younger patients, and they may be discharged from the rehabilitation program sooner. Some studies designed to examine age as an independent prognostic factor have not found a correlation between age and functional ADL outcome in 6 months.

Coexisting heart disease and diabetes represent comorbidities that are likely to increase the chance of recurrent stroke and may limit a patient's full participation in an intensive program. These comorbidities affect survival, that is, increase the likelihood of recurrence or death, but it is not known to what degree their presence influences functional recovery from stroke. Such measures of the severity of the stroke as reduced sitting balance, visuospatial impairment, mental changes, and incontinence all influence functional outcome. Intuitively, it would seem reasonable to assume that patients with more severe neurological deficits would have worse functional outcomes, but this is not necessarily the case when isolated neurological impairments are considered. For example, analyses of predictive variables have failed to show that patients with sensory deficits have a poorer ultimate outcome. The severity of the neurological deficit is reflected in the overall ADL score, and most authors have reported that the initial ADL score is a good predictor of ultimate ADL function. Patients admitted for rehabilitation with lower ADL scores do not have as good a functional outcome as patients who initially had higher admission ADL scores.

TABLE 41.10 Factors Predicting Poor ADL Outcome

Advanced age
Comorbidities
Myocardial infarction
Diabetes mellitus
Severity of stroke
Severe weakness
Poor sitting balance
Visuospatial deficits
Mental changes
Incontinence
Low initial ADL scores
Time interval: onset to rehabilitation

ADL, activities of daily living.

It is now generally accepted that therapy should be started as early as possible. Early rehabilitation minimizes secondary complications such as contractures and deconditioning, and helps motivation. The Post-Stroke Rehabilitation Outcomes Project demonstrated that shorter intervals between symptom onset and admission to rehabilitation resulted in better functional outcomes at discharge and shorter length of stays. That study also showed that higher-intensity levels of therapy, as an independent variable, improve ultimate functional recovery.

Social Variables

The discharge destination of a patient, home or institutional placement, living arrangements, and social integration are all important in reflecting the social status of patients following recovery. Patients most likely to require long-term institutional care are those with severe disabilities who need maximum physical assistance in ADL and who have bowel or bladder incontinence. However, psychosocial variables, especially prestroke family interaction and the presence of an able spouse, also influence whether the patient returns home. A supportive family whose members are willing to provide significant physical care may be able to manage a severely disabled patient at home. By contrast, a patient with much less disability but no family support may require institutional care if not fully independent.

When a clinician is confronted with the challenge of evaluating an individual patient, guidelines for predicting functional outcome are useful but are not precise because multiple variables interact. A patient who might be judged as having a good prognosis for functional outcome may do poorly because of a negative psychosocial factor. The best estimate of prognosis can be made only after a thorough and comprehensive evaluation of the patient's medical, neurological, functional, and psychosocial status. The clinician at the bedside is in the best position to formulate a prognosis and provide an answer to the question, "Is this patient a good candidate for rehabilitation?"

MEDICAL MANAGEMENT IN THE POSTACUTE PHASE

There is a high incidence of coexisting medical disorders among patients recovering from stroke, reflecting the age of the patient population and the fact that cerebrovascular disease is part of a generalized disease process. If severe, or if poorly managed, these disorders may interfere with the patient's participation in the rehabilitation program and may adversely affect outcome. It is imperative, therefore, that the attending physician assesses the patient thoroughly and monitors the medical status closely, being prepared to intervene promptly when required. Some of the important and more frequent disorders are discussed briefly.

Medical Comorbidities

In a large majority of patients, a stroke is an acute event in the course of a systemic disease (e.g., atherosclerosis, hypertensive vascular disease, or cardiac embolism). These patients frequently exhibit other clinical features of the underlying systemic disorder, especially heart disease. Up to 75% of stroke patients may show evidence of coexisting cardiovascular disease, including hypertension (estimates range from 50% to 84%) and coronary artery disease (up to 65%). Another group of heart diseases causes a stroke through cardiogenic cerebral embolism. These diseases include atrial fibrillation and other arrhythmias from multiple causes—valvular disease, cardiomyopathy, endocarditis, recent myocardial infarction, and left atrial myxoma.

Concomitant heart disease has a negative impact on short- and long-term survival and probably on functional outcome of stroke patients. Acute exacerbations of heart disease occur frequently during postacute stroke rehabilitation. Common problems include angina, uncontrolled hypertension, hypotension, myocardial infarction, congestive heart failure, atrial fibrillation, and ventricular arrhythmias. Development of one of these complications may have minimal or no impact on the patient's progress or outcome if the problem is promptly diagnosed and appropriately treated. However, these complications often do impact the patient's capacity to participate fully in the therapeutic program. Congestive heart failure and angina decrease exercise tolerance and reduce capacity to roll over in bed, transfer, and walk.

All patients should be monitored carefully during postacute rehabilitation for evidence of cardiac disease. The classical features of coronary artery disease and congestive heart failure may be present, but often they are not. Ischemia may be silent. The clinical clues to significant coexisting heart disease may be subtle (e.g., slower than expected progress, excessive fatigue, lethargy, or mental changes). Patients should undergo appropriate cardiac investigation with electrocardiography, Holter monitoring, echocardiography, and other diagnostic techniques and should receive optimal therapy. These cardiac complications can be successfully treated and are not contraindications for rehabilitation.

The rehabilitation management of patients with identified cardiac complications should include formal clinical monitoring of pulse and blood pressure during physical activities. Brief electrocardiac monitoring during exercise can add more specific information. A useful set of cardiac precautions in patients undergoing rehabilitation was developed by Fletcher et al. and are listed in Table 41.11. It should be noted that in deconditioned patients, the resting heart rate may be high, and in an elderly patient the estimated limit for heart rate based on 50% above resting may be too high. For patients on β-blockers, a reasonable limit might be a heart rate at around 20 beats above the resting level.

TABLE 41.11 Cardiac Precautions

Activity should be terminated if any of the following develops:

1. New onset cardiopulmonary symptoms
2. Heart rate decreases >20% of baseline
3. Heart rate increases >50% of baseline
4. Systolic BP increases to 240 mm Hg
5. Systolic BP decreases >30 mm Hg from baseline or to <90 mm Hg
6. Diastolic BP increases to 120 mm Hg

BP, blood pressure.

Data from Fletcher BJ, Dunbar S, Coleman J, et al. Cardiac precautions for nonacute inpatient settings. *Am J Phys Med Rehabil* 1993;72: 140–143.

Medical Complications

Medical complications frequently occur during the postacute phase of rehabilitation, affecting up to 60% of patients and up to 94% of patients with severe lesions. Common medical and neurological complications are listed in Table 41.12.

Pulmonary Aspiration and Pneumonia

Dysphagia is a frequent and serious complication of stroke. It is a usual feature in brainstem lesions or bilateral hemisphere lesions, but it also occurs in patients with unilateral hemisphere lesions. Difficulty in swallowing may occur in the oral preparatory phase or in the pharyngeal phase. There is usually delay in or absence of the swallowing reflex. Evaluation of a patient includes observation of the muscles of the lips, tongue, cheeks, and jaw, and elevation of the larynx during swallowing. Poor muscle control results in trickling of saliva or liquids into the valleculae or inability to handle solids. There is poor protection of the airway, with high risk for aspiration.

Aspiration usually causes coughing, but some studies report a significant number of patients with silent aspiration. Careful bedside evaluation should be performed in all patients before oral feeding is started. Muscles of the lips and tongue should be tested and the patient observed when taking sips of water and during eating. If the patient has a poor cough response, or if there is any question about the safety of swallowing, a videofluoroscopy using a modified barium swallow should be performed to assess swallowing and to detect aspiration. Numerous therapeutic interventions can improve swallowing. Techniques include stimulation to increase arousal, sitting the patient upright in a chair with head forward, closely supervising the patient, modifying the consistency of food to pureed solids and thickened liquids, and exercising. If swallowing is not safe, an NG tube is indicated for enteral feedings. It should be noted that patients fed via an NG tube are still at risk for aspiration because of gastroesophageal reflux, especially when lying flat in bed. Dysphagia rapidly improves in patients with unilateral stroke, and by 1 month postonset, only about 2% of these patients still have difficulty. In patients with brainstem lesions or bilateral hemisphere lesions, dysphagia may progress more slowly and will usually require gastrostomy.

TABLE 41.12 Medical Complications during Postacute Stroke Rehabilitation

Complication	Frequency (%)
Medical	
Pulmonary aspiration, pneumonia	40
Urinary tract infection	40
Depression	30
Musculoskeletal pain, RSD	30
Falls	25
Malnutrition	16
Venous thromboembolism	6
Pressure ulcer	3
Neurological	
Toxic or metabolic encephalopathy	10
Stroke progression	5
Seizure	4

RSD, reflex sympathetic dystrophy.

Data from Feigenson JS, McDowell FH, Meese P, et al. Factors influencing outcome and length of stay in a stroke rehabilitation unit Part 1. *Stroke* 1977;8:651–656; Gresham GE, Fitzpatrick TE, Wolf PA, et al. Residual disability in survivors of stroke: the Framingham Study. *N Engl J Med* 1975;293:954–956; Wade DT, Langton-Hewer R. Functional abilities after stroke; measurement, natural-history and prognosis. *J Neurol Neurosurg Psychiatr* 1987;50:177–182; and Wade DT, Langton-Hewer R, David RM, et al. Aphasia after stroke: natural history and associated deficits. *J Neurol Neurosurg Psychiatr* 1986;49:11–16.

Urinary Tract Infection

Urinary tract infections are common because of the neurogenic bladder and the need for catheterization in the acute phase. Immediately postonset, the sacral reflexes mediating micturition are depressed, and the bladder will overdistend and, if not drained, empty by overflow incontinence. Overdistention is best avoided in the acute stage by intermittent catheterization every 4 or 6 hours, depending on the rate of urine flow. The objective is to prevent the bladder from filling beyond about 500 mL and to stimulate physiological emptying. There is a modest risk of urinary tract infection with catheterization, but the risk is greatly increased if an indwelling Foley catheter is used. Intermittent catheterization is preferred, especially as the need for catheter drainage may be very brief, for a few days or less. As soon as spontaneous voiding begins, the intermittent catheterization can be reduced in frequency and may be stopped when postvoid residual bladder volumes are <100 to 150 mL. The patient can be helped to achieve better bladder control by using a posture that increases intra-abdominal pressure; that is, sitting on a commode or toilet or standing to use a urinal.

In the postacute phase of stroke rehabilitation, the problem is not one of bladder overdistention but one of uninhibited bladder with incontinence. The patient has a sense of urgency to micturate and cannot postpone voiding. Bladder volumes and voided volumes are often rather small. At least some improvement in bladder function during the day can be achieved through deliberate training or pharmacologically, using anticholinergics such as oxybutynin chloride (Ditropan) to inhibit bladder contraction. Tricyclic antidepressants such as imipramine may also be useful because they exhibit both peripheral anticholinergic and a-adrenergic agonist activity, relaxing the bladder and increasing urethral pressure and sphincter tone. Bladder infections must be promptly recognized and treated. Management of incontinence can be quite difficult, and usually involves one or all of the following: intermittent catheterization (self-catheterization whenever possible), medication, fluid restriction, and use of special diapers.

Malnutrition

A surprising number of patients admitted for stroke rehabilitation are malnourished, and in one report, 22% of patients showed nutritional deficiencies. Elderly patients may be admitted to the hospital following a stroke already in a marginal nutritional status, and their condition is exacerbated by the low calorie intake during initial acute care. If not closely monitored during postacute rehabilitation, a patient's nutritional status may be further compromised because of dysphagia, reliance on others for oral or tube feedings, lack of interest in food, depression, and problems with communication. The risk of malnutrition and/or dehydration should be recognized, and the intake of fluid, protein, and total calories should be monitored closely in all patients. Oral nutritional supplements may have to be prescribed, and if a patient continues to have inadequate intake, enteral tube feeding may be necessary.

Musculoskeletal Pain and Reflex Sympathetic Dystrophy

Pain in the shoulder and arm is a frequent complaint of patients undergoing postacute stroke rehabilitation. It tends to develop early—several weeks to 6 months postonset—and may affect up to 72% of individuals, especially those with more severe hemiplegia.

Although some patients may have preexisting shoulder problems such as rotator cuff tendinitis, most hemiplegic patients with shoulder pain have varying combinations of glenohumeral subluxation, spasticity, and contracture. The role of subluxation in generating a painful shoulder has been debated, but it often precedes and then accompanies a painful shoulder. Subluxation of the glenohumeral joint is a clinical diagnosis that can be quantified by X-ray. It occurs in 30% to 50% of patients and is probably caused by the weight of the arm pulling down the humerus at a stage when the supraspinatus and deltoid muscles are flaccid and weak and by weakness of the scapular muscles, which allow the glenoid cavity to rotate facing downward. The shoulder is best managed in the early phases of rehabilitation through proper positioning of the arm and hand and through avoidance of pulling on the arm during assisted transfers. Whenever the patient is sitting, the arm should be supported in an arm trough or lapboard. Therapy should be directed at facilitating return of active movement of the shoulder and should include techniques such as stretching to minimize spasticity, especially in shoulder depressors and internal rotators. Chae et al. have shown that intramuscular electrical stimulation of shoulder muscles can correct glenohumeral subluxation and reduce shoulder pain. When spasticity becomes severe and cannot be controlled with stretching, consideration may be given to reducing the tone in the subscapularis muscle with intramuscular phenol neurolysis or with botulinum toxin.

Reflex sympathetic dystrophy syndrome, also known as complex regional pain syndrome, occurs quite commonly in the hemiplegic arm (shoulder–hand syndrome). A clinical diagnosis was made in 12.5% of patients with hemiplegia and 25% of patients studied with a bone scan as reported by Davis et al. The clinical features usually develop between 1 and 4 months postonset and, once established, run a rather predictable, protracted course. Pain dominates the clinical picture. The hand is swollen, and contractures develop at the shoulder, wrist, and hand, and these contractures will persist as permanent sequelae unless the syndrome is treated early and aggressively. Treatment is most effective when begun early and consists of medical and physical measures. Some authorities have reported good results with prompt resolution of the clinical features with an intra-articular injection of steroids or a short course of relatively high-dose prednisone, tapering and discontinuing the drug over several weeks. A series of stellate ganglion blocks is also advocated in acute cases. The blocks are repeated every few days. Analgesics or nonsteroidal anti-inflammatory drugs are necessary for pain control. The most important intervention, however, is therapy to the limb to maintain range of motion of all joints, reduce swelling, and desensitize the limb through physiological stimulation such as massage and hot and cold contrast baths.

Venous Thromboembolism

Immediately postonset, stroke patients are at high risk for DVT, the risk being greater when the leg is paralyzed. The risk of DVT may be as high as 75% in hemiplegic patients not receiving prophylaxis. The thrombosis begins early, sometimes as soon as the second day postonset of symptoms and usually within the first week, although some new DVT events are recorded weeks after onset in the postacute rehabilitation phase.

All patients with stroke should receive DVT prophylaxis. Low-dose subcutaneous heparin and low molecular weight heparin (LMWH) are effective in reducing the incidence of DVT. External pneumatic compression stockings are an alternative to heparin when the risk of bleeding is high (e.g., patients with peptic ulcer disease or intracerebral hemorrhage). Prophylaxis should continue well into the postacute phase and preferably until the patient is walking, although there are no studies to indicate the optimal duration of DVT prophylaxis.

The clinical signs of DVT are not reliable, being absent in about 50% of cases with proven DVT. However, the development of clinical signs suggesting DVT should always prompt laboratory investigation. The test of choice for diagnosis of DVT is venous duplex scanning, which has a high degree of sensitivity and specificity in patients with clinical features suggesting DVT. A positive scan is sufficient to justify treatment for DVT with anticoagulation.

The diagnosis of a new-onset DVT is a medical emergency, and immediate full-dose anticoagulation should be started with heparin infusion or full-dose LMWH. Warfarin can be started on day 1, and once the prothrombin time is therapeutic, usually within 5 days, the heparin infusion can be stopped. To minimize the risks of pulmonary embolism (PE), it is advisable to keep a patient with an acute DVT on bed rest for at least 24 hours and until the heparin is therapeutic. In patients who are at risk for hemorrhage, for example, those with hemorrhagic stroke, DVT may be treated by installing a vena cava filter to prevent PE. The reader is referred to recent reviews on venous thromboembolism in stroke.

REHABILITATION MANAGEMENT

Therapy for Hemiplegia

Early Phase

In the early poststroke phase, the hemiplegic limbs are often paralyzed and flaccid. At this stage, which may last for a few hours to days, the limbs and joints are prone to development of contractures. Through poor positioning, a stuporous patient may develop nerve pressure palsies. If the patient sits up or stands with a flaccid weak arm, the weight of the arm may stretch the capsule of the shoulder joint, leading to development of subluxation and painful shoulder.

Therapy during this early phase should consist of proper positioning of the patient in bed and support of the arm in a wheelchair trough when sitting. Traction on the arm should be avoided when the patient is moved in bed or transferred to a wheelchair. All joints of the affected limbs should be passively moved through a full range of motion at least once daily to prevent contractures. Within hours or a few days, muscle tone returns to the paralyzed limbs, and spasticity progressively increases. Therapists use different approaches during this phase of motor recovery. The most widely accepted method, the neurodevelopmental technique (NDT) advocated by Bobath, stresses exercises that tend to normalize muscle tone and prevent excessive spasticity. This is achieved through the use of special reflex-inhibiting postures and movements. If spasticity becomes severe, the tone can be reduced by slow, sustained stretching, which neurophysiologically reduces muscle spindle Ia afferent discharge rate as the muscle spindles accommodate to their elongation.

Vibration of an antagonist muscle will also reduce tone in a spastic muscle through reciprocal inhibition, although the effect does not persist after the vibration stops.

Development of Motor Control

Movements in a hemiparetic limb show typical features of a UMN lesion. Muscles show increased tone and are weak. Initiation and termination of muscle activation are prolonged, and there is a variable degree of co-contraction of agonists and antagonists, making movements slow and clumsy. Studies of recruitment patterns of individual motor units in affected muscles show slower firing rates and impersistent firing; that is, there are more gaps in long motor unit firing trains.

Conventional methods of rehabilitation to regain motor control consist of stretching and strengthening, attempting to retrain weak muscles through reeducation. Use of sensory feedback is often stressed to facilitate muscle activation (e.g., stroking the overlying skin, sudden stretching of the muscle, and vibration of the muscle or its tendon). Some of these latter facilitation techniques are incorporated into well-defined systems of therapy. The system developed by Rood involves superficial cutaneous stimulation using stroking, brushing, tapping, and icing, or muscle stimulation with vibration, to evoke voluntary muscle activation. Brunnstrom emphasized the synergistic patterns of movement that develop during recovery from hemiplegia. She encouraged the development of flexor and extensor synergies during early recovery, hoping that synergistic activation of muscle would, with training, transition into voluntary activation. Proprioceptive neuromuscular facilitation (PNF) was developed by Kabat, Knott, and Voss. This relies on quick stretching and manual resistance of muscle activation of the limbs in functional directions, which often are spiral and diagonal. The PNF methods are more useful when muscle weakness is not due to UMN lesions. As described earlier, the NDT (by Bobath) approach aims to inhibit spasticity and synergies, using inhibitory postures and movements, and to facilitate normal automatic responses that are involved in voluntary movement. As yet, no clinical trial has shown that application of any of these approaches improves patient outcome over conventional therapy.

Therapy for the Hemiparetic Arm

As outlined in the previous section, early intervention is important to support the arm, preserve joint range of motion, and maintain shoulder integrity. If the arm becomes quite spastic, frequent slow stretching can help reduce tone. Spasticity usually dominates in the flexors and may hold the wrist and fingers in a constant position of excessive flexion. A static wrist-hand orthosis is often helpful in maintaining these joints in a functional position.

The challenge of poor function in the hemiparetic hand has prompted therapists to develop new forms of therapy. One approach that has undergone considerable study is focused neuromuscular reeducation supplemented by electromyogram (EMG) biofeedback. Results of trials have been mixed, some showing benefit but others no better results than control therapy. One review of clinical trials of biofeedback did appear to show that biofeedback was an effective treatment method. The EMG biofeedback involves recording surface EMG from the test muscle and using auditory and/or visual display of the EMG signal as feedback to the patient on the ongoing activity status of the muscle. The EMG signal supplements conventional reeducation given by the therapist. Another form of therapy uses functional electrical stimulation (FES) to provide sensory-motor reeducation. The most promising technique for the hemiparetic arm appears to be FES when it is initiated by the EMG signal of the test muscle. Recently, EMG-triggered FES has been refined using intramuscular electrodes. The initial case reports appear promising. These techniques may be useful in individual patients. They should be viewed as supplemental to all the other forms of therapy given to the patient.

When severe weakness of the hemiparetic arm persists, attention of the therapist and patient is directed toward functional retraining, using the unaffected limb to achieve independence in self-care skills, and so forth. Several recent reports indicate that some individuals who begin to use the unaffected limb early and ignore the paretic limb succumb to what is called *learned nonuse* of the weak limb. These individuals have latent potential for improved motor function but do not improve because of failure to use the limb. Forcing patients to use the weak limb by repeated encouragement or even restraint of the unaffected hand produces measurable improvement in function in the weak hand. Trials of constraint-induced movement therapy have shown significant increases in speed and strength of contraction. These studies appear to confirm the belief that improved function may occur with vigorous and intensive therapy, strong motivation, and good cognition, providing some selective hand movement is present.

Therapy for Mobility

An important rehabilitation goal for almost all hemiplegic patients is to achieve independent ambulation. In the early stages of recovery, or if recovery is limited to weak synergy patterns only, walking will not be possible because of poor upright trunk control, inability to achieve single-limb support during stance, and inability to advance the leg during swing phase. Patients should receive initial therapy to develop gross trunk control and training in pregait activities such as posture, balance, and weight transfer to the hemiparetic leg. As recovery progresses, patients develop better gross motor skills and trunk balance and greater strength in the leg. At Brunnstrom stage 3 recovery (described earlier), characterized by strong synergies and spasticity but no selective muscle activation, most patients will walk, although many will require an ankle-foot orthosis and cane and will walk slowly. Ambulation improves as motor recovery provides for selective phasic activation of muscles during the gait cycle. For details on evaluation of hemiplegic gait and therapeutic interventions, see recent reviews.

There have been recent reports of the benefit of intensive gait training in hemiplegic patients who received gait training on a treadmill with body weight partially supported with a harness. The harness substitutes for poor trunk control, and the motor-driven treadmill forces locomotion. During early training the patient is assisted by two therapists in controlling the trunk and pelvis, and weak leg. Treadmill training with body weight support is superior to conventional therapy. It was found that with treadmill training, some nonambulatory hemiplegic patients learned to walk, and those who were already walking significantly increased their gait speed.

Communication Therapy

Language therapy is based on the detailed evaluation of the patient's cognitive and linguistic capabilities and deficits. In general, speech pathologists attempt to improve communicative ability by circumventing or deblocking the language deficit, or by helping the patient to compensate. In the early stages of rehabilitation it is important for the therapist to help the patient establish a reliable means for basic "yes/no" communication. The therapist then progresses to specific techniques based on the patient's deficits. Even though spontaneous recovery is responsible for early improvement, speech therapy plays an extremely important role in minimizing patient isolation and encouraging the patient to actively engage in the program. Although communication may be difficult, simple childish phrases or tasks should be avoided, as patients perceive them as infantile, and may withdraw and reject the therapy. Specific techniques have been described for improving comprehension, word or phoneme retrieval, and gestures to supplement verbal communication. There have been reports of patients showing continued slow recovery between 6 and 12 months and beyond. It is difficult to predict which patients will show late recovery, but it seems quite justified to continue speech therapy while patients are showing measurable gains in communication.

Disorders of Cognition and Behavior

Cerebrovascular lesions produce a wide spectrum of cognitive and behavioral clinical features. At the extreme end is dementia, which may preclude functional recovery and render efforts at rehabilitation futile. Less severe impairments of higher level function may be observed frequently in patients undergoing rehabilitation (e.g., poor attention, decreased memory, ignoring the food on one side of a plate, or bumping into one side of a doorway). Other more subtle changes may not be apparent until the patient returns home, and family members notice mild behavioral changes such as decreased judgment or insight. All of these conditions affect performance of functional activities, sometimes profoundly. Therefore, the professional should be able to recognize significant cognitive and behavioral disorders and anticipate how therapeutic strategies may be employed to ameliorate them.

Lesion and Cognition/Behavior

In general, the absolute size of a brain lesion determines the severity of behavioral and psychological changes poststroke. For example, large cortical lesions produce more psychological changes than smaller subcortical lesions. Behavioral and organic mental changes occur most often in association with frontal lesions and less often with parietal, temporal, or occipital lesions. Patients with multiple lesions, especially when bilateral, are more likely to show features of dementia. Numerous studies have shown that in patients with a history of stroke, those with more extensive white matter changes are at higher risk for dementia.

It has been reported that patients with left hemisphere lesions, especially when they are anterior, are more likely to be depressed, although this has been disputed. Patients with right hemisphere lesions are more likely to be unduly cheerful. Emotional lability occurs in up to 20% of patients poststroke, and is more common in patients with right hemisphere lesions. It is a typical feature of the syndrome of pseudobulbar palsy. The clinical features of emotional lability tend to improve with time and often respond to tricyclic antidepressants.

Unilateral Neglect

Many patients with a nondominant parietal lobe lesion neglect and ignore the opposite side of the body or hemispace. Inattention also occurs with impaired sensation or homonymous hemianopia. Patients with persistent inattention perform functional tasks less well, and various therapies have been tried to remediate the inattention. Therapy is directed at retraining, with repetitive exercises or use of compensatory techniques, to teach new methods of task completion. These therapies include training patients to visually scan from side to side, offering stimuli to draw attention to the left hemispace, and environmental adaptations. An example of environmental adaptation is orientation of the patient's neglected hemispace toward the side most frequently stimulated (e.g., entrance to the room). Specific therapy is usually given to remediate visual neglect and/or hemianopia, which almost always includes visual scanning. Another strategy for improving vision in patients with complete hemianopia is the use of Fresnel prisms applied to eye glasses. These devices shift images in the affected hemivisual field toward the center of the retina and hence into the field of view.

Depression

Depression is very common following stroke and, depending on diagnostic criteria, has been reported in up to 50% of patients. Although there is some dispute about lesion location and depression, there is apparently a relationship between left frontal lesions and major depression, though this relationship may operate only in the early phase poststroke. It has been hypothesized that the depression in these cases may be induced by catecholamine depletion through lesion-induced damage to the frontal noradrenergic, dopaminergic, and serotonergic projections. Many authors have pointed out the important psychological factors that can lead to depression following stroke. These include psychological responses to the physical and personal losses caused by the stroke and the state of helplessness and loss of control that often accompanies severe disability.

The diagnosis of poststroke depression is often difficult because some of the diagnostic criteria used may simply reflect sequelae of the stroke (e.g., vegetative symptoms such as sleep disturbance, fatigue, and psychomotor retardation). Of particular importance in the diagnosis is depressed mood and loss of interest in participating in daily activities such as the rehabilitation program.

Persisting depression correlates with delayed recovery and poorer ultimate outcome. Active treatment should be considered for all patients with significant clinical depression. There is general acceptance that psychosocial intervention is important for all professional staff, with individual psychotherapy supplemented by positive reinforcement of the progress being made in rehabilitation. Many patients respond to drug therapy. Antidepressants improve depression in a majority of patients, desipramine or the selective serotonin reuptake inhibitor group being favored because of fewer side effects. Some practitioners prescribe methylphenidate (Ritalin [CibaGeneva]) with the antidepressant, as this drug will often bring about an abrupt improvement in arousal and motivation to participate in the therapeutic program.

Sexuality

It has been well documented that the majority of elderly persons continue to enjoy active and satisfying sexual relationships. By contrast, however, there is considerable sexual dysfunction following stroke. Pre- and poststroke have reported a marked decline in sexual activity, involving both men and women. There is a marked reduction in libido with a corresponding decrease in coital frequency. In one study, male patients reported that before the stroke 95% had erections, but only 38% reported normal erections poststroke, and 58% believed that after the stroke they had a sexual problem. These and most other poststroke sexual problems are related to emotional factors, such as fear, anxiety, or guilt about the stroke itself. Patients have a loss of self-esteem, and they may fear rejection or abandonment by their partner. They are, therefore, reluctant to make emotional demands. Health care professionals should be sensitive to relationship issues and be prepared to ask questions about intimacy, sexual attitudes, needs, and behavior. Most will require supportive psychotherapy to provide them with better mechanisms to cope with the sequelae of the stroke.

Psychosocial Aspects

The psychological, social, and family aspects of stroke rehabilitation are extremely important. The abrupt change in the life situation of the stroke survivor impacts all phases of care. The patient fears loss of independence and the disabilities reduce self-esteem and self-worth. Patients are often concerned about the capacity of their spouse to sustain them following discharge, and whether they will both be able to make the appropriate role adjustments. The response of some patients to the stroke may be catastrophic with subsequent maladaptive behavior. All members of the rehabilitation team should contribute to a positive and supportive milieu to promote appropriate coping strategies on the part of the patient, and to assist the patient and family prepare for discharge and reintegration into the home and community. This will involve early discussions around planning for discharge, education about stroke and its consequences, and detailed discussions around potential problems and opportunities that patient and family will encounter in the future.

Late Rehabilitation Issues

There are important issues that make postdischarge follow-up mandatory. From a medical perspective the majority of patients have ongoing medical problems requiring monitoring and therapeutic intervention such as hypertension, heart disease, and diabetes. Appropriate management will reduce the risk of stroke recurrence and prolong survival. A seizure disorder develops in about 8% of stroke survivors, and this requires conventional monitoring and treatment.

There are also rehabilitation issues that are ongoing. The rehabilitation program does not finish when the patient leaves the hospital, and almost all patients benefit from continued therapy. There are many reports describing continued improvement over many months postdischarge, and many patients require formal therapy to achieve that continued progress. The physician overseeing the rehabilitation program should regularly reevaluate the patient to document physical progress and define ongoing therapeutic goals. Specific problems that may become prominent following discharge from the hospital, during the outpatient therapy phase of care, include the following: psychological maladjustment and depression, reduced sexuality, poor role adjustment in the home and family, equipment needs, transportation and driving, and secondary physical problems such as excessive spasticity in the arm, reflex sympathetic dystrophy, changing pattern of ambulation, and so forth. Management of spasticity requires careful evaluation, goal setting, and selection of appropriate therapies. Dantrolene (Proctor & Gamble Pharmaceuticals) has been used for many years for pharmacological treatment of hemiplegic spasticity caused by stroke, but early use of dantrolene did not improve function in a recent double-blind study. A small number of patients are bothered by spontaneous spasms occurring mostly at night in bed. These can usually be adequately controlled by small doses of diazepam before bedtime. For localized spasticity, such as biceps, forearm flexors or the calf muscles, intramuscular neurolysis with phenol or chemodenervation with intramuscular botulinum toxin injections can be very effective.

For all of these reasons, the rehabilitation physicians should continue to monitor the progress of the patient as long as necessary to be satisfied that the patient has reached a stable, optimal level of function.

SELECTED REFERENCES

Bard G, Hirshber CG. Recovery of voluntary motion in upper extremity following hemiplagia. *Arch Phys Med Rehabil* 1965;46:567–572.

Bohannon RW. Correlation of lower limb strengths and other variables with standing performance in stroke patients. *Physiother Can* 1989;41: 198–202.

Bohannon RW. Is the measurement of muscle strength appropriate in patients with brain lesions? *Phys Ther* 1989;69:225–230.

Bohannon RW, and Smith MB. Interrater reliability of a modified Ashworth scale of muscle spasticity. *Phys Ther* 1987;67:206–207.

Brandstater ME, deBruin H, Gowland C, et al. Hemiplegic gait: analysis of temporal variables. *Arch Phys Med Rehabil* 1983;64:583–587.

Brandstater ME, Siebens H, Roth EJ. Venous thromboembolism in stroke: Part I. Literature review and implications for clinical practice. *Arch Phys Med Rehabil* 1992;73:S379–S391.

Brunnstrom S. *Movement Therapy in Hemiplegia: A Neurophysiological Approach.* New York: Harper & Row; 1970.

Chae J, Yu DT, Ng A, et al. Intramuscular electrical stimulation for hemiplegic shoulder pain: a 12-month follow-up of a multiple-cener, randomized clinical trial. *Am J Phys Med Rehabil* 2005;84:832–842.

Davis SW, Petrillo CR, Eichberg RD, et al. Shoulder-hand syndrome in a hemiplegic population: 5-year retrospective study. *Arch Phys Med Rehabil* 1977; 58:353–356.

Feigenson JS, McDowell FH, Meese P, et al. Factors influencing outcome and length of stay in a stroke rehabilitation unit Part 1. *Stroke* 1977;8:651–656.

Fletcher BJ, Dunbar S, Coleman J, et al. Cardiac precautions for nonacute inpatient settings. *Am J Phys Med Rehabil* 1993;72:140–143.

Foulkes MA, Wolf PA, Price TR, et al. The Stroke Data Bank: design, methods and baseline characteristics. *Stroke* 1988;19:547–554.

Fugl-Meyer AR, Jaasko L, Leyman I, et al. The post-stroke hemiplegic patient. I: A method for evaluation of physical performance. *Scand J Rehab Med* 1975;7:13–31.

Ganesan V, Ng V, Chong WK, et al. Lesion volume, lesion location, and outcome after middle cerebral artery territory stroke. *Arch Dis Child* 1999; 81:295–300.

Gresham GE, Duncan PW, Stason WB, et al. *Post-Stroke Rehabilitation. Clinical Practice Guideline, No 16.* Rockville, MD: US Department of Health and Human Services, Public Health Service, Agency for Health Care Policy and Research. AHCPR Publication No. 95-0662, May, 1995.

Gresham GE, Fitzpatrick TE, Wolf PA, et al. Residual disability in survivors of stroke: the Framingham Study. *N Engl J Med* 1975;293:954–956.

Hammond MC, Kraft GH, Fitts SS. Recruitment and termination of EMG activity in the hemiparetic forearm. *Arch Phys Med Rehabil* 1988;69:106–110.

Harvey RLand Green D. Deep venous thrombosis and pulmonary embolism in stroke. *Top Stroke Rehabil* 1996;3(1):54–70.

Hesse S, Bertelt C, Jahnke M, et al. Treadmill training with partial body weight support compared to physiotherapy in nonambulatory hemiparetic patients. *Stroke* 1995;26:976–981.

Hesse S, Bertelt C, Schaffrin A, et al. Restoration of gait in nonambulatory hemiparetic patients by treadmill training with partial body weight support. *Arch Phys Med Rehabil* 1994;75:1087–1093.

Horn SD, DeJong G, Smout RJ, et al. Stroke rehabilitation patients, practice, and outcomes: Is earlier and more aggressive therapy better? *Arch Phys Med Rehabil* 2005;86(12 Suppl 2):S101–S114

Horner J, Massey EW, Riski JE, et al. Aspiration following stroke: clinical correlates and outcomes. *Neurology* 1988;38:1359–1362.

Jongbloed L. Problems of methodologic heterogeniety in studies predicting disability after stroke. *Stroke* 1990;21(Suppl II):II-32–II-34.

Jorgensen HS, Nakayama H, Raaschou HO, et al. Stroke rehabilitation: outcome and speed of recovery. Part II: speed of recovery. The Copenhagen Stroke Study. *Arch Phys Med Rehabil* 1995;76:406–412.

Katrak PH, Cole AMD, Poulos CM, et al. Objective assessment of spasticity, strength, and function with early exhibition of dantrolene sodium after cerebrovascular accident: a randomized double-blind study. *Arch Phys Med Rehabil* 1992;73:4–9.

Kertesz A. *Western Aphasia Battery.* New York: Grune & Stratton; 1982.

Kraft GH, Fitts SS, Hammond MC. Techniques to improve function of the arm and hand in chronic hemiplegia. *Arch Phys Med Rehabil* 1992;73: 220–227.

Monga TN, Lawson JS, and Inglis J. Sexual dysfunction in stroke patients. *Arch Phys Med Rehabil* 1986;67:19–22.

Moulden SA, Gassaway J, Horn SD, et al. Timing of initiation of rehabilitation after stroke. *Arch Phys Med Rehabil* 2005;86(12 Suppl 2): S34–S40.

Nakayama H, Jorgensen HS, Raaschou HO, et al. Recovery of upper extremity function in stroke patients: the Copenhagen Stroke Study. *Arch Phys Med Rehabil* 1994;75:394–398.

Perry J. *Gait Analysis: Normal and Pathological Function.* Thorofare, NJ: Slack; 1992.

Robinson RG, Szetela B. Mood change following left hemisphere brain injury. *Ann Neurol* 1981;9:447–453.

Roth EJ. Medical complications encountered in stroke rehabilitation. *Phys Med Rehab Clin North Am* 1991;2(3):563–578.

Roth EJ. Heart disease in patients with stroke. Part II: impact and implications for rehabilitation. *Arch Phys Med Rehabil* 1994;75:94–101.

Sarno MT. *The Functional Communication Profile: Manual of directions. Rehabilitation monograph 42.* New York: Institute of Rehabilitation Medicine; 1969.

Schleenbaker RE, Mainous AG, III. Electromyographic biofeedback for neuromuscular reeducation in the hemiplegic stroke patient: a meta-analysis. *Arch Phys Md Rehabil* 1993;74:1301–1304.

Skilbeck CE, Wade DT, Langton-Hewer R, et al. Recovery after stroke. *J Neurol Neurosurg Psychiatr* 1983;46:5–8.

Strub R, Black F. *The Mental Status Examination in Neurology.* 2nd ed. Philadelphia, PA:FA Davis; 1995.

Taub E, Miller NE, Novack TA, et al. A technique for improving chronic motor deficit after stroke. *Arch Phys Med Rehabil* 1993;74:347–354.

Taub E, Wolf SL. Constraint induced movement techniques to facilitate upper extremity use in stroke patients. *Top Stroke Rehabil* 1997;3(4): 38–61.

Twitchell TE. The restoration of motor function following hemiplegia in man. *Brain* 1951;74:443–480.

Van Onwenaller C, LaPlace PM, Chartraine A. Painful shoulder in hemiplegia. *Arch Phys Med Rehabil* 1985;67:23–26.

Wade DT, Langton-Hewer R. Functional abilities after stroke; measurement, natural-history and prognosis. *J Neurol Neurosurg Psychiatr* 1987;50: 177–182.

Wade DT, Langton-Hewer R, David RM, et al. Aphasia after stroke: natural history and associated deficits. *J Neurol Neurosurg Psychiatr* 1986;49: 11–16.

Wade DT, Wood VA, Langton-Hewer R. Recovery after stroke—the first 3 months. *J Neurol Neurosurg Psychiatr* 1985;48:7–13.

World Health Organization (WHO). Recommendations on stroke prevention, diagnosis, and therapy: report of WHO Taskforce on Stroke and Other Cerebral Vascular Disorders. *Stroke* 1989;20:1407–1431.

CHAPTER

42 Stroke And Discharge Planning

REBECCA BRASHLER

OBJECTIVES

- What constitutes good discharge planning and why is it important?
- What health policy and financial and personal concerns drive discharge planning in hospitals?
- What kind of assessment is needed to construct a good discharge plan?
- What does a good discharge plan include?

Satisfaction with the discharge planning process is highly correlated with patients' overall satisfaction with medical care and future loyalty to physicians and hospitals. Clearly, a poorly executed discharge plan leaves families feeling unsupported and abandoned no matter how excellent their actual medical treatment might have been during hospitalization. The discharge planning process provides the final and most lasting impression of the entire stay, and when done poorly it can undermine long-term health outcomes for the patient. Achieving satisfaction with discharge planning, however, is no easy task. The literature indicates that frequently patients and their caregivers feel unprepared for the transition into the community and that health care providers often underestimate the need for education and support at this critical juncture.

BACKGROUND AND RATIONALE

Discharge planning is a biopsychosocial task. It starts with careful consideration of the medical needs of the patient yet also demands a thorough appreciation of psychosocial factors. However, both the medical and the psychosocial needs often take a back seat to financial pressures because discharge planning is so intimately tied to lengths of hospitalization, bed use, and ultimately to reimbursement. The Medicare prospective payment system in the United States, in which hospitals are paid a predetermined amount based on a patient's condition or diagnosis, places a huge emphasis on treating patients efficiently and quickly during hospital stays. It is often toward the end of the hospital stay, the days immediately preceding discharge, when these pressures are felt most intensively, and therefore, the process of discharge planning is sometimes rushed. While it is important to acknowledge these external policy pressures, discharge planning remains essentially a clinical task. It should be driven by principles of evidence-based practice and should involve the same attention to assessment, treatment, and monitoring as any other patient-related function.

Discharge planning, the process of preparing a patient and family for the transition from one health care setting to another, occurs repeatedly during the treatment of stroke. Patients encounter discharge planners and transitions in care each time they move from the emergency department, to an intensive care unit, to a step-down unit, to an inpatient rehabilitation unit, to a skilled nursing home, and eventually back home. Each one of these transitions can be considered a discharge. For the purposes of this chapter, the focus is on the final transition—the discharge from an acute hospital or rehabilitation facility to home.

CLINICAL APPLICATIONS AND METHODOLOGY

Psychosocial Assessment

The process of discharge planning begins with a comprehensive psychosocial assessment that provides the treatment team with background information on available resources and identifies barriers to a smooth community transition. A good psychosocial assessment includes the following elements:

- *Family composition* (including marital status, ages of family members in the home, the quality of these familial relationships, parenting responsibilities, geographic availability)
- *Housing* (including the wheelchair accessibility if appropriate)
- *Economic resources* (including income maintenance concerns for patients unable to return to work, available resources for hiring attendant care, entitlement eligibility, and the capacity to afford posthospital health care needs such as medications)
- *Community services* (including the availability of respite, transportation, support groups, home health programs, and other community-based programs)
- *Educational needs* (including the level of formal education, English language proficiency, literacy levels, and present understanding of the health care needs of the patient)

- *Religious/cultural factors* (including health beliefs)
- *Psychological, social, and interpersonal factors* (including presence of substance abuse, criminal or abusive history, presence of mental illness)
- *Vocational concerns* (including work history and goals for both the patient and the primary caregivers, childcare responsibilities, and recreational interests)

A comprehensive psychosocial summary leads to a full understanding of the patients' personal goals as well as the meaning they have assigned to this health care event. Gaining an understanding of an individual's personal interpretation of what it means to have sustained a stroke is what often helps in constructing a successful discharge plan. Two individuals with similar backgrounds, having closely matched demographic profiles and comparable financial resources, may frame their situations very differently. One may see the stroke as an opportunity to retire early and spend more time with family while maintaining a healthy lifestyle. Another patient with similar demographics may see the stroke as one of life's many challenges, and it may trigger a strong desire to quickly return to work and resume normal activities to demonstrate that the health crisis has not altered prestroke plans. Both patients may do well in the community, but they have defined success differently and will need different elements in their discharge plan to feel that the health care team was responsive and supportive.

Timing and Readiness

"Good discharge planning starts on the day of admission" is a phrase very familiar to experienced hospital case managers. However, it is important to acknowledge that while the treatment team needs to consistently think ahead and anticipate the transition back to the community, often patients and family members are not emotionally prepared to engage in conversations about discharge early in the stay when anxiety about medical issues and fears about loss of function are understandably of primary concern. Hospital stays have continued to shorten over the last decade, which has increased the need to begin discharge planning much earlier. Yet everything we know about adjustment to illness and disability tells us that patients and families need time to integrate information and reestablish emotional equilibrium before they can begin to address future plans.

Introducing the concept of discharge planning to patients and families must be handled in a sensitive manner so that they do not feel that the treatment team is ignoring their immediate needs or "kicking them out." This can be accomplished best when discharge planning is embraced by all members of the team and is not seen as solely the function of a utilization nurse or social worker. Every health care provider on the stroke team has the opportunity to integrate future planning in their daily conversations with patients. The respiratory therapist while providing treatment can introduce the idea that family members will be instructed to provide suctioning at home if it is anticipated that this care will be needed after discharge. When a physician orders intravenous (IV) medications, options for home infusion or the possibility of switching to oral medications can be addressed before the patient is discharged from the hospital. Physical therapists should always discuss the home environment when practicing mobility skills so that patients and family members begin to think about needed modifications. Integrating the preparations for discharge into each care task throughout the day provides stroke patients and their families with the message that the team will provide the necessary information, education, and assistance required to safely transition from the hospital to the community and encourages a future orientation that is predicated on patient's interests rather than fiscal constraints.

In addition to providing a consistent interdisciplinary approach to discharge planning, it is important to remain cognizant of the fact that preparing for the transition to the community involves emotional work as well as pragmatic elements. Building a ramp to the front door, for example, is largely a concrete task. However, it may also trigger specific conversations about the likelihood of permanent paralysis, which may be intricately tied to issues of loss, altered body image, and concerns about dependence. Teams unprepared to address the emotional and adjustment components of these pragmatic tasks may find that patients and families resist planning and begin to view any move toward leaving the hospital as something to be delayed or avoided.

PRACTICAL RECOMMENDATIONS

Identifying Care Requirements

The first step in good discharge planning is ensuring that the treatment team has clearly outlined the daily needs of the patient. This includes physical (nonskilled) need for assistance with activities of daily living, mobility, personal care, communication, and supervision. It also includes skilled care such as tracheostomy care, bowel and bladder management, skin care, feeding tube management, wound care, medication administration, and other tasks normally provided by nursing in a hospital setting.

Identifying Available Caregivers and Family Support

Once physical and medical needs have been identified, caregivers must be located. Frequently family members, if available, able, and willing, fill this need. However, it is this step in the process—the identification of family caregivers—that is often rushed, leading to complications and dissatisfaction after discharge. Health providers may assume that family members who have been present at the bedside will become primary caregivers after discharge. Assumptions are also made on the basis of familial relationships—all wives will care for their husbands or all adult children will care for their elderly parents. These assumptions are sometimes colored with unspoken judgments that are communicated at times as "good" wives will care for their husbands or good children will care for their parents. While many health providers who work on stroke units hold strong beliefs about familial responsibility and the benefits of being cared for by a loving relative, it is important that our personal opinions do not intrude on the patient's or family's right to make an informed decision about how they will arrange care for the stroke patient after the hospital stay.

If we think about caregiver decisions using the same model as other informed medical decisions we can avoid these pitfalls. When providing informed consent the patient/family must have information about the suggested treatment (providing care for the patient at home), the possible risks (e.g., caregiver burnout, loss of caregiver independence, loss of caregiver income outside the home), and the possible benefits (ability to control the quality of care being provided, the emotional satisfaction of meeting the patient's needs). They need to know the availability of alternative treatments (nursing home placement, hired attendant care) and the possible risks and benefits of these alternatives. It is only after this discussion that patients and family members can truly decide whether a relative is best suited to becoming a primary caregiver.

Once a family caregiver(s) is identified, the team can begin to assess the capacity of the caregiver to perform the necessary tasks. At times the caregiver, while eager to provide care, is limited physically, emotionally, or cognitively. The caregiver may need the strength to safely transfer the patient or use a mechanical lift, the fine motor coordination to perform intermittent catheterization, the vision to draw up a syringe, or the cognitive ability to keep track of a complex schedule of medications. Each of these tasks, and many others, must be demonstrated and taught, with careful attention given to the caregivers who need to practice these skills in a safe and supportive environment.

Stroke professionals, when teaching family caregivers, should remain cognizant of the fact that, providing care to a relative brings special challenges that we do not necessarily face in our own work routines. Catheterizing a patient—even one that we care about deeply—is an inherently different task than catheterizing one's parent. In addition to teaching the technique and procedure, we need to check on the caregiver's emotional response and reactions based on his or her unique relationship.

When the family caregiver has demonstrated competence in performing the task, we must also begin to assess the frequency and time demands that accompany the care. A family member may be able to perform all necessary care tasks in a supportive environment, but can he or she perform these tasks at home 24 hours a day, 7 days per week, without outside assistance? Families are set up for failure when practitioners fail to acknowledge that turning somebody in bed every 2 hours at night leads to considerable fatigue and the need for respite the next day. Providing a single return demonstration in the hospital is different from providing care every day at home.

Identifying Available Resources within the Community

Locating home health agencies, community-based services, and other attendant care programs to support the home care plan are essential parts of the discharge process. This step demands that discharge planners have a thorough understanding of available privately and publicly funded resources in the patient's community. Patients without family caregivers or supportive relatives may be completely dependent on community resources for assistance. In these circumstances it becomes critical to ensure that the hired caregivers and involved agencies can fully support the needs of the patient.

Implementation and Documentation

Implementation involves finalizing referrals, communicating the plan to everyone involved, and reviewing the information with the patient and family/caregivers. A final written document that outlines the discharge plan and includes all relevant information should be provided to every individual and each participating agency. This often involves making multiple copies of the final document to be sent to the primary care physician, a home health or personal care agency, an outpatient therapy clinic, and so on. The final document should include the following elements:

- Patient's demographics and family contact (including information on advance directives)
- Insurance information (including policy/group numbers, and a benefit's phone contact)
- Brief summary of the current illness, medical history (including dates of hospitalization/procedures), and functional status
- Primary care physician (including address/phone and next appointment)
- Other follow-up medical appointments (including specialty, physician's name, address, phone number, and the next booked appointment)
- Lab requirements (including dates for next blood draw/procedure and the name/contact number of the physician who should receive the results)
- Therapy orders (including the agency that will provide any ongoing physical, occupational, speech, or other therapies along with the schedule of appointments and the duration of the program)
- Medication list (including reconciliation forms, the name/address/phone of the community pharmacy, information on medication administration/side effects, and whom to contact for renewals)
- Durable medical equipment information (name/contact of the company supplying the wheelchair, bed, bath equipment, other devices)
- Disposable supply information (name/contact of the company supplying bowel and bladder supplies, wound care supplies, oxygen etc. and the specific items/quantities ordered)
- Skilled nursing provisions (name/contact of home health or other agencies that will provide skilled nursing after discharge if needed)
- Nonskilled attendant care provisions (name/contact of the agency or individual providing assistance in the home for nonskilled help)
- Transportation (resources for routine and emergency transportation in the area)
- Support (name/contact of counselors, mental health professionals, support groups, hotlines, and other resources to assist the patient and family with adjustment after discharge)

Following Up

The best-laid plans will need to be reassessed periodically and sometimes revised. Periodic reassessment should be incorporated into the regular medical recheck and follow-up protocol. If the patient will be returning to see the physician 2 weeks postdischarge, the protocol should include time and space to ask about adjustment at the next level of care and the well being of the caregivers. Whether this is done by a nurse in the clinic, the physician, or a social worker is not as important as the fact that it is routinely integrated into the follow-up procedures.

When it becomes clear that the discharge plan must be reworked because of changes in the patient's circumstances, the best approach is to revert to step one (reassessing the patients physical needs) and run through the DC process anew. This should not to be framed as a failure of the original plan but as the appropriate response to changing circumstances and a hallmark of quality stroke care.

SELECTED REFERENCES

Clark, PA. *Patient Satisfaction and the Discharge Process: Evidence-Based Best Practices.* HCPro, Inc and Press Ganey Associates; 2006.

Hardwig J. What about the family? *Hastings Center Report* 1990;20:5–10.

Joint Commission on Accreditation of Healthcare Organizations. *Comprehensive Accreditation Manual for Hospitals: The Official Handbook.* 2007.

Levine, C. *Always on Call.* United Hospital Fund of New York. 2000.

Rolland, J. *Families, Illness and Disability: An integrative treatment model.* New York: Basic Books; 1994.

Schild DR, Sable MR. Public health and social work. In: Gehlert, S and Browne, TA, eds. *Handbook of Health Social Work.* Hoboken, NJ: John Wiley & Sons, Inc; 2006.

United Hospital Fund. *Rough Crossings: Family Caregivers' Odysseys through the Health Care System.* New York: United Hospital Fund of New York; 1998.

Weed RO, ed. *Life Care Planning and Case Management Handbook.* 2nd ed. Boca Raton, FL: CRC Press; 2004.

CHAPTER 43

Practical Recommendations for Oral Anticoagulant Therapy Management

HEATHER P. WHITLEY

OBJECTIVES

- Which patient-specific factors might influence initial oral anticoagulant dosage selection?
- What is the frequency of titrating oral anticoagulants following initiation based on the onset of action?
- What are the differences between the utility of prothrombin time and international normalized ratio for monitoring anticoagulation?
- What are the most important aspects of oral anticoagulant therapy that should be discussed with a patient upon initiation?
- What questions should be asked at every follow-up anticoagulation visit and how is an appropriate assessment and plan constructed after an anticoagulation follow-up visit?
- What is the appropriate frequency of patient follow-up?
- Which point-of-care testing devices should be used in managing anticoagulation therapy?

There are three classes of antithrombotic agents: anticoagulants, antiplatelet agents, and thrombolytic agents. Thrombolytic agents act directly by dissolving thrombi through activation of the thrombolytic system. Conversely, anticoagulant and antiplatelet therapy provide primary prophylaxis, as they prevent new clot formation where none previously existed, or secondary prophylaxis by preventing extension of developed blood clots.

BACKGROUND

For the last several decades, the most commonly prescribed oral anticoagulant in North America has been warfarin. Anticoagulation through warfarin therapy is widely used to prevent thrombotic events for a variety of medical conditions. One of the most common indications for warfarin therapy is for the prevention of cardioembolic stroke secondary to atrial fibrillation. The risk of atrial fibrillation increases with age. Therefore, as the older population in America continues to expand, so will the number of patients with cardiac arrhythmia, and thus, those requiring anticoagulation.

Issues about warfarin therapy initiation and maintenance stem from the narrow therapeutic window and great intrapatient variability. Warfarin dosing is sensitive and is patient specific. Slightly elevated doses quickly result in supratherapeutic anticoagulant effects that can produce undesirable side effects, such as internal hemorrhage. Conversely, too small a dose, for a given patient, can result in subtherapeutic anticoagulation and possibly clot formation, which can result in devastating events. Warfarin dosing is highly patient specific, but anticoagulant effects of warfarin vary widely within each patient. Therefore, it is essential that every patient using warfarin therapy be followed up frequently and regularly to maintain therapeutic effects and prevent unwanted consequences.

Much of anticoagulation therapy management in the United States is provided by the primary care physician. Therefore, the primary care physician must coordinate the initiation, maintenance, and complication management of anticoagulation therapy alongside all other daily patient care responsibilities. Several U. S.-based studies have shown that many physicians choose not to initiate oral anticoagulant therapy when indicated predominately because of fear of complications and difficulty with management.

To the practitioner, warfarin management may appear time consuming, cumbersome, frustrating, or even daunting. In fact, it does require exceptional attention to detail for the protection of the patient and the practitioner. This chapter discusses practical aspects of managing the oral anticoagulation therapy and the anticoagulation clinic in efforts to minimize practitioner error, improve patient care, and streamline therapy management.

METHODOLOGY

Anticoagulation and the Clotting Cascade

The clotting cascade is composed of two intertwined pathways. The intrinsic or content activation pathway is activated by the presence of a foreign body and involves factors VIII, IX, XI, and XII. Alternatively, the extrinsic or tissue factor pathway is activated by the tissue factor and involves only factor VII. These two pathways merge into the common pathway with the activation of factor X into factor Xa. Factor Xa cleaves prothrombin (factor II) forming thrombin (factor IIa). In turn, thrombin converts fibrinogen into fibrin, which stimulates clot synthesis.

Particularly significant to the action of oral anticoagulation therapy are the vitamin K–dependent clotting factors (II, VII, IX, and X) and the coagulation inhibitors (proteins C and S), all of which are produced in the liver. These proteins require vitamin K from the diet, which functions as a cofactor with glutamic acid residues on *N*-terminal portions of the profactors to become activated through carboxylation. In turn, carboxylation of the profactors results in oxidized epoxide vitamin K. Vitamin K must be processed through two steps to regenerate the reduced form required for the production of active clotting factors.

Warfarin sodium, discovered at the University of Wisconsin in the 1940s, inhibits the production of vitamin K–dependent clotting factors and coagulation inhibitors by prohibiting the recirculation of reduced vitamin K from the oxidized form. When vitamin K is not present in the diet or the reduced forms of vitamin K are not available because of warfarin administration, uncarboxylated, and therefore, inactivated profactors are produced. When warfarin is administered in the correct dose sufficient for a specific patient for 5 to 7 days, an anticoagulant effect is achieved. The half-lives of the vitamin K–dependent coagulation factors vary from 4 to 60 hours (see Table 43.1). Therefore, depletion of these clotting factors and a therapeutic anticoagulant effect, induced by warfarin administration, requires several days of therapy before onset is reached.

Prothrombin Time versus International Normalized Ratio

For decades, health care providers have relied on prothrombin time (PT) to evaluate the efficacy of warfarin therapy. Although acceptable, the innovation of the international normalized ratio (INR) has improved on this old standard. PT results vary depending on laboratory thromboplastin reagents used. Therefore, laboratories report different PT values on the same blood specimen depending on the sensitivity of the reagent. This prohibits the transfer of information between laboratories (e.g., from inpatient to outpatient) and jeopardizes PT result reliability.

The INR has standardized PT results such that all laboratories may communicate anticoagulation reports more easily. A mathematical correction normalizes the PT by adjusting for the variability in the sensitivity of different thromboplastin reagents. The calculation incorporates a sensitivity index specific for the reduction of vitamin K–dependent clotting factors by different thromboplastin reagents. It is therefore preferred to monitor warfarin therapy by INR rather than by the older standard of PT, and for this reason the remainder of this chapter discusses warfarin titration based on INR. However, like many laboratory tests, it is also subject to error. Incorrect sensitivity index assignments by the manufacturer or incorrect control of PT influences calculations and provides unreliable INR results.

TABLE 43.1 Half-lives of Vitamin K–Dependent Coagulation Factors

Coagulation Factor	Half-life (h)
VII	4–6
IX	24
X	48
II (prothrombin)	60 (42 to 72)
Protein C	6
Protein S	30–60

PRACTICAL RECOMMENDATIONS

Initiating Warfarin Therapy

Although warfarin dosing is highly patient specific, in general for patients who require therapy, the dose should be started at approximately 5 mg per day. Some patient-specific factors, however, support initiating therapy at alternate doses. Lower doses of 2, 2.5, 3, or 4 mg per day are more appropriate for older patients (>65 years), those with poor nutritional status or hepatic function, those concurrently using warfarin-enhancing medications, and those at risk for bleeding. Larger doses of 6 or 7.5 mg per day may be selected for younger patients, chronic alcoholics, and those who use cytochrome P-450 (CYP) 2C9-inducing medications, such as aprepitant, carbamazepine, phenobarbital, phenytoin, rifampin, rifapentine, ritonavir, or St. Johns wort. Other patient-specific factors, such as gender and ethnicity, appear to contribute mildly to daily warfarin dosage requirements, with men and African Americans requiring slightly larger doses than women and whites.

Owing to the long half-life of some clotting factors, the onset of anticoagulation by warfarin takes a full 5 to 7 days to achieve therapeutic levels (Table 43.1). Owing to this long onset of anticoagulation, the initial dose should be maintained for several days before increasing it, while daily monitoring should begin no later than the third day of therapy. It is important to begin monitoring for anticoagulation efficacy of warfarin daily, despite the time to steady state, for safety purposes. If subtherapeutic levels remain after the fifth day of continuous therapy the dose may be increased mildly to facilitate achievement of the target anticoagulation level. This may be done by adding an extra half or two halves (dosed on different days) of tablet therapy per week. Titrating using one tablet strength is better for the patient because of convenience and lower monthly medication cost, both of which may increase patient compliance.

Some practitioners prefer loading warfarin therapy with 10 mg initially or after several days of unachieved, desired anticoagulation; however, practical experience has proved this to be more dangerous than effective. Initiating therapy with large loading doses quickly depletes factor VII because of its short half-life; however, factors II, IX, and X remain at physiological levels, maintaining coagulation, until after 5 to 7 days of continuous therapy. In addition, coagulation factor protein C also gets rapidly depleted because of its short half-life of only 6 hours. Removal of functioning protein C may inadvertently produce a procoagulant state before full anticoagulation. For these reasons, clinical guidelines recommend against initiating therapy with loading doses. Finally, although the initiation of warfarin therapy may take place in an inpatient service, it is acceptable to have the patient followed up in an outpatient service if the individual is willing to return frequently until therapeutic anticoagulation is achieved.

Initial Patient Interview

On initiation of anticoagulation for patients, caregivers should be educated at length about the efficacy and safety of warfarin therapy. Because extensive information must be provided to the patient, it is important to assess the amount of information retained immediately after providing the instruction and review various aspects at each patient encounter.

Using layman's terms, begin by informing the patients and caregivers as to why warfarin was added to their drug regimen. To provide comfort, educate them about the high prevalence of warfarin usage and safety when taken exactly as prescribed and followed closely. The importance of frequent follow-up should be disclosed to patients during this first educational visit. They will need to present to clinic or the laboratory every few days until therapeutic anticoagulation is achieved. After this point less frequent appointments may be scheduled for once a month or every 2 weeks as recommended by their anticoagulation specialist.

Educate patients about INR monitoring, including the method and frequency of phlebotomy. A few laboratories require phlebotomy via venipuncture, while others may use point-of-care testing (POCT) devices that use less blood from a finger tip.

An INR of a non–warfarin-treated blood sample is ≤ 1. As warfarin anticoagulates the blood, the INR will increase. Inform the patients of their desired target INR range. Discuss the risk of warfarin therapy, specifically bleeding with substantially elevated INRs. Because their INR will be elevated >1 they will experience increased incidence of bruising, but they should seek medical attention for bruises that appear following no trauma or cuts, which do not stop bleeding over an extended period. This may indicate that their INR is too high and that their blood may be too thin. Advise patients to inform all health care professionals including dentists, physical, occupational, or massage therapists, and chiropractors in addition to physicians, nurses, and pharmacists about their use of warfarin therapy at every visit. This should remind prescribers of potential drug interactions, therapists of increased risk of injury with physical exertion, and dentists and physicians of increased bleeding risk with surgeries.

Obtain a complete and accurate medication history, including not only prescriptive but also over-the-counter (OTC) products, vitamins, and herbals. Many products induce drug interactions when added to or discontinued from medication regimens that include warfarin. Patients need to realize that all drugs, whether prescription, OTC, or herbals, may interact with their warfarin therapy. Initiating or discontinuing drugs may increase or decrease a patient's INR, thus resulting in unintentional bleeding or thrombosis, respectively. Patients should become proactive and always inquire about potential INR fluctuations when medications are added to or discontinued from their regimen. The same precaution should hold true for ingestion of OTC and herbal products. Along the same lines, advise patients to avoid using nonsteroidal anti-inflammatory agents when possible. Aspirin therapy may be indicated for other various reasons, and therefore, may be appropriate for use in combination with warfarin. But for general aches and pains advise patients to try acetaminophen instead.

Explaining the need for consistent dietary vitamin K intake is typically a tough concept for patients to grasp. Vitamin K reverses the effect of warfarin. Suddenly increasing the amount of dietary vitamin K intake will sharply decrease the INR. Conversely, abruptly eliminating vitamin K from the diet will raise the INR and increase the patient's bleeding risk. Although vitamin K is found to some degree in almost all dietary products, it is most prevalent in leafy green vegetables, mayonnaise, and some oils. There is no need for patients to completely avoid intake of all green vegetables. Rather they should maintain a consistent number of leafy green vegetable servings per week. A helpful list of vitamin K–rich foods can be found in the Coumadin patient leaflet. Another useful tool may be found at the ClotCare online resource (www.clotcare.com/clotcare/include/vitaminkcontent.pdf).

Follow-up Patient Visits

During each follow-up visit certain basic questions should always be asked to the patient. Collectively, patients' answers to these questions help assess the anticoagulation status and determine the most appropriate plan of action. Begin by verifying the patient's dose, tablet strength, and tablet color. It is not uncommon for a patient to misunderstand new warfarin dosing instructions or revert to the previously prescribed dosing schedule. This quickly identifies patients who are supra- or subtherapeutic because of incorrect doses. Each strength of warfarin tablets, whether brand-name or generic, are dyed consistently. Clinical experience has shown that quick verification of the tablet strength, by way of color, has halted consumption of inappropriately prescribed or dispensed strengths of warfarin. In addition, education of the prescribed tablet strength and color may help patients become proactive in preventing receipt of the incorrect strength from the pharmacy.

After verifying use of the correct dosing schedule and tablet strength, question the patient about medication adherence. Ask each patient to quantify the number of missed doses over the last week. Doses missed earlier than approximately 10 days before have little effect on present INR values. A subtherapeutic INR due to missed doses would not require an increase in dose schedule. Unfortunately, when not asked, prescribers may inappropriately increase the dose to treat a subtherapeutic INR; concurrent follow-up visits with medication adherence then provide supratherapeutic anticoagulation.

Because many drugs interact with warfarin, enquire about recent changes in medication therapy at every patient visit. It is during this time that a medication review should be performed. Prescription, OTC, and herbal products added or discontinued since the previous visit should be reported, as well as changes in product doses or frequency of usage of current medications. Depending on the drug, the change in therapy, and the mechanism of interference with warfarin, anticoagulation may fluctuate up or down.

Like other medications, changes in eating habits of foods rich in vitamin K will also affect anticoagulation status. Ask patients if their diet has remained stable over the last 7 to 10 days. Extraordinary splurges of mustard greens, spinach, or collards will decrease the INR. Typically, when patients become ill because of minor issues their general dietary consumption decreases. This often results in less vitamin K consumption and therefore an increase in INR. Similarly, if patients desire to alter their diet in efforts to lose body weight they often decrease total food intake and/or increase consumption of vegetables. Depending on the action taken, anticoagulation may alter in either direction. Regardless of the circumstances, continue to remind patients to consume consistent amounts of vitamin K–rich foods on a weekly basis. It is important to note that patients should not be instructed to remove all vegetables or even only all leafy green vegetables from their diet.

As with most patient visits, ask if the patient has any concerns or complaints. This should immediately allude to increased incidence of bruising or bleeding, which when combined with an elevated INR may necessitate more extreme plans of action. In addition, ask patients whether they are anticipating any impending surgeries or procedures. In the event of future surgeries or procedures, the health care provider should assess the need for bridge therapy based on each patient's past medical history, indication for warfarin therapy, and the type of procedure to take place. Find several selected readings that will help assess need and methods for selecting, dosing, and implementing bridge therapy in the reference section of this chapter.

It is prudent to document all patient responses to each of the issues mentioned in the preceding text at every anticoagulation follow-up visit in the patient's medical record with diligence. Not only will this serve as important information for medication assessment, but it will also protect against litigation.

Anticoagulation Assessment and Plan

As in the case of management of all other disease states, one should treat the patient rather than the number. This is especially true when monitoring and titrating medications with narrow therapeutic windows, such as warfarin. For these reasons it is essential to address all the questions discussed in the preceding sections before making an assessment and planning for management. The most important piece of information to determine in the face of sub- or supratherapeutic anticoagulation is the explanation behind the inappropriate value. In addition, review the patient's past several INRs to determine a trend. Some trends, such as gradually decreasing or rising INRs may be relatively obvious. Conversely, others are more ambiguous because of periodic poor medication adherence, fluctuations in diet, or use of prn medications that affect anticoagulation status. Often, these are only discernable through thorough patient inquiry and accurate documentation. Explanations for inappropriate anticoagulation are listed in Table 43.2. Therefore, investigation and documentation of patient responses are imperative and will guide the plan of action.

Therapeutic Anticoagulation

Warfarin regimens that produce therapeutic INRs rarely require alterations; however, there are always exceptions. Reports of several missed warfarin doses in the past week with a therapeutic INR may require a mild weekly dosage reduction. In general, therapy alterations should not be prophylactically altered to account for newly added or discontinued interacting medications; consider monitoring the patient's anticoagulation status more frequently until the INR restabilizes. Addition of some interaction medications is known to require average dosage reductions of 20% to 50%. While some may elect to dramatically reduce the dose initially, others prefer to follow patients closely and alter therapy as needed.

Subtherapeutic Anticoagulation

Patients with subtherapeutic INRs due to missed doses or acute increases in vitamin K intake do not require long-term increases in therapy. Rather it is more reasonable to continue the current dose or simply boost therapy with a one-time extra half or whole tablet, depending on the extent of INR depression. However, these patients' anticoagulation status should be re-evaluated in approximately 2 weeks.

By convention, the reference thromboplastin INR is standardized to 1.0 for untreated samples. Therefore, patients who are prescribed warfarin and who present to a clinic with an INR of 1.1 or less are likely nonadherent to their warfarin therapy dosing schedule. Under these circumstances, rather than boosting or altering warfarin therapy, discuss the importance of medication adherence with the patients and follow up again in 2 weeks.

When a patient presents with subtherapeutic anticoagulation repeatedly or following addition or discontinuation of a maintenance medication, warfarin therapy should be increased. To determine the appropriate dosage change, begin by calculating the total weekly warfarin maintenance dose (TWD). Increase therapy based on percent change of TWD anticipated to produce a therapeutic INR. While mildly subtherapeutic INRs would require small TWD changes of approximately 5%, INRs more distant from the target range would require larger TWD alterations between 15% and even 20%. See Critical Pathway for dosage adjustments.

Supratherapeutic Anticoagulation

Acutely elevated INRs are most commonly due to temporary illness or unintended diet change; both result in decreased consumption

TABLE 43.2 Explanations for Inappropriate Anticoagulation

Subtherapeutic INRs	Supratherapeutic INRs
Missed warfarin doses	Acute or chronic illness
Increase in vitamin K intake	Recent reduction in vitamin K intake
Incorrect prescription or dispensing of lower tablet strength	Accidental extra dose
Discontinuation or addition of interacting medication	Incorrect prescription or dispensing of higher tablet strength
Hyperthyroid exacerbation	Discontinuation or addition of interacting medication
	Exacerbation of chronic heart disease

INR, international normalized ratio.

of vitamin K. As in acute, mild, subtherapeutic INRs, therapy need not be altered indefinitely. Rather, omission of the next warfarin dose, or only half of the dose, may be enough to allow the INR to decrease to the therapeutic range. On the other hand, elevated INRs that result from longstanding illness or purposeful diet changes will require alterations in TWD.

When the INR is substantially higher than the upper target limit, omit one to several doses of therapy. Follow the patients' INR closely and reinitiate therapy, usually at a lower TWD, once the INR has decreased to the target range. Use the Critical Pathway to help direct the most appropriate TWD change.

Patient Follow-up

The frequency of patient follow-up is highly dependent upon the patient's current and past control of anticoagulation therapy. Patients who are stable with anticoagulation should be followed up every 4 weeks. Because of the long onset of action, those who present with slightly sub- or supratherapeutic INRs should return to clinic in approximately 10 to 14 days. If nontherapeutic anticoagulation remains at this time, the need for additional TWD alterations should be considered. Patients who present with exceptionally elevated INRs, yet are asymptomatic and do not require hospitalization, should be followed up more closely. Schedule these patients to return to clinic in 3 to 4 days depending upon extent of anticoagulation. Regardless of the period of follow-up, when possible, provide patients with new clearly written dosing instructions at the completion of each appointment. This helps remove communication errors and clearly describes the plan. Figure 43.1 is an example of written dosing instructions for patients.

Managing the Warfarin Clinic

As mentioned earlier, warfarin has a narrow therapeutic index, a small window of therapeutic effectiveness, and must be carefully dosed and managed. Therefore, anticoagulation management is best achieved in the setting of an anticoagulation management service, frequently called *anticoagulation clinics*. These clinics should be staffed by clinicians who function solely to improve patient safety and outcomes of oral anticoagulants and improve appropriate prescribing and care.

Practitioner Selection

An anticoagulation clinic is best managed by a highly skilled and organized individual. Those clinically trained practitioners qualified to coordinate or staff such a specialized and high-risk patient population should be hired only after they are given substantial training in outpatient care settings. Managing complicated aspects of warfarin therapy, such as bridge therapy or pregnancy, requires knowledge and skill. Allowing non–residency-trained practitioners to function within such a discipline only places the patients at risk for negative consequences.

Because of the importance of systematic and thorough documentation, it is essential to use practitioners with high organizational skills in providing anticoagulation services. Incomplete documentation may result in inappropriate plans at concurrent visits and harm to the patient. Furthermore, due to the significant amount of documentation, it is imperative that the workload be streamlined, is efficient, and made manageable.

System Control

Consider streamlining patient visits by developing preformulated computer-generated or hard-copy templates. This will allow the development of subjective, objective, assessment, and plan (SOAP) notes to be less redundant and accident prone. The implementation of anticoagulation clinics frequently and rapidly evolves into an overwhelming supply of patients. In situations where there are more patients than patient appointments, be cognizant of the importance of maintaining order and reasonably schedule patients' visits. Some medical facilities may elect to shorten patient visits in an effort to increase daily practitioner load. Realize that this comes at the expense of patients' safety. To maintain accurate documentation and ensure patients' safety, schedule patients no more frequent

Name: ________________ Date: ________________

Today's INR: ________________ Goal INR range: ________________

Warfarin (Coumadin®) tablet strength: ________________

Warfarin (Coumadin®) tablet color: ________________

Special Instructions: ________________

____

____

____

Day	Sunday	Monday	Tuesday	Wednesday	Thursday	Friday	Saturday
Dose	mg	mg	mg	mg	mg	mg	mg
Number of Tablets							

Next appointment: ________________

FIGURE 43.1. Dosing handout to be distributed to patients using warfarin sodium therapy following each patient encounter to improve communication of new or continued anticoagulation regimen.

than every 15 to 20 minutes. In the presence or provision of students or residents, schedule patients no more frequent than every 20 to 30 minutes. Simple visits of anticoagulation-stable patients may be conducted and documented within 10 or 15 minutes; however, the need for assessment and plan for bridge therapy may require up to 45 minutes for a single patient. Compromising such situations by limiting duration may hinder the quality of care provided. In response to increased patient care load it is more prudent to hire the services of an additional clinically trained and competent practitioner. When formulating the new patient schedule, it is most practical to assign patients to one practitioner to enhance continuity of care. The knowledge one practitioner develops about each patient is valuable expertise to the assessment and plan.

Point-of-care Testing Devices

Phlebotomy during anticoagulation evaluations is performed by either venipuncture or POCT devices. While anticoagulative services have been provided for many years by venipuncture, this method has several drawbacks. Venipuncture requires larger amounts of blood, may be more painful, and if provided in central laboratories typically increases patient's wait time. In addition, if the assessment and plan are not conducted by the phlebotomist, the patient interview must be conducted via telephone or after waiting to meet with a second practitioner.

The use of POCT devices has dramatically improved anticoagulative patient services and patient satisfaction. Not only do most patients prefer this method of testing for several reasons, but this method also usually results in better continuity of care due to face-to-face interactions before, during, and after receipt of the laboratory test results. When establishing an anticoagulation clinic, seriously consider investment in a POCT device to improve patient and practitioner satisfaction.

SELECTED REFERENCES

Absher RK, Moore ME, Parker MH. Patient-specific factors predictive of warfarin dosage requirements. *Ann Pharmacother* 2002;36:1512–1517.

Ansell J, Hirgh J, Poller L, et al. The pharmacology and management of the vitamin K antagonists. The seventh ACCP conference on antithrombotic and thrombolytic therapy. *Chest* 2004;126:204S–233S.

Du Breuil AL, Umland EM. Outpatient management of anticoagulation therapy. 2007;75(7):1031–1042.

Dunn AS, Turpie AGG. Perioperative management of patients receiving oral anticoagulants. *Arch Intern Med* 2003;163:901–908.

Eisen GM, Baron TH, Dominitz JA, et al. Guideline on the management of anticoagulation and antiplatelet therapy for endoscopic procedures. *Gastrointest Endosc* 2002;55(7):775–779.

Harrison L, Johnston M, Massicotte MP, et al. Comparison of 5-mg and 10-mg loading doses in initiation of warfarin therapy. *Ann Intern Med* 1997;126:133–136.

Hirsh J, Fuster V, Ansell J, et al. American Heart Association/American College of Cardiology Foundation Guide to warfarin therapy. *J Am Coll Cardiol* 2003;41:1633–1652.

International Committee for Standardization in Haematology and International Committee on Thrombosis and Haemostasis. ICSH/ICTH recommendations for reporting prothrombin time in oral anticoagulant control. *J Clin Path* 1985;38:133–134.

Jafri SM, Mehta TP. Periprocedural management of anticoagulation in patients on extended warfarin therapy. *Semin Thromb Hemostas* 2004; 30(6):657–664.

Kearon C, Hirst J. Management of anticoagulation before and after elective surgery. *N Engl J Med* 1997;336(21):1506–1511.

Lotke P, Palevsky H, Keenan A, et al. Aspirin and warfarin for thromboembolic disease after total joint arthroplasty. *Clin Orthop* 1996;1(324): 251–258.

Torn M, Rosendaal FR. Oral anticoagulation I surgical procedures: risk and recommendations. *Br J Haematol* 2003;123:676–682.

Weibert R. Management of oral anticoagulation therapy. *Clin Trend Pharm Pract* 1999;(2):42–55.

CRITICAL PATHWAY
Clinical Guideline for Dosage Adjustments

International Normalized Ratio (INR) 2–3

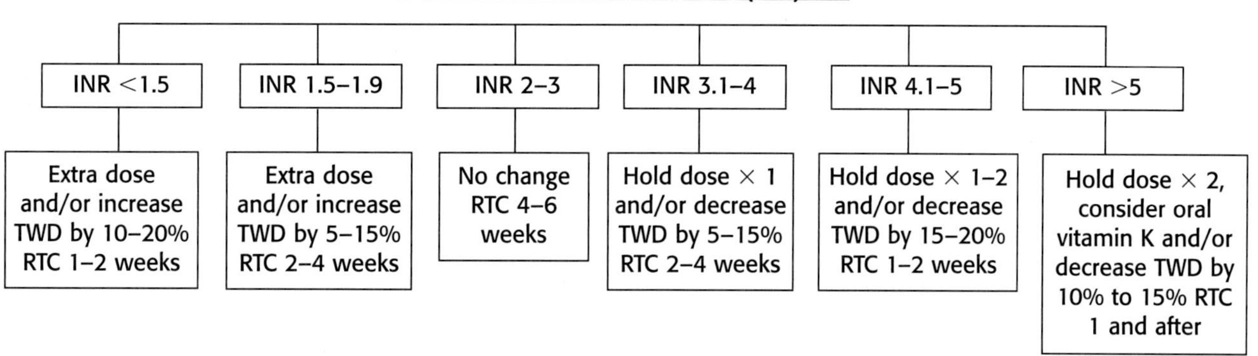

INR Target 2.5–3.5

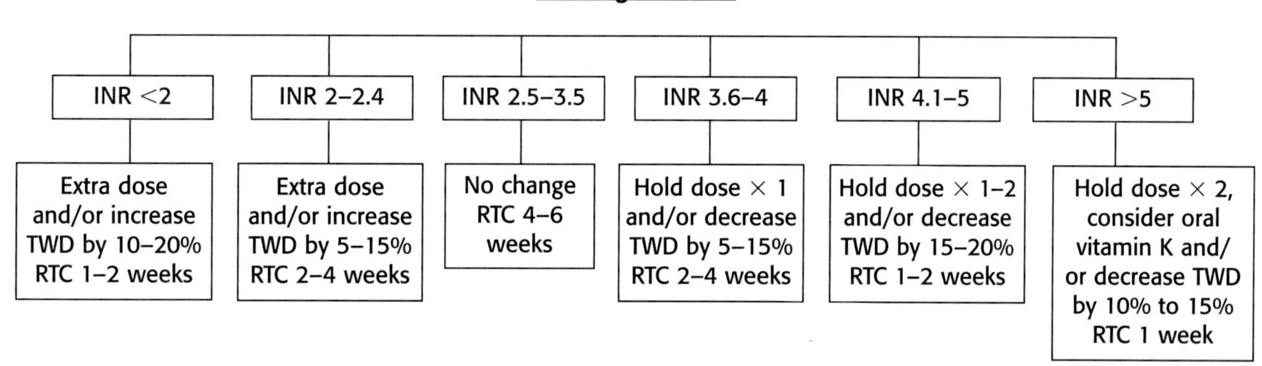

TWD, total weekly warfarin, maintenance dose; RTC, return to clinic.

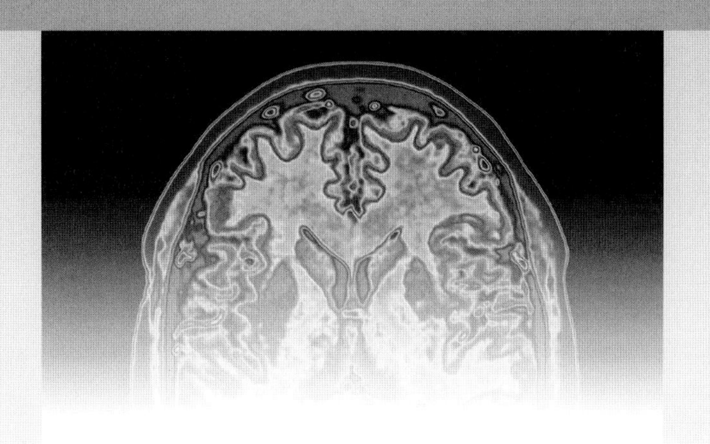

Appendices

APPENDIX

The Medical Examination

JAMES D. GEYER, CAMILO R. GOMEZ, A. ROBERT SHEPPARD, AND NADEEM AKHTAR

The general appearance of the patient provides insight into underlying chronic medical conditions. The smell of alcohol obviously suggests intoxication, which has implications on response to therapy and increased risk of complications during the hospitalization. The smell of fetor hepaticus suggests hepatic dysfunction, which can increase the risk of either intracranial hemorrhage or hypercoagulable state. Tongue, lip, and cheek trauma suggest the possibility of seizure activity (a contraindication to thrombolytic therapy). Ecchymoses may be caused by a number of etiologies including falls (possible head trauma), medication effects, and bleeding diatheses.

Even a cursory assessment of the skin can provide clues to the etiology of a stroke and to conditions that might complicate the stroke and its treatment. Systemic lupus erythematosis often has a facial butterfly rash. Dermatomyositis also has a stereotypical rash. Cyanosis of the extremities and/or lips suggests the possibility of congestive heart failure, chronic obstructive pulmonary disease, or congenital heart disease. Localized pallor indicates the possibility of arterial obstruction, such as embolic disease or vasospasm. Trophic skin changes may be seen in a number of disorders but can be associated with cardiovascular and peripheral vascular disease.

The cardiac evaluation requires special attention during the screening physical examination. Cardiovascular assessment includes cardiac auscultation, precordial palpitation, and evaluation of the peripheral pulses and edema.

Chest auscultation may reveal rhonchi, rales, or wheezing. Abnormalities on chest auscultation can provide evidence of heart failure, pneumonia, asthma, chronic obstructive pulmonary disease, and other disorders that could complicate treatment or affect the long-term prognosis.

The head and neck should be assessed for evidence of trauma. A rapid assessment of the patient would reveal raccoon eyes, a Battle sign, or other evidence of trauma.

APPENDIX 2

The Neurological Examination

JAMES D. GEYER, CAMILO R. GOMEZ, A. ROBERT SHEPPARD, AND NADEEM AKHTAR

Not all neurological symptoms are caused by stroke; they may be caused by nonneurological disorders or other diseases of the nervous system. Numbness and tingling may be secondary to vascular insufficiency, peripheral neuropathy, or demyelinating diseases among others. Generalized weakness may be caused by overall systemic illness or neuromuscular disease. Altered mental status may represent an aphasia or may be due to systemic illness, medication effect, or other conditions.

It is imperative that all patients be approached from a broad perspective, beginning with a detailed history. Most diagnoses are made using the history. The history allows you to direct your physical examination and make it more time effective, a consideration that is extremely important in the acute stroke setting.

The cognitive and mental status portion of the neurological examination is complicated and time consuming when performed in detail. In the acute stroke patient, the mental status should be assessed in a relatively superficial manner.

Speech and language abnormalities are readily assessed. Speech abnormalities are related to problems with articulation (e.g., dysarthria, hypophonia). The examiner should listen to spontaneous speech and have the patient repeat phrases/sentences. Dysarthria is the most common abnormality of speech and is poorly localizable (can occur with lesions in multiple areas of the central and peripheral nervous system). The degree of dysarthria may imply an increased risk of aspiration. Regardless of the degree of dysarthria, all stroke patients should be considered at high risk for aspiration and if possible nothing should be administered by mouth.

Language abnormalities are related to problems with communication (dysphasia, most commonly referred to as *aphasia*). The evaluation of language includes listening to spontaneous speech (fluency), checking repetition, and asking the patient to follow a three-stage command. In contradistinction to dysarthria, aphasia is localizable (dominant hemisphere). Expressive (Broca) aphasia is nonfluent language with poor repetition but with retained ability to follow commands. Conductive aphasia is fluent speech with poor repetition and the retained ability to follow commands. Receptive (Wernicke's) aphasia is a fluent aphasia with abnormal content, poor repetition, and the impaired ability to follow commands. Most clinical presentations consist of global aphasia, with a weighting more toward receptive or expressive. In general, abnormalities of verbal communication parallel abnormalities of written communication. The emotional content of language is provided by corresponding areas of the nondominant hemisphere, and abnormalities of these areas are referred to as *aprosodias*.

Other abnormalities of higher cortical function include neglect, which can manifest in several different ways. Neglect of specific sensory stimuli is referred to the involved hemisphere (tactile stimulation, visual perception, etc.), which when more severe can involve the entire side of the body. The patient may even neglect the neurological impairment, in a condition known as *anosognosia*.

Cranial nerve examination can be done quickly but is best performed in a standard order. Olfactory testing is not typically performed in the acute stroke setting.

When visual fields testing is performed in the optic nerve lesions, look for monocular visual field abnormalities; binocular field abnormalities are more common and indicate lesions behind the optic nerve. Test each eye separately with gross confrontation using fingers in the periphery of all four quadrants. Patients may have difficulty cooperating with this and be unable to fix their gaze.

The pupillary light reflex is performed by shining a light into each eye separately. Unreactive or asymmetric pupils may be seen in a number of disorders including cranial nerve ischemia, aneurysms, and brainstem strokes.

Fundoscopic examination allows visualization of the optic nerve head (disc) and nerve fiber bundles. The retina examination can provide information on hypertension, diabetes, and other conditions. The retina should also be examined for evidence of cholesterol emboli.

A rapid evaluation of extraocular movements should be assessed by having the patient follow a finger vertically and horizontally. Abnormalities in ocular motion can represent peripheral lesions, cranial nerve abnormalities, and brainstem lesions.

Facial sensation, supplied by the ophthalmic, maxillary, and mandibular divisions of the trigeminal nerve should be tested with light touch and pinprick.

Facial symmetry is an important component of the physical examination since a code stroke may be called for a patient with Bell's palsy. Typically, facial weakness related to a stroke will involve the lower facial muscle and spare the forehead. Conversely, Bell's palsy will usually involve the upper and lower portions of the face. To test the muscles of facial expression, have the patient wrinkle the forehead, close eyes, smile, and grimace.

Hearing is tested crudely with finger rub or whispered sounds in each ear. More elaborate testing is usually not required in the acute stroke setting.

The patient should be asked to protrude the tongue. Tongue deviation on this simple test suggests weakness in the motor pathway of the hypoglossal nerve. In some strokes, the patient may not even attempt to protrude the tongue.

The motor examination is one of the most important components of the neurological examination in the acute stroke setting. First assess the appearance of the musculature noting any asymmetries, atrophy, or fasciculations. The muscle tone may be decreased in the hyperacute stroke and then becomes increased over time. Tone is assessed by passive range of motion in the upper and lower extremities. Strength is graded as follows:

Power/strength
1: twitch
2: movement of joint with gravity eliminated
3: movement of joint against gravity
4: movement of joint against resistance
5: normal strength
(Note: *normal* can vary considerably, and the examiner must learn by experience what to expect from an individual patient.)

The pattern of weakness can indicate the neurological lesion localization. Central lesions usually result in contralateral (hemispheric) weakness. Brainstem lesions may produce a confusing crossed pattern of weakness. Spinal cord lesion usually results in weakness below the spinal level. Weakness is associated with increased tone (if chronic), hyper-reflexia, and pathological reflexes.

Peripheral patterns of weakness are localizable to nerve root or peripheral nerve, are proximal generalized (myopathy), or are variable (neuromuscular junction). Peripheral patterns of weakness are often associated with hyporeflexia and/or hypotonia.

The sensory examination should be a rapid cursory examination in the acute stroke setting. It is not in the best interest of patient care to spend inordinate amounts of time on the details of the sensory examination. A screening sensory examination should include light touch or pin-prick in all extremities.

Cerebellar examination includes evaluation of speech (a scanning dysarthria), eye movements (ocular dysmetria, nonsmooth pursuits, nystagmus, ocular flutter, etc.), and appendicular ataxia or dysmetria. The limbs are rapidly assessed by testing rapid alternating movements or finger–nose–finger.

Deep tendon reflexes include biceps (C5-C6), brachioradialis (C6), triceps (C7), quadraceps (L-2,3,4), and achilles (S1) and are rated as follows:

0: absent
1: OK, but less than average
2: average
3: OK, but greater than average
4: sustained clonus

Again, the pattern of abnormality is more important than the actual number assigned. In general, a lesion of the central nervous system will cause an increase in deep tendon reflexes, and a lesion of the peripheral nervous system will cause a decrease. This is not always the case, especially in the hyperacute phase of stroke, where the reflexes may actually be decreased. Pathological reflexes, such as a positive plantar reflex (Babinski), are also indicators of central nervous system dysfunction.

Finally, gait testing is not a component of the acute stroke assessment since the patient should be kept in bed to maintain the optimal hemodynamic condition.

INDEX

Note: Page numbers followed by *f* denote figures, while those followed by *t* denote tables.